Childhood Epilepsy
Language, Learning, and Behavioral Complications

More than one-half of children with epilepsy have interrelated language, learning, and/or behavior complications. By adulthood, these problems can interfere with socialization and employment. The seizures may be controlled, but the developmental distortions can continue to present problems for health and education systems and carers. In this comprehensive and fully referenced book, William Svoboda distills a lifetime of clinical experience with childhood epilepsy into three areas that address each of the main areas of difficulty. In each, he looks at why the problems arise and assesses diagnostic and remedial approaches. The focus is on the whole care of the child rather than on diagnosis, classification, and medication alone.

Clinicians, mental health practitioners, educators, and speech and language pathologists will find this book invaluable.

William B. Svoboda was Associate Clinical Professor of Pediatrics at the University of Kansas School of Medicine. He was also founder and director of the Via Christi Epilepsy Center Program. He has received grants for his work on institutionalized individuals with epilepsy, and he was appointed to the Federal Commission on Epilepsy and its Consequences, also serving on the subsection on institutionalized care. He is a former president of the Kansas branch of the Epilepsy Foundation of America.

Childhood Epilepsy
Language, Learning, and Behavioral Complications

William B. Svoboda M.D.
Founder and Former Director
Via Christi Comprehensive Epilepsy Center
Wichita, KS, USA

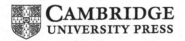
CAMBRIDGE
UNIVERSITY PRESS

CAMBRIDGE UNIVERSITY PRESS
Cambridge, New York, Melbourne, Madrid, Cape Town, Singapore,
São Paulo, Delhi, Dubai, Tokyo, Mexico City

Cambridge University Press
The Edinburgh Building, Cambridge CB2 8RU, UK

Published in the United States of America by Cambridge University Press, New York

www.cambridge.org
Information on this title: www.cambridge.org/9780521530293

First published 2004
First paperback printing 2010

A catalogue record for this publication is available from the British Library

Library of Congress Cataloguing in Publication data
Svoboda, William B.
  Childhood epilepsy: the language, learning, and behavioral complications / by
William B. Svoboda.
      p.   cm.
  Includes bibliographical references and index.
  ISBN 0 521 82338 2 (hardback)
  1. Epilepsy in children. 2. Language disorders in children. 3. Behavior disorders in children.
4. Learning disabilities. 5. Learning disabled children – Education. I. Title.

RJ496.E6S89 2003
618.92′853–dc21   2003046032

ISBN 978-0-521-82338-8 Hardback
ISBN 978-0-521-53029-3 Paperback

Not all children with epilepsy have the associated
problems of language and/or learning and/or behavior . . .
but some do . . .
and some will.

It is especially to help those that this book is dedicated.

The purpose of this text is to promote awareness and
help for such problems.

Contents

Part III   Behavior problems

Preface

I am struck by the debates over issues in epilepsy. The literature suggests that for every article, there is an equal and opposite article, and for every finding of the existence of a problem, there is one denying the existence. With therapies, there are three sides to the argument: those claiming that a drug produces a problem, those denying any relationship between the therapy and the problem, and those proclaiming that the drug may help with the problem. Some spend more time criticizing the efforts of others than contributing insight or explanations. Thus, the reader is left with more references arguing about than explaining the reason for such problems.

The emotional biases often show up in both authors and readers, both of whom tend to find what they seek. Those who deny the existence of a complication tend not to find it. Those who worry about the coexistence of complications often find it or else create it in their own view.

The reality is that many individuals do not have the problems that are ascribed to epilepsy. However, the incidence is sufficient enough to state that some do beyond mere chance. Why do some children have the problem? What can be done to prevent or to overcome such difficulties?

Glossary

The following are simplified, working definitions, not technical definitions. For each deficit of function, generally there may be a near-total loss, or a partial loss/distortion of the skill being described, the prefix "a" signifying the former (as in aphasia, anomia, agnosia) and the prefix "dys" signifying the latter (as in dyslexia, dysphasia, dyscalculia).

Modifiers

Cause: An impaired or lost function may be "acquired," i.e. the result of an insult or damage to the brain, or may be "congenital" or "developmental," i.e. an impairment of the ability to develop the function.

Degree: The prefix "a" (as in aphasia) usually implies a loss of function, but in the developing child it may also mean a lack of the ability to develop the skill.

Timing: A disturbed function may be episodic, as with an episodic aphasia. If such an episode is due to a seizure, then it is a paroxysmal aphasia.

Terms

Absence seizures: A generalized seizure manifest predominately by a brief pause and staring, sometimes with minor rhythmic movements. There is no warning and the child usually resumes the preceding activity at the end of the attack.

Acquired: A loss of a function due to brain damage, as opposed to congenital or developmental.

Agnosia: Inability or impairment in recognition of incoming sensory stimuli.

Anarithmia: A deficiency in mathematic skills that can affect any of multiple areas, including calculation (dyscalculia), math table memory, reading, recognition of mathematical symbols (numbers, operational signs, words), and perceptual-spatial awareness, such as in borrowing and carrying.

Anomia: Memory problems for proper names, names of items, etc.

Anosognosia: Unawareness or denial of a neurologic dysfunction or handicap.

Aphasia/dysphasia: Loss or lack of understanding of meanings of speech or of what is said, or difficulty in expressing one's thoughts through spoken or written language.

Aphasia, acquired: Loss of understanding of meanings of speech or of what is said, or difficulty in expressing one's thoughts through spoken or written language due to damage or destruction of a vital language-processing center.

Aphasia, congenital: Lack of acquisition of speech skills due to a developmental inability to understand or lack of expression of speech due to the underdevelopment of a vital language-processing center, usually bilaterally.

Aphasia, expressive: Loss of understanding of meanings of speech or of what is said, or difficulty in expressing one's thoughts through spoken or written language due to damage or destruction of Broca's area in the posterior inferior frontal lobe involving the dominant hemisphere.

Aphasia, receptive: Loss of understanding of meanings of speech or of what is said, or difficulty in expressing one's thoughts through spoken or written language due to damage or destruction of Wernicke's area in the temporal-parietal junction of the dominant hemisphere.

Aphasic dyslexia: An impairment in attaching meanings to words when reading, often linked with a more generalized aphasia.

Apraxia/dyspraxia: Loss of the ability to translate a response concept into a motor act, such as speech, writing, or gesturing.

Arrest, speech: The abrupt, transient interruption of the neurologic function of speech.

Astatic seizures: An old term for generalized seizures characterized by a loss of balance.

Atonic seizures: Generalized seizures in which the patient's head or body drops.

Auditory agnosia: The state of being confused and unable to recognize speech sounds or other familiar sounds.

Broaca's aphasia: See *expressive aphasia*.

Choreoathetoid: Twisting, turning, and jerking movements.

Complex partial seizures: Partial seizures usually involving the frontal or temporal lobes, presenting with initial partial loss of consciousness and automatic behaviors, followed by amnesia for the event.

Congenital neurologic problem: A deficient development of a neurologic function due to a perinatal (around the time of conception through neonatal period) brain insult, usually bilateral. The term is often used interchangeably with developmental neurological problem.

Corpus callosotomy: A surgical procedure in which the corpus callosum connecting the two brain hemispheres is cut partially or completely to prevent seizure spread.

CSWS: Continuous spike-wave status in sleep.

Deafferentation: The disconnection of incoming nerve connections from a site in the brain.

Developmental neurologic problem: A deficient development of a neurologic function due to a perinatal (around the time of conception through neonatal period) brain insult or deficiency, usually bilateral. The term is often used interchangeably with congenital neurologic problem.

Developmental (or congenital) dyslexia: A developmental impairment in reading, which may be inherited and seen in other family members.

Dextral: Right-handed.

Dysarthria/anarthria: A neurologic difficulty in the formation and pronunciation of speech sounds and words.

Dysarticula, articulation problems: A mechanical impairment of clear formation and pronunciation of speech sounds and words, usually due to a muscular or structural problem of the mouth or throat.

Dyscalculia/acalculia: Deficient or lack of ability to calculate, as in math. See also *Anarithmia*.

Dysfluency: A neurologic impairment resulting in the break-up of the normal flow of speech, such as with stuttering or stammering.

Dysfunction: The partial loss or distortion of a language or cognitive function as opposed to a complete loss, as with dysphasia/aphasia, dyslexia/alexia, etc.

Dysgraphia/agraphia: Deficient or distorted ability to write.

Dyslalia: Impairment of utterances, with abnormality of the external speech organs.

Dyslexia/alexia: Deficient, distorted ability in reading for comprehension. Commonly expanded in definition to imply an inability to read, spell, and write words despite the ability to see and recognize letters. There are many types of dyslexia, the most common of which are *aphasic dyslexia, developmental dyslexia,* perceptual dyslexia and *verbal, phonic or, auditory dyslexia.*

Dysorthographia: Deficient or distorted ability to spell.

Dysphasia: A partial loss or distortion of understanding or expression of language.

Episodic dysfunction: A brief episode of dysfunction, as with an episodic aphasia, dyslexia, etc. due to some insult the brain that temporarily impairs function of the related brain area.

Generalized tonic–clonic seizures: Generalized seizures with loss of consciousness at the onset, manifesting tonic stiffening and/or clonic repetitive jerking movements.

Hemidecorticectomy and hemispherectomy: Related surgical procedures in which much or all of the cortex or hemisphere is removed from one side of the brain in order to halt progressive degenerative seizures.

Infantile myoclonic spasms: A seizure syndrome of infancy marked by the onset of repetitive brief flexing or stiffening movements, at which time intelligence declines and the EEG shows a hypsarrhythmic pattern (high-amplitude, disorganized appearance, with multifocal spikes and occasional brief generalized suppression of activities).

Learning disability: A specific learning disability is a disability of one or more of the basic learning processes involved in the understanding or using of spoken or written language, manifest by an inadequate ability to listen, think, speak, read, write, spell, or do mathematical calculations. This includes disorders such as perceptual handicaps, brain injury, minimal brain dysfunction, dyslexia, and developmental aphasia. Such terms do not include children who have learning problems that are primarily the result of visual, hearing, or motor handicaps, mental retardation, emotional disturbances, or environmental disadvantages. (Such children demonstrate a discrepancy between expected and actual achievement expected for their overall mental age, commonly interpreted as meaning two standard deviations below normal.) (Adopted from Public Law 91-230, Section 602-15, Federal Department of Health, Education & Welfare, USA.)

Learning handicap, specific:

A seldom applied concept that indicates that the child who has a specific learning disability is handicapped in efforts to perform the task impaired by the learning disability, such as reading, writing, spelling, math, etc.

Learning problem: A non-specific term applied to any child who has difficulty in performing in school.

Lennox–Gastaut syndrome: A seizure syndrome of childhood onset marked by the appearance of mixed generalized seizures, mental deterioration, and a generalized slow spike-wave EEG appearance.

Mutism: Lack of speech or speech efforts.

Myoclonic seizures: Generalized seizures manifest as a jerk of a part or all of the body.

Neologism: The inadvertent creation of new words.

Paraphasia: A form of aphasia in which the patient uses wrong words or uses words in wrong and senseless combinations.

Paroxysm: A sudden occurrence of a symptom, such as with a spasm or a seizure.

Paroxysmal disturbance: A severe interference with a language or cognitive processing function associated with seizures. This may include transient aphasias and transient reading disorders.

Perceptual dyslexia: Confusion of similar letters and words, impairing the reading process.

Positron emission tomography (PET) scan: An isotopic brain scan that measures positrons emitted by a variety of radioisotopes injected into the bloodstream to measure chemistry and metabolism of areas of the brain.

Pragmatism: The use of language in terms of rules of usage, word meanings, and fitting together of words so as to communicate in an understandable, acceptable way.

Prosody: The character of spoken language that reflects the emotional aspects of speech, characterized by changes in pitch, tempo, inflection, and stresses in spoken efforts.

Pyramidal signs: Signs such as spasticity, hyperreflexia, and Babinski signs caused by impairment of the pyramidal tracts of the spinal cord.

Regression: The loss of a previously attained skill, such as a speech or language regression.

Retardation, mental: Overall intelligence of at least three standard deviations (borderline) below the average. Retardation may be borderline (overall intelligence at least two standard deviations below average but less than three standard deviations below normal), mild (overall intelligence roughly one-half to two-thirds normal), moderate (overall intelligence roughly one-quarter to one-half normal), or severe (overall intelligence below one-quarter normal).

Simple partial seizures: Seizures beginning in a part of the brain with intact consciousness at the onset, usually presenting with a movement, sensation, emotion, or memory. These may be auras progressing on to another seizure type.

Sinistral: Left-handed

Syntax: The way words are traditionally assembled into phrases and sentences.

Utterances, vocal: Uncontrolled uttering of non-speech sounds or single words, as during a seizure.

Verbal agnosia: Confusion or inability to recognize words.

Verbal, phonic, or auditory dyslexia: Confusion of letter or word sounds or problems in developing phonetic approaches to the recognition and understanding of words and their meanings.

Verbosity: An excessive use of words.

Wernicke's aphasia: See *receptive aphasia.*

Looking ahead

For many centuries, seizures and epilepsy were thought of in terms of magic and mysticism, demons and dread. Were the seizure events a divine blessing or a demonic curse? Even into the mid twentieth century, epilepsy, idiocy, and insanity were often spoken of as interrelated, for managements often dulled the mind and disturbed the functioning. Epilepsy, mental illness, and falling IQs were thought to be the product of a deteriorating brain, possibly inherited. The prejudices gave rise to such terms for epilepsy as "demoniac" and "lunacy" (moonstruck).

Advocates responded with denial that epilepsy was anything more than a brief interruption of normal function due to a sudden uncontrolled burst of abnormal electrical activity in the neural network of the brain, occurring in otherwise normal people who had no related intellectual or emotional disturbances.

The dawn of the modern age came with the findings of the Federal Commission on Epilepsy and Its Consequences of 1977. This exhaustive study spearheaded the emerging awareness that epilepsy is seldom "just seizures." Roughly half of the individuals with epilepsy experience significant emotional problems and nearly half experience learning difficulties. Such associated problems often lead to later problems in employment and socialization, thus becoming more handicapping than just seizures, spikes, and medications.

The medical world now approaches epilepsy in terms of electroencephalograph (EEG) interpretations, medications, and antiepileptic blood levels, to which have been added surgery, stimulators, and diets. This is the medical model of epilepsy. The educational model portrays a child with epilepsy as one with academic struggles, epilepsy-related absenteeism, and class disruptions. The psychiatric model debates a picture of epileptic personalities and psychotic diagnoses. The employer model presents an insurance-risk, underproductive, and too often absent employee with epilepsy. Little is said of a language model of epilepsy. Few speak of the whole-person view of epilepsy and even less of the child model. Yet comprehensive epilepsy care needs to address the language, learning, emotional and later employment problems as well as the medical aspects of the condition.

Problems associated with epilepsy in children

The brain is a dynamically growing, changing, and developing organ, especially in the early years of life. Seizures can inhibit, alter, or distort brain development as well as the related functions. The child's inherent potentials as well as handicaps can be altered dynamically by early interventions if given the chance (Svoboda, 1979; Svoboda, 1989).

The developing child

Seizures and seizure therapy interfere with brain functions by overactivation, interruption, inhibition, and destruction of vital functional pathways. Long or frequent attacks may alter neural circuits and neurotransmitter balances. This is seen especially in the limbic system.

In childhood, the brain and brain functions are developing over the first decades of life. Seizures and seizure care may interfere with the essential emerging skills at the age of epilepsy onset and thereafter. The immature brain has the capability of reorganizing around insulted areas, thus rendering the damage less impairing. This diminishes with maturation.

Epilepsy dysfunctions
Language

The incidence of speech and language problems in epilepsy is not known, for this area is often overlooked. Language problems are most apt to develop in individuals with epilepsy involving the left hemisphere and especially the temporal-frontal areas. Such problems may precede, occur simultaneously with, or follow seizures. The problems may be episodic or ongoing; if ongoing, they may result in a gradual loss of language abilities. The manifestations of such problems depend on the location of the seizure disturbance. Such manifestations may present as difficulties in recognizing speech sounds, in understanding what is being said, in expressing ideas, in remembering key words, or in speaking clearly and smoothly. Communication impairments often result in behavioral reactions. The manifestations may be subtle or may appear only under stress.

Learning

Roughly half of children with epilepsy have learning difficulties. Learning problems may show up as retardation, regression, specific learning disabilities, or underachievement. Retardation is most apt to appear in individuals with symptomatic generalized or multifocal seizures. Intellectual regression is most apt to be seen with medication reactions, or in symptomatic epilepsy, especially in epileptic syndromes, with progressive causes, or with overlooked seizures, such as with nighttime events. Specific learning disabilities are more apt to be seen with partial seizures and medication reactions, showing up as delays and distortions in reading, spelling, math, writing, and other academic areas. Attention and memory are most vulnerable, as is academic performance. Underachievement may result from overlooked problems, missed seizures, and adverse attitudes of those around the individual. Attention problems often relate to small subclinical discharges interfering with attention.

Behavior

One in every four children with epilepsy is reported to have behavior problems. Some estimates are at least twice that. Emotional and behavior problems may relate to both extrinsic factors and intrinsic factors. Extrinsic factors include the attitudes of the parents and siblings, the teachers and peers, and the resultant self-concept of the individual, which often reflects the experiences with other individuals. Intrinsic factors may result from the nature and location-lateralization of the epilepsy and related complications. Problems in understanding may result in any of autistic, avoidant, attention, or activity problems, whereas problems in expression may result in withdrawal, anger, and parental overprotectiveness. These may interfere with the development of socialization skills.

Vocation may be impaired more by the lack of adequate remediation of language, learning, and emotional factors than by the seizure stigma, the epilepsy restrictions, or the medications.

Factors and modifiers

Seizure type and location

The location and degree of brain involvement of the seizure pertains to the dysfunctions seen.

Generalized seizures involve the entire brain and all brain functions at the onset. Usually the individual is of relatively normal IQ, but often recurring generalized seizures or prolonged attacks may lead to some deterioration or depression of intelligence. Little bursts may interrupt attention.

Partial seizures are more often related to learning disabilities and language impairments than to retardation, although the majority of individuals with this group of seizures are relatively normal. Frequently recurring or prolonged partial seizures can be damaging to the nerve cells, leading to loss of specific functions, a dropping of intellectual processes, and emotional problems.

The laterality of the partial seizure discharge is important. Dominant-hemisphere discharges can impede language processing, while non-dominant-hemispheric discharges may impede non-verbal functions such as perceptual motor skills. Frontal involvement, especially early, may interfere with planning and organization skills and the development of executive functioning. Limbic involvement impairs memory and distorts emotional reactions.

Epileptic syndromes may present in idiopathic and symptomatic forms, all with some degree of related impairment. The symptomatic syndromes such as West's syndrome and Lennox–Gastaut syndrome are usually associated with severe impairments of language and learning with related severe behavior problems. Even the benign syndromes have been associated with subtle interruptions of function by special testing procedures.

Reflex epilepsies are those seizures triggered by specific sensory stimuli to the brain, such as flashing lights, video games, hearing speech, reading, concentration, etc. Academic efforts may occasionally trigger such events, resulting in brief seizures that interrupt the academic effort.

Transient cognitive impairments may result from epileptiform discharges in vital brain areas that may be neither large enough nor long enough to produce clinical symptoms but can interrupt, distort, or obliterate cognitive and emotional functions. The result may be interrupted attention, impaired recall, or distorted behaviors.

Appearance

Little seizures, like stares or small jerks, may easily be overlooked. Nocturnal events may be missed. By comparison, grand mal attacks are the center of attention, aversion, and fear by curious yet anxious onlookers. The stigma over the seizure spreads to include the child and all functioning attempts thereafter, with failures often blamed on the epilepsy if not on the medications used to treat the seizures.

Idiopathic versus symptomatic

All seizures are subject to the adverse attitudes and interactions of their environment. Consequently, language, learning, and behavior problems may be seen with all seizure types. However, people with symptomatic seizures are more apt to have problems and more apt to have more severe difficulties due to both the seizures and the underlying damage. Those with idiopathic epilepsy have only the effects of the seizures to cope with.

Gender

The male brain tends to be more lateralized in brain functions and more vulnerable to the insults that result in cognitive difficulties and language impairments. Gender differences appear to play a major role in how emotions are expressed, such that boys tend to act out and girls tend to withdraw. Teachers and parents display differences in expectations depending on the gender.

Age at onset

A major difference between childhood epilepsy and adulthood epilepsy is the factor of brain (and brain function) development. Children are not just little adults. The earlier-onset seizures interfere more with the developing brain and brain functions, as well as perhaps distorting reparative efforts of plasticity. Yet earlier seizure insults may allow more recovery by utilizing alternative brain sites. This effect lessens with age.

To fully understand pediatric epilepsy is to understand developmental differences in children. This entails understanding the developing brain, the developing child, the developing language skills, the developing learning abilities, and the developmental stages of emotions and behaviors. The seizures, the medications, and the approaches differ according to the stage of development, as do the parents, the school, and the peers.

The common age divisions of childhood are divided into neonatal (0–2 months), infancy (2 months–2 years), toddlers (2–5 years), childhood (5–12 years), and adolescence (13–18/21 years of age). Adolescence is often alluded to as the typical onset of puberty. Infancy may be subdivided into early infancy and late infancy, correlating with the first and second years of life. Similarly, adolescence has been divided into early adolescence, implying the first three or four years, and late adolescence. There is some effort to carve out a preadolescence period of 9–12 years of age, representing the hormonal preparation for puberty. These stages parallel the development surges of the brain and the maturation of the neurotransmitter system, as they are manifest in seizure presentation, in cognitive approaches, and in related emotional reactions.

The International Classification of the Epilepsies movement in syndrome classification, speaking of neonatal seizures, early and late infantile-onset seizures, early childhood seizures (toddler period on into childhood), childhood seizures, and adolescent (juvenile) seizures, follows these same age periods. Some seizures, such as atypical absence, may emerge in the preadolescent period. Infantile spasms represent the infant brain's style of reacting to a variety of insults. Landau–Kleffner syndrome begins after infancy, when language has become sufficiently established to be noticeably lost. This syndrome is an early-childhood emerging seizure type occurring when language is being established. The various juvenile epilepsies tend to reflect the hormonal changes of puberty as well as the continuing maturation of the brain.

These periods also characterize major periods of development of the brain and of brain functions. They relate to stages of emotional development in children. Infancy is a perceptual-motor period, late infancy to the toddler age is one of language acquisition and establishment, childhood is a concrete age, and adolescence marks the onset of abstract thinking. Once begun, the developmental processes continue on into the next age. Similarly, one can see stages of emotional developmental challenges at each age. The trusting infant changes into the independent young toddler ("terrible twos"), to the friendly but hero-worshipping early childhood, to the more social-centered later childhood stage. In adolescence, there is a repetition of this evolution, including the terrible twos, as the child moves away from family dependence to self and society dependence.

The epileptic factors may distort developmental processes in the developing brain, yet the developing brain may be able to overcome such distortions by alternate development processes. The developed brain is essentially matured and thus not apt to experience developmental distortions. However, any damage done at this age is a loss, since the mature brain is limited in its ability to recover functions.

The brain is especially sensitive to insults in the earliest years of life. Recovery may be gained with age but in part this may be more of compensation and rewiring of the developing nervous system. Children with severe seizures in infancy are often more functionally handicapped than those with seizures of onset later in childhood and those with early-childhood-onset seizures may be more handicapped than those with adolescent-onset seizures. This is seen with other medical conditions; for example, children under three to five years of age with leukemia and other cancers are more sensitive to chemotherapy or radiation therapy than children over the age of seven.

Anticonvulsants can be affected by age. Metabolism can be more erratic in younger children. The so-called "safe" anticonvulsants like phenobarbital may impair nerve cell growth in infancy, although this is more in the balance centers (cerebellum) than in the thinking brain. Phenytoin can also have adverse effects in the younger child. The treating physician needs to weigh the risks of treatment versus the risks of non-treatment; if treatment is the choice, the physician must monitor the risks carefully and, if needed, provide early interventions.

Timing

Seizures and even seizure bursts during the performance of important tasks may result in failures and frustrations. Seizures at night may go unnoticed but render the child sleep-deprived the next day, thus impaired in function and behavior.

Frequency

Frequent seizures do not allow time for the brain to recover between episodes. Frequent seizures over a period of time may lead to changes in the neuronal circuitry and neurotransmitter balance, resulting in functional losses and delayed emergence of some psychiatric complications.

Length

Lengthy seizures, as with status epilepticus, through the metabolic and circulatory changes in the brain as well as the release of neural excitatory amino acids, can be destructive to vital learning areas of the brain. Changes in cognitive functions (especially memory) and in behavior may be seen following a lengthy bout of epileptic status. The child appears less susceptible than the adult to the devastation of status.

Therapy

All antiepileptic drugs may help or hinder brain functions and emotions. This can occur if the blood–brain levels of the medication are excessive, if multiple drugs are used, or if the patient is overly sensitive to the drug. In children, the effect is not only on the brain but also on brain development. With new medications and seizure surgery, the seizures may be controlled but the associated language, learning, and behavior problems often remain.

Attitudes and interactions

Children do not experience seizures; they experience the reactions to the seizures. This is what shapes their self-concept, their learning experience, their communicative efforts, their social skills, and their preparation for adulthood. It is the experiences with parents and peers, educators and employers. From the time of the diagnosing of the epilepsy, the child's parents go through an evolution of their feelings and responses to the seizures, which affects their parenting as well as their view of the child. Teachers tend to expect less and blame all on the medications. Reduced expectations may result in reduced help for problems, which are then often overlooked or blamed on the medication. Children with epilepsy are still expected not to learn as well, not to tolerate as much stress, and not to be able to participate as fully as their classmates. Medical personnel interact with the young patient as an entity to be poked, prodded, punctured and pounded upon, and then ignored, as the physician addresses all questions and explanations to the worried parents, with the back often turned to the child. Whose seizures are they anyway? The parents'?

The whole-child model

Epilepsy in modern times is no longer only the control of seizures; it is the helping of the individual with epilepsy to gain his or her whole potential and abilities in terms of learning, socialization, communicating, earning, and enjoying. The need is to look beyond the epilepsy and see not only the seizure problems but also the child's potential.

The physician expert in epilepsy treats the whole child, detecting early signs of emerging problems in education, behavior, earning preparation, and socialization; such a physician is very vigilant to clues of potential problems and responds rapidly. The treating team is not just the medical personnel, but also the parents and family, the educators, the community, and others involved in remediative services. The true management approach draws together all aspects of functional living into a unified therapy to help the child and ultimately to help the child help themselves. Treat the child, not the EEG, not the spikes, not the pills, not the seizure classification.

REFERENCE

Commission for the Control of Epilepsy and Its Consequences (1977). *Plan for Nationwide Action on Epilepsy*. Bethesda, MD: National Institutes of Neurological and Communicative Disorders and Stroke.

Svoboda, W. B. (1979). *Learning about Epilepsy*. Baltimore, MD: University Park Press.

Svoboda, W. B. (1989). Kansas Task Force on Epilepsy and Other Seizure Related Disorders: Report and Reference Documents. Topeka, KS: Kansas Department of Health.

Part I

Speech and language problems

Language: the challenge

Communication is the exchange of ideas and feelings. The main avenue of communication is language, in many forms, both verbal and non-verbal. Verbal language is the code of learning and underlies much of emotional development. If there is no means of communication, there exists limited learning and scant socialization. Language is among the highest of evolutionary skills. The developing brain may sacrifice other higher cognitive abilities to preserve the ability to communicate.

So intricate and fragile is this ability that many worldly woes emanate from gender differences, age dissimilarities, societal variants, and national differences in mother tongues. Far greater is the betrayal of an ability that is distorted or lost due to a brain insult or to epilepsy. The individual is frustrated, as are the parents, teachers, and social contacts.

Are speech and language problems a part of epilepsy?

Dr Frank M. C. Besag, noted, "If children have seizures, then they are particularly liable to language deficits." He asked, "What is it about having seizures that should determine that language deficits specifically occur?" In the same discussion, Dr Bruce Hermann commented, "There is not much work on language" (Besag & Hermann, 2001).

Failure to communicate accurately or adequately underlies many of the problems experienced in families, in school, in social interactions, and in employment. Some children with epilepsy do not communicate well. They experience subtle and often variable language problems. They may misunderstand or they may be misunderstood. Such misunderstandings distort emotional development, educational efforts, and later earning. Some try to communicate but not clearly or smoothly, resulting in taunts and frustrations.

Amid the shock and confusion following the occurrence of a seizure, the turmoil of EEGs, scans, and other tests, the follow-up pills and blood tests, problems of speech and language are overlooked, although they may well be a part of the whole seizure problem.

Speech–language problems occur in the population of children with epilepsy. In one clinic study, 20% were found to have language problems and 4% were referred for further evaluation. (Williams *et al.*, 1992). Is brain damage causing both the seizures and the speech–language problems? Do recurrent seizures lead to brain damage and subsequent language problems? Does the epilepsy directly cause the language dysfunction? The types of speech–language problems may be temporary, ictal or postictal, paroxysmal or temporary that may become permanent.

The international experience

One of every four children with epilepsy may have speech–language problems, according to a presentation on speech and language dysfunctions of epilepsy given at the International Epilepsy Conference in Oslo, Norway in July 1993. It was found that 51 of 200 children with seizures had speech–language problems in screening. The types of problems seen included loss of speech, receptive or expressive language problems, problems in recall, motor speech disturbances, and, most commonly, mixed problems.

The national experience

Language problems of epilepsy include word-finding difficulties, memory disturbances, as well as ictal and interictal language problems (Gordon, 1991). These may be of lateralizing and localizing value, especially in epilepsy surgery evaluations. Word-finding problems (43%) and forgetting names (31%) are the most common language findings in individuals with temporal lobe epilepsy. These problems may relate to the cause or the interactivity of non-traditional language areas in the anterior and inferior temporal lobe. The incidence is more than twice that found in a control population. Such individuals should at least be screened if not tested formally, for they can be helped.

The Kansas Epilepsy Center experience

At the St Francis (Wichita, KS) Epilepsy Symposium of 1987, David Henry and Marilyn Brown reviewed the findings of language and auditory processing deficits in mostly children referred to the Kansas Epilepsy Center. The referral population was 96% children, seen by a team of multidisciplinary specialists especially trained in epilepsy. The patients comprised 11% preschoolers, 54% grade scholars, 31% adolescents, and 4% adults. Although initially 85–89% were felt to have generalized seizures in referral, the evaluation showed that the incidence was reduced to 60% by adolescence. Partial seizures were diagnosed in 36–40% from the onset.

The types of speech–language problems included problems in language processing (53%), problems in articulation (3%), auditory memory problems (especially in short-term memory) in (61%), and problems other than memory (16%).

Fluency and voice prosody problems were detected in this group. The problems were subtle to profound in presentation. Relationships to seizure frequency, age of onset, and seizure intensity were noted. Alternations in the intelligibility of the speech (80%) and vowel prolongations (20%) were noted. Errors bore some relationship to the lateralization and localization of the seizure and the discernment of the physician examiners. Problems observed in these children included abnormal speech discrimination (23%), which was usually bilateral (18%). Other difficulties included problems in auditory processing (41%), which could be unilateral (20%) or bilateral (13%). The most common auditory-processing problems included peripheral auditory deficits of hearing and articulation, auditory attention, auditory memory, language-processing problems, and native cognitive abilities.

Audiometry examinations were performed for those with the slightest indication for such by history or by screening. Thus, new testing was performed most often in school-age children and least often in preschoolers. Middle-ear infections were common. In those tested, problems found included flat tympanogram in one or both ears (14%), and the placement of ear tubes in one or both ears (8%). Of the 60% of the entire group tested, 23% had reduced hearing in one or both ears, and 14% had moderate reduction in both ears. High-frequency problems were common and appeared to contribute to some reduction in understanding of speech in 70%; problems in discrimination in a noisy background were seen in 24% who had problems with one ear and in 9% who had problems with both ears.

Overall conclusions

The following section is based on Svoboda (1979).

Speech–language problems are more common than suspected yet often overlooked

Language problems may be seen with nearly all types of seizures but especially those involving the frontal-temporal lobes and adjacent areas.

Following a generalized tonic–clonic seizure, speech deficiencies and distortions may be part of the postictal confusion state. This gradually clears. Occasionally, children with uncontrolled frequent absence seizures, especially atypical forms, may present with blocks, halts, and jerky speech efforts. They may exhibit humming or they may get stuck on words. There are omissions in understanding. Rarely, their speech efforts may seem confused, slurred, or even deficient. This can be seen more commonly with excess stress. Jerky speech with momentary halts or inflections may be seen with minor motor seizures (the akinetic drops or myoclonic jerks).

With some simple partial seizures, blocks, halts, utterances, or distortions of pronunciation may be seen. Complex partial seizures, especially those involving the dominant temporal lobe, are more apt to disturb language processing with problems of anomia and auditory memory noted. Learning disabilities involving the auditory sphere, often with secondary perceptual motor problems, may be seen. Aphasias, arrests, and anomias may be noted, as well as problems in word fluency. There may be a deficiency or a loss of language. Speech utterances may occur ictally. Some individuals have a flat, emotionless style of speech, with a loss of prosody.

Reflex seizures may occur, such as in individuals who experience seizures when they try to read aloud. There may be a history of stuttering when reading as a child.

Epileptiform discharges of a subclinical nature involving language-processing areas may contribute to language-processing impairments.

All aspects of language have been associated with epilepsy-related problems

The five most common problems are (1) the loss of a smooth flow of spoken ideas, (2) a slow, slurred, labored, tick-tock speech pattern, (3) trouble with understanding others, (4) difficulties expressing ideas clearly, leading to misunderstandings by others, and (5) problems with remembering the names of people or items. However, still other problems have been seen in children with epilepsy.

There are multiple causes for language problems in epilepsy

With seizures, there are four ways in which language can be impaired, including (1) the underlying brain insult that causes both the seizures and language disturbance, (2) the seizures themselves, (3) episodic, epileptic short-circuits disturbing language processing, and (4) medication reactions. A negative environment in which the child with epilepsy struggles to develop may aggravate these.

The underlying brain insult may produce both seizures and language problems. The insult may be an underlying brain irritant, such as a focal chronic virus infection, an autoimmune problem, a tumor, or a vascular malformation. If the child has an active process of the brain, the speech may continue to deteriorate. However, if the seizures eventually improve or become controlled, the language function also may then improve or recover. Occasionally, the speech problem may develop before the seizure difficulties.

The seizures, especially if prolonged or repeated, may cause a loss of a language skill (especially in an adult) or a distortion or depression of language development (in a child) with or following the seizure. Speech and language problems may be seen with obvious seizures or with a left-hemispheric disturbance, especially involving the left frontal-temporal area, with or without any epileptic symptoms.

The seizure discharges themselves may short-circuit language processes and, if larger or longer in duration, may produce more recognizable seizure symptoms. The electrochemical seizure potential discharges, not great enough to produce seizures, still short-circuit language processes without a history suggestive of epilepsy.

The antiepileptic drugs used to control the seizures may impair speech and sometimes also language, especially if used at higher doses or if more than one drug is used. Some patients are sensitive at therapeutic blood levels. Sometimes, the seizures appear to be controlled but the speech problem persists. Occasionally, an increase or an alteration of the anticonvulsant within the normal therapeutic range may overcome the speech difficulties.

The course of the language problem may be variable

Speech and language problems may precede the onset of seizures, may develop along with the seizures, or may develop some time later after the onset of the seizures. Such problems may be ongoing or they may occur in episodes, often linked with the appearance of seizures clusters. If they are an ongoing problem, the severity may wax and wane. Speech and language problems, like learning problems and emotional problems, can be brought out by stress, by poor seizure control, or by inappropriate use of anticonvulsant medications. Nocturnal seizures may result in daytime struggles. Of all these, stress is the most apt to bring out a speech or language problem. The child with a seizure coming from the left half of the brain is at the most risk for such problems.

The onset may be before, during, or following the onset of the seizure disorder. The symptoms may be temporary, lasting hours to weeks, may recur as brief episodes, or may present as a progressive problem. Symptoms may present as an aura to seizure, as part of seizure, or as an aftereffect of seizure, or they may emerge as a problem between seizures.

A group of special language-regression syndromes exist as a special challenge

There are a group of seizure syndromes that are especially prone to emerging in the first decade of life. The onset of seizures, sometimes fairly resistant to medication, may be accompanied by the loss, often severe, of language. The frustrated patient often develops major behavior problems. The seizures may be outgrown, after which language may or may not return. Specific epilepsy language combination syndromes include the acquired agnosia/aphasia with epilepsy syndrome of Landau-Kleffner, the sleep spike-wave status syndrome, absence/minor motor status, protracted partial complex status, and Rasmussen's encephalitis, the latter often having a dire outcome.

Language problems may underlie some learning and behavior problems of epilepsy

A variety of emotional reactions to the frustration of language problems are noted. Children with a receptive aphasia may be described as autistic, as having attention deficit/hyperactivity disorder (ADHD), or as withdrawing, whereas children with expressive aphasia are more apt to be shy or to display temper reactions. Similar tendencies are seen in elderly people after strokes. Problems of communication may underlie social difficulties and learning problems (Cantwell *et al.*, 1980, 1981; Gordon, 1991).

The challenge

Considering three aspects, i.e. language as the base for learning, language as related intimately to emotions, and epilepsy as a potential distorter of language, the physician, teacher, or therapist should consider the relationships between speech–language and epilepsy.

This leads to three questions to be considered in approaching the child with epilepsy: how does epilepsy interfere with language, what type(s) of epileptic language problems are potentially present, and how may abnormal language functioning affect overall functioning as well as seizure control?

REFERENCES

Besag, F. M. C. & Hermann, B. (2001). Panel discussion 2. In *Epilepsia and Learning Disabilities*, ed. G. F. Ayala, M. Elia, C. M. Cornaggia and M. M. Trimble. *Epilepsia* **42**: 28.

Cantwell, D. P., Baker, L. & Mattison, R. E. (1980). Psychiatric disorders in children with speech and language retardation. *Arch. Gen. Psychiatry* **37**: 423–6.

Cantwell, D. P., Baker, L. & Mattison, R. E. (1981). Prevalence, type, and correlates of psychiatric diagnosis in 200 children with communicative disorders. *J. Dev. Behav. Pediatr.* **2**: 131–5.

Gordon, N. (1991). The relationship between language and behavior. *Dev. Med. Child Neurol.* **33**: 86–9.

Svoboda, W. B. (1979). Epilepsy and learning problems. In *Learning About Epilepsy*, pp. 186–200. Baltimore, MD: University Park Press.

Williams, J., Sharp, G. B. & Griebel, M. I. (1992). Neuropsychological functioning in clinically referred children with epilepsy. *Epilepsia* **33** (suppl 3): 17.

3

Speech, language, and communication

Communication is the exchange of ideas and feelings between two or more persons. The main method of communication is language, spoken or written. Failure to communicate accurately or adequately may lead to misunderstandings. Subtle language problems often underlie many of the problems people experience at home, at school, in society, and in employment.

Some epileptic children do not communicate well. They experience subtle language problems. They may misunderstand what others say. They may not be able to express themselves so that others can understand. One adolescent complained, "They don't understand me." The parents complained, "She doesn't seem to listen." Her teachers noted, "We teach her one day and the next day she has learned nothing." These problems may vary from day to day. Such misunderstandings may impair emotional development, learning, and later earning.

There are numerous types of speech–language problems reported in children who have epilepsy. Speech problems include difficulties in pronunciation, in the rate and in the flow of speech. Language problems include difficulties in understanding speech sounds, words, and word meanings, as well as problems in expressing ideas in words and in forming the actual words. This may be related to impairments in memory, in remembering what was heard recently as well as what was previously learned. Problems in remembering names is also a common difficulty.

Communication disorders

MacDonald Critchley defined language as "the expression and reception of ideas and feelings." This does not say how the ideas and feelings are expressed or understood. Spoken language is not the only method of communication, for other means of communication include reading and writing, body language, telegraphy, sign language, Braille, visual symbols, not to mention drum messaging, whistled language, smoke signaling, semaphore, flagging, and flashing-light signals. The emphasis herein will be restricted to the spoken word. Speech is the expression of ideas and feelings by way of verbal sounds and words (Critchley, 1979).

Language is a dynamic yet complicated system of symbols, spoken and written, used in various ways for thought and for communication. The historical, social, and cultural environment in which it is used shapes the language. Language governs behavior. Influential factors in learning and using language include biologic, cognitive, psychosocial, and environmental factors. Effective use of language in communication requires understanding of human interactions beyond just the spoken words, for just as important are non-verbal cues (body language), motivation, and social-cultural roles.

In 1982, the American Speech and Hearing Association (1982) attempted to clarify confusions and disagreements regarding speech and language disorders by developing a statement defining the various aspects of communication, as follows:

A communication disorder is impairment in the ability to understand and/or process spoken (or written) language. The problem may be in the handling of the sounds and words themselves, or their meanings. The problem may be difficulties in transmitting and using the sounds, words, and language. The impairment is observed in disorders of hearing, language, and/or speech processes. Such problems can be slight to severe. The cause may be developmental or acquired. The problem may be episodic or ongoing. Individuals may manifest one or any combination of the three aspects of the disorder, i.e. a speech disorder, a language disorder, or problems in the communication of ideas by other methods.

Language disorders

A language disorder is the impairment or abnormal development of understanding and/or use of a spoken, written and/or other symbol system. The disorder may involve the form of language (phonologic, morphologic and syntactic systems), the content of language (semantic system), or the function of language in communication (pragmatic system) in any combination.

Phonology is the study, of vocal sounds including articulation. Morphology is the making and shaping of speech. Syntax is the arrangement of words in speech. Semantics is the meanings of words and the rules for their use. Pragmatics addresses the practical aspects of how words fit together to convey an acceptable concept.

Speech disorder

Speech is not the same as language. Children may know what they want to say and try to say the right words only not be able to pronounce the words clearly. This frustrates them and those trying to understand what they are trying to say.

A speech disorder is an impairment of voice, articulation (making of speech sounds), and/or fluency (the smooth flow of speech sounds), as observed in spoken efforts. A voice disorder is the absence or abnormal production of vocal quality, pitch, loudness, resonance, and/or duration. An articulation disorder signifies the abnormal production of speech sounds. A fluency disorder is defined as the abnormal flow of verbal expression, characterized by impaired rate and rhythm, which may be accompanied by struggling effort as with stuttering.

Other communicative disorders

Communicative differences, i.e. dialects, refer to a variation of a symbol system used by a group of individuals, who reflect and are defined by shared regional, social, or cultural/ethnic factors. These variations should not be considered a disorder of speech or language.

Speech is only one of the ways that language can be expressed. Written language is another way. Gestures, sign language, and body language are still other ways of communicating. Augmented communication is a system used to supplement the communicative skills of individuals for whom speech is temporarily or permanently inadequate to meet communicative needs.

Hearing disorders

A hearing disorder is altered auditory sensitivity, acuity, function, processing, and/or damage to the integrity of the physiological auditory system. A hearing disorder may impede the development, comprehension, production, or maintenance of language and speech. Hearing disorders are classified according to difficulties in detection, perception, and/or processing of auditory information. Young children with epilepsy may be more prone to ear infections and subsequently hearing problems. Such acute infections may trigger seizures. However the focus often is on the resultant seizure only and the ear infection may be overlooked.

Language processing

Incoming auditory sensations are perceived and discriminated primarily in the temporal lobes. Language stimuli are then transferred to Wernicke's area in the posterior temporal parietal area on the dominant side to be understood. Connections to the limbic system and diffuse cortical memory areas draw upon related associations to form concepts, which are projected forward either to Broca's area on the dominant posterior inferior frontal lobe to be expressed in spoken efforts, or just above that area to be expressed in a written or gestured manner.

Organization and language in the brain

The brain is neither anatomically nor functionally symmetrical. The dominant hemisphere, the hemisphere that handles the majority of basic language functions, is usually the left side. The non-dominant hemisphere, usually the right, processes non-language functions such as perceptual-motor skills but also contributes the emotional flavor to language, adding feelings and the melodious features that prevent speech from being a flat monotone. In a young child whose dominant hemisphere is damaged, vital functions may be moved to an adjacent area or to the other hemisphere. This recovery alibility lessens with age (Milner *et al.*, 1966;

Schulhoff & Goodglass, 1969; Berlin *et al.*, 1972; Luria, 1974; Heilman *et al.*, 1975; Drewe, 1976; Benson, 1979; Ojelmann, 1979).

Localization

Barry Gordon (1996) reviewed the organization and localization of language in the brain at the American Epilepsy Conference. Classically, in the dominant hemisphere, language has been located to the anterior Broca's area for expression and the posterior Wernicke's area for receptive understanding. Auditory discrimination, the distinguishing between various speech sounds, is performed in the posterior superior temporal lobe. On the left, in the temporal parietal occipital junction, is Wernicke's area, where the word and phrase sound clusters are given meaning. In the inferior temporal and pre-occipital area, interpretation of the meanings of sounds and of pictures occurs on the left and right sides, respectively. The information is then sent forward to be expressed. Production of sound and language is in the classic Broca's expressive area in the lower premotor frontal area. These concepts address reception (comprehension), transmission, and production (expression). There are many more components for language, such as acoustic analysis, visual analysis of normalization, and other related functions.

Language may be represented more diffusely in the left hemisphere of left-handed people than in right-handers. Some left-handers have bilateral speech representation. Hemispheric speech representation tends to be more variable in left than in right-handers. Bilateral representation of speech functions in left-handers may lessen the effectiveness of the right hemisphere in perceptive studies (Todd & Satz, 1977). The non-dominant hemisphere may contribute to the recognition of high-frequency, concrete thoughts or nouns that create mind images (Bradshaw, 1980).

The anatomic concepts of Wernicke's and Broca's areas are overly simplified. In most people, the Broca's expressive areas are in the lower premotor frontal location in the brain, but one in six have an aberrant location. Other language areas have been identified through cortical-stimulation studies and functional imaging studies. Areas of importance include the parietal, anterior-lateral temporal, and frontal areas, the latter playing importance in initiating speech and language. The function of the lateral inferior temporal area is not yet understood. In picture naming, the entire temporal lobe to inferior temporal areas as well as Broca's and Wernicke's areas are activated.

Patients with basal-temporal language localization due to damage or an insult are fluent in language but anomic during confrontation naming. They do not differ in response to semantic or phonemic cues in overcoming naming defects, but they tend to be paraphasic and spontaneously describe attributes of objects that they cannot name, suggesting relatively intact access to semantic stores. They display impoverished vocabulary skills and perform poorly on delayed verbal memory. Often, they have impaired semantic clustering. The basal-lateral temporal region thus assumes a more critical role after injury to the primary cortical language zone (Fedio *et al.*, 1992).

Normal function variability exists. This is least in low-level relatively anchored functions, such as speech perception, and greatest for highest-level functions, such as processing. Higher functions such as naming are more variable in exact localization. The influences for variability in epilepsy include early injury (especially in the neonate) and the lesion presence, size and location. The seizure focus in terms of lesion location and pathology is important but alone does not shift language to another part of the brain. The age and the nature of the injury are the greatest cause of shift.

An area devoted to a function expands and contracts either momentarily or lastingly over years. An area devoted to a function may be shifted by millimeters to centimeters as related to functional shifts and the pathology. Static maps of location may need to be modified. Bilateralism and variability allow more aggressiveness in operative approaches than might first be thought, but this requires sufficient studies to be localized. The outcomes are better, especially in children, when a full evaluation has been done.

Lateralization

Gordon (1996) also reviewed lateralization. Most individuals are predominantly right-handed. Roughly one-third of all right-handed people are strongly right-sided dominant in hand–foot–eye–ear function; the remainder are of variable mixed dominance, depending on what they are doing. In the general population, slightly more than 97% of people have speech development in the left hemisphere (Balthazar, 1963; Goodglass and Quadfasel, 1954).

Males tend to be more functionally lateralized than females, especially for verbal processes (McGone, 1977). Individuals who reach puberty at an earlier age, as do females, appear less lateralized (Weintraub, 1981). In both boys and girls, the language ability improves during the phase of increasing neural connections. Language ability decreases or remains at a plateau during a phase of decreased connections, the pruning stage. The rates and times for growth and pruning cycles for the same brain network differ in boys and girls. Boys favor vocabulary subskills needed for comprehension, while girls favor fluency and phonic subskills needed for the mechanics of reading.

Right-handers

About 90–92% of individuals are naturally right-handed, with speech strongly in the left hemisphere; the remaining 8% may have speech either on the right or bilaterally. In right-handed individuals, the language centers are associated with the left hemisphere language in 99%. However, up to 30% may have some language in the right hemisphere and 9% will have significant right hemispheric language.

Left-handers

Only about 10% of individuals are left-handed, often, there is a family history of left-handedness. A totally left-sided person is rare; most left-dominant people are a mixture of right- and left-sided dominance, depending on the task. In naturally left-handed individuals, the problems are more complicated. For left-handed and ambidextrous patients without brain damage, 60–70% have speech predominantly in the left hemisphere and 20% have it in the right hemisphere with some degree of mixture not uncommon. Those left-handed individuals with a strong family history of left-handedness are more apt to have a language function shared between the two brain halves or lateralized to the right side. Those with little or no family history of left-handedness may have had their language shifted to the right hemisphere because of some early brain insult. Such an insult may also have shifted the handedness and caused other problems, such as seizures, learning disabilities, mental retardation, and speech defects. One tries to differentiate between those born to be left-handed and those who are left-handed because of an early insult to the left side of the brain.

Language development

At 30 weeks into pregnancy, the speech centers of the brain are already prominent. Language is not set firmly until nearly ten years of age. In a young child, an epileptic brain insult must affect both sides of the brain to impair language development severely. The process of language development and lateralization play a major role in the nature of the language impairment of children with epilepsy and language disorders.

Prenatal

Language potentials, originally bilateral, tend to develop predominantly on the left side. As early as 29 weeks into the pregnancy, the portion of the brain over the posterior temporal lobe between Herschel's gyrus and the posterior margin of the Sylvian fissure near the lower parietal lobe, the area known as the plenum temporale, is already becoming asymmetrically prominent on the left in 90% of fetuses. This area is destined to serve receptive language functions. This area enlarges more than the similar area on the right brain. Such asymmetries existed up to 40,000 years ago. The asymmetries are less marked, are absent, or sometimes are reversed in left-handed patients (Geschwind, 1972).

Infancy

Within days to weeks after birth, the newborn can distinguish different sounds. Within months, the infant is identifying and categorizing sounds. The young child's receptive understanding precedes the expressive language skills in development. Receptive language is continually being shaped and developed in the first year of life (Geffen, 1976). Children as young as three weeks age favor the right ear, perhaps reflecting the left hemisphere dominance for speech, in dichotic listening. Ninety percent of fetuses have a larger left hemisphere in regions important for speech and language (LeDoux et al., 1978). Inter-hemispheric differences in auditory evoked potential amplitude to speech and music in newborns also suggest lateralization to the right-ear advantage for dichotically presented speech sounds at that age.

The first half-year of life is associated with emotional vocalization, self-entertaining coos, and babbling. The infant practices through repetition. Then, over the ensuing half-year, the infant echoes back what is heard. Repetitive sounds are initiated and practiced. Jargon nonsense language emerges as imitative efforts in the growing efforts to communicate. By around one year and certainly below two years, the infant begins to experiment with single words. By two years of age, the infant is into phrases, mainly nouns and verbs.

Early childhood

Language development is an important activity from two years of age until the onset of puberty. Receptive language develops ahead of expressive language. Girls tend to develop language skills more rapidly than boys. Gordon (1996) notes that by age two and a half, children have the beginning of the adult language pattern, with words, language, syntax, and grammar basically developed.

By three years of age, the child uses pronouns, adjectives, and adverbs. By this age, the toddler uses sentences, including descriptive terms and pronouns. In this two- to three-year range, speech deteriorates if the child has not made the leap from imitative word efforts to initiated phrases and sentences. A child who lacks language may lose interest in repeating words and brief phrases and thus be thought to regress in language when the problem is the failure to development language processes.

The child's capacity to learn to control what is heard and what is rehearsed probably begins early in life but appears not to be a major control factor until the late third to fourth year of life. The relationship between what the child hears and how the child processes this information is very important in development (Hardy, 1965). From this age onwards, certain seizure syndromes are associated with a regression-loss of language skills, the sites having become established and thus vulnerable to attack.

The left-hemispheric established dominance for language emerges by three to five years of age. The right hemisphere plays less and less of a role in language processing.

From the sentence stage of true language, the child goes through a physiologic stuttering stage at about four years, due to the feedback system now developing. Continued significant stuttering after five to six years of age is a concern. In the sixth to seventh years, complex sentences and full grammar are almost developed as the language centers approach maturity. By the eighth year of age, articulation is fully developed.

By five to seven years of age, the functionally mature language lateralization is essentially established, although in older individuals intensive rehabilitation may bring about an amazing yet incomplete recovery. With the development of the lateralization of language processing to the left hemisphere, the right ear continues to be more sensitive than the left to spoken language when competing verbal stimuli are presented simultaneously to both ears. This right-sided advantage emerges fully at around four years of age and increases through at least 12–15 years of age (Geffen, 1976). The onset of puberty appears to signal the end of the lateralization process, suggesting hormonal influences.

Late childhood

By the school years, girls are nearly a year ahead of boys in speech and language skills. Even as adults, language skills are often better developed in the female than in the male. The maturing of those areas of the brain that serve the language functions parallels this development of language skills.

The myelination of the speech centers is not completed until near the end of the first decade of life, which is about the same time that the basics of language are finally established. The language areas become fully developed by around seven years of age, when the myelination is essentially completed. In children older than eight years, the configuration of the language cortex is similar to adults. Children tend to make fewer language errors. Auditory comprehension is interrupted more frequently in children than in adults. The frontal language cortex is more circumscribed than the temporal language areas and is most often characterized by speech arrest during seizures in 67% of children and most adults (Risse *et al.*, 1999). Although relatively limited as compared with the recoverability of the younger child, in therapy the human brain continues to be able to recover some lost speech and language functions far into adulthood.

Damage versus plasticity

Damage to established language centers may result in a loss of language abilities, as seen in adults and older children. Damage to undeveloped centers, as in younger children, may allow the shift of development of language to other capable areas of the brain, resulting in non-classical localizations or unexpected lateralization for language. The younger child may be able to compensate, after a slight developmental delay, by developing alternative sites for language functions. If early damage occurs, about 55% have speech development in the right hemisphere and 30% still have speech in the left hemisphere. In a younger child, both brain hemispheres may need to be involved to affect language significantly. If language is affected in the adult or older child after the language sites have been established, usually the language centers in the left brain must be involved.

Gordon (1996) notes that after an insult in early life, those that recover may have shifted the developmental lateralization to other regions retaining language potential. Problems may not appear until four to five years of age, even with insults at a much earlier age. This is a developmentally quiescent period, possibly related to some yet unidentified biological factor. Perhaps this is a delayed onset of a developmental problem in that autism emerges in infancy whereas these acquired aphasias develop in early to mid childhood.

The right hemisphere has the capacity to comprehend some speech and, if necessary, has the ability to assume the language functioning in the brain that would normally have speech on the left; or it can contain one speech area while the left hemisphere follows the other. Even when the major language processing is performed in the left hemisphere, the right hemisphere is not silent to language functions. The right hemisphere processes the melodious tone variations, accents, and inflections that give emotional feeling to language. It assists in some recognition of single words but not phrases. Damage to the right hemisphere renders a person unable to understand or to express the emotional aspects and inflections of language. The resultant language may seem a flat and featureless monotone. Understanding may be affected similarly, as the person may fail to heed meanings of emotional content and inflections of what others say. The language of the left hemisphere is the language of thought and logic; the language of the right hemisphere is the language of emotions and feelings (Weintraub *et al.*, 1958; Geets & Pinon, 1975; Heilman *et al.*, 1975; Searleman, 1978; Benson, 1979; Ross & Mesulam, 1979; Smith, 1980; Ross *et al.*, 1981).

Plasticity and function transfer

In 2000 at the Cleveland Clinics Epilepsy Conference, Duchaney reviewed the transfer of neural functions. The ability of the immature human brain to adjust for insults is called plasticity. If any vital language centers are damaged, the brain may shift the developing function to an adjacent area of the brain or to the other side of the brain. Whether this is a true shifting of function from one side to the other, or whether it is the development of the function in the undamaged site, is not known. If a very young child experiences an insult to one brain side, speech and language are apt to be affected, suggesting that initially language begins to develop bilaterally but eventually settles to the left side. The child with an insult to the right hemisphere is far more apt to recover language function than a child with an insult to the left hemisphere.

Early damage may result in new anatomic connections through collateral sprouting and synaptogenesis. New strategies may be acquired through reorganization of intrinsic functions of residual structures. After a lesion, positron emission tomography (PET) studies show limited inter-hemispheric reorganization of the involved area. Cortical areas are specified genetically and by extrinsic factors relating to at least three distinct processes: radial specification of the cortex, development of internal microcircuitry, and development of external connectively. Lesions in utero may lead to anomalous loci and aberrant cortical connections. In humans, the cortex is capable of undergoing remodeling after intrauterine and early childhood insults.

In individuals with early insults without hemiparesis, cortical dysplasias and aberrant connections may be found. The language cortex in patients with developmental pathology remains localized to the expected areas. The cortical surface devoted to language is similar to adult patients with epilepsy. Language may be shifted to the other hemisphere, especially with lesions acquired before age five years.

Children with congenital or infantile hemiplegia are verbal. No aphasia occurs after very early hemispherectomy. Children with temporal lobe epilepsy caused by a focal dysplasia of the left temporal lobe may have speech represented in the right hemisphere. The language cortex shows few changes.

The ability to shift functions decreases with age. An insult to either hemisphere before 15 months of age may be accompanied by a transient lag in speech development, but no major defects are seen once speech begins. This suggests that early language functions reside in both hemispheres, with either hemisphere being able to assume the language-processing role. The emergence of a major language deficit suggests a bilateral insult.

Up to five or six years of age, the child is often able to recover language fairly well after an insult to left-hemisphere language centers, although there may be a recovery lag. The child may begin to recover some of the prior speech skills as late as three months after the insult and continue to improve for another year or two. If the original insult has been overcome, the child usually will essentially have recovered a good command of the language within about two years of the insult. Left-hemisphere damage after five years of age but before puberty does not necessary result in irreversible loss of functioning, even though the left hemisphere has basically differentiated for language. Intermediate degrees of recovery are still possible (Bishop, 1981; Lenneberg, 1966).

By 11–14 years of age, damage to the speech centers may result in only partial recovery. Permanent speech and language problems become apparent around puberty. By adolescence, recovery from such insults to speech centers is poor. However, even the teenager can be taught to use what skills they have regained more efficiently and effectively.

Language is a developmental task vulnerable to adverse factors, such as seizures, seizure causes, and seizure-management approaches, especially in the younger child. If language is forced to develop in an alternate site, especially if shifted contralaterally, it uses brain centers that otherwise would have served other brain functions. The result is that the child may show only minor language handicaps and perhaps only a subtle learning disability, but also will exhibit perceptual motor handicaps, although the damage was to the left brain. Verbal intelligence may be depressed more with a dominant hemisphere focus, which, although performance intelligence remains relatively intact, pulls down the overall intelligence. Early acquired brain damage is usually bilateral to some degree, but the left hemisphere appears more vulnerable (Milner, 1975; Knaven, 1980).

Epilepsy

Gordon (1996) has reviewed laterality in patients with epilepsy. In right-handed people, many (80%) have left-hemisphere speech or bilateral representation (19%), with pure right-hemisphere localization being rare (1%). In left-handed individuals, the distribution is different, with 50% showing left-hemispheric dominance, 40–42% having right-hemispheric dominance, and 8–10% being mixed. The Wechlser Performance IQ may be selectively reduced relative to verbal IQ in boys, but not girls, with right-hemisphere speech dominance in association with childhood-onset left-hemisphere complex partial epilepsy (Novelly & Naugle, 1985).

The child with a partial seizure problem, especially one involving the left hemisphere, is at risk for language problems, especially if the onset is early in life and if it is due to an underling brain insult. Boys appear more vulnerable than girls to such insults. Early insults to the brain may not be associated with as severe a language impairment as expected, for the brain may have shifted functions as part of the recovery. In an individual with left-hemisphere seizures, particularly those of early onset or due to brain damage, the localization of language to the left hemisphere is less certain. Major language impairment in a young child usually implies bilateral brain damage.

Unlike the usual epilepsy patients whose intelligence, verbal memory, and memory scores are similar to the general population, there is a group with more scattered and more diffuse language sites than traditionally seen. In such individuals, the IQ tends to be depressed, with decreased language and memory skills, especially if the sites are outside the traditional Wernicke's area. Language may be displaced more interiorly and inferiorly. A wider dispersion may result in a disruption of normal language development due to a pathologic lesion, epileptogenic dysplasia, or both.

Parietal representation of language is more extensive in patients with seizure foci extending to the posterior temporal lob. The verbal IQ may be depressed (Devinsky *et al.*, 2000).

The effects of early-life temporal-lobe seizure foci on language development may differ for frontal-parietal foci. If early seizure foci are restricted to the left temporal lobe, motor dominance will not shift to the right hemisphere because the left sensory motor areas are intact. With left-hemisphere motor dominance, language functions almost always remain on the left side. The effects of left-temporal seizure foci during early development may produce a displacement of language functions either interiorly or inferiorly (Devinsky *et al.*, 2000).

Early onset of dominant temporal-lobe epilepsy is associated with more anteriorly disturbed temporal naming and reading functions. Dominant temporal-lobe seizure foci during language acquisition may cause a wider distribution of language, including a larger incidence of right-hemispheric dominance. Early left frontal and temporal insults, not just temporal injury, can displace language functions partially or completely to the right hemisphere. Right-hemisphere displacement is more likely in left-handers without a family history of left-handedness. Language lateralization may be determined by both the direct effects of left frontal parietal injury and a tendency for motor aspects of language to develop in the same hemisphere dominant for other motor functions (Devinsky *et al.*, 2000).

The non-dominant right hemisphere has a considerable capacity for language. Under certain neuroanatomical conditions, the right hemisphere becomes functional and thus measurable as seen in right-handed patients undergoing temporal lobectomy of the right hemisphere for medically intractable seizures. The right hemisphere is found to contribute to language even in individuals whose seizures are acquired in adulthood (Andy, 1984). Epileptic focus in the right hemisphere of children with early-onset seizures (preschool) leads to aphasia and, in some cases, alalia, in children with Lennox–Kleffner or Lennox–Gastaut syndromes. Correlations between the speech impairment (aphasia, alalia, dysphasia) and deficiencies in imaginative functions in drawings bring out differences between the two hemispheres in verbal and imaginative functions. The role of the hemisphere is increased in the development of speech and intellectual functioning. Milder speech and drawing impairments are noted and reflect essentially the psychoeducational sphere and the level of adaptation to speech insufficiency (Sorokina & Selitsky, 1999).

REFERENCES

American Speech and Hearing Association (1982). Definitions – communicative disorders and variations. *ASHA* **24**: 949–50.

Andy, O. J. (1984). Right-hemispheric language evidence from cortical stimulation. *Brain Lang.* **23**: 159–66.

Balthazar, T. E. (1963). Cerebral unilateralization in chronic epileptic cases: the Wechsler object assembly subtest. *J. Clin. Psychol.* **19**: 169–71.

Benson, D. F. (1979). Associated neurobehavioral problems *Aphasia, Alexia, and Agraphia*, pp. 158–73. New York: Churchill Livingstone.

Berlin, C. I., Lowe-Bell, S. S., Jannetta, P. J. & Kline, D. G. (1972). Central auditory deficits after temporal lobectomy. *Arch. Otolaryngol.* **96**: 4–10.

Bishop, D. V. M. (1981). Plasticity and specificity of language localization in the developing brain. *Dev. Med. Child Neurol.* **23**: 545–6.

Bradshaw, J. L. (1980). Right hemisphere language: familial and non-familial sinistrals, cognitive deficits and writing hand position in sinistrals and concrete-abstract imageable-nonimageable dimensions in word recognition: a review of interrelated issues. *Brain Lang.* **10**: 172–88.

Critchley, M. (1979). Physiology and other aspects of language. In *Aphasiology.* London: Edward Arnold.

Devinsky, O., Perrine, K., Hirsch, J., McMullen, W., *et al.* (2000). Relation of cortical language distribution and cognitive functions in surgical epilepsy patients. *Epilepsia* **41**: 400–404.

Drewe, E. A. (1976). An experimental investigation of Luria's theory on the effects of frontal lobe lesions in men. *Neurophysiology* **13**: 421–9.

Duchaney, M. (2000). The transfer of function in dysplastic contex. Cleveland Clinic Conference, Cleveland, OH, June 2, 2000.

Fedio, P., August, A., Sato, S. & Kufta, C. (1992). Neuropsychological characteristics of patients with basolateral temporal language. *Epilepsia* **33** (suppl 3): 120.

Geets, W. & Pinon, A. (1975). Crises agnosiques avec troubles du languge et anomalies asmetricques de EEG. *Acta Psychiatr. Belg.* **75**: 160–72.

Geffen, G. (1976). Development of hemispheric specialization for speech perception. *Cortex* **12**: 337–46.

Geschwind, N. (1972). Cerebral dominance and anatomic asymmetry. *N. Engl. J. Med.* **287**: 194–5.

Goodglass, H. & Quadfasel, F. A. (1954). Language laterality and left-handed aphasiacs. *Brain* **77**: 521–84.

Gordon, B. (1996). Organization and localization of language in the brain. Presented at the American Epilepsy Society Conference, San Francisco, December, 1996.

Hardy, W. G. (1965). On language disorders in young children: a reorganization of thinking. *J. Speech Hear. Disord.* **30**: 3–16.

Heilman, K. M., Scholes, R. & Watson, R. T. (1975). Auditory affective agnosia: disturbed comprehension of affective speech. *J. Neurol. Neurosurg. Psychatry* **38**: 69–71.

Knaven, F. (1980). Cognitive functioning in adults – discussion notes. In *Epilepsy and Behavior '79*, ed. E. M. Kulig, H. Meinardi & G. Stores, pp. 43–6. Lisse: Swet & Zeitlinger.

LeDoux, J. E., Barclay, L. & Premuck, A. (1978). The brain and cognitive sciences. *Ann. Neurol.* **4**: 391–98.

Lenneberg, E. H. (1966). Speech development: its anatomical and psychological concomitants. In *Brain Function III Proceedings of the Third Conference (Nov. 1963) Speech, Language and Communication*, ed. E. C. Carterette. Berkeley: University of California Press.

Luria, A. R. (1974). Language and brain: towards the basic problems of neurolinquistics *Brain Lang.* **1**: 1–4.

McGone, J. (1977). Sex differences in the cerebral organization of verbal functions in patients with unilateral brain lesions. *Brain* **100**: 775–93.

Milner, B. (1975). Psychological aspects of focal epilepsy and its neurosurgical management. In *Advances in Neurology*, ed. D. P. Purpura, J. R. Penry & R. D. Walter, Vol. 8, pp. 299–321. New York: Raven Press.

Milner, B., Branch, C. & Rasmussen, T. (1966). Evidence for bilateral speech representation in some non-right handers. *Trans. Am. Neurol. Assoc.* **91**: 306–8.

Novelly, R. A. & Naugle, R. I. (1985). Neuropsychological prediction of hemisphere speech dominance in childhood onset complex partial epilepsy. *Epilepsia* **26**: 539.

Ojelmann, G. A. (1979). Individual variability in cortical localization of language. *J. Neurosurg.* **50**: 164–9.

Quinn, P. J. (1972). Stuttering: cerebral dominance and the Dichotic Word Test. *Med. J. Austr.* **2**: 639–45.

Risse, G. L., Hempel, A., Farnham, S. J., Penovich, P. E., *et al.* (1999). A comparison of cortical language areas in adults vs. children based on electrical stimulation with subdural electrode array. *Epilepsia* **40** (suppl 7): 53.

Ross, E. D. & Mesulam, M. M. (1979). Dominant language functions of the right hemisphere: prosody and emotional gesturing. *Arch. Neurol.* **36**: 144–8.

Ross, E. D., Harney, J. H., deLaCosta-Utemssing, C. & Purdy, P. D. (1981). How the brain integrates affective and prepositional language into a unified behavioral function. *Arch. Neurol.* **38**: 475–8.

Schulhoff, G. & Goodglass, H. (1969). Dichotic listening, side of brain injury and cerebral dominance. *Neuropsychogia* **7**: 149–60.

Searleman, A. (1978). A review of right hemisphere linguistic capabilities. *Psychol. Bull.* **83**: 503–28.

Smith, B. L. (1980). Cortical stimulation and speech timing: a preliminary observation. *Brain Lang.* **10**: 89–97.

Sorokina, N. & Selitsky, G. A. (1999). Impairment of verbal and imaginative function in childhood epilepsy. 23rd International Epilepsy Congress, Prague, Czech Republic. *Epilepsia* **40** (suppl 2): 68.

Todd, J. & Satz, P. (1977). WAIS performance in brain-damaged left and right handers. *Ann. Neurol.* **2**: 422–4.

Weintraub, P. (1981). The brain: his and hers. *Discover* 15–20.

Weintraub, S. Mesulam, M.-M. & Kramer, L. (1958). Disturbances in prosody, a right hemisphere contribution to language. *Arch. Neurol.* **368**: 742–4.

4

Speech and language problems in epilepsy

Children with epilepsy may not use language as well as non-epileptic children (Green & Hartlage, 1971). Language functions are especially sensitive to transient disturbances of thought, such as would appear with seizure discharges. Imaginative fluency may be affected significantly (Davies-Eysenick, 1952). Transient language disturbances in children with focal epilepsy may be ictal or postictal phenomena (Serafetinides & Falconer, 1963). In school-age children, epilepsy may cause language disorders in syntactic and semantic processes that are similar to disorders observed in frontal-lobe dysfunction and in dyslexic children (Kossciesza *et al.*, 1998).

Children are not adults, and they respond differently to language disturbances. The adult is more apt to talk excessively, to use trite or stereotyped phrases, or to repeat certain words, phrases, or sentences. The child does not confuse words of a similar nature as often as the adult does. A child's speech may be slow and stumbling, difficult to understand, or peppered with unexpected and sometimes peculiar word selections that are similar to, but not correct for, the idea. More subtle signs of delayed or deviant development are seen. The child may not be able to speak or may speak with a slow, labored, slurred, and often vague speech pattern, as if attempting to compensate for the language difficulties. The speech may clear markedly for periods of time, corresponding to the introduction of certain anticonvulsants or even a bout of illness. Sometimes, however, medication or illness may aggravate the speech problem.

Processing problems

Reception language is organized more formally and develops earlier than expressive language. In left-handed individuals, language representation is often bilateral and thus all language function is organized more diffusely in either hemisphere than in the case of right-handed individuals (Hecaen & Percy, 1956). When lateralization of paroxysmal brain activity occurs, the laterality of language is not necessarily the side suggested by handedness and eye preference as being the dominant hemisphere. In adults, handedness and speech dominance are practically independent variables (Lee *et al.*, 1980).

When an epileptic event occurs as the result of unilateral discharge, it is more likely to be associated with a paroxysmal dysphasia in a left-handed individual than in a right-handed person, irrespective of the side of the function. In right-handers, the side of the focus is much more related to the incidence of paroxysmal dysphasia than it is in left-handers (Hecaen & Piercy, 1956).

Agnosia

Agnosia is the state of being confused by and unable to recognize speech sounds (or other familiar sounds). Recognition of various sound combinations is an important early stage to understanding what is said. Noting subtle differences in the tone, emphasis, and pitch, as well as discriminating between similar sounds, underlies understanding. In speech agnosia, the individual has problems in recognizing the word sounds and sound clusters. What is heard may seem to be gibberish or meaningless. Rarely, brief episodes of such problems have been observed to occur at the time of seizure discharges involving both sides of the brain (Cooper & Ferry, 1978; Geets & Pinion, 1975; Hardy, 1965; Rapin *et al.*, 1977).

An epileptic agnosia may present as part of a seizure when the child is unable to recognize speech sounds. This may be acute or chronic, transient or persistent. Children with an epilepsy-associated agnosia may seem deaf despite normal audiometric and brainstem evoked potentials. This has been referred to as central word deafness. The EEG shows epileptiform discharges in the dominant temporal lobe. Antiepileptic drugs may control clinical seizures and may help the agnosia (Borkowski & Lotz, 1986; Cooper & Ferry, 1978; Geets & Pinion, 1975; Hardy, 1965; Rapin *et al.*, 1977).

Aphasia

Aphasia is the loss of understanding of what is said or a difficulty in expressing one's thoughts through language. Aphasia may be receptive or expressive. Receptive (sensory) aphasia implies a defect in the ability to understand spoken or written language. Expressive (motor) aphasia implies a defect in the ability of language expression by speech, by written effort, by gesture, or by signing. Aphasia is associated with an insult to vital brain centers serving these functions, an insult often resulting in the loss of functions.

Aphasia may present as part of a seizure, although consciousness is sustained. These episodes may be brief but recurrent, or they may be prolonged. The appearance of such problems with associated findings of marked EEG abnormalities may represent an underlying brain insult.

In chronic aphasia from a brain insult, the disturbed language is a combination of the damage and efforts to compensate by undamaged areas of the brain. The repair is imperfect. When radical relearning of language skills is needed, it is more difficult if prior language skills are not well organized or well established. Learning that has not yet become a well-organized skill is much more likely to break down under temporary stress (Hecaen & Piercy, 1956).

The use of the term "aphasia" in the young child is debated. Can a child lose that which is not yet developed? To avoid this argument, consider aphasia as a disturbance of an individual's inherent potential for language comprehension and usage (Hardy, 1965).

Characteristically, childhood aphasia usually presents as an impairment of spontaneously spoken language. A reduction of understanding alone is uncommon. Most common is a reduction of language efforts, both spoken and written. Even gesturing is reduced. Incentives with much encouragement are needed to get an aphasic child to speak. When the child finally speaks, pronunciation problems and difficulties in articulation, as well as a frank dysarthria, may become apparent (Alajouanine & Lhermitte, 1965).

Child aphasia and adult aphasia tend to differ in presentation. In children with aphasia, logorrhea, an uninhibited torrent of speech, is rare. Jargon aphasia, a fluent, quick utterance of nonsense words, is uncommon, as are naming deficits as in anomia. Dysarthria is common but differs from that seen with aphasia in adults. The child's dysarthria tends to be a dyslalia or even an idioglossia, representing an avoidance of difficult sounds or substitution of easier ones. Reduplicating simple sounds is common, as are rare speech iterations, the latter taking the form of a word, a phrase, or a neologism (Alajouanine & Lhermitte, 1965; Critchley, 1970).

Aphasic children may overreact emotionally to environmental noises. Attention deficits may be apparent as the child either becomes fixated on a stimulus or pays only fleeting attention to it. Such children tend to be unpredictable, swinging rapidly from ignoring the environment to a frantic overactivity, possibly related to the child's difficulties in handling incoming language stimuli. Other children appear to be gregarious but easily become puzzled and frustrated as they try to fit in the sound clusters they hear and to remember what they have heard (Hardy, 1965).

Unlike the aphasic adult, the young aphasic child has no means of knowing what is expected and cannot fall back on pretraumatic experiences. Often, the child is thought to be stupid, deaf, psychotic, or at least emotionally disturbed. In the beginning, distinguishing between a hearing impairment, an intellectual impairment, or a psychiatric problem is important, for therapy and prognoses differ markedly (Hardy, 1965).

The EEG is not useful in distinguishing between aphasia, deafness, retardation, or emotional disturbances in children. Abnormal EEGs are not uncommon, often having focal or diffuse non-temporal slowing. Occasionally, left temporal or bitemporal spiking is seen. Focal abnormalities and a history of a convulsive disorder are more apt to be present in an aphasic population than in a population of hearing-impaired children.

Aphasia may be an ictal or postictal symptom or a symptom of the underlying cause of the seizure. Rarely, a brief aphasia may be the only symptom of a seizure. Seizure discharges may interrupt the processing of language in the brain, resulting in the aphasia. This may occur with simple and partial complex seizures, during absence seizures, and as part of the postictal period following a generalized tonic–clonic seizure. Most seizure aphasias are limited to the period of the seizure itself or to the immediate postictal period (Haecaen & Piercy, 1956; Geets, 1975; Geets & Pinon, 1975; Gastaut, 1979; Hamilton & Matthews, 1979; Vollbracht, 1979; Lecours & Joanette, 1980).

In children, episodic brief but repeated aphasias with retained alertness have been seen. The child may be able to attend to but not understand sounds. The child's spoken efforts may be slurred. Audiologic studies usually are normal. The EEG shows epileptiform discharges, often bitemporal in location. These respond to antiepileptic medications, although subtle learning and memory problems may be noted between the episodes.

Isolated episodic aphasias

Aphasic seizures are infrequent. Serial appearance as in a partial epileptic status is quite rare (De Pasquet *et al.*, 1976). Some patients exhibit focal status with dysphasic symptoms but will recover between the epileptic symptoms; others will not recover. In the latter, the seizure may last for a longer time, i.e. a period of several days. This has been called an epileptic aphasic status (Hamilton & Matthews, 1979). Aphasia may be the sole manifestation of a focal status with a left frontal discharge. This can be confirmed by an EEG and terminated by intravenous anticonvulsant therapy. Focal epilepsy with aphasia only, without motor or psychomotor manifestations, can be seen with frontal or temporal cortical seizures (De Pasquet *et al.*, 1976). Anticonvulsants can eliminate these seizures (Baratz & Mesulan, 1982).

Paroxysmal dysphasias may present either as an expressive aphasia, referring to a severe interference with speech efforts presenting as a near complete speechlessness, or as a receptive aphasia, with a severe defect of auditory comprehension. A severe reading disturbance may be seen. An isolated paroxysmal reading disturbance as an ictal phenomenon is reported rarely (Hecaen & Piercy, 1956).

Receptive aphasia

Paroxysmal receptive aphasia as part of an aura is far less frequent than paroxysmal expressive aphasias, or at least it is harder to recognize. A paroxysmal receptive aphasia is rare, occurring most often in right-handed patients with a left-sided epileptic focus. Even in the right-handed, the incidence is about half that of expressive aphasia. In a right-handed patient, the frequency of a receptive dysphasia is related to the side of the lesion and is usually seen with a left-sided seizure discharge. The incidence of the aphasia is not necessarily related to the side of the lesion in left-handers (Hecaen & Piercy, 1956).

A paroxysmal receptive aphasia is very rare in a left-hander, whether it be a paroxysmal or a permanent defect. Receptive language is more focally organized than expressive language. In left-handers, representation is more apt to be bilateral and tends to be organized more diffusely within either hemisphere than in the case of right-handers, and thus it is less apt to be impaired by a focal seizure discharge.

There is a certain resemblance between the cerebral organization of language in left-handed people and that in children. Aphasias following a right-hemispheric lesion are more common in children than in adults. Aphasias of childhood characteristically recover more rapidly and expressive defects occur far more frequently than receptive defects. This parallels the differences that distinguish left-handers from right-handers. A lesser degree of functional lateralization for language in left-handed individuals may be associated with a greater vulnerability to an acute disturbance and with a greater potential for spontaneous recovery following brain injury (Hecaen & Piercy, 1956).

Expressive aphasia

Paroxysmal expressive problems are much more frequent in left-handers than in right-handers, which is the reverse of comprehension tendencies. With left-handers, it makes no difference which side the seizure focus is on. Expressive dysphasias in right-handers are usually seen when the discharge comes from the left cerebral hemisphere (Hecaen & Piercy, 1956).

Presentation

Aphasia is known to occur as part of a seizure or in the immediate postictal period. Usually, this occurs in patients with documented seizures (Racy *et al.*, 1980). Rarely, aphasia may be the only symptom of the seizure (De Pasquet *et al.*, 1976; Holmes *et al.*, 1981). The seizure discharge disrupts the language processing, which results in the aphasic symptoms (Gilmore & Heilman, 1981). All types of expressive and receptive aphasias, either as isolated symptoms or not, may occur. These may resemble a transient amnesic type of aphasia. Such spells are usually brief in duration, lasting for only a few minutes (Lecours & Joanette, 1980).

The most obvious sign of an ictal aphasic seizure is when the patient is unable to speak due to a complete expressive aphasia (Vernea, 1974). Other types of aphasia may be mistaken for confusional symptoms associated with the seizures.

Basic characteristics identify an aphasic seizure. The patient may or may not fully comprehend what is going on. The patient's spoken replies must be evaluated carefully to exclude the possibility that they may originate from confusion and disorientation. The patient either stops talking or talks in an incorrect manner. In recall, it may be determined that the patient was conscious but was not able to find the correct word to express themselves, so either they stopped talking or they talked in an incorrect manner. The spells present as an expressive aphasia, a receptive aphasia, or both. The timing is important. The ictal aphasia may occur as an aura with or without subsequent loss of consciousness. If the patient is unconscious, the patient must be nudged immediately upon reawakening to differentiate the spell from confusion. The spells characteristically are brief. The spells may be the only clinical manifestations of the seizure (Serafetinides & Falconer, 1963).

Simple brief attacks

Episodes of aphasia associated with epilepsy have been seen both in children and in adults. Rarely, aphasia may be the only symptom of a seizure. In a paroxysmal aphasia, there is a transient impairment of speech and language functions, which can be recalled by the patient (Serafetinides & Falconer, 1963). Some aphasic spells occur without change in consciousness or behaviors other than those related to oral or written speech and language. They may be accompanied by a headache. Other paroxysmal aphasias may be accompanied by some change in consciousness or may follow an initial alteration of consciousness. More often, the spells coexist with non-aphasic symptoms and signs, often minor, including sensory, motor, or behavioral changes, which may suggest a seizure relationship. Such attacks are brief, usually lasting for only a few minutes. During the time of the episode, the patient is unable to speak and may or may not understand what is occurring. The language impairment is greater than would be expected if due to the confusion of a seizure or a speech arrest. Patients recall that during the attack they could not speak the right words or seemed unable to understand what others said (Lecours & Joanette, 1980).

Complex presentations

Paroxysmal dysphasic episodes of longer duration and comprising more complex manifestations may occur. These often appear with the appearance of global, receptive, conduction, and amnestic aphasias, with severe problems involving both understanding and expression of language, and lasting three to five minutes. Then, for minutes to hours, a cluster of regressive dysphasic symptoms much like a receptive aphasia, often with an overlooked anomia, may emerge. The patient may appear confused. Both written and spoken language are impaired. The EEG during this time shows little if any abnormality, often with related but incorrect word choices (paraphasias) manifest in both speech and writing. Deviant spelling may be seen. Even after resolution of these symptoms, word-finding difficulties and spelling problems may persist, with wrong word choices manifest in both speech and writings. This may involve all types of language, including naming, reading, and writing, with oral language more distorted than written language (Lecours & Joanette, 1980). .

Aphasic status

Aphasia may be seen with partial epileptic status, a rare condition. The aphasic symptoms often will resolve between the bursts of abnormal epileptic activity. In some patients, however, the seizure status and concurrent aphasia may last for days. This has been called aphasic epileptic status. Very rarely, an aphasic episode may be the only sign of a focal epileptic status of the frontal or temporal brain surface. Such a state has been known to last for weeks. The use of anticonvulsant drugs improves or normalizes the aphasia by bringing about control of the seizure discharges (Hamilton & Matthews, 1979).

Postictal aphasia

In some children, a transient loss of speech may occur following a seizure, particularly a focal seizure, although this is often overlooked as it is obscured by other phenomena of the postictal state (Watters, 1974). In children, temporary aphasias are known to occur in association with certain types of epilepsy, particularly temporal lobe complex partial epilepsy. They usual follows a series of seizures. Such aphasia usually recovers within a variable interval, but it may recur after further seizures (O'Donohoe, 1979).

Persistent episodic aphasia

Occasionally, an episodic aphasia may be lasting. In some individuals, there is a history of seizures with episodic aphasias. These episodes become worse, with the emergence of a persistent aphasia. The aphasia changes from time to time and from type to type. Sometimes, the person seems to have more problems in understanding; at other times, incorrect word choices predominate. The aphasia is of changing intensity, sometimes appearing as a receptive aphasia but more often appearing like a central or conduction type of aphasia. Mild problems with reading may also be seen. The source appears to involve the left temporal structures, with little spread to the parietal lobe. After the severe phase settles down, a moderate degree of aphasia may persist. If this permanent aphasia appears abruptly, the concern is that there may be an underlying brain lesion causing both the seizure and the aphasia (De Pasquet *et al.*, 1976).

Related seizure types

Transient episodic aphasia of epilepsy may occur during partial seizures (usually complex partial epilepsy) or during simple partial seizures involving either the left lower motor strip or the supplementary motor area. Episodic aphasia episodes have been noted with generalized seizures, such as during absence seizures or during the postictal period following a generalized tonic–clonic seizure. These aphasias are essentially limited to the seizure period itself or to the immediate postictal period (Holmes *et al.*, 1981).

In children, a temporary loss of speech may follow a seizure, especially a focal seizure, but it is often obscured by other postictal symptoms. Such temporary aphasias most often follow seizures involving the temporal lobe, especially after a series of seizures. The child recovers from the aphasia but the aphasia may recur with future seizures. The seizure usually originates in the language areas of the temporal lobe and adjacent brain tissue. Left-handed adults, like young children, tend to have the language centers more shared between the brain sides. Thus, a young child, like a lefthander, is more apt to have aphasias, even with a right brain discharge, than a right-handed older child or adult.

Such ictal aphasias usually originate in the dominant temporal lobe or at least in that hemisphere. Three sites have been suggested: the posterior temporal parietal area of Wernicke's area, Broca's area, and the supplementary motor area just anterior to the foot area on the medial surface of the cerebral hemisphere. The latter area is associated more with speech production than with speech processing. An anterior temporal lobe site on the dominant side has been incriminated (Serafetinides & Falconer, 1963).

Diagnosis

Previously, the diagnosis of a paroxysmal aphasia as an epileptic aura or ictal symptom was made on the basis of a unilateral focus of epileptiform activity in a language-processing cortical site. Reliable diagnosis of ictal aphasia can now usually be made based on well-identified speech disturbances in complex partial seizures with an adequate description of the witnessed spells accompanied by EEG confirmation (Racy *et al.*, 1980).

Cause

Temporary aphasias have been documented with idiopathic epilepsies, especially with complex partial seizures (Serafetinides & Falconer, 1963; Worster-Drought, 1971; Foerster, 1977; Lecours & Joanette, 1980), following a single episode or a series of seizures. Such aphasia recovers after various intervals, but the aphasia may recur following further epileptic attacks (Worster-Drought, 1971; Foerster, 1977). The epileptiform discharges usually come from the left temporal lobe and adjacent area in the perisylvian region, especially the posterior temporal language areas (Ingvar, 1976; Baratz & Mesulan, 1982), perhaps involving the associative areas of the cortex where different language inputs are combined into a thought (Lecours & Joanette 1980).

An episode of epileptic aphasia is of abrupt onset and usually of too short duration to permit any kind of cerebral adaptation to the interferences. In cases of a permanent dysphasia, the disturbance of language may be the product of both the defect produced by the lesion and of any resultant restitution of function resulting from compensatory activity of undamaged cerebral areas. The initial examination reveals the immediate breakdown symptoms, whereas the following observations may show a more or less imperfect repair. Learning that has not achieved the status of a well-organized skill and is organized more diffusely may be more resistant to acute inferences, but more likely to break down under temporary stress, than a function organized in an established site that is less capable of recovering spontaneously after an insult. With aphasia and epilepsy combined, the concern is less with how the skills of language are integrated and more with where the skills are located. Left-handed and right-handed individuals may differ in localization (Hecaen & Piercy, 1956).

It is important to differentiate true epileptic dysphasia from a speech arrest or from verbal utterances induced by a seizure. The localizing value of each is different. Speech arrests and repetitive vocalizations originate in prefrontal cortical areas and are not uncommon in some forms of simple partial seizures. Language disturbances are of greater localizing value and are usually referable to a disturbance in the dominant temporal or posterior frontal area (Racy *et al.*, 1980).

Differential diagnosis

Epileptic aphasia is a rarely described syndrome in adults and is recognized even more rarely in children. Patients with true paroxysmal aphasia may show a dramatic response to anticonvulsant therapy. Many are misdiagnosed as having a vascular episode. Twenty-four-hour ambulatory EEG monitoring can demonstrate that in some cases the aphasia is of epileptic origin, whereas the initial EEG showed the left temporal slowing but did not reveal evidence of paroxysmal activity (Vollbracht, 1979).

In children, one must differentiate temporary aphasias of seizure origin from other causes. Temporary aphasias may be seen following a head injury in a child, i.e. "cerebral shock." They may be seen after an acute vascular accident, such as an arterial thrombosis of the dominant hemisphere, or a hemorrhage. Slow recovery ensues with both instances (O'Donohoe, 1979). With vascular etiologies, the aphasia may begin with or before the onset of a seizure disturbance. A prolonged period ranging from months to years may be seen between the onset of the aphasia and the first seizure. There are cases in which the aphasia and the concurrent or delayed onset of seizures are both symptoms of a cerebral insult (Benson, 1979).

Brain tumors of the dominant hemisphere may also produce aphasia, but these are rarely temporary. Seizures may be concomitant symptoms of such insults in a child. Strokes result in aphasia in children, just as in adults. These may be accompanied by seizures at the time of the insult or may develop months to years later. Speech may also be lost permanently in certain cerebral degenerative disorders. All of the above may also have seizures as symptoms. With the appearance of an episodic aphasia, these other causes must be ruled out by diagnostic studies, including an EEG and scan (O'Donohoe, 1979). Maintaining a high index of suspicion in cases of fluctuating symptoms remains crucial for early diagnosis and management, especially in terms of differentiating an epileptic aphasia from some other problem (Racy *et al.*, 1980).

Speech–language regression

Speech regression with seizures may be seen. A young child may have episodes of subtle regression of speech and language lasting days to weeks after preceding normal language development. The primary presentation is of expressive language impairment. An associated generalized spike-wave discharge, maximum over the dominant temporal lobe, is seen on the EEG in the drowsy state. Cerebrospinal fluid (CSF) and computed tomography (CT) studies are normal. The episodes may end spontaneously, or they may be recurrent. Anticonvulsant therapy if tolerated, may also control the episodes. The speech regression is longer than the typical episodic aphasia but may represent a variant of the usual ictal aphasias. It has been thought that a seizure discharge in the developing language centers of the immature brain can produce a prolonged impairment response. Unlike the acquired aphasia syndrome, there is not usually the abrupt onset of such a speech disturbance. These episodes are longer than a mere postictal or ictal attack, unless these attacks represented an aphasic or dysphasic epileptic status. It could be that a temporary ictal disturbance affecting the developing language centers of a young child could precede a prolonged inhibition response (Deonna *et al.*, 1982).

A focal infection such as meningitis, abscess, or cerebritis may be associated with aphasia and seizures. Encephalitis in neonates and younger children may result in speech and language deficits. Those with encephalitis in the first year or two of life are often found to have depressed intelligence and delayed language development. Their heads may be smaller than normal. Seizures are not characteristically a part of the sequelae, although they may be prominent in the initial presentation.

Progressive neurologic symptoms including speech and language regression and loss may be seen with focal encephalitis. Therapy-resistant or progressive focal seizures, often accompanied by a deterioration of intellectual function and speech/language skills as well as hemiparesis and other neurologic deficits are seen frequently. These progressive focal neurologic findings suggest a chronic viral infection of the brain (Aquilar & Rasmussen, 1960), possibly a chronic or less focal encephalitis occurring in infancy or childhood, resulting in focal symptoms and signs (Deonna *et al.*, 1982).

Apraxia of speech

Apraxia is the inability to form speech or even speech sounds although the patient knows what they want to say. This is a very rare state. A speech apraxia implies a problem in the transforming of a language concept into the motor act of expressing the thought through speaking. Seizures may interrupt such language processing, resulting in an apraxia of speech as a seizure symptom with or without other symptom (Gilmore & Heilman, 1981).

Anomia

Anomia is a memory deficit in which an individual cannot remember proper nouns, especially the names of people and items. It is associated primarily with complex partial epilepsies involving the dominant temporal lobe. This condition is not uncommon. The individual may be seen to pause or hesitate in search of the word or a similar word. This is rarely recognized as an isolated item or even as a complication in childhood epilepsy (Cohn, 1970; Marin & Saffran, 1975; Ojemann, 1975). Children with complex partial seizures may have anomia as part of the subtle memory problems noted.

Performance problems

Speech arrest

Speech arrests are characterized by the speech being interrupted abruptly for a brief period of time. This may show up as brief hesitations in the conversation, as a halting flow of language, or as episodes in which the individual is unable to talk. They may be seen with absence, minor motor (myoclonic, atonic) seizures, and complex partial seizures. The child with a convulsive disorder may develop a non-fluent aphasia that persists with an associated severe comprehensive defect, whereas the adult with focal seizures may be more apt to develop a paroxysmal transient speech arrest.

As the manifestation of an epileptic discharge, a patient may be unable to speak or vocalize (Baratz & Mesulam, 1981). The types of speech arrests seen include an isolated arrest or speech arrest as a prodrome to an impending secondarily generalized seizure, a temporal or temporal insular seizure, a right seizure focus, a discharge involving the supplementary motor area, or as part of a complete expressive aphasia (Vernea, 1974). The seizure discharge disrupts normal speech–language processing, resulting in an expressive aphasia or a disruption of the translation of the language concept into a spoken word, as with an apraxia. The seizure may interfere with deeper brain centers that activate the brain surface to speak. There may also be seizure activation or interference with the intention centers that prepare the cortex to carry out a motor activity (Gilmore & Heilman, 1981).

Speech arrests occurring with complex partial seizures are usually brief and accompanied by stereotypic confusion and automatic behaviors (Belafsky *et al.*, 1978; Hamilton & Matthews, 1979). The seizure can come from either side of the brain, but if a transient aphasia is also noted, the discharges usually come from the left frontal-temporal to central-temporal areas of the brain (Hamilton & Matthews, 1979; Gilmore & Heilman, 1981). The speech arrest may be the only symptom of the seizure. Occasionally, the patient may complain of a headache (Vernea, 1974; Hamilton & Matthews, 1979; Gilmore & Heilman, 1981).

Rarely, speech arrests may be seen with absence seizures or in epileptic stupors from minor seizure status (Holmes *et al.*, 1981). Speech arrests and stereotyped automatisms are common in epileptic stupors, although they may be absent in the final hours of the stupor. The patient stares in an unresponsive manner (Belafsky *et al.*, 1978).

Early treatment is desirable to shorten the patient's distress and to prevent the development of permanent deficits caused by continued cortical discharges. Improvement or elimination of such discharges occurs with the use of antiepileptic drugs (Hamilton & Matthews, 1979; Baratz & Mesulam, 1982).

Vocal utterances

Vocalizations, sometimes dramatic, present with the uttering of non-language sounds or single words, which may occur with non-dominant complex partial seizures. Paroxysmal word utterances are episodes during which the patient utters a seemingly irrelevant statement, sometimes repeatedly. Palilalia is characterized by the repetition of a phrase or word with increasing rapidity. Patients may also make irrelevant statements, sometimes in repeated paroxysms. During these events, the patient is not alert; nor are such utterances recalled.

Utterances may be preictal, ictal, or postictal. Five types of utterances are noted, including (1) warning utterances at the onset of a seizure, (2) recurrent, seemingly relevant words or phrases spoken during the seizure, (3) irrelevant spoken efforts that are conversational in pattern but are out of context with the situation or conversation, (4) emotional utterances as if in response to an emotional feeling or hallucinatory experience as part of the seizure, and (5) utterances of a confused nature in the immediate period following the seizure spoken as if the person were trying to reorient themselves. Such utterances are usually grammatically correct. Discharging lesions from either temporal lobe may produce seizure automatisms of this type. Most often, they tend to involve at least the non-dominant temporal lobe if they are not present bilaterally (Serafetinides & Falconer, 1963).

Dysarthria and articulation problems

These problems refer to poorly formed or unclear speech efforts. Dysarthria and disarticulated speech efforts are characterized by words and word sounds that are not pronounced clearly or properly. Disturbances in the pronunciation and formation of speech are rarely a seizure symptom.

Articulation problems

Articulation problems imply a muscular or structural problem in the oral and throat speech mechanisms that interferes with clear pronunciation of the speech sounds and words. This is called a disarticulation. Occasionally, articulation problems can be seen with simple partial seizures, usually associated with more obvious ictal symptoms. Most often, slurred or poorly pronounced speech is an undesirable side effect of antiepileptic medication, especially if the blood levels of the anticonvulsant are high. Paroxysmal disturbances of articulation and dysarthria are associated with seizures rarely (Lecours & Joanette, 1980). A temporary articulation problem may be a postictal symptom of oral damage suffered during a major seizure.

Dysarthria

An anarthria or dysarthria implies a neurologic interference with the pronunciation of words and the making of the speech sounds due to a problem within the central nervous system. This usually implies too much or too little tone. Thus, one can talk about spastic (harsh, strangled, imprecise) speech; flaccid (breathing-imprecise) speech; irregular speech emphasis with choreoathetotic speech; stifled, muffled, tremulous speech as with the speech pattern of tremors or parkinsonism; or the variable speech with a tick-tock compensatory rhythm of a cerebellar dysarthria. Dysarthria, in which the patient cannot speak clearly, may be seen with simple partial seizures and with some medications for seizures, especially at high dosage (Lecours & Joanette, 1980).

Dysfluency

Dysfluency is a condition in which the speech does not flow smoothly. There is stuttering, jerky or stammering speech efforts, as with absence seizures, partial seizures, and rarely reading reflex seizures. The loss of smooth speech flow may be a characteristic of left complex partial seizures in some individuals who present a jerky or staccato speech, flat speech, as an interictal or postictal finding. Stuttering and stammering are speech dysfluencies.

Stuttering

Stuttering may be divided into dysarthric stuttering, apractic stuttering, and dysnomia stuttering, as acquired stuttering problems. Dysnomia stuttering is a disturbance of word retrieval seen in patients with dominant complex partial seizures, especially when stressed. The speech flow comes to an abrupt and inappropriate halt as the individual fails to come up with the appropriate word to express the thoughts. There also exists a congenital word-retrieval problem, which may manifest by full-blown stuttering behavior characterized by anxiety and other secondary symptoms.

Childhood developmental stuttering usually emerges between the ages of two to six years, but it is often more severe than the normal degree of stuttering and stammering at this age, and it persists. It is found most often in males. The stuttering is characterized by hesitations or blocks in speaking, repetitions of the initial sounds and syllables of words, and occasionally prolongation of the initial sounds and syllables. With children, secondary mechanisms such as facial grimacing and limb swinging are often seen with the stuttering. This is rare in adult stutterers. Adult-acquired stuttering such as that following a brain insult differs. It is characterized by repetitions, prolongations, and the blocks falling anywhere in the words, not just in the beginnings of sounds and syllables. Any class of words may be involved. Secondary features such as grimacing and limb movements occur rarely in adults (Baratz & Mesulam, 1982).

In children with seizures, recurring speech arrests are often misdiagnosed as stuttering or stammering. Stuttering was once thought to be epileptic interruptions of automatic control of speech (West, 1958). Paroxysmal epileptiform discharges from the left temporal lobe region have been associated with stuttering. This stuttering resembles the childhood form of stuttering, with hesitations, repetitions of initial word sounds and syllables, and occasional prolongation of the initial word sound or syllable (Baratz & Mesulam, 1982). Some patients with seizures triggered by reading, speaking, or writing give a history of stuttering from childhood, but there are no accompanying EEG disturbances recorded with such stuttering (Geschwind & Sherwin, 1967).

Automatic flow of speech

Some individuals with dominant complex partial epilepsy may exhibit a particularly speech pattern. The speech may be characterized by a tendency to slur words together in a flat, monotone effect with a labored speech flow, as if the person is searching for words. The content is often overly detailed in manner, as if the speaker is seeking desperately to be understood, at times referring to equally detailed notes. If interrupted, the speaker returns to the beginning rather than picking up where the interruption came.

Verbosity

Patients with chronic dominant complex partial seizures may tend to be verbose, with the content described as trivial, subjectively detailed, and consistent with circumstantiality. They display more dysfluency and shifting of topics than normal. This is unrelated to intelligence, anomia, or memory, although patients may recall fewer words. No hypergraphia is displayed, although some patients may keep a diary. Although verbosity is infrequent, it occurs in up to half of those with chronic left complex partial seizures. The individuals seem internally driven to talk. They may notice or give more than usual significance to details, commenting about subjective and illusory details to which they give more significance, regardless of the relevance. A combination of linguistic and perceptual anomalies is consistent with the notion of a sensory-limbic disconnection, i.e. an epileptic focus leads to enhancement of affective associations (Hoeppner *et al.*, 1987).

Mutism

Occasionally, individuals with mixed dominance and multifocal to generalized cerebral damage, and who undergo a two-stage and full corpus callosum sectioning for control of drug-refractory multifocal seizures, display a marked decrease in spontaneous speech with repetition abilities intact postoperatively after the second-stage sectioning of the posterior portion. Paraphasias are rare. This improves with time but does not resolve entirely. Patients stabilize with lengthy verbal response latency and short phrase length. When speech is elicited, it may be excessive rather than slow or labored. No receptive deficits are seen. This is not seen in individuals with right-sided dominance (Rayport *et al.*, 1984).

Prosody

Prosody refers to the affect or emotional aspects of language, i.e. the melodiousness of speech. This refers to the modulation of the pitch, tempo, inflection, and stresses of language as a person speaks. The person who lacks prosody speaks in a flat, emotionless monotone. Such aspects impart emotional feeling to a spoken sentence. The inflection may be all that differentiates a question, a statement, a demand, or an exclamation. This helps differentiate various dialects and languages (Heilman *et al.*, 1975).

Prosody tends to be primarily a right brain function (Weintraub *et al.*, 1958; Searleman, 1978). This relates to emotional language, including gesturing (Ross & Mesulam, 1979). The minor hemisphere is known to play a role in understanding affective and intoned speech, in emotional behavior, and in musical functions.

Others have reported, infrequently, ictal disturbances of prosodic features of speech with a weak, unmodulated, monotonous speech devoid of inflection and coloring (Deonna *et al.*, 1987). No isolated seizure prosody symptom has been described in either children or adults, but when addressed, prosody problems are often referred to as a complication of some other speech deficit. There are disturbances of prosody of both receptive and expressive types. A person may present with a receptive prosodic defect in which the patient fails to perceive the affect contained in another's speech (Heilman *et al.*, 1975). Prosody expressive problems may present as a distortion or loss of the melodious qualities of speech that give it an emotional flavor. The speech is often slowed and monotonous but without any aphasic disturbance in comprehension and expression. In seizure patients, transient as well as ongoing disturbances of prosody, like other language deficits, are largely overlooked (Deonna *et al.*, 1987).

Some children with complex partial epilepsy seem to lack this prosody, speaking in a monotone style. The ictal speech disturbance may be limited to only the prosodic (or so-called suprasegmental or non-segmental) features of speech, i.e. intonation, tempo, rhythm, and pauses, resulting in a speech effort characterized by marked slowness and irregularity with exaggerated pauses and hesitations and a lack of intonation. The slow, monotonous speech of an epileptic child may be mistaken for mental dullness and not studied further (Deonna *et al.*, 1987).

Several types of transient language disturbances have been identified in children, similar to those of more permanent types of aphasia, but usually the attention has been focused on the symbolic (semantic-syntactic) aspects of language, with little attention to prosody (intonation, stress, tempo, and rhythmi city, with their physical acoustic counterparts of pitch, loudness, duration, and rhythm). An important part of childhood epileptic aphasia is that of a prolonged, isolated, yet rapidly reversible language disorder (Deonna *et al.*, 1987). Some children with the acquired agnosia–aphasia with epilepsy syndrome, with or without clinical seizures, but with an abnormal EEG, may develop a highpitched voice lacking the natural quality and inflections, resembling the voice of a deaf child. They lack normal prosody (Cooper & Ferry, 1978).

Speech content

Other areas of speech to be considered include the speech content, including syntax, semantics, phonology, morphology, and grammar. Speech content in epilepsy is largely overlooked, and little is written or said about it. Problems of speech content, such as grammar and syntax, may occasionally be noted in children with epilepsy.

Pragmatism is the study of language usage, considering the rules of usage, meaning, and the practical aspects of how words fit together to convey a concept. The social and language background of the subject need to be determined. Pragmatic deficits may differ, i.e. in the appropriate use of speech-supportive motor acts, verbal constructs, communication interactions, voice usage, etc. By age five years or older, pragmatic basics have emerged. One can judge the intelligibility, voice quality and intensity, specificity and accuracy, cohesiveness, quantity, conciseness, intelligibility and repair–revision aspects, as well as the facial expressions and pause times. In the adult, one can also note the variety of speech acts, as well as the eye contact and contiguity (Prutting & Kirchner, 1987). Occasional problems in the pragmatic aspects of language have been noted in children with epilepsy.

Children with articulation disorders exhibit struggles in intelligibility and vocal quality and intensity, as well as in fluency, pauses, and associated facial expressions. Children with language disorders have obvious difficulties in specificity and accuracy, but they also have difficulties in cohesiveness, repair/revisions, quantity, and conciseness with difficulties of fluency. Adults with left-hemispheric problems have major difficulties with specificity and accuracy, as well as quantity and conciseness, with pausing, fluency, and the variety of speech actions also noted. Adults with right-hemispheric problems often have problems with eye gaze, prosody, contingency, adjacency, quantity, and conciseness (Prutting & Kirchner, 1987).

Antiepileptic drug bonuses

Sometimes, a change in anticonvulsant drug therapy may overcome the speech problems and yield improved seizure control. Occasionally, a child with known complex partial seizures may gain control of the seizures with the institution of a more effective antiepileptic drug. Concomitantly, the chronic language problems, for which the child is in speech therapy, disappear. This is an unexpected bonus of seizure therapy.

REFERENCES

Alajouanine, T. & Lhermitte, F. (1965). Acquired aphasia in children. *Brain* **88**: 653–63.

Aquilar, J. M. & Rasmussen, J. (1960). Role of encephalitis in pathogenesis of epilepsy. *Arch. Neurol.* **2**: 663–6.

Baratz, R. & Mesulam, M.-M. (1981). Adult-onset stuttering treated with anticonvulsants. *Arch. Neurol.* **38**: 132.

Belafsky, M. A., Rosman, N. P., Miller, P., Waddell, G., *et al.* (1978). Prolonged epileptic twilight states: continuous recordings with naso-pharyngeal electrodes and videotape analysis. *Neurology* **28**: 239–45.

Benson, D. F. (1979). Associated neurobehavioral problems. In *Aphasia, Alexia, and Agraphia*, pp. 158–73. New York: Churchill Livingstone.

Borkowski, W. J., Jr & Lotz, W. K. (1986). A case of verbal auditory agnosia with subsequent loss of speech treated successfully with anticonvulsants. *Ann. Neurol.* **20**: 417.

Cohn, B. (1970). Amnestic aphasia and other disturbances in naming. *Arch. Neurol.* **22**: 515–20.

Cooper, J. A. & Ferry, P. C. (1978). Acquired auditory verbal agnosia and seizures in childhood. *J. Speech Hear. Disord.* **43**: 176–84.

Critchley, M. (1970). True acquired aphasia as occurring in childhood. In *Aphasiology and Other Aspects of Language*, pp. 278–81. London: Edward Arnold.

Davies-Eysenick, M. (1952). Cognitive factors in epilepsy. *J. Neurol. Neurosurg. Psychiatry* **165**: 39–44.

Deonna, T., Chevrie, C. & Hornung, E. (1987). Childhood epileptic speech disorder: prolonged isolated deficit of prosodic features. *Dev. Med. Child Neurol.* **29**: 96–109.

Deonna, T., Fletcher, P. & Voumard, C. (1982). Temporary regression during language acquisition: a linguistic analysis of a $2\frac{1}{2}$ year old child with epileptic aphasia. *Dev. Med. Child Neurol.* **24**: 156–163.

De Pasquet, E. G., Gaudin, E. S., Bianchi, A. & De Mendilaharsu, S. A. (1976). Prolonged and monosymptomatic dysphasic status epilepticus. *Neurology* **26**: 244–7.

Foerster, G. (1977). Aphasia and seizure disorders in childhood. In *Epilepsy, the Eighth International Symposium*, ed. J. Penry, pp. 305–6. New York: Raven Press.

Gastaut, H. (1979). Aphasia: the sole manifestations of focal status epilepticus. *Neurology* **29**: 1938.

Geets, W. (1975). Le language de l'inconisceint. *Acta Psychiatr. Belg.* **75**: 273–9.

Geets, W. & Pinon, A. (1975). Crises agnosiques avec troubles du language et anomalies asmetriques de l'EEG. *Acta Psychiatr. Belg.* **75**: 160–72.

Geschwind, N. & Sherwin, I. (1967). Language-induced epilepsy. *Arch. Neurol.* **16**: 25–31.

Gilmore, R. L. & Heilman, K. M. (1981). Speech arrest in partial seizures: evidence of an associated language disorder. *Neurology* **31**: 1016–19.

Green, J. B. & Hartlage, L. C. (1971). Comparative performance of epileptic and non-epileptic children and adolescents on tests of academic, communicative and social skills. *Dis. Nerv. Syst.* **32**: 418–21.

Hamilton, N. G. & Matthews, T. (1979). Reply to Gastaut M re Aphasia: the sole manifestation of focal status epilepticus (letter to the editor). *Neurology* **29**: 1638.

Hardy, W. G. (1965). On language disorders in younger children: a reorganization of thinking. *J. Speech Hear. Disord.* **30**: 3–16.

Hecaen, H. & Piercy, M. (1956). Paroxysmal dysphasia and the problem of cerebral dominance. *J. Neurol. Neurosurg. Pyschiatry* **19**: 193–201.

Heilman, K. M., Scholes, R. & Watson, R. T. (1975). Auditory affective agnosia: disturbed comprehension of affective speech. *J. Neurol. Neurosurg. Psychiatr.* **38**: 69–72.

Hoeppner, J. B., Garron, D. C., Wilson, R. S. & Koch-Weser, M. P. (1987). Epilepsy and verbosity. *Epilepsia* **28**: 35–40.

Holmes, G. L., McKeever, M. & Saunders, Z. (1981). Epileptiform activity in aphasia of childhood: an epiphenomenon. *Epilepsia* **22**: 631–9.

Ingvar, D. H. (1976). Functional landscapes of the dominant hemisphere. *Brain Res.* **107**: 181–97.

Kossciesza, M., Stelmasiak, Z. & Kosciesza, A. (1998). Characteristics of language in children with epilepsy, 3rd European Congress of Epileptology. *Epilepsia* **39** (suppl 2): 120.

Lecours, A. R. & Joanette, Y. (1980). Linguistic and other psychological aspects of paroxysmal aphasia. *Brain Lang.* **10**: 1–23.

Lee, S. I., Sutherling,W. W., Persing, J. A. & Butler, A. B. (1980). Language-induced seizure – a case of cortical origin. *Arch. Neurol.* **37**: 433–6.

Marin, O. S. M. & Saffran, E. M. (1975). Agnosic behavior in anomia: a case of pathologic verbal dominance. *Cortex* **11**: 83–9.

O'Donohoe, N. V. (1979). Learning disorders in children with epilepsy. In *Epilepsies of Childhood*, pp. 186–9. London: Butterworth.

Ojemann, G. A. (1975). Language and the thalamus: object naming and recall during and after thalamic stimulation. *Brain Lang.* **2**: 101–20.

Prutting, C. A. & Kirchner, D. M. (1987). A clinical appraisal of the pragmatic aspects of language. *J. Speech Hear. Disord.* **52**: 105–19.

Racy, A., Osborn, M. A., Vern, B. A. & Molinari, G. I. (1980). Epileptic aphasia: first onset of prolonged monosymptomatic status epilepticus in adults. *Arch. Neurol.* **37**: 419–22.

Rapin, I., Mattis, S., Rowan, A. J., *et al.* (1977). Verbal auditory agnosia in children. *Dev. Med. Child Neurol.* **19**: 192–207.

Rayport, M., Ferguson, S. M. & Corrie, W. S. (1984). AES society proceedings. *Epilepsia* **25**: 5.

Ross, E. D. & Mesulam, M.-M. (1979). Dominant language functions of the right hemisphere: prosody and emotional gesturing. *Arch. Neurol.* **36**: 144–8.

Searleman, A. (1978). A review of right hemisphere linguistic capabilities. *Psychol. Bull.* **83**: 503–28.

Serafetinides, E. G. & Falconer, M. A. (1963). Speech disturbances in temporal lobe seizures. A study in 1000 epileptic patients submitted to anterior temporal lobectomy. *Brain* **86**: 333–46.

Vernea, J. J. (1974). Partial status epilepticus with speech arrest. *Proc. Aust. Assoc. Neurol.* **11**: 223–8.

Vollbracht, R. (1979). Epileptic aphasia (letter to the editor). *Arch. Neurol.* **37**: 787.

Watters, G. V. (1974). The syndrome of acquired aphasia and convulsive disorder in children. *Can. Med. J.* **1101**: 611–12.

Weintraub. S., Mesulam, M.-M. & Kramer, L. (1958). Disturbance in prosody, a right hemisphere contribution to language. *Arch. Neurol.* **38**: 742–4.

West, R. (1958). An agnostic's speculation about stuttering. In *Stuttering, A Symposium*, ed. J. Eisenson, pp. 169–222. New York: Harper.

Worster-Drought, C. (1971). An unusual form of acquired aphasia in children. *Dev. Med. Child Neurol.* **13**: 563–71.

5

Seizure types and speech and language risks

Specific speech and language problems, such as speech arrests, aphasias, paroxysmal word utterances, palilalia, dysarthrias, and unformed vocalizations, are more apt to occur with specific seizure types. Speech and language problems may appear simultaneously with, later than, or occasionally before the onset of the epilepsy. They may occur as part of or as the aftereffects of a seizure. At times, they may be the only manifestation of the seizure. Children appear to be less susceptible than adults to these rarely recognized disturbances, yet a child's speech and language are also susceptible to the effects of a seizure disorder.

Language problems may be brought out by stress, by uncontrolled seizures, by medications, or as seizure aftereffects in a postictal period. Surgery in the area of language functioning may sacrifice language and thus must be carefully localized preoperatively. Language problems are often unrecognized yet they may underlie later learning and behavior problems blamed on the epilepsy. Medication, especially at high doses, may bring out some of these problems.

Symptoms of an ongoing disturbance of speech and language, varying from day to day, must be differentiated from the brief episodic disturbed speech function due to actual seizure attacks and from the aftereffects seen during a recovery period. In chronic speech and language problems, there may be deterioration in the clarity or the smooth flow of speech, in word selection, and in understanding or word order or word sounds when the patient tries to express thoughts. These are apt to be associated with dominant temporal lobe epilepsy. Such problems may appear as isolated disturbed speech patterns, as receptive or expressive aphasias, or as difficulties remembering names and retrieving desired words.

Epilepsy types

Henry and Browne (1987) detailed the language and auditory processing complications of various seizure types for the Via Christi Epilepsy Center Conference (Wichita, KS).

Generalized epilepsies

With generalized seizures, the whole brain and all its functions are impaired and the patient is unconscious at the seizure onset.

Generalized tonic–clonic

The patient is unconscious with the attack. Therefore, speech and language functions are not in action. If a speech disturbance precedes the seizure, most likely the seizure is a secondary generalized partial seizure rather than a true primary generalized tonic–clonic seizure. A postictal aphasia or other speech or language problem may occasionally follow a generalized tonic–clonic seizure due to the seizure itself or due to the medication used to stop the attack.

Status epilepticus

Patients with a secondary generalized epileptic status, especially with a left-sided complex seizure disorder, may show unrecognized changes in verbal fluency lasting up to several weeks after the status. A deteriorative cognitive status may follow a generalized tonic seizure for severe days (Fewick, 1981).

Status epilepticus may produce a reversible receptive aphasia. The diagnosis is difficult. Often, there are other neurologic findings, usually with a non-fluent expressive aphasia or a mixed aphasia presentation. This is often confused with psychiatric problems, attention difficulties, or depression. The EEG may show a polyspike wave in the Wernicke's area that responded to diazepam, but the language does not change. The language, a fluent, perseverative, literal style with paraphasic errors, anomia but intact matching skills, may clear in about ten days. Vining (1996), at the American Epilepsy Society Conference section on language function in epilepsy, noted that this might recur periodically.

Absence

Absence seizures may be accompanied by various speech disturbances. The absence attack consists of a partial to complete out-of-consciousness state, with minimal to complete lack of responsiveness and, if lasting more than a few seconds, often with minor stereotyped repetitive movements (automatisms) such as blinking or rhythmic head or hand movements. Vining (1996) noted that the absence speech problems reported with absence seizures include speech arrest, slowing, or partial to complete loss, receptive and expressive language, i.e. an aphasia. When speech problems occur during absence seizures, the disturbances may be overlooked (Lennox, 1951; McKeever et al., 1983).

Speech arrests may occur as part of these automatisms. Occasionally, a child may be clear-minded during the attack but unable to respond. A change in the rate of speaking may be noted, characterized by a slow, drawn-out pattern, hesitancy, or a halting rate, often with brief pauses or stammering noted. Some children become stuck on a word or phrase, persevering on this throughout the attack. Humming may be part of the attack. Rarely, if ever, is speech normal during the seizure. Reduced to absent understanding or expression may be noted if partial consciousness is retained. These deviations are usually, but not always, associated with generalized spike-wave discharges (Belafsky *et al.*, 1978; Holmes *et al.*, 1981). Early stimulation during the burst onset may abbreviate or stop the burst duration. Responses to questions asked within seconds of the bursts may be delayed, but if the delay was extended beyond a few seconds no response may be obtained.

Absence status

Some children experience a prolonged absence status, with waxing and waning consciousness, during which language is confused and sparse. The child may seem confused or even psychotic. Speech attempts appear confused, hesitating, or deficient, and the child seems not to understand. This is seen most often with atypical absences and may recur. It responds rapidly to intravenous diazepam.

Atypical absence attacks

With atypical absences, a child experiences less demarcated and often longer staring episodes with confusion. Atypical spike-wave bursts are seen. These children tend to be slowed in intelligence and in language skills, with behavior problems noted more often. A brief aphasic state may occur with or immediately after a seizure. Brief episodes of reduced comprehension or expression of language have been noted when the absence attack does not result in complete loss of consciousness. Other symptoms include slurring of speech during the seizure discharge, decreased speaking rate, hesitations, blocking, or humming. When the seizures ceases, speech and language function returns to that which is normal for the child. This must be differentiated from the acquired aphasia with epilepsy syndromes. The response to antiepileptic medication for atypical absence episodes is often incomplete (Shoumaker *et al.*, 1974).

Absence versus complex partial stares

Absence seizures and complex partial seizures may be confused. Speech changes are common with both, including problems in understanding (53–56%), problems in expression (90–94%), speech slowing (25–26%), dysarthria (31–32%), and perseverative efforts (11–13%). Complex partial epilepsy may be associated with groaning (31%) and a tendency to change topics (31%). With absences, often patients are not noted to have formed speech during a seizure, although humming may occur. However, some have noted speech to occur during absence seizures (Penry *et al.*, 1975; McKeever *et al.*, 1983; Bancaud *et al.*, 1981).

Minor motor (atonic, akinetic, myoclonic) seizures

Atonic, akinetic, and myoclonic seizures are often associated with developmental delays and occasionally with intellectual deterioration. The seizure attacks are usually so brief that the seizure is not characteristically associated with any speech or language problems, although momentary halts or hesitations in the speech may be noted. Delays in speech and language may be seen as part of the overall developmental delay. With some myoclonic syndromes, the myoclonic discharges may show up initially as hiccoughs. As the disorder progresses, the speech may become frail and tremulous, matching the appearance of gait and hand movements.

Syndromes

Vining (1996) noted that many of the epilepsy syndromes produce language problems.

Infantile spasms

Infantile myoclonic spasms are usually associated with delays in communication skills seen as part of the overall developmental delays, including severe mental retardation.

Lennox–Gastaut syndrome

In this syndrome, children experience longer atypical absences and are more often in a confused state than completely out of it. Tonic, atonic, and myoclonic seizures are also common. The EEG shows generalized slower spike-wave discharges and the child's intellectual functioning is slowed. Distractibility, inattentiveness, and impulsivity are common. Auditory memory deficits may be present. Other diagnostic considerations would include acquired aphasia with epilepsy syndrome or even sleep status epilepsy. Speech and language problems are common in such children.

Partial seizures

Vining (1996) noted that localization-related seizure syndromes might produce language dysfunction, such as with seizures originating in the lateral temporal lobe, the frontal lobe including the motor and opercular areas (Broca's expressive language area), and the posterior temporal parietal lobe (Wernicke's area for receptive area).

Transfer of speech functions to the right-hemisphere in right-handed individuals is suggested by an ictal focus in the usual left speech area without evidence for ictal or postictal aphasic speech, or there may be suggestions of an ictal or postictal aphasic component to the patient's attacks with a right hemisphere, especially if there are signs of motor damage from infancy. Such different lateralization should be confirmed by carotid amobarbital testing (Ojemann, 1980) or by functional imagery utilizing rapid magnetic resonance imaging (MRI) or isotopic recordings.

Children with language impairments accompanying progressive seizure disorders may present symptoms different from those with a simple lateralized seizure disorder. Such children may exhibit fluent speech with frequent jargon but with severely impaired auditory comprehension. Severe language comprehension disorder in children usually requires bilateral involvement of the temporal lobes and it is difficult to explain such acquired deficits otherwise in light of plasticity (Ludlow, 1980). Usually, a seizure discharge originates in the left brain half if language is disturbed.

Simple partial epilepsies

Simple partial seizures are usually brief, with the patient conscious at the onset. Seizures originating in the dominant hemisphere may disturb language, especially if language centers are involved. Aphasia may occur during or after the seizure. When the speech and language areas are involved, episodes of halting or pausing of speech (speech arrests), bursts of poorly pronounced or even unformed speech (utterances), slurring or imprecision of speech or a deterioration of pronunciation (dysarthria), the repeating of words or phrases with increasing rapidity (palilalia), as well as the hearing of formed or most often unformed sounds (auditory hallucinations) may occur (Lecours & Joanette, 1980). Speech arrests may occur with focal seizures from either side, especially those involving the frontal and temporal lobes of the brain. Such episodes, with a transient receptive or expressive aphasia, are more apt to come from the left or dominant hemisphere, whereas a pure speech arrest may be seen coming from the right (non-dominant) hemisphere. A speech arrest or aphasia may be the primary or sole seizure symptom. Usually, these episodes are brief (Gilmore & Heilman, 1981; Hamilton & Matthews, 1979). If seizure activity is allowed to persist, the defect may become permanent.

Frontal

Simple partial seizures involving the left frontal lobe may present with a pure expressive aphasia. The patient is unable to come up with the words of speech. Left frontal lesions in a non-aphasic patient may produce a deficit in verbal fluency, similar to that seen following a partial frontal lobectomy for the control of epilepsy. In addition to diminished spontaneous speech, there is a markedly diminished ability to form a word list. The medial frontal supplementary motor area may be part of a more primitive system involved in a starting mechanism of speech and also in the maintenance of speech fluency (Alexander & Schmitt, 1980). Frontal speech dysfluency is seen in the non-dominant frontal lobe (McDaniel & McDaniel, 1976).

Supplemental motor

Motor speech disturbances can originate from discharges in either the Rolandic or the supplementary motor area of either hemisphere. Partial stimulation of either supplementary motor area produces repetitive vocalization, speech arrests, and/or bilateral mouth movements (Gilmore & Heilman, 1981). Surgical ablation of the supplementary motor area may produce a transient failure in the initiation, a motor aphasia, or autistic-like speech. Permanent speech disorders include difficulty in the initiation of speech and anomia. A transient to near-complete aphasia may be noted. Transcortical motor aphasia may present with an absence of spontaneous speech, difficulties in initiating speech, limitations in the ability to name, or a limited ability to make brief responses. Auditory comprehension, reading comprehension, and reading aloud remains relatively intact. The ability to repeat back what is heard remains prompt, well articulated, grammatically intact, and free of any difficulty in imitation that marks all other speech problems (Alexander & Schmitt, 1980).

Benign Rolandic (centrotemporal) epilepsy

Some children with benign Rolandic epilepsy, presenting with speech delays and typical central-temporal spikes, may show a more or less prolonged focal neurologic deficit referable to the Sylvian region. They may experience a transient impairment of oral movements of speech and swallowing, correlated with increased seizure frequency with EEG findings of an active left or bilateral centrotemporal typical Rolandic spike focus. There may be periods of dysarthria as a rare ictal phenomenon. These episodes may be accompanied by a speech deterioration manifested by anomia and slurred speech as well as associated drooling and difficulties in swallowing (Staden et al., 1998; Croona et al., 1999). The question is whether the dysfunction is related to the seizures or the anticonvulsants, and if it is seizure-related, whether it is ictal or postictal; these are not so benign (Deonna et al., 1997).

A speech evaluation may reveal oral motor deficits, including facial weakness, excessive salivation, difficulties in chewing and swallowing, reduced speech fluency, and difficulties in pronunciation and articulation. A mild deficit in production of oral pressure with tight lips and a mild deficit in tongue movements as well as naming and word retrieval deficits may be seen; these may persist (Staden et al., 1998; Croona et al., 1999). The transient oromotor deficits may relate to an increased interictal epileptic activity as part of an inhibitory mechanism affecting functions of the lower motor strip (Engel, 1996; de Saint Martin et al., 1999) or it may be an ictal phenomenon. Rarely after the episodes of oral motor deficits, a word-retrieval difficulty or a permanent speech dysfluency may remain (Roulet *et al.*, 1989; Deonna *et al.*, 1997; Kramer *et al.*, 2001). Subtle cognitive, attention, visuomotor, as well as a variety of specific language deficits have been noted. These include recall of auditory verbal materials, auditory perception, reading, spelling, expressive grammar, and verbal fluency problems (Staden *et al.*, 1998; Croona *et al.*, 1999). Verbal tasks are influenced particularly by left-sided discharges (Rugland *et al.*, 1987). The deficit varies between patients, lasting hours to weeks. An alteration of antiepileptic medication may lead to a rapid improvement (Staden *et al.*, 1998; Croona *et al.*, 1999).

There is a similar disorder presenting with a speech dyspraxia either in childhood when the disorder is active or at some time afterward. This is a familial disorder with an autosomal dominance inheritance pattern, presenting with Rolandic epilepsy when the disorder is active (Scheffer *et al.*, 1996).

Temporal–parietal

Some patients may hear sounds or speech (auditory hallucinations) as part of a simple special sensory partial seizure.

Complex partial epilepsies

Children with complex partial seizures involving the dominant anterior temporal lobe are more apt to present with learning disabilities involving the auditory channel. Language performance also tends to be below normal (Hermann *et al.*, 2001). Verbal cognitive dysfunctions do not ordinarily manifest as aphasia but instead manifest as reading and spelling problems and reduced language efficiency and expression. Speech may be slowed and hesitant as if it is no longer automatic. A loss of learning skills might result from the development of a functional aphasia (Keating, 1960). Word-finding difficulties, including word substitutions, paraphasias, and mild anomias, may be noted. There may be a relationship to personality disturbances and deteriorations in temporal lobe epilepsy (Quadfasel & Pruyser, 1955). These are seen especially with anterior temporal lobe spikes. In EEG-monitored testing, some subjects occasionally show verbal confusion such as misusing common words or talking incoherently before ultimately giving an answer. Such expressions of confusion may be associated with concomitant bursts on the EEG.

Speech and language disturbances in complex partial seizures often go unnoticed (Racy *et al.*, 1980). More common complications include speech arrests, aphasias, anomias, and paroxysmal utterances. Slowing of the speech rate, changes in what is being talked about, dysarthrias, preservative speech automatisms (such as the uttering of identifiable words and phrases repeatedly), and even groaning, humming, or moaning sounds may be seen (Lennox, 1951; Serafetinides & Falconer, 1963; Hecaen & Piercy, 1956; Bingley, 1958; McKeever *et al.*, 1983). Changes in the fluency and appropriateness of speech and language may go unrecognized yet persist for several weeks following a complex partial seizure, especially if the seizure becomes generalized. An aphasic component to the problem suggests that the discharge most probably involved the left brain half. If it is on the left, there may be a wide range of problems, including anomia, dysfluency, monotony of the voice, auditory language-processing deficits, reduced initiation of speech, fewer spontaneous verbalizations, simplified syntax, short-term auditory memory deficits, and subtle pragmatic deficits. Emotional behavioral disturbances due to language impairment are common. Paroxysmal speech disturbances are of considerable significance in complex partial epilepsy, often constituting either the origin itself or one of its elements, although much more research is needed to discover the correlates between the irritative lesion and a speech–language disturbance (Porrazzo & Mayersdorf, 1980).

Anterior temporal lobe seizure defects have been associated with verbal auditory learning disabilities, including speech deficits. The discharges most often involve the temporal to lower frontal portion of the brain, especially the limbic system (Cherlow & Serafetinides, 1976). Three potential sources of speech disturbances include the posterior temporal-parietal area of Wernicke's area, Broca's area, and the supplementary motor area on the mesial portion of the hemisphere, most anterior to the area serving the foot (Serafetinides & Falconer, 1963). Another area in the anterior lower external temporal lobe also appears to be related to speech production.

Children with complex partial seizures use less self-initiated repair mechanisms to correct errors during a conversation compared with children with primarily generalized absences and controls. Redundant use of referential and syntactical correction makes speech sounds unusual, providing additional evidence that complex partial seizures impact the ongoing development of children's communications. They make significantly more self-initiated corrections of references and syntax. Children with poor seizure control have to correct referential and syntactic items unlike those with good seizure control. Children with complex partial seizures of temporal origin make more corrections than those of frontal origin.

Language-processing deficits

In brainstem auditory evoked response testing of central hearing, when a novel stimulus is given the P300 is the late event that results. This waveform is influenced by the initial cognitive activity and is thought to be linked to the hippocampus and amygdala. With left temporal EEG seizure disorders, the P300 latency is longer with lower amplitudes derived, a phenomenon not seen with generalized seizures. This seems to relate to a disturbance of cognitive processing seen with temporal lobe dysfunction (Syrigou-Papavasiliou *et al.*, 1985). This may be seen in individuals with left temporal lobe memory difficulties. The P300 changes may also relate to the intolerance to noisy situations seen in some left temporal lobe seizure patients.

Agnosia

Agnosias are rarely recognized as a separate entity associated with some types of epilepsy. More often, they are a part of or are confused with an acquired aphasia syndrome, such as the acquired aphasia with epilepsy syndrome.

Aphasia

Aphasias are seen with complex partial epilepsy as part of a single attack or following a series of seizures. Such a temporary aphasia usually resolves after a variable interval, but it may recur with further seizures (O'Donohoe & Naill, 1979). In children, receptive aphasias with confusion or non-understanding can come from either brain side, whereas expressive aphasias, like speech arrests, tend to come from the left side. The seizure discharge usually begins in the left hemisphere. One of the more likely areas of involvement, especially in an expressive aphasia, is the temporal-frontal area of the brain (Serafetinides & Falconer, 1963). However, others feel that it may originate in the associative areas within the language areas of the brain and especially the posterior temporal receptive area (Lecours & Joanette, 1980). This is more likely with a receptive aphasia.

The aphasia usually follows an initial change in consciousness. Often, other symptoms or signs are present, usually of a sensory, motor, or psychic nature, suggesting the diagnosis of a complex partial seizure disorder (Lecours & Joanette, 1980). Ictal speech automatisms and, in focal seizures of the dominant temporal lobe, a paroxysmal aphasia that may be expressive or both receptive and expressive, may occur. The nature of the patient's neologistic jargon would suggest a problem in the auditory association area and arcuate fasciculus (Wilson *et al.*, 1983).

Nearly half (48%) of patients with lateralized epileptiform discharges manifest paroxysmal aphasia when a dominant-sided focus is present, but few (12%) do so with a non-dominant-sided discharge. Speech abnormalities thus occur in 67% of patients with complex partial seizures, with dysphasia seen in about half, primarily those with dominant-hemisphere epileptiform discharges (Hecaen & Piercy, 1956; Bingley, 1958; Serafetinides & Falconer, 1963; McKeever *et al.*, 1983).

In children, complex partial seizures are often more complicated, especially if the dominant hemisphere is involved. Intelligence may be depressed, language development may be slowed, and specific reading problems are common, especially in children whose seizures began before five to six years of age. Preadolescent children with childhood-dominant temporal lobe discharges differ from adults in that the discharges may be seen from either or both sides or, rarely, only from the right side.

Rather than obvious aphasic problems, children may show a reticence to speak, a simplified grammatical structure, and diminished spontaneous speech pattern. Less spontaneous spoken efforts are noted. Word-finding problems occur more commonly than is recognized. Often, the child is introverted, supporting the concept that a specific but minimal cognitive impairment during development is associated with specific epileptic foci, which can result in specific sequelae in the personality of the adult with complex partial seizures (Novelly, 1982).

Some children, particularly at times of stress or of seizure activity, may develop aphasic problems that can be detected if looked for. These problems may be associated with social and school catastrophes due to misunderstandings. Such a tendency may not be detected in a routine speech–language evaluation unless the child is stressed during the testing.

Children with temporal lobe seizures may have learning problems as a part of their seizure disorders, especially involving the verbal-language channel of learning. Interictal discharges may disturb temporal lobe functioning as reflected in deficits in verbal cognitive tasks, a disturbance not ordinarily manifested clinically as an overt aphasia (Quadfasel & Pruyser, 1955).

Anomia

Anomia may be seen as a part of a seizure and also between seizures with complex partial epilepsy. Anomia is often a component of aphasia, but it may appear as an independent problem. Patients complain of difficulties in remembering specific words, especially names of items and people. Such a problem is most apt to occur under stress or when infrequently used words are being recalled. Some individuals will show verbal confusion, such as misusing common words or talking incoherently. Their speech pattern may be halting or interrupted by their searching for the word. Patients with dominant temporal lobe complex partial epilepsy who manifest anomia may note difficulties in remembering a specific word at times of stress or when an infrequently used word is required. This tends to occur during periods of impaired alertness, distractions, time pressure, or stress, or if the given item is unfamiliar. This may become obvious only by tests that include some stress factors and may require use of lower-frequency words (Mayeus *et al.*, 1980).

Paroxysmal word utterances

Paroxysmal word utterances may include warning statements of a seizure onset, recurring phrases, irrelevant words or phrases, emotional outbursts, or perplexed statements. The patient is out of contact at the time and usually does not recall the utterances. Discharges may be seen from either or both temporal lobes, although the non-dominant right temporal lobe is usually involved (Serafetinides & Falconer, 1963).

Arrests

Speech arrests may be seen with complex partial seizures (Gilmore & Heilman, 1981). These are seldom prolonged and are usually accompanied by confusion and automatisms. Motor and psychomotor manifestations may not be present. The seizure discharge usually comes from the frontal and temporal brain surface. A speech arrest may be part of the seizure or it may be a postictal symptom. Speech arrests and stereotypic automatisms are common in an epileptic stupor, although the speech problem often clears up in the final hours of the episode (Belafsky *et al.*, 1978).

Fluency

Conversations with dominant complex partial epilepsy patients may be free of gross dysphasic errors but may be characterized by reticence, a simplified grammatic structure, and diminished spontaneity. Speech fluency may be disturbed in some individuals with a left temporal lobe seizure problem. In some patients, the speech may be characteristically slowed, slurred, and often effortful. It is as if the normal automatic flow of speech does not occur. This pattern is present even when the seizures are controlled, but it becomes more obvious before the onset of overt seizures. Changes in medication may normalize this pattern, suggesting that this is a subtle, subclinical seizure effect.

Verbosity

Verbosity is a rare trait seen uniquely in individuals with left-sided complex partial epilepsy, and especially in those with more severe or a longer duration of seizures and medication usage. The speech is characterized by non-essential and sometimes peculiar details, which resemble the triad of obsessive patterns, circumstantiality, and viscosity. Such patients tend to refer to non-essential details, including subjective, peculiar details, or elaborations. They may bring to the surgery extra long written notes. These patients do not differ in terms of memory or intelligence. Hypergraphia, or a tendency for right temporal lobe epileptics to write spontaneously, frequently, and at great length, have been described (Hoeppner *et al.*, 1987).

Left temporal lobe patients tend to be anomic, with memory difficulties. Their loquaciousness and circumstantiality may represent in part attempts at getting around the problems. However, these patients tend to be rather detailed in their recall. They also appear to be driven to talk, to notice things not noticed by others, and to give particular significance to things that others see but do not emphasize (Hoeppner *et al.*, 1987). The adolescent may say much but never get to the point, always talking around the subject despite frequent reference to copious notes. Speech may be a flat, monotonous, tick-tock effort, overly detailed in content but boring to the listener.

Neologisms

The uttering of neologisms accompanied by an extreme emotional liability (like a mania) and hallucinations have been noted as a part of a seizure. The neologisms resemble those of a fluent aphasia. The neologisms of the right temporal seizure discharge do not have the overly condensed and saturated with-meaning quality sometimes attributed to schizophrenic neologisms but rather resemble paraphasic distortions described in the context of fluent aphasias, although this distinction is controversial (Hoffman *et al.*, 1986).

The concurrent EEG suggests that the right hemisphere might play a role in the expression of this language content. The right hemisphere seems related functionally to emotional and melodic qualities of language and to general expressions of affect. There may be a loss of the usual variations of pitch, rhythm, and stress of emotional meaning (speech prosody) without dysarthria or apraxia in patients with supra-Sylvian lesions of the right hemisphere. The organization of affective language in the right hemisphere seems to mirror the organization of language in the left hemisphere. The right hemisphere is probably involved in the acquisition of musical sequences in the musically naive.

Periods of extreme emotional behavior during seizures may be related to propagation of the discharges to subcortical structures (Floor-Henry, 1972). Cortical and subcortical structures (Crosson, 1985) in the right hemisphere add the affect and emotional aspects to spoken language, perhaps through favorable connections to basilar limbic systems. The patient may be more emotionally labile. An adolescent with a right temporal focus later developed prominent emotional swings between a keyed up, giddy state and a depressed state.

Partial epileptic aphasic status

Some patients with focal status recover between the epileptic burst symptoms, but some do not. Rarely, such seizures may be prolonged, lasting hours to days, during which time the patient may be in and out of the state. This has been called aphasic seizure status. Aphasia due to partial status epilepticus is rare, especially in the absence of any history of epilepsy. Aphasia may be the only manifestation of a focal epileptic status involving the left frontal lobe. To diagnose a partial ictal aphasic status, the patient must have language production that shows aphasic features during the seizures. Consciousness should be preserved, at least partially. Seizures should be correlated with the aphasia, as documented by EEG monitoring and behavior testing (Hamilton & Matthews, 1979).

In adults and children presenting with an episode of hours to days of reduced speech, often with confusion, the initial diagnosis is usually that of a vascular problem, even if the person is able to perform non-verbal tasks. Because acute aphasia more commonly results from such a cause, recognizing the possibility of an ictal event in a patient without a previous seizure history can be difficult but should always be considered. Diagnosis may be delayed up to three weeks. EEG can confirm the diagnosis rapidly and the attack can be terminated by giving intravenous anticonvulsant medication. Delay in treatment has the potential to affect the final outcome. Early treatment is important to shorten the patient's considerable functioning impairment and to prevent development of a permanent deficit caused by incessant cortical discharges (Hamilton & Matthews, 1979).

Complex partial epileptic status may be confused with a psychiatric problem (Belafsky *et al.*, 1978). Numerous types of speech disturbances, including the cessation of language, may accompany left temporal lobe seizure status. Other problems include the recall of familiar words and difficulties with reading and writing. None of the more common language disturbances of word deafness, dysarthria, or jargon aphasia are seen. Occasionally, some patients do present with word deafness and/or with jargon aphasia (Gastaut, 1979).

A patient might have periods of agitated speech efforts that do not make sense, seeming to be a jumble of unrelated phrases and sentences interspersed with periods of sitting in a rather confused state, perhaps rocking or aimlessly playing with their hands. It is unusual for a patient to appear to be deaf to words, to exhibit poorly pronounced slurred speech, or to utter only nonsensical jargon sounds. The status may occur in two phase states, alternating back and forth. One state is a continuous twilight state with partial responsiveness. The patient demonstrates various automatic reactions to the environment, including periods of partial responsiveness and rather automatic reactions to the environment. Eventually, the individual gives a correct response. The EEG at this time looks diffusely slow. This state is periodically interrupted by episodes of blank staring, at which time the patient is not responsive. Stereotyped automatisms may be seen. About half of the time the EEG will show anterior temporal lobe spike bursts when these periods of confusions occur, although clinically no seizure is apparent. Between the seizures, the patient may function relatively normally. Faster paroxysmal activities develop over the temporal head regions, during which speech arrests and stereotyped automatisms may be seen (Belafsky *et al.*, 1978).

Acquired agnosia/aphasia with epilepsy

A rare problem, acquired aphasia with epilepsy syndrome often involves both temporal lobes in the seizure discharge, although often the seizure discharge is more generalized (see Chapter 6).

Language-induced reflex seizures

Seizures can induce speech and language disorders. The reverse is seen also, as language can induce seizures. Seizures can be triggered by any or all of three language modalities, i.e. reading, speaking, and writing (Geschwind & Sherwin, 1967). Attempts to speak, to read silently or aloud, or to write may introduce paroxysmal discharges. Calculations do not necessarily induce these seizures (Lee *et al.*, 1980). There appears to be no relationship to word familiarity, the form (poetry or prose) of the written material, the comprehension of the reading content, or the organization of the written word on the page (Bennett *et al.*, 1971). Concentration on the spoken word, such as when being spoken to directly or when specific words pertinent to the patient's concerns are uttered, appear to trigger some discharges (Tsuzuki & Kasuga, 1977). The seizures are more apt to occur if the patient is speaking rapidly or is fatigued (Bennett *et al.*, 1971). Even whispering can precipitate some attacks. Once a seizure has been induced, the patient appears more susceptible to repeat seizures if the stimulus is given again. In some, the speaking of memorized materials may produce seizures (Geschwind & Sherwin, 1967; Bennett *et al.*, 1971; Foerster, 1977). The singing of unfamiliar songs may also produce seizures (Foerster, 1977). When actual seizures are recorded during attempts to speak or write, the discharges originate in the left temporal lobe. The seizure presentation is of myoclonic or clonic jerks, or jerking of the mouth, face, or jaw (Bennett *et al.*, 1971; Geschwind & Sherwin, 1967).

Many EEG findings have been described. Often, there are generalized rather than focal disturbances, generalized spike or polyspike wave discharges being recorded most commonly. However, some patients display clinical partial seizures with focal random spike activity in the contralateral central or frontal-central areas; with other patients, random focal spikes may be seen more often around the central motor strip. Attempts to speak, read, or write have been associated with paroxysmal discharges in the left temporal or central area when reading aloud, and in the left central areas when writing (Geschwind & Sherwin, 1967; Lee *et al.*, 1980). Others may show discharges from the right posterior-frontal and central regions when reading more than when speaking or writing (Bennett *et al.*, 1971). Concern and concentration on the task appear to bring out this discharge tendency. Some patients may have a history of stuttering in childhood without accompanying EEG changes noted (Geschwind & Sherwin, 1967).

Although patients may or may not respond to anticonvulsants (Lee *et al.*, 1980), clonazepam and valproate have benefitted some.

Surgery has been considered in adults with antiepileptic-medication-resistant seizures. In adults with a left temporal (superior posterior temporal and inferior posterior frontal) focus, seizures often occur when the individual is communicating

verbally with others or reading. Typical seizures often begin with auditory hallucinations and tend to occur in clusters. These trigger complex partial seizures. EEG
studies have shown the seizures to be easily induced by the use of language, including reading. The focus is on the left side. Another type of epilepsy with seizures
induced by language activity appears with myoclonic jerking of the jaw, face, or
upper extremities as the main seizure type. A lesion may occasionally be found and
excised, leading to seizure remission (Inoue *et al.*, 1998).

Spikes but no clinical seizures

Language functions appear sensitive to transient cognitive impairments (Bates,
1953; Shimazono *et al.*, 1953; Goldie & Green, 1961; Jus & Jus, 1962; Tizard &
Murgerson, 1963; Binnie, 1980). An EEG may be performed for reasons other than
suspicions of possible epilepsy. Occasionally, a child with a speech or language
problem will have an EEG that is unexpectedly abnormal, i.e. sharp waves, spikes,
or spike-wave discharges in the language-processing areas of the brain, yet the child
has never had any symptoms to suggest a seizure. This does not indicate that the
child has epilepsy and needs to be on medication. The EEG abnormality of spikes,
sharp waves, or spike-wave discharges may represent an irritation or an inherited
tendency that may never go on to produce seizures or potential seizures.

When a spiking is found but no seizure history is elicited, some will assume
that the child is having seizures that are overlooked and thus diagnose and treat
the mythical seizure. A good history-taking will usually bring out descriptions of
actual seizures and also some seizure-like behaviors (e.g. staring when the child is
overwhelmed by a task). It is generally felt that anticonvulsant therapy will help with
clinical seizures but will not help with the language problem if there are no seizures.
Studies have been done in which a child with an abnormal EEG was monitored
with an ongoing EEG and videotaping as speech and language examinations were
performed. No demonstrated relationship between the occurrence of the speech
abnormalities and the epileptic-like abnormalities on the EEG was detected.

Children with subclinical epileptic discharges and developmental language disorders may be more impaired in their ability to process complex language functioning
(grammar processing). There appears to be a relation between EEG subclinical discharges and the grade of dyslalia. Memory performance is inconsistent and often
abnormal. This measure is most obvious with focal EEG discharges as compared
with those with generalized discharges. Patients with abnormalities of the EEG tend
to show more malfunctions in the articulation of sibilants (Kutschkke *et al.*, 1999).

Children who have a speech delay and no history to suggest a prior brain insult or
seizure-like episodes very rarely show any EEG abnormalities and rarely, if ever, respond to antiepileptic medications. Children who experience a regression in speech

and language skills may need to have an EEG performed. If the EEG is negative, the child should undergo an overnight videotelemetric EEG study performed to investigate possible seizure discharge during sleep.

With an abnormal EEG and a language deficit but nothing to suggest seizures, control with a safe anticonvulsant at therapeutic levels for several months may be tried. If a striking improvement does not appear within two to three months, the problem is most probably not epileptic.

The chances of such a therapeutic trial producing a beneficial response is one in 1000. The chances of the medication interfering with speech and language efforts, learning, and behavior are probably more likely to result.

Modifiers

Types of seizure disorders may cause other problems if combined with a variety of factors.

Causes

Symptomatic epilepsy suggests the cause of the language problems is more than just the epileptic activity, i.e. the underlying damage is to be considered. However, if the seizures are of early onset, language may have been moved to adjacent areas or corresponding areas in the opposite hemisphere, resulting in recovery of functions but perhaps at the sacrifice of non-verbal perceptual motor functions after a lag of about six months. Such language functions may be far less impaired than the damage might suggest, but subtle verbal learning impairments may remain that can be brought out by stress or by seizure activity. This plasticity recovery lessens with increasing age of onset. Symptomatic epilepsy is also more apt to be associated with interictal impairments.

Gender

Generally, males are more at risk than females for a language impairment resulting from an insult. The male brain develops at a slower rate than the female brain, but with the difference in onset of puberty the male still has a few more years to lateralize language function. The female may be more apt to have temporary language impairment following an insult but is more apt to recover than a male exposed to a similar insult.

Age of onset

The child with early onset of seizures is more apt to experience learning and language impairments but is more apt to recover, at least partially, due to the plasticity of brain development. This recovery capability lessens with age.

Frequency

Frequent seizures may impair a language or learning ability, as the events do not allow the brain to recover between events. Normal developmental processes may be inhibited.

Timing

Seizures at night may be missed, resulting in daytime impairments, as evidenced in the sleep spike-wave status syndrome of childhood.

Epileptic status

Status is damaging. The child is more apt to recover than the adult. Minor status as with absence, minor motor, or complex partial status inhibits language functioning as part of the symptoms.

REFERENCES

Alexander, M. P. & Schmitt, M. A. (1980). The aphasia syndrome of stroke in the left anterior cerebral artery territory. *Arch. Neurol.* **37**: 97–100.

Bancaud, J., Henricksen, O., Rubio-Donnadieu, F., *et al.* (1981). Proposal for revised clinical and electroencephalographic classification of epileptic seizures. *Epilepsia* **22**: 489–501.

Bates, J. A. V. (1953). A technique for identifying changes in consciousness. *Electroencephalogr. Clin. Neurophysiol.* **5**: 445–6.

Belafsky, M. A., Carwille, S., Miller, P., *et al.* (1978). Prolonged epileptic twilight states: continuous recordings with nasopharyngeal electrodes and videotape analysis. *Neurology* **28**: 239–45.

Bennett, D. R., Mavor, H. & Jracho, L. W. (1971). Language induced epilepsy: report of a case. *Electroencephalogr. Clin. Neurophysiol.* **30**: 159.

Bingley, T. (1958). Mental symptoms in temporal lobe epilepsy and temporal lobe gliomas. *Acta Psychiatra et Neurol. Suppl.* **120**: 95–101.

Binnie, C. D. (1980). Detection of transitory cognitive impairments using epileptiform EEG dischargers: problems in clinical practice. In *Epilepsy and Behavior '79*, ed. P. M. Kulig, H. Masseinardi & G. Stores, pp. 91–7. Lisse: Swet & Zeitlinger.

Cherlow, D. G. & Serafetinides, E. A. (1976). Speech and language assessment in psychomotor epileptics. *Cortex* **12**: 11–26.

Croona, C., Kihlgern, M., Lundberg, S., *et al.* (1999). Neuropsychological findings in children with benign childhood epilepsy with centrotemporal spikes. *Dev. Med. Child Neurol.* **41**: 813–18.

Crosson, B. (1985). Subcortical functions in language: a working model. *Brain Lang.* **25**: 257–92.

Deonna, T. W., Roulet, E., Fontan, D., *et al.* (1997). Speech and oromotor deficits of epileptic origin in benign partial epilepsy of childhood with Rolandic spikes (BPERS): relationship to the acquired aphasia-epilepsy syndrome. *Neuropediatrics* **35**: 84–7.

De Saint Martin, A., Petiau, C., Massa, R., *et al.* (1999). Idiopathic Rolandic epilepsy with interictal-facial myoclonia and oromotor deficit (a longitudinal EEG and PET study). *Epilepsia* **40**: 614–20.

Engel, J. R. (1996). Excitation and inhibition in epilepsy. *Can. J. Neurol. Sci.* **23**: 167–74.

Fewick, P. (1981). Precipitation and inhibition of seizures. In *Epilepsy and Psychiatry*, ed. E. H. Reynolds & M. R. Trimble, pp. 306–21. New York: Churchill Livingstone.

Floor-Henry, P. (1972). Ictal and inter-ictal psychiatric manifestations in epilepsy: specific or non-specific. *Epilespia* **13**: 733–83.

Foerster, F. M. (1977). Epilepsy evoked by higher cognitive functions: communication evoked epilepsy (language epilepsy: reading epilepsy). In *Reflex Epilepsy, Behavior Therapy and Conditioned Reflexes*, pp. 94–153. Springfield, IL: Chas C. Thomas.

Gastaut, H. (1979). Aphasia, the sole manifestation of focal status epilepticus. *Neurology* **29**: 1938.

Geschwind, N. & Sherwin, I. (1967). Language induced epilepsy. *Arch. Neurol.* **16**: 25–31.

Gilmore, R. L. & Heilman, K. M. (1981). Speech arrest in partial seizures: evidence of an associated language disorder. *Neurology* **31**: 1016–1019.

Goldie, L. & Green, U. M. (1961). Spike and wave discharges and alterations of conscious awareness. *Nature* **191**: 200–201.

Hamilton, N. G. & Matthews, T. (1979). Aphasia, the sole manifestation of focal status epilepticus. *Neurology* **29**: 745–48, 1636.

Hecaen, H. & Piercy, M. (1956). Paroxysmal dysphasia and the problem of cerebral dominance. *J. Neurol. Neurosurg. Psychiatry* **19**: 194–201.

Henry, D. & Browne, M. (1987). Language and auditory processing deficits. Presented at the St Francis Epilepsy Symposium, Wichita, KS, September 17, 1987.

Hermann, B. P., Bell, B., Seidenberg, M., *et al.* (2001). Learning disabilities and language function in epilepsy. *Epilespia* **42** (suppl 10): 21–3.

Hoeppner, J. B., Garrons, D. C., Wilson, R. S., *et al.* (1987). Epilepsy and verbosity. *Epilepsia* **28**: 35–40.

Hoffman, R. E., Stopek, S. & Anderasen, N. C. (1986). A comparative study of manic vs. schizophrenic speech disorganization. *Arch. Gen. Psychiatry* **43**: 831–8.

Holmes, G., McKeever, P. I. & Saunders, Z. (1981). Epileptiform activity in aphasia of childhood: an epiphenomenon? *Epilepsia* **22**: 631–49.

Inoue, Y., Miahara, T., Fukao, K., *et al.* (1998). Ictal paraphasia induced by language activity. 3rd European Congress of Epileptology, Warsaw, Poland, May 1998. *Epilepsia* **39** (suppl 2): 71.

Jus, A. & Jus, K. (1962). Retrograde amnesia in petit mal. *Arch. Gen. Psychiatry* **6**: 163–7.

Keating, L. E. (1960). A review of the literature on the relationship of epilepsy and intelligence in schoolchildren. *J. Mental Sci.* **106**: 104–59.

Kramer, U., Ben-Zeev, B., Harel, S., *et al.* (2001). Transient oromotor deficits in children with benign childhood epilepsy with central-temporal spikes. *Epilepsia* **42**: 616–20.

Kutschkke, G., Brodbeck, V., Boor, R., *et al.* (1999). Do subclinical epileptic discharges (SED) influence language functions in children with developmental language disorders (DLD)? 23rd International Epilepsy Congress. *Epilepsia* **40** (suppl 2): 20.

Lecours, A. R. & Joanette, Y. (1980). Linguistic and other psychological aspects of paroxysmal aphasia. *Brain Lang.* **10**: 1–3.

Lee, S. I., Sutherling, W. W., Persing, J. A., *et al.* (1980). Language-induced seizure: a case of cortical origin. *Arch. Neurol.* **37**: 433–6.

Lennox, W. G. (1951). Phenomena and correlations of the psychomotor triad. *Neurology* **1**: 357–71.

Ludlow, C. L. (1980). Children's language disorders: recent research advances. *Ann. Neurol.* **7**: 497–507.

McDaniel, J. W. & McDaniel, M. L. (1976). Visual and auditory cognitive processing affected by epilepsy. *PDM* **7**: 38–42.

Mayeus, R., Brandt, J., Rosen, J., *et al.* (1980). Interictal memory and language impairment in temporal lobe epilepsy. *Neurology* **30**: 120–25.

McKeever, M., Holmes, G. L., Russman, B. S. (1983). Speech abnormalities in seizures: a comparison of absence and partial complex seizures. *Brain Lang.* **19**: 25–32.

Novelly, R. A. (1982). Minimal developmental dysphasia: constraints on specificity of expressive language with early onset left hemisphere epilepsy. *Epilespia* **23**: 438–9.

O'Donohoe, N. V. (1979), Learning disorders in children with epilepsy. The acquired aphasia syndrome. In *Epilepsies of Childhood*, pp. 186–9. London & Boston: Butterworth.

Ojemann, G. A. (1980). Brain mechanisms for language: observations during neurosurgery. In *Epilepsy, A Window to Brain Mechanisms*, ed. J. S. Lockard & A. A. Ward, Jr, pp. 243–60. New York: Raven Press.

Penry, J. K., Porter, R. J. & Dreifuss, F. E. (1975). Simultaneous recording of absence seizures with video tape and electreoencephalography. *Brain* **98**: 427–40.

Porrazzo, S. & Mayersdorf, A. (1980). The measurement of interictal speech and language disturbances in complex partial seizures. In *Advances in Epileptology, the Xth Epilepsy International Symposium*, ed. J. A. Wada & J. K. Penry, p. 528. New York: Raven Press.

Quadfasel, A. F. & Pruyser, P. S. W. (1955). Cognitive deficits in patients with psychomotor epilepsy. *Epilespia* **4**: 80–90.

Racy, A., Osborn, M. A., Veern, B. A., *et al.* (1980). Epileptic aphasia, first onset of prolonged monosymptomatic status epilepticus in adults. *Arch. Neurol.* **37**: 419–22.

Roulet, E., Deonna, T. & Despland, P. A. (1989). Prolonged intermittent drooling and oromotor apraxia in childhood epilepsy with centrotemporal spikes. *Epilepsia* **30**: 564–8.

Rugland, A. L., Bjoanes, H., Henrickson, O., *et al.* (1987). The development of computerized tests as a routine procedure in clinical EEG practice for the evaluation of cognitive changes in patients with epilepsy. 17th Epilepsy International Congress. *Epilepsia* **28**: 102.

Scheffer, I. E., Jones, L., Pozzebon, M., *et al.* (1996). Autosomal dominant Rolandic epilepsy and speech dyspraxia: a new syndrome with anticipation. *Ann. Neurol.* **38**: 663–42.

Serafetinides, E. G. & Falconer, M. A. (1963). Speech disturbances in temporal lobe seizures: a study in 100 epileptic patients submitted to anterior temporal lobectomy. *Brain* **8**: 333–46.

Shimazono, Y. Hirai,T., Okuma, T., *et al.* (1953). Disturbances of consciousness in petit mal epilepsy. *Epilepsia* **2**: 498–55.

Shoumaker, R. D., Bennett, D. R., Bray, P. F., *et al.* (1974). Clinical and EEG manifestations of an unusual aphasic syndrome in children. *Neurology* **24**: 10–14.

Staden, U., Isaacs, E., Boyd, S. G., *et al.* (1998). Language dysfunction in children with Rolandic epilepsy. *Neuropediatrics* **29**: 242–8.

Syrigou-Papavasiliou, A., LeWitt, P. A., Green, V., *et al.* (1985). P300 and temporal lobe epilepsy. AES Society Proceedings. *Epilepsia* **26**: 528.

Tizard, B. & Murgerson, J. M. (1963). Psychological function during wave-spike discharges. *Br. J. Soc. Clin. Psychol.* **3**: 6–15.

Tsuzuki, M. & Kasuga, I. (1977). Paroxysmal discharges triggered by hearing spoken language. *Electroencephalogr. Clin. Neurophysiol.* **43**: 499.

Vining, E. (1996). Epilepsy syndromes associated with language dysfunction. Presented at the American, Epilepsy Society Conference, San Francisco, CA, December 1996.

Wilson, A., Petty, R., Perry, A., *et al.* (1983). Paroxysmal language disturbance in an epileptic treated with clobazam. *Neurology* **33**: 652–4.

6

Language regression with epilepsy syndromes

The acquired aphasias (or agnosias) with or without epilepsy are a group of disorders in children presenting in the first decade of life with the loss of understanding, followed by the loss of expression of language with some depression of intelligence. Behavior problems emerge. In a number of such children, seizures may emerge or the EEG may become abnormal, especially at night in slow sleep. The seizures are controllable with medication, but the language deficit continues, although partial recovery is seen in adolescence. The Landau–Kleffner syndrome (LKS) is the primary model of acquired aphasia with epilepsy, but there are other similar syndromes that are possibly related if not variants of the same basic disorders. Treatment is controversial. The cause is unknown.

Landau–Kleffner syndrome

LKS of acquired aphasia with epilepsy is a childhood syndrome that occurs in previously normal children. This is a triad consisting of a loss of language functions, the usual emergence of a variety of seizures with EEG abnormalities in the temporal-parietal-occipital areas, and a resultant deterioration of behavior. The condition stabilizes for years and then, often in adolescence, begins to recover (Ballaban-Gil & Tuchman, 2000).

LKS has aslo been called the acquired childhood aphasia (or agnosia) with epilepsy syndrome and the acquired aphasia and epileptiform EEG syndrome (Roger *et al.*, 1985). It is related to, if not the same as, such entities as continuous spike-wave status in sleep, epileptic status epilepticus in sleeps, and similar syndromes. These may be variants of a common insult.

Clinical

The child, often aged four to five years and usually during the preadolescent years, begins to lose language skills, often with the development of seizures. This age is a period when active synaptic formation contributes to the establishment of language centers. The active regression is followed by years of stabilization and then, often in adolescence, a partial recovery (Foerster, 1977; Bishop, 1985). Occasionally, the onset may be followed by a prompt recovery but later recurrences in a fluctuating course (O'Donohoe, 1979; Mantovani & Landau, 1980; Holmes *et al.*, 1981).

Acute regressive stage

The syndrome begins in childhood with the emergence of the typical triad of language regression, seizure emergence, and behavior reactions.

Language regression

After the period of normal development, the child experiences the progressive loss of receptive and then expressive language over weeks to months without comparable intellectual deterioration (Roger *et al.*, 1985).

The disorder usually begins as an auditory verbal agnosia (Gascon *et al.*, 1973; Watters, 1974). The child ceases to comprehend and respond to speech and speech sounds, with difficulties differentiating between familiar words, non-speech sounds, and even environmental sounds (Roger *et al.*, 1985; Pearl *et al.*, 2001), resembling deafness or autism (Landau & Kleffner, 1957; Worster-Drought, 1971; Shoumaker *et al.*, 1974; O'Donohoe, 1979; Ballaban-Gil & Tuchman, 2000). A hearing deficit would not be sufficient to explain the language-comprehension loss, since deafness on a cortical basis from a unilateral lesion would be unexpected because the primary auditory areas are bilateral (Gascon *et al.*, 1973; Watters, 1974). This "hearing loss," initially severe, often subsists but may improve, resembling a central brain deafness, i.e. a "cortical deafness" (Landau & Kleffner, 1957; Stein & Curry, 1968; Worster-Drought, 1971; Gascon *et al.*, 1973; Watters, 1974; Duel & Lenn, 1977; Lou *et al.*, 1977a; Lou *et al.*, 1977b; Rapin *et al.*, 1977; Cooper & Ferry, 1978; Mantovani & Landau, 1980). Frustration leads to the emergence of behavior problems.

A receptive aphasia with a gradual loss in comprehension of spoken language usually follows the agnosia, although the two may merge to the degree that the agnosia is not recognized or is overlooked (O'Donohoe, 1979). Often, the child has problems in understanding even when visual cues and lip-reading are possible. Some can understand only simple statements, whereas others cannot understand anything (Landau & Kleffner, 1957; Gascon *et al.*, 1973; Worster-Drought, 1971; Watters, 1974; Duel & Lenn, 1977; Lou *et al.*, 1977a; Lou *et al.*, 1977b). Impairment in sequencing verbal materials is prominent (Kim *et al.*, 1980).

A rapid reduction of oral expression then appears (Roger *et al.*, 1985), with a severe loss in 90% (Landau & Kleffner, 1957; Worster-Drought, 1971; Gascon *et al.*, 1973; Watters, 1974; Duel & Lenn, 1977; Lou *et al.*, 1977a; Lou *et al.*, 1977b; Ballaban-Gil & Tuchman, 2000). Initially, the child makes little effort to speak spontaneously. What is said tends to be stereotyped and repetitive, with perseverations and paraphasias, but far less than with an adult. The child tends to talk around the subject rather than explain an idea. Disarticulations become increasingly apparent. Output may be abbreviated. Eventually, a telegraphic speech or a fluent jargon may be heard. What spoken efforts remain may be high-pitched and distorted. The child, especially the younger patient, frequently becomes totally unresponsive (Rapin *et al.*, 1977; O'Donohoe, 1979; Wioland *et al.*, 2001). There may be a loss of the ability to voluntarily express facial movements. Even the ability to use sign language can be lost. Some children may express themselves with grunts, crude sign systems, or gestures (Rapin *et al.*, 1977). This expressive aphasia persists.

The language disorder can be progressive or incremental, characterized by remissions and exacerbations. In a younger child without advanced language development, the effect is more devastating as the normal auditory route leading to the acquisition of language is blocked (Bishop, 1985). In the older child, after the age of seven to nine years, the effect is less severe as language has already been learned partially (Pearl *et al.*, 2001). Logorrhea, verbal stereotypies, perseverations, and paraphasias are uncommon in children, as compared with adults. The child's nervous circuits subservient to language are still developing and thus less established than in adults (Lou *et al.*, 1977a; Lou *et al.*, 1977b).

The abnormalities of speech are characterized by severe articulatory disorders (58%), syntactical transformations (17%), jargon paraphasias (22%), and combined receptive and expressive aphasia (89%), although a pure expressive aphasia has been noted in 11% (Watters, 1974). The speech problems do not correlate with the EEG abnormal bursts.

Seizures

Concomitant with or a within a few months to years after the language problem emerges, often at five to ten years of age (Pearl *et al.*, 2001), the child may experience a few of many types of seizures, which usually are controlled easily (Worster-Drought, 1971; Foerster, 1977; O'Donohoe, 1979; Mantovani & Landau, 1980; Holmes *et al.*, 1981).

The seizures begin as a single seizure or as status, especially at the onset (33%) (Hirsch *et al.*, 1990). One or several types (Roger *et al.*, 1985) of seizures emerge (70–80%), often with atypical absence (16%) or complex partial seizures (16%) with psychomotor automatisms (Dugas *et al.*, 1982; Sawhney *et al.*, 1988; Deonna, 1991; Gascon *et al.*, 2000), although eventually generalized tonic–clonic attacks (33%) are noted. Nocturnal simple partial motor seizures (33%) resembling benign central-temporal epilepsy, sometimes with a transient postictal facial weakness, may be seen (Dugas *et al.*, 1982; Deonna, 1991). Minor motor attacks with akinetic (5%), and occasionally facial or arm myoclonic seizures or myoclonic-astatic attacks may occur (Gomez & Klass, 1983; Roger *et al.*, 1985). Tonic attacks are not seen

(Dugas *et al.*, 1982; Deonna, 1991). Some patients may have very infrequent seizures (30%), or no seizures (22%), although the typical EEG abnormality is present (Landau & Kleffner, 1957; Shoumaker *et al.*, 1974; Watters, 1974; Foerster, 1977; Lou *et al.*, 1977a; Lou *et al.*, 1977b; O'Donohoe, 1979; Mantovani & Landau, 1980; Holmes *et al.*, 1981; Gomez & Klass, 1983). Attacks occur more often during sleep (Roger *et al.*, 1985).

The seizures are usually infrequent, isolated attacks. Infrequent repetitive seizures do not correlate with the neurologic deficits, the language dysfunction, or the prognosis (Landau & Kleffner, 1957; Gomez & Klass, 1983), although the fluctuations in language skills may suggest the underlying epileptiform disorder (Ballaban-Gil & Tuchman, 2000). The impairment may be progressive, especially when the EEG seizure activity occupies over 80% of the slow-wave sleep stages for more than years (Wasterlain *et al.*, 1993).

Treatment with antiepileptic monotherapy is generally effective for seizure control but not for the aphasia, as only an occasional patient (6%) improves in this respect with antiepileptic therapy (Mantovani & Landau, 1980; Holmes *et al.*, 1981; Sawhney *et al.*, 1988; Deonna, 1991; Gascon *et al.*, 2000). After ten years, only 20% of patients continue with sporadic seizures, and by age 15 seizures rarely persist, even in the absence of any antiepileptic medication treatment (Roger *et al.*, 1985; Pearl *et al.*, 2001).

Behavior

Behavioral disturbances are common (50–70%) (Roger *et al.*, 1985; Sawhney *et al.*, 1988; Gascon *et al.*, 2000), especially at the onset of the disorder. The behavior deterioration usually parallels the language deterioration and does not relate to intelligence (Barrett, 1910). The behavior may relate to an acute anxiety of the child with impaired capability of understanding what is going on. The initial emotional tensions gradually fade (Roger *et al.*, 1985).

Behavior problems include hyperactivity and attention deficits, aggressiveness, anger with tantrums, withdrawal, social deficits, frustration outbursts, and, if severe, autistic and psychotic-like presentations (Roger *et al.*, 1985), all known to be reactions to a loss of communication skills (Landau & Kleffner, 1957; Foerster, 1977). Global attention disorders and hyperactivity, seen in at least half of these patients, suggest that the reticular activating-inhibitory systems may also be involved in the disorder, either as a manifestation of a primary disinhibition at the temporal lobe–limbic level or even perhaps at the diencephalic or upper brainstem levels, or as a secondary behavioral reaction (Worster-Drought, 1971; Gascon *et al.*, 1973; Duel & Lenn, 1977; O'Donohoe, 1979; Mantovani & Landau, 1980; Holmes *et al.*, 1981).

Stabilization period

The disorder progresses from weeks to months or longer, then stabilizes without further progression for months to years, waxing and waning as a prolonged aphasia (Landau & Kleffner, 1957; Worster-Drought, 1971; Gascon et al., 1973; Watters, 1974; Duel & Lenn, 1977; Lou et al., 1977a; Lou et al., 1977b; O'Donohoe, 1979). Occasionally, the onset, recurrence, and fluctuations may coincide with the clinical seizures (O'Donohoe, 1979; Mantovani & Landau, 1980; Holmes et al., 1981).

Recovery period

The condition then improves gradually. The seizures cease and the EEG often normalizes, usually before age ten (80% of patients), and always before 15 years of age (Roger et al., 1985). Then, over several years, the aphasia improves, with gradual partial recovery of language functions usually over weeks to years. The outlook is anywhere from near-recovery to a persistent severe language handicap. About 33–42% are left with a severe residual deficit, 24–25% remain with a mild to moderate residual deficit, and 35–40% make a relatively good recovery (Cooper & Ferry, 1978). Very few patients recover to the point of completely normal speech (Gascon et al., 1973; Watters, 1974; Cooper & Ferry, 1978; Ballaban-Gil & Tuchman, 2000).

The degree of recovery of language depends on the age of onset, with the best outlook after seven years of age. The younger the onset, the poorer the outlook (Ballaban-Gil & Tuchman, 2000). The provision of early rehabilitative intervention is also a strong prognostic factor. If aphasia onset is after the child has acquired handwriting skills, re-education is facilitated (Roger et al., 1985).

Examination

The examination is usually normal except for the major language impairment and marked behavior problems (Gascon et al., 1973; Sawhney et al., 1988; Roger et al., 1985). There may be evidence of other minor neurologic abnormalities on examination (Mantovani & Landau, 1980; O'Donohoe, 1979; Worster-Drought, 1971).

Epidemiology

The family history is often negative for epilepsy or significant speech delays. In children who develop seizures, the family history for epilepsy is 12%; in those who do not develop seizures, the family history is 5% (Roger et al., 1985). The pregnancy, birth history, and preceding development are normal (Worster-Drought, 1971; Landau & Kleffner, 1957; Gascon et al., 1973; Watters, 1974; Duel & Lenn, 1977; Lou et al., 1977a; Lou et al., 1977b). The syndrome is two to four times more likely to occur in boys than girls, possibly related to an increased language lateralization difference in males or a sex-lined inherited predisposition (Foerster, 1977).

Diagnostics

Electroencephalography

The Landau–Kleffner syndrome appears to be partial seizures originating in the temporal cortex, most often on the left posterior, producing both the localized epileptic discharges during wakefulness and the sleep pattern resembling the continuous spike-wave status of sleep (Shoumaker *et al.*, 1974; Metz-Lutz & Massa, 1999). The seizures are associated with severe bilateral yet asymmetric paroxysmal EEG abnormalities (Hirsch *et al.*, 1990; Sat & Dreifuss, 1973). The picture varies in both degree and location during the evolution (Roger *et al.*, 1985). Three types of EEG abnormalities are noted: generalized, often slow-spike or polyspike wave bursts (56%) or sharp waves (6%), posterior temporal spikes, more prominently left-sided, or a combination of both (Stein & Curry, 1968; Geets & Pinon, 1975; Holmes *et al.*, 1981; Roger *et al.*, 1985; Sawhney *et al.*, 1988; Gomez & Klass, 1990; Ballaban-Gil & Tuchman, 2000; Gascon *et al.*, 2000). The posterior temporal spikes, which may be unilateral (6%), bilateral (11%), or multifocal (11%), spread forward to the mid-temporal and motor areas or occasionally to frontal, occipital, or parietal areas, with a tendency to become bilateral or generalized (Landau & Kleffner, 1957; Worster-Drought, 1971; Gascon *et al.*, 1973; Watters, 1974; Duel & Lenn, 1977; O'Donohoe, 1979; Holmes *et al.*, 1981). The generalized spike discharges may be an epiphenomenon rather than the cause of the aphasia (Roger *et al.*, 1985). When intravenous diazepam suppresses the generalized discharges, a left temporal spike focus may still be seen (Landau & Kleffner, 1957; Worster-Drought, 1971; Gascon *et al.*, 1973; Shoumaker *et al.*, 1974; Watters, 1974; Duel & Lenn, 1977; O'Donohoe, 1979; Holmes *et al.*, 1981; Roger *et al.*, 1985). This is also seen with methohexital suppression tests and intracarotid amobarbital injections (Metz-Lutz & Massa, 1999).

The EEG background activity between the discharges is often normal or borderline, but it may be abnormal. Activation by hyperventilation or photic stimulation is rare (Roger *et al.*, 1985).

These EEG findings vary in severity, lateralization, and location, especially with sleep (Roger *et al.*, 1985). The EEG abnormalities are severe and tend to be nearly continuous, although seizures are infrequent (Landau & Kleffner, 1957; Worster-Drought, 1971; Gascon *et al.*, 1973; Watters, 1974; Duel & Lenn, 1977; Lou *et al.*, 1977a; Lou *et al.*, 1977b). The abnormal EEG is usually (90%) found in the first ten years of life, especially around age three to five years (Roger *et al.*, 1985).

Sleep spike-waves of sleep

There is significant activation of generally continuous or near-continuous bilateral slow spike-waves localized to the central-parietal region (Deonna, 1991) during nearly 85% of non-rapid eye movement (REM) deeper stages of sleep, which may resemble sleep status, as in continuous spike-wave status in sleep (CSWS) and epilepsy with status epilepticus in sleep (ESES), but not to the extent seen in the latter syndrome (Roger *et al.*, 1985; Hirsch *et al.*, 1990). There may or may not be clinical seizures. The abnormalities may be restricted to sleep with a relatively normal wake record (Sawhney *et al.*, 1988; Gascon *et al.*, 2000). There may be a shift in laterality, at times predominating over the temporal lobe with posterior spread, suggesting possible activation of subcortical mechanisms, primarily or secondarily (Foerster, 1977; Gascon *et al.*, 1973). The bilateral discharges may appear asynchronous with a unilateral predominance, especially to the left, suggesting the possibility of a focus with bilateral synchrony despite a unilateral preponderance (Rapin *et al.*, 1977). Multiple spike and slow waves are seen in a few cases (Gascon *et al.*, 2000; Sawhney *et al.*, 1988).

Video-electroencephalography monitoring

With recording of a seizure, there is a left temporal mono-rhythmic theta build-up, with rapid discharging of spike-wave discharges, maximum from the left as the patient begins to stare with oral automatisms. The EEG may seem generalized from the onset at times (Roger *et al.*, 1985; Ming *et al.*, 1996).

Relationships

The EEG abnormalities may be epiphenomena of underlying pathology of the cortex related to speech rather than the cause of the aphasia (Holmes *et al.*, 1981). There is a debated tendency towards correlation of the language deficit and the EEG abnormalities, particularly the continuous spike-wave discharging of sleep, in onset, severity, and recovery (Landau & Kleffner, 1957; Gascon *et al.*, 1973; Watters, 1974; Foerster, 1977; van Dongen & Loonen, 1977; Mantovani & Landau, 1980; Sawhney *et al.*, 1988; Deonna, 1991; Ming *et al.*, 1996; Gascon *et al.*, 2000).

The focus is apparent on the initial EEG at around three to nine years of age (90%) and is often most prominent at three to five years of age (Roger *et al.*, 1985). Occasionally, the EEG abnormality may resolve by the time of onset of the verbal agnosia (Rapin *et al.*, 1977). The EEG may normalize by age 15 years (Roger *et al.*, 1985), although a left-temporal occipital spike focus has been reported to remain years later (Shoumaker *et al.*, 1974; Lou *et al.*, 1977a; Lou *et al.*, 1977b). Partial resolution of the aphasia does not occur until after the epileptic discharges disappear (Foerster, 1977; O'Donohoe, 1979; Sawhney *et al.*, 1988; Gascon *et al.*, 2000). In some patients, the deficits may persist (Watters, 1974; Mantovani & Landau, 1980; Deonna, 1991).

Magnetoencephalography

Magnetoencephalography has shown a temporal lobe focus, especially in the dorsal third of the supratemporal gyrus with a reduced-frequency modulated steady-state response (Swarton, 1995).

Brain mapping

Field-potential mapping and power-spectrum analysis of digitalized EEGs localize the focal and generalized epileptiform abnormalities to the posterior perisylvian region, suggesting an epileptic focus on the dorsal surface of the superior temporal gyrus in the depth of the Sylvan fissure (Hoeppner et al., 1992; Hoeppner et al., 1993). Spectral and topographic mapping reveal variability in the mode of propagation of paroxysmal discharges (Nakano et al., 1989; Hirsch et al., 1990). The perisylvian spikes often project to homologous regions on the other hemisphere and may project to the frontal regions. Spike and wave discharges in sleep originate from the same perisylvian site but spread more rapidly (Hoeppner et al., 1992; Hoeppner et al., 1993).

Other diagnostics

Radiologic brain imaging

Pneumoencephalograms, angiograms, CT scans, and MRI scans obtained to exclude treatable lesions are usually normal (Nakano et al., 1989; Hirsch et al., 1990; Deonna, 1991; Feekery et al., 1993; Morrell, 1995; Otero et al., 1989; Hirsch et al., 1990; Solomon et al., 1991; Solomon et al., 1993; Bhatia et al., 1994; Nass et al., 1993; Nass et al., 1999). Occasionally, the abnormalities found are felt to be secondary to the chronic epileptic process (Pearl et al., 2001), such as CT/MRI white-matter changes (Otero et al., 1989; Solomon et al., 1991; Solomon et al., 1993; Bhatia et al., 1994; Nass et al., 1993; Nass et al., 1999) or asymmetry of the temporal horns (Cole et al., 1988; da Silva et al., 1997).

Functional imaging studies

Single photon emission computed tomography (SPECT) and PET studies have shown focal abnormalities, predominantly in temporal or infratemporal locations, in brain perfusion and glucose metabolism (O'Tuama et al., 1992; Rintahaka et al., 1995; Guerreiro et al., 1996), with asymmetrically increased blood flow ictally and decreased blood flow interictally. PET scans with a variety of chemicals have shown focal cerebral hypometabolism at the epileptic focus in one or both temporal lobes (Swarton, 1995), especially in the middle temporal gyri and occasionally in extratemporal areas, with activation of the temporal focus in sleep (da Silva et al., 1997).

Audiometric evaluation and evoked potentials

Conventional audiometry, used to separate the syndrome from a peripheral acquired deafness, is difficult to perform and gives inconsistent responses. Routine hearing tests, including pure tone audiograms, are normal (Landau & Kleffner, 1957; Watters, 1974). Dichotic listening shows permanent, one-ear extinction contralateral to the affected temporal cortex (Wioland *et al.*, 2001; Pearl *et al.*, 2001). Auditory evoked potentials may verify the central deafness by showing normal early components of auditory evoked potentials to test stimuli, which would be against lesions below Heschl's gyrus (Gascon *et al.*, 1973; Watters, 1974; O'Donohoe, 1979). Delays and abnormalities of long-latency cortical evoked responses suggest localization to the posterior temporal regions (O'Donohoe, 1979; Zovan & Choyakh, 1977; Swarton, 1995). The P300 component of auditory evoked potentials is delayed (Squires & Hecox, 1983), as may be somatosensory and visual evoked potentials (Gascon *et al.*, 1973; Watters, 1974). Studies of the long-latency auditory evoked potentials in children who have recovered from Landau–Kleffner syndrome suggest a long-term dysfunction of the auditory associative cortex persists (Wioland *et al.*, 2001; Pearl *et al.*, 2001).

Other tests

Studies including CSF examination are usually normal (Worster-Drought, 1971; Watters, 1974; McKinney & McGraw, 1974; Lou *et al.*, 1977a; Lou *et al.*, 1977b; Cole *et al.*, 1988; Pascual-Castroveiuo *et al.*, 1992; Gascon *et al.*, 2000). Mild elevations of CSF protein have been noted occasionally (Lou *et al.*, 1977a; Lou *et al.*, 1977b; Pascual-Castroveiuo *et al.*, 1992; Perniola *et al.*, 1993).

Functional diagnostics
Psychological evaluation

Although the patients are often thought to be retarded or psychotic (Gascon *et al.*, 1973), if tested by non-language tests intelligence is found to be basically not impaired.

Intelligence testing

Intelligence in the acute stages when the syndrome is initially identified is generally relatively preserved and may be above average (Gascon *et al.*, 1973; Worster-Drought, 1971). Verbal channels may be depressed. These children tend to do well on non-verbal testing (Gascon *et al.*, 1973; Landau & Kleffner, 1957; O'Donohoe, 1979; Worster-Drought, 1971). The Hiskey-Nebraska Test of Learning Aptitude, the performance subtests of the Wechsler Preschool and Primary Scale of Intelligence (WIPPSI) or Weschler Intelligence Scale for Children – revised WISC-R, and the Leiter International Performance Scale are recommended (Cooper & Ferry, 1978).

Psycholinguistic testing

Psycholinguistic testing shows that there may be a severe short-term auditory sequential memory span deficit as well as visual perceptual problems (Stein & Curry, 1968).

Academic testing

Academic testing frequently demonstrates reading and writing problems, including problems in writing to dictation. Spelling errors may be a problem for some children. Many children can copy written matter and can arrange pictures normally, but drawings may be primitive. They may be rapid in the association of printed and written materials with normal story-sequencing skills (Worster-Drought, 1971).

Speech and language evaluation

Attempts to elicit verbal communication and to improve receptive skills are unsuccessful in 42% of patients (Cooper & Ferry, 1978). An early speech–language evaluation for both diagnostic and rehabilitative purposes is important.

Differential diagnosis

Developmental language disorders with abnormal EEGs include Landau-Kleffner syndrome, developmental dysphasia, and ESES, as well as ictal aphasia (Ballaban-Gil & Tuchman, 2000). Landau–Kleffner syndrome shows a much more variable aphasic to mute state, whereas in ESES only 50% of patients have problems. The sleep nocturnal spike-wave discharge is present for more than 85% of the time in the non-REM sleep stage with ESES, but usually less with Landau–Kleffner syndrome, suggesting a relationship between Landau–Kleffner syndrome and ESES syndrome (Hirsch *et al.*, 1990).

Pathogenesis

The etiology remains unknown. The nature of the disorder has been a matter of speculation (Foerster, 1977; Lou *et al.*, 1977a; Lou *et al.*, 1977b; O'Donohoe, 1979). Possible causes include a tumor or vascular problem, a genetic or developmental disorder, low-grade encephalitis, an infectious or immune problem, and epileptic disruptions, with the latter being the most popular theory (Sawhney *et al.*, 1988; Gascon *et al.*, 2000). Landau–Kleffner syndrome may be a final common pathway with multiple potential etiologies, acquired or genetic, most likely insulting the temporal-parietal areas of the developmental brain (Pearl *et al.*, 2001).

Epileptic disruption

Persistent epileptic discharges in the primary cortical centers of language may functionally ablate these centers, precluding them from participation in normal language processing, essentially a disconnecting and resultant isolation of one part of the brain from another (Landau & Kleffner, 1957; Foerster, 1977; Lou *et al.*, 1977a; Lou *et al.*, 1977b; Rapin *et al.*, 1977; O'Donohoe, 1979; Beaumanoir, 1985). The EEG discharges may be a manifestation of lower-level subcortical differentiating processes, possibly involving auditory pathways and disturbing auditory input into Wernicke's area (Gascon *et al.*, 1973). Seizures during a critical period of circuit development may cause the emergence and fixation of permanent aberrant connections (Holmes *et al.*, 1998; Holmes *et al.*, 1999).

Developmental problem

An immaturity or developmental disturbance of the nerve input bringing signals to key brain centers or possibly a sectional disorganization consequent to deafferentation may exist (Roger *et al.*, 1985), perhaps with a genetic predisposition in light of the male preponderance and an increased incidence of developmental language problems in other family members (Landau & Kleffner, 1957; Nakano *et al.*, 1989; Feekery *et al.*, 1993). There may be impairment of the pruning of synaptic contacts and collaterals in an otherwise normal cortex, resulting in deterioration of higher cerebral functions subserved as well as hampering new acquisitions. The same imbalance would predispose to synchronous firing of local neuron populations, leading to the development of discharges, especially with the reinforced synchronization of neuronal firing of non-REM sleep (Maquet *et al.*, 1999).

Infectious/autoimmune disorder

An infectious etiology (Mantovani & Landau, 1980; Maichalowicz *et al.*, 1989; Otero *et al.*, 1989; Ansink *et al.*, 1989; Perniola *et al.*, 1993; Bhatia *et al.*, 1994; Bicknese *et al.*, 1996; Fayad *et al.*, 1997), possibly a chronic encephalitis, or secondarily triggered autoimmune reaction (Worster-Drought, 1971) has been suggested based on occasional findings, but these have not been substantiated in further studies including CSF tests and biopsies (Worster-Drought, 1971; Gascon *et al.*, 1973; Watters, 1974; Lou *et al.*, 1977a; Lou *et al.*, 1977b; O'Donohoe, 1979; Duel & Lenn, 1977; Mantovani & Landau, 1980; Pearce & Darwish, 1984).

Brain lesion

Rare findings include a temporal astrocytoma (Soloman *et al.*, 1991; Solomon *et al.*, 1993), temporal ganglioma (Nass *et al.*, 1993; Nass *et al.*, 1999), small-vascular abnormalities of the temporal or adjacent parietal lobe (Mantovani & Landau, 1980), and bilateral Sylvian region infarctions (Gascon *et al.*, 1973). Younger children with such findings may present with initial left-sided focal epileptiform discharges becoming generalized as continued spikes and waves aggravated by sleep. An MRI scan rapidly differentiates these patients from those with Landau–Kleffner syndrome, allowing a surgical approach (Soloman *et al.*, 1991; Solomon *et al.*, 1993).

Miscellaneous reports

Rare considerations include gliosis and abnormal zinc metabolism, suggesting a zinc deficiency (Lerman-Sagie *et al.*, 1987).

Pathology

In the Children's Hour at the 1995 American Epilepsy Society Conference, Donald Shields (1995) reviewed possible causes. Micropathological reports suggest abnormal synaptic arrangements. The disorder appears during synaptogenesis or the circuit-building process of language development, creating abnormal synaptic arrangements.

Diagnostic considerations

In early stages, Landau–Kleffner syndrome may be mistaken for ADDH (Beaumanoir, 1985), autism, personality disorders, aggressiveness, and depression (White & Sreenivasan, 1987), as well as deafness, elective mutism, and acute psychiatric disorders (Pearl et al., 2001). A degenerative disorder, tumor, or static lesions with focal seizures with related aphasias (Deonna, 1991) are often considered. Other epilepsy syndromes to be considered include slow spike-wave status of sleep (Roger et al., 1985).

Treatment

Children with Landau–Kleffner syndrome and continuous spike-wave status in sleep syndrome are often treated aggressively initially with antiepileptic medications. A trial of steroids or other medical approaches or gamma globulin may be considered. If this fails, then surgery is considered.

Anticonvulsants

If seizures are present, they should be treated (Cooper & Ferry, 1978; O'Donohoe, 1979). The goal of treatment is to control the seizures and seizure discharges, although usually this does not lead to improvement in language, even if there is EEG normalization (Foerster, 1977; Rapin et al., 1977; Mantovani & Landau, 1980; Holmes et al., 1981; Pearce & Darwish, 1984; Hirsch et al., 1990; Pearl et al., 2001). In some patients, the language worsens with seizure control (Billard et al., 1982; Roger et al., 1985). The seizures may cease without medication. The aphasia may or may not return when the medications are slowly tapered (Gastaut, 1979). The older antiepileptics are often ineffective and may aggravate the situation. Phenytoin and carbamazepine may increase the duration of the spike-wave activity in sleep. Valproate, ethosuximide, clonazepam, and clobazam may be partially helpful for the seizures, at least for a brief time, but will not help the aphasia, even if given intravenously (Gordon, 1964; Marescaux et al., 1990; Genton et al., 1992). Vigabatrin (Appleton et al., 1993) and felbamate may be effective (Glauser et al., 1995).

Immunologic therapy

Based on the theory that Landau–Kleffner syndrome is an autoimmune disorder, a trial of two to three months on corticosteroids, monitored closely for objective improvements, has been reported to help both clinical and EEG abnormalities (McKinney & McGraw, 1974; Watters, 1974), especially if used early on (Lerman-Sagie *et al.*, 1987). If prednisone is not beneficial, adrenocorticotropic hormone (ACTH) is not apt to work either. There may be re-emergence of an epileptiform EEG and aphasic relapse with the tapering of the steroids (Marescaux *et al.*, 1990; Morrell *et al.*, 1995). Chronic therapy or intermittent therapy may be warranted if a significant improvement of neuropsychological function is obtained (Deonna, 1991; Marescaux *et al.*, 1990).

Intravenous immunoe globulins have also been reported to be of transient benefit, both clinically and by EEG with each infusion, with deterioration of both about two months post-infusion (Fayad *et al.*, 1997; Lagae *et al.*, 1998; Mikati & Saab, 2000).

Neurosurgical approaches

Surgery may be beneficial. Surgical approaches include temporal lobectomy in both lesional (Solomon *et al.*, 1991; Solomon *et al.*, 1993; Nass *et al.*, 1993; Nass *et al.*, 1999) and non-lesional (Cole *et al.*, 1988) conditions, resulting in improvements in language and seizure control.

Subpial transection

Subpial transection surgery ablates the prime spike and the contralateral mirror focus. It is considered in light of the effect of the epileptiform lesion on the adjacent cortex. The result of the surgery on one side stops seizures and recovers speech. Many patients have had preceding trials on antiepileptic medications and on steroids, often with transient benefits for about two years (Morrell *et al.*, 1995).

The subpial operative approach is most desirable for patients who have acquired speech and have a relatively normal IQ but who have lost speech abilities due to epileptiform activity in the speech area, although other cognitive abilities remain intact. The EEG may show diffuse features, bilateral and posterior with a horizontal dipole, posterior in the superior temporal lobe. Further studies show a unilateral origin driving bilateral spiking.

Multiple subpial transections (Morrell *et al.*, 1995; Mikati & Saab, 2000) result in recovery (28–50%), improvement (28–44%), or no change (12–22%). The improvements may be temporary (Nass *et al.*, 1993; Nass *et al.*, 1999). Some deficits in attention and expressive language remain (Hoeppner *et al.*, 1992; Hoeppner *et al.*, 1993). In follow-up to multiple transpial transections for Landau–Kleffner syndrome, the behavior ratings by parents were normal, and the children were back in regular school classes (Morrell *et al.*, 1995).

Remediative support

Children with Landau–Kleffner syndrome do best in special schools dealing with aphasic patients (Landau & Kleffner, 1957; O'Donohoe, 1979; Shoumaker *et al.*, 1974; Worster-Drought, 1971). A school or class for deaf children is not appropriate.

Learning

The child is inhibited in learning by auditory methods so alternatives utilizing a multisensory remediative approach become most important. The children can be taught to read and to write (Deonna *et al.*, 1989; Tharpe *et al.*, 1991). If the aphasia onset occurs after the child has acquired handwriting, re-education is more successful (Roger *et al.*, 1985).

Impaired comprehension secondary to background noise in adolescents and adults who have recovered from Landau–Kleffner syndrome suggests that improvements in the acoustic environment may enhance speech recognition (Mantovani & Landau, 1980). Increasing speech volume over ambient noise may assist listening. The child needs to be trained to tolerate background noises, but initially a quieter setting may reduce the acting out of frustrations.

Language

Speech and language therapy is indispensable with periodic language and neuropsychological re-evaluations. Some children have problems even in controlling their voice. The child may begin to react to environmental noises, although the need for training in the association of the noise with the meaning may include use of manual communication, written efforts, and communication boards. Often, the children need to resort to alternate methods of communication, such as sign language. The child who regains verbal language will drop the use of signs (Deonna *et al.*, 1989; Tharpe *et al.*, 1991).

Using a multisensory approach, including signing (hand language, gestures, finger letters) lip-reading, writing language, and communication boards (Cooper & Ferry, 1978), may help the child with a severe communication problem. A child successful in these areas may begin to be willing to learn and to engage in personal relations. The formation of syntax, concepts, and person relations parallels the initiation of learning sign language and writing language willingly (Hashima *et al.*, 1987). Some individuals may remain dependent on sign language into adulthood. Functional MRI may reveal strong activation of the auditory cortex on the right more than the left to heard speech, little response to silent lip-reading, and strong activation of right temporal-parietal-occipital association cortex after viewing sign language (Sieratzki *et al.*, 2002).

Behavior

Adverse behavioral manifestations may partially reflect frustration caused by the aphasia. The inhibition of language learning with anosognosia and a behavioral regression to infantilism and dependency is noted (Hashima *et al.*, 1987). Introduction of an effective communication system may help to alleviate such negative behaviors (Deonna *et al.*, 1989; Tharpe *et al.*, 1991). In light of the frustration behaviors that often emerge, behavior approaches and parental counseling and guidance become important factors.

Prognosis

The prognosis of children with the syndrome of acquired aphasia with epilepsy is poor. Years later most continue to show severe language deficits, which appear to be persistent (Watters, 1974). The variability of outcome of similarly affected children remains a puzzle. There is nothing about the age of onset, the focus of the EEG abnormality, or the clinical features to give any prognosis (Mantovani & Landau, 1980).

There are two types of epilepsy aphasia syndrome, transient and chronic, although they vary widely in severity and duration. Some children experience a brief, self-limited episode with good recovery. Those with a chronic form may have an earlier onset and continue after the EEG recovery with a lack of speech, with language impairments inhibiting academics. Behavior remains infantile and dependent (Hashima *et al.*, 1987). After a fluctuating course, the process improves as the seizures cease, the EEG normalizes, and antiepileptics if used, are no longer needed. The aphasia may be less severe but remains until it too tends to improve, although in some children the loss is permanent (Landau & Kleffner, 1957; Worster-Drought, 1971; Gascon *et al.*, 1973; Watters, 1974; Lou *et al.*, 1977a; Lou *et al.*, 1977b; O'Donohoe, 1979).

The prognosis may be influenced by several variables, including age of onset, pattern of language deficit, frequency and topography of EEG discharges, duration of epilepsy, and efficacy as well as side effects of antiepileptic drugs (Deonna *et al.*, 1989). Moderate residual language deficits remain in many patients (Mouridsen, 1995), especially if EEG abnormalities persist. Over a near-decade of follow-up, few patients (18.2%) achieved complete language recovery (Mantovani & Landau, 1980). Depressed intellectual ability was found in many (63.6%). Adverse factors include onset before four years of age, duration of aphasia greater than one year, and the duration and continuity of sleep spike-wave epileptic status. Whether or not the patient has clinical seizures does not appear to be a decisive factor regarding the therapeutic response or in determining the ultimate outcome. A bilateral EEG disturbance limits the prognosis of language function (van Dongen & Loonen, 1977; Mantovani & Landau, 1980). The verbal IQ channel depression persists, especially in vocabulary and short-term auditory memory skills (Metz-Lutz & Massa, 1999). The severity of the auditory comprehension deficit is an important prognostic indicator.

Complications

Cognitive, language, and behavioral recovery may be incomplete (Roger *et al.*, 1985). At age four to seven years the child has not acquired sufficient reading and writing skills, whereas the older child may lose these skills. Comprehension of written language precedes the comprehension of oral language (Gascon *et al.*, 1973). Partial retention of writing skills suggests a better prognosis in the re-educative phase (Beaumanoir, 1985). Children with a younger age of onset may appear normal until their entry into school demonstrates language deficits. Most children are left with some language-processing problems, although the problems may be limited to academic areas such as reading and spelling. Many of the children will require special education throughout their schooling.

Neurologic recovery

All the children in follow-up essentially have a normal neurologic examination, except for impairments of language and learning functions (Mantovani & Landau, 1980).

Language recovery

Neuropsychologic assessments usually show a wide spectrum of residual defects, mainly of language functions, but often affecting other learning skills (Lou *et al.*, 1977a; Lou *et al.*, 1977b). Some of those with the best language output display decreased visual perceptual abilities, whereas those with the more impaired language residua have relatively good visual perceptual abilities (Mantovani & Landau, 1980). The outcomes can generally be summarized into three groups: those with the recovery of relatively normal speech (36–44%), those with moderate improvements (24–28%), and those with minimal to no improvements (26–40%) (Holmes *et al.*, 1981). The prolonged duration for recovery suggests that compensatory mechanisms in the young child are also disabled in both hemispheres and the brain must utilize remaining intact cortical or lower-level pathway (Gascon *et al.*, 1973).

In the early stages, most of the children are unable to sing or to control their phonation. The voice may be quite tremulous. In several cases, the children merely exhibit uncontrolled vocal noises until, with therapy, they begin to imitate speech movements and some word sounds. They react immediately to bells, whistles, gongs, and sibilants, but they are slower to appreciate musical sequences. They do not associate appropriate animal sounds until after training. In less severe cases, auditory memory for words and their written values, once acquired, is retained. Articulation in both initiation and in spontaneous speech is more difficult to recover. Children usually first learn to associate the written word with the object shown, then to select and to associate the auditory and the visual pattern with the written word and object (Worster-Drought, 1971).

Learning disabilities

Subsequent learning deficiencies are also seen that may lead to poor school performance. A residual decline in intellectual abilities may be seen. Some children with continued severe language impairment may retain a relatively intact non-verbal performance (visuomotor) channel of learning. Others may recover their language skills but be left with a severe non-language perceptual motor learning channel impairment. A variety of learning disabilities have been reported, including auditory memory problems, slowed visuomotor reaction time, auditory perceptual problems, and impaired motor processing problems.

Related acquired epilepsy and aphasia syndromes

There are other epilepsy syndromes that are associated with prominent language deficits. Some of these may be related to, similar to, or a variant of Landau–Kleffner syndrome, such as epileptiform status epilepticus in sleep, developmental language disorders, and autistic regression. Other syndromes are entirely different in origin and in manifestations, except for the presence of language impairments (Ballaban-Gil & Tuchman, 2000). The EEGs are similar although often non-specific, including some with sleep activation when seizures are present (Swarton, 1995).

Developmental dysphasia with epilepsy

The lack of developmental language ability has been referred to as a congenital or developmental aphasia. Some developmental aphasias may be associated with epilepsy, although the prominent feature is the lack of the development of language abilities. In young children, interference with language development requires both temporal lobes to be involved.

Clinical

Children with delays of speech and language development from birth usually achieve other developmental milestones (motor development) normally, including non-verbal skills. Often, a mixed developmental language deficit is found, with receptive language more impaired, although in some children a pure expressive deficit that improves with age has been identified. These children may have problems in adapting to a group, with later difficulties in social interactions. Although few have seizures, such children frequently are diagnosed as retarded, deaf, autistic (Maccario *et al.*, 1982), or as having a central deafness or pseudobulbar palsy (Sat & Dreifuss, 1973).

Some children have a language delay from the beginning of language efforts, but others may have relatively normal language until after the onset of seizures. Both may have similarly marked EEG abnormalities involving both sides of the brain, but not all patients have seizures. Yet another group of children may have significant developmental language problems from birth, with a marked worsening noted at the time of seizure appearance (Maccario *et al.*, 1982; Swarton, 1995).

Developmental aphasia (dysphasia) shows an 8% cumulative incidence of epilepsy in aphasic children that is increased with a history of language regression. There is a 58% cumulative incidence of epilepsy in children with verbal acquired agnosias and aphasias (Ballaban-Gil, 1995; Tuchmnan & Rapin, 1997; Ballaban-Gil & Tuchman, 2000).

Some children with a congenital epileptiform dysphasia may exhibit recurrent utterances in a monophasic manner. Some can utter emotional expletives and little more. Such children are not annoyed by their inability to talk and show little if any frustration behaviors (Sat & Dreifuss, 1973).

Diagnosis

Delayed development of speech is more frequent than is recognized. Complete speechlessness itself is very rare in mentally retarded patients, and is essentially unheard of in retarded individuals who are capable of self-care (Sat & Dreifuss, 1973).

Cause

A cause for developmental dysphasia with epilepsy is not often found. Considerations include perinatal factors, a genetic defect, or a specific enzyme deficit (Maccario *et al.*, 1982).

Examination

In pure congenital aphasias, abnormal bilateral neurologic findings on examination are often found. There is no consistency of findings. Bilateral involvement is usually found in a young child who fails to acquire hemispheric dominance in either hemisphere of normal language-learning abilities (Sat & Dreifuss, 1973).

Diagnostics

The diagnostics are to exclude treatable causes.

Electroencephalography

Children with both developmental and acquired aphasias may display bilateral EEG abnormalities, often bitemporal sharps and spikes and waves, shifting from side to side (Maccario *et al.*, 1982; Ballaban-Gil & Tuchman, 2000). If known epileptic patients are excluded, slightly more than one third of patients with an expressive developmental dysphasia have epileptiform EEGS. Only a few such children had actual seizures. Further studies suggest that an abnormality may be found on one side but the EEG may show secondary bilateral synchrony with a unilateral focus. With developmental dysphasia, epileptiform EEGs may be found on all-night recordings (Sat & Dreifuss, 1973; Ballaban-Gil & Tuchman, 2000).

Radiologic diagnostics

CT and isotopic scans are usually relatively normal, although occasionally a focal lesion is found (Maccario *et al.*, 1982).

Pathology

The pathology, if any, appears to be that of bilateral temporal lobe disturbances, with degenerative lesions, sometimes with spread to the medial geniculate bodies (Sat & Dreifuss, 1973).

Therapy

Anticonvulsants have been tried in children with such developmental language deficits and abnormal EEGs, but no improvements have been reported in language skills. Rare subjective improvements have been suggested, although most experts do not feel that any improvements occur.

Autism with epilepsy

Autism is a disorder of onset before 18 months of age that consists of delayed and deviant language development, deviant social interactions, and a strong desire for sameness. These children, like other handicapped children with difficulties in handling sensory input, manifest rhythmic movements when stressed. It is important to differentiate between autism and autistic. There are far more children, such as those with developmental aphasia, that manifest some but not all of the behaviors seen in autism and thus are referred to as "autistic." The diagnosis of autism should not be made unless one has excluded the possibility of a developmental aphasia. In Landau–Kleffner syndrome, the abnormalities of reciprocal social relatedness and restricted stereotypical patterns of interests and behaviors seen with autism are not present (Ballaban-Gil *et al.*, 1991).

Autism is associated with an increased frequency of seizures, especially in patients with associated motor and cognitive deficiencies. EEG abnormalities are common (Volkmar & Nelson, 1990). The risk for developing epilepsy is highest in the first year of life. The incidence is around 13% at five years of age. The incidence decreases gradually until around age seven to eight. The incidence of epilepsy thereafter rises to peak at around 17 to 18 years of age, and is around 35% at 20 years of age. Thereafter, the incidence decreases gradually (Ballaban-Gil *et al.*, 1991). The most common site of seizure discharge is the temporal lobe, especially the left.

Communication deficits in autism spectrum disorders include abnormal development of spoken language and impaired ability to initiate or sustain conversation. The child's language is often stereotyped, repetitive, and idiosyncratic, with echolalia and neologisms (Dunn & Rapin, 1997). One-third of autistic toddlers demonstrate a history of neurodevelopmental regression involving language, sociability, play, and cognition (Rapin, 1995). There are no differences in paroxysmal discharges in autism with or without speech regression (Swarton, 1995). Around 38% of autistic children have a history of speech regression, which may be severe; 30% without severe mental retardation have a history of regression (Ballaban-Gil *et al.*, 1991). Those children with autism who show language regression do so before age three years (Tuchman & Rapin, 1997), whereas the mean age of language regression in Landau–Kleffner syndrome is five to seven years. Only 10% of children with Landau–Kleffner syndrome regress before three years (Bishop, 1985).

In children with autism without epilepsy, an epileptiform EEG is identified in 14% of children with language regression compared with 6% of those without regression (Tuchman & Rapin, 1997). Overnight studies show epileptiform potentials in 19%, but continuous spike-wave status in sleep is not seen. Overnight EEG appears to be warranted only in autistic children with regression or fluctuation in their clinical course (Rapin, 1995; Pearl *et al.*, 2001). Not all children with abnormal EEG discharges have seizures (Swarton, 1995).

Electrical status epilepticus in sleep

Electrical status epilepticus during sleep, also known as continuous spike-waves of sleep, presents with regressions in behavior, cognition, and language complicated by a variety of epileptic seizures, including atypical absence attacks (Roger *et al.*, 1985).

This is a mixed focal and generalized seizure syndrome (Roger *et al.*, 1985). Some believe that it is related to Landau–Kleffner syndrome, and some cases have been described that evolve from one to the other (Ballaban-Gil & Tuchman, 2000). Any child who loses language skills for no other apparent reason should have overnight monitoring (Besage, 2001).

Epidemiology

This is a rare disorder seen more often in boys (58%) than girls, without any evidence of any inheritance (Roger *et al.*, 1985). It sometimes starts in infancy and is likely to remit spontaneously in adolescence, peaking at four to five years of age (Roger *et al.*, 1985; Stores, 1990). It is seen in up to 1% of children with epilepsy, with various seizure types, but especially in those with a combination of generalized and partial motor seizures (Stores, 1990).

Clinical

Thysanura (1998) noted that when the disorder emerges, there appears to be some mental regression. The child, often of previously normal development, begins to exhibit a widespread regression of intelligence, behavior, and especially language. Speech efforts may slow and drooling may occur. The child may manifest word-finding difficulties, paraphasia, slow speech, misuse of different consonants, distortion of vowels, and motor articulatory disturbances, or an expressive aphasia but no oral dyspraxia (Yamashita *et al.*, 2000). There is a concurrent intellectual deterioration but language or memory and orientation may be affected more severely (Stores, 1990). If the child is of school age, reading difficulties may be noted. The child may also not copy correctly due to poor hand–eye coordination (Yamashita *et al.*, 2000).

Behavior changes include attention defects with limited attention and inattentiveness, as well as hyperactivity and occasionally a psychotic state during the ESES stage (Stores, 1990; Ballaban-Gil & Tuchman, 2000; Yamashita *et al.*, 2000).

Seizures

Seizures occur in a majority of cases and often precede the ESES. The seizures may be nocturnal initially in sleep (50%) (Rogers *et al.*, 1985) and then occur upon awakening as partial seizures involving the face (Yamashita *et al.*, 2000). At the onset, the initial seizures may be partial, often unilateral (20%), or generalized as clonic attacks (40%). Unilateral status is rare (Roger *et al.*, 1985). Facial myoclonic seizures occur in 16%, with mandibular contractions and an associated loss of consciousness. Myoclonic seizures may be seen in 4%. Tonic seizures do not occur (Roger *et al.*, 1985). Atypical absence seizures are seen especially at the onset of the ESES (Roubertie *et al.*, 1998; Ballaban-Gil & Tuchman, 2000).

There are three subtypes: those with rare nocturnal motor seizures outgrown by adolescence; those who go on to exhibit absence attacks at the time of the ESES emergence; and those who also may exhibit atonic and clonic components at the onset of ESES. All children tend to outgrow the seizure problem by adolescence (Roger *et al.*, 1985).

Examination

The examination is essentially normal unless earlier problems are noted as part of a preceding developmental delay (Roger *et al.*, 1985). All the children are functionally impaired, presenting with depressed intellectual skills, language impairments, and behavioral disturbances (Yasuhara *et al.*, 1991).

Differential diagnosis

These patients are to be differentiated from those with benign epilepsy with Rolandic spikes, Lennox–Gestalt syndrome and Landau–Kleffner syndrome (Roger *et al.*, 1985; Stores, 1990). Children with continuous spikes and slow waves during sleep appear to comprise a spectrum of entities including electrical status epilepticus during sleep, nonvconvulsive status epilepticus with epileptic negative myoclonus, atypical benign partial epilepsy, and Landau–Kleffner syndrome (Yamashita *et al.*, 2000), as well as infantile autism and developmental dysphasia. In those children with a sleep spike-wave index between 20 and 50%, many (86%) have an early-onset cognitive disorder without further deterioration but with severe mental deficiency. In children with an index from 50 to 85%, and in those with a spike-wave index above 85%, the patients manifest neuropsychological and intellectual regression in the first years of life (Roubertie *et al.*, 1998).

Diagnostics

Possible tests include EEG, auditory evoked potentials, and anatomic imaging studies such as a CT, SPECT, or especially MRI, the latter to exclude the possibility of a lesion (Swarton, 1995).

Electroencephalography

Patients with otherwise classical seizures of Rolandic epilepsy may develop atypical seizures, including generalized tonic–clonic seizures, atonic and atypical absences, as well as ESES and cognitive and behavior disturbances (Pearl *et al.*, 2001). An overnight EEG study may be needed to observe all stages of sleep.

Prior to the CSWS emergence in the wake state, generalized spike-wave bursts may be seen, sometimes associated with clinical attacks. Focal unilateral isolated interictal spikes or slow spikes from either side may also be noted over the frontal-temporal areas, the central temporal areas, or both. These increase in sleep (Roger *et al.*, 1985).

At the onset of ESES, the syndrome presents with sleep activation, with diffuse complexes of spike and wave activity at a rate of 1.5 to two per second occurring in more than 85% of EEG tracings in non-REM slow sleep, which occurs every time the child sleeps. The discharges continue for hours (Tassinari *et al.*, 1985; Stores, 1990; Yasuhara *et al.*, 1991). Less common are continuous focal discharges with frontal predominance, including frontal-central discharges or nearly continuous diffuse bisynchronous sharp waves. Normal sleep morphologies are obscured (Ballaban-Gil & Tuchman, 2000). REM sleep halts the generalized spike-wave status, although rare bursts of diffuse spike-wave fragments and focal frontal-central rhythmic discharges may be seen (Roger *et al.*, 1985). Arousal may be difficult, with ongoing slow waves associated with slowed waking up. Thysanura (1998) reported that in the wake state, there might be an increase of the previously noted interictal abnormalities, often diffuse. Focal disturbances including frontal and central temporal spikes, as well as diffuse spike-waves, are noted in less than 25% of patients in the wake state. The background is normal. Brain mapping shows a focal onset that may be parietal, central-frontal, or located elsewhere. A few years into the syndrome, the spike-wave very regular sleep pattern tends to break up in rhythmic discharges with some brief few-second pauses. Intravenous diazepam can stop this, but the phenomena tend to reappear in ten to 20 minutes.

Left-sided spikes have been associated with errors in verbal tasks, whereas right-sided spikes produce errors in non-verbal tasks (Aarts et al., 1984). Subclinical epileptiform discharges interfere with academic skills and subtests of IQ to testing involved in short-term memory (Siebelink et al., 1988). The longer the discharge lasts, the greater is the resultant effect (Ballaban-Gil & Tuchman, 2000).

After the end of ESES, both the seizures and the EEG improve in adolescence. The EEG findings eventually resolve, although they may wax and wane before this occurs. The seizures resolve at about the same time as the EEG (Roger et al., 1985). Normalization of the EEG correlates with an increase in many areas of the IQ (Stores, 1990; Ratmelli et al., 1998).

Other studies

There is no mention of any consistent structural lesions or other abnormal findings (Roger et al., 1985). A PET scan shows a focal increase of isotopic activity; if this is on the dominant side, it is associated with an acquired aphasia; if it is on the right (non-dominant) side, it is associated with an apraxia (Thysanura, 1998). Features of an immature brain characterize the cerebral metabolic pattern of CSWS, with the deterioration of cognitive functions, focal or regional dysfunction of one or more associative cortices, and the absence of significant thalamic diaschisis (Maquet et al., 1995).

Cause

The pathophysiology is not known (Roger et al., 1985). Thysanura (1998) found that 50% of patients might have had a pre-existing brain insult, but no consistent cause has been found. Isolated reports include mild gliosis, a left temporal lobe ganglioglioma, a left temporal lobe neurocysticercosis, isolated cerebral arteritis, an astrocytoma of the left temporal lobe, and demyelinating lesions in the left frontal lobe white matter and right parietal centrum semi-ovale (Ballaban-Gil & Tuchman, 2000).

Course

The seizures often emerge at about eight to 8.5 years of age (range 4–14 years). The ESES appears about one to two years later and begins to disappear at about ten to 12.5 years of age. Seizures are self-limited, disappearing by age 10–15 years (Roger *et al.*, 1985).

Prognosis

The seizures usually respond well to therapy and disappear, but cognitive, behavioral, and learning disabilities may persist as the major handicap (Roger *et al.*, 1985).

Complications

Some children are normal before the syndrome onset, but others are previously not normal (Roger *et al.*, 1985; Yasuhara *et al.*, 1991). Those children with prior normal psychomotor development experience a severe deterioration of IQ to a resultant borderline IQ level. Severe associated impairments include regression of language function (54%), often associated with marked impairments of memory and temporal spatial orientation. There may be a history of prior speech delays. Behavior problems emerge in most (90%) patients, including a reduced attention span, hyperactivity, aggressiveness, difficulties in social contact, inhibition, and some times psychotic states (18%). When the ESES state ends, recovery is slow and usually incomplete, with only 28% of patients becoming normal (Roger *et al.*, 1985).

Those children with prior abnormal psychomotor development often had a severe encephalopathy complicated by a motor impairment, such as a hemiplegia or quadriplegia. Atypical forms of this disorder have been reported. There are children with a CSWS clinical picture but with spike-wave incidence of less than 85% (Yamashita *et al.*, 2000). Some have a duration lasting from a few months to one year plus. A small number of children with ESES have no neuropsychological impairment (Roger *et al.*, 1985).

Therapy

Treated patients tend to show some improvement in language, cognition, and seizures. In some, the EEG improves without functional improvement (Ballaban-Gil & Tuchman, 2000). In others, functional improvement is seen when the ESES is controlled (Besage, 2001). Sometimes, combinations of carbamazepine, valproate, ethosuximide, and clonazepam seem to control the seizures, stop the nocturnal status, and lead to a decrease in signs and symptoms of ESES (Yasuhara *et al.*, 1991). When the seizures are controlled, there is an improvement in emotional stability.

ACTH occasionally may produce occasional miracle cures. It may suppress the ESES, improve cognitive and language functions, and even stop negative myoclonus, but only while the patient is on the steroid (Roger *et al.*, 1985). Several months after discontinuation of ACTH, moderate difficulties and word-problems finding return, and the EEG deteriorates (Yamashita *et al.*, 2000).

Thysanura (1998) reported that subpial resections have been used targeting the area around the Sylvian fissure with some benefits, including normalization of the EEG. Post-procedure, the entire EEG is suppressed, but within about ten minutes rhythmic activity reappears. Speech may begin to return in a week or two after the surgery.

Landau–Kleffner syndrome/continuous spike-wave of sleep variants

Children are seen who present with a skill regression and with findings of continuous spike-waves during slow sleep (Metz-Lutz & Massa, 1999). However, the predominant associated features involve non-language skills, primarily perceptual motor processes.

Acquired visual agnosia with epilepsy

Some previously normal children have lost the ability to recognize objects although their visual acuity remains intact. This often appears around six to eight years of age and may follow a febrile illness. Generalized tonic–clonic seizures appear, which are found to be associated with localized cortical disturbances in the occipital temporal regions. Visual perceptual-motor skills deteriorate, including object recognition, shape discrimination, and reduced copying abilities, as well as writing difficulties, without any verbal intelligence or memory impairments. Auditory recognition and verbal communication skills remain intact, although expressive language efforts tend to be slowed. Some patients show a mild deterioration of intelligence, and later short-term memory impairments, both visual and auditory, may be noted. The wake EEG shows frequent subclinical bilateral spike-wave discharges over the frontal Rolandic area, shifting from side to side. Months later, a continuous spike-wave pattern emergs in sleep. Video encephalography demonstrates continuous spike-wave activity in 80% of non-REM sleep, maximum bilaterally over the occipitotemporal areas, with left-sided onset, and resistant to antiepileptic therapy. The right frontal temporal area is more disturbed than the left on nuclear magnetic resonance imaging (NMRI). Clonazepam may help with the seizures. Auditory short-term memory, if depressed, improves but visual spatial memory tends to remain low. Other regions of the brain can be affected in the same way, causing a specific, profound neuropsychological problem that is easily overlooked in children without manifest motor seizures (Roulet-Perez, 1995; Eriksson et al., 2000).

Acquired apraxia with continuous spike-waves in sleep

The patient previously normal, at around eight years of age begins to experience complex partial seizures, after which a severe apraxia–agraphia emerges. Dressing and object-manipulation apraxia, predominantly of the left hand, emerges, and a left motor hemineglect and attention deficit is noted. A visual spatial short-term memory deficit is confirmed as part of depressed performance intelligence. Language functions remain intact. The waking EEG shows bilateral spike-wave discharges with right frontal predominance, with the appearance of a continuous generalized spike-wave picture. PET shows increased fluorodeoxyglucose (FDG) uptake in the right middle and superior temporal regions as well as in the inferior and superior parietal cortices (Maquet *et al.*, 1995; Metz-Lutz & Massa, 1999).

Acquired frontal dysfunction with epilepsy

A child at age seven years developed behavior disturbances with attention and auditory comprehension difficulties. Within a year, complex partial seizures emerged, with right-sided temporal spikes and waves seen on the EEG. Behavior then presented with irritability, disinhibition, and inappropriate postures and speech, suggestive of a childhood mania. Treatment with valproic acid, clobazam, and pipamperone controlled the seizures but gave only mild behavior improvements. Sleep-associated CSWS then appeared. The IQ was normal but low in coding and digit-span subtests, which required sustained attention (Metz-Lutz & Massa, 1999).

REFERENCES

Aarts, J. H. P., Binnie, C. D., Smith, A. M., *et al.* (1984). Selective cognitive impairments during focal and generalized epileptiform EEG activity. *Brain* **107**: 292–308.

Ansink, B. J., Sarphatie, H. & VanDongen, H. R. (1989). The Landau–Kleffner syndrome: case report and theoretical considerations. *Neuropediatrics* **20**: 132–8.

Appleton, R., Hughes, A. Beirae, M., *et al.* (1993). Vigabatrin in the Landau–Kleffner syndrome. *Dev. Med. Child Neurol.* **35**: 457–8.

Ballaban-Gil, K. (1995). Spectrum of acquired language regression. Presented at the American Epilepsy Society Conference, Baltimore, MD, December 1995.

Ballaban-Gil, K. & Tuchman, R. (2000). Epilepsy and epileptiform EEG: association with autism and language disorders. *Ment. Retard. Dev. Disabil. Res. Rev.* **6**: 300–308.

Ballaban-Gil, K., Rapin, I., Tuchman, R., *et al.* (1991). The risk of seizures in autistic individuals: occurrence of a secondary peak in adolescence. *Epilepsia* **32** (suppl 3): 84.

Beaumanoir, A. (1985). The Landau–Kleffner syndrome. In *Epileptic Syndromes in Infancy, Childhood and Adolescence*, ed. J. Roger, M. Dravet, C. Bureau, F. E. Dreifuss & P. Wolf, pp. 81–91. London: J. Libbey Eurotext.

Besag, F. M. C. (2001). Treatment of state dependent learning disabilities. In *Epilepsy and Learning Disabilites*, ed. G. F. Ayala, M. Elia, C. M. Cornaggia & M. M. Trimble. *Epilespia* **42**: 46–9.

Bhatia, M. S., Shome, S., Chadda, R. K., *et al.* (1994). Landau–Kleffner syndrome in cerebral neurocystercosis. *Indian Pediatr.* **31**: 584–7.

Bicknese, A. R., Preston, J., Ettinger, A. B., *et al.* (1996). Epileptic aphasia (Landau–Kleffner syndrome) secondary to progressive encephalitis. *Ann. Neurol.* **40**: 305–7.

Billard, C. S., Autret, A., Laffront, F., *et al.* (1982). Electrical status epilepticus during sleep in children. In *Sleep and Epilepsy*, ed. B. M. Sterman, M. N. Shouse & P. Passoquant, pp. 481–94. New York: Academic Press.

Bishop, D. V. M. (1985). Age of onset and outcome in "aquired aphasia with convulsive disorder" (Landau–Kleffner syndrome). *Dev. Med. Child. Neurol.* **27**: 705–12.

Cole, A. J., Andermann, F., Taylor, L., *et al.* (1988). The Landau–Kleffner syndrome of acquired epileptic aphasia: unusual clinical outcome, surgical experience, and absence of encephalitis. *Neurology* **38**: 31–8.

Cooper, J. A. & Ferry, P. G. (1978). Acquired auditory verbal agnosia and seizure in childhood. *J. Speech Hear. Disord.* **43**: 176–84.

Da Silva, E. A., Chugani, D. C., Muzik, O. P., *et al.* (1997). The Landau Kleffner syndrome: metabolic abnormalities in temporal lobe are a common feature. *J. Child Neurol.* **12**: 489–95.

Deonna, T. W. (1991). Acquired epileptiform aphasia in children (Landau–Kleffner syndrome). *J. Clin. Neurophysiol.* **9**: 288–98.

Deonna, T., Peter, C., & Ziegler, H. I. (1989). Adult follow-up of the acquired aphasia-epilepsy syndrome in childhood: report of seven cases. *Neuropediatrics* **20**: 132–8.

Duel, R. K. & Lenn, N. J. (1977). Treatment of acquired epileptic aphasia. *J. Pediatr.* **90**: 959–61.

Dugas, M. M., LeHeusey, M. F. & Reginer, N. (1982). Aphasic acquise de l'enfant avec epilpesie (syndrome de Landau–Kleffne): douze observations personelles. *Rev. Neurol. (Paris)* **138**: 755–80.

Dunn, M. & Rapin, I. (1997). Communication in autistic children. In *Behavior Belongs to the Brain: Neurobehavioral Syndromes*, ed. P. J. Accardo, B. K. Shapiro & A. J. Caputo, pp. 97–111. Baltimore, MD: York Press.

Eriksson, K., Kylliainen, A. & Hirvonen, K. (2000). Visual agnosia with occipital CSWS-A Landau Kleffner Equivalent? *Epilepsia* **41** (suppl 7): 195.

Fayad, M., Choveiri, R. & Mikati, M. (1997) . Landau–Kleffner syndrome: consistent response to repeated intravenous gamma-globulin doses: a case report. *Epilepsia* **38**: 489–94.

Feekery, C. J., Parry-Fielder, B. & Hopkins, J. J. (1993). Landau–Kleffner syndrome: six patients including discordant monozygotic twins. *Pediatr. Neurol.* **9**: 49–53.

Foerster, G. (1977). Aphasia and seizure disorders in childhood. In *Epilepsy, the Eighth International Symposium*, ed. J. K. Penry, pp. 305–6. New York: Raven Press.

Gascon, G., Victor, D., Lombroso, G. & Goodglass, H. (1973). Language disorder, convulsive disorder, and electroencephalographic abnormalities. *Arch. Neurol.* **28**: 156–62.

Gascon, G., Victor, D. & Lombroso, C. T. (2000). Language disorder, convulsive disorder and EEG study of five cases. *Epilepsia* **32**: 756–67.

Gastaut, H. (1979). Aphasia: the sole manifestation of focal status epilepticus. *Neurology* **2**: 1938.

Genton, P., Maton, B., Ogihara, M., *et al.* (1992). Continuous focal spikes during REM sleep in a case of acquired aphasia (Landau–Kleffner syndrome). *Sleep* **15**: 454–60.

Glauser, T. A., Olberding, L. A. S., Titanic, M. K., *et al.* (1995). Felbamate in the treatment of acquired epileptic aphasia. *Epil. Res.* **20**: 850–89.

Gomez, M. R. & Klass, D. W. (1983). Epilepsies of infancy and childhood. *Ann. Neurol.* **13**: 113–24.

Gordon, N. S. (1964). The concept of central deafness. In *Clinics in Developmental Medicine*, Vol. 13, pp. 62–4. London: Spastics Society and Heinemann.

Guerreiro, M. M., Camargo, E. E., Kato, M., *et al.* (1996). Brain single photon emission computed tomography imaging in Landau–Kleffner syndrome. *Epilepsia* **37**: 60–7.

Hashima, Y., Endo, M., Yagimuchi, T., *et al.* (1987). Epilepsy aphasia syndrome (word deafness) – course and prognosis over 10 years. *Brain Dev.* **9**: 166.

Hirsch, E., Maresceauex, C., Paquet, P., *et al.* 1990). Landau–Kleffner syndrome: a clinical and EEG study of five cases. *Epilepsia* **31**: 756–67.

Hoeppner, J. A. S., Grotz, C. L. & Morrell, F. (1993). Long- term follow-up of cognitive and behavioral function after surgery for Landau–Kleffner syndrome. *Epilepsia* **34** (suppl 6): 72.

Hoeppner, T. J., Morrell, F., Smith, M. C., *et al.* (1992). The Landau–Kleffner syndrome: a peri-Sylvian epilepsy. *Epilepsia* **33** (suppl 3): 122.

Holmes, G. L., Gairsa, J.-L., Chevassus-Au-Louis, N., *et al.* (1998). Consequences of neonatal seizures in the rat: morphological and behavioral effects. *Ann. Neurol.* **44**: 845–57.

Holmes, G. L., McKeever, M. & Saunders, Z. (1981). Epileptiform activity in aphasia of childhood: an epiphenomenon. *Epilepsia* **22**: 621–39.

Holmes, G. L., Sarkisian, M., Ben-Ari, Y., *et al.* (1999). Mossy fiber sprouting following recurrent seizures during early development in rats. *J. Comp. Neurol.* **404**: 537–53.

Kim, Y., Royer, F., Bonstselle, C., *et al.* (1980). Temporal sequencing of verbal and nonverbal materials: the effect of laterality of lesion. *Cortex* **116**: 135–43.

Lagae, L. G., Silberstein, J., Gilliss, P. L., *et al.* (1998). Successful use of intravenous immuno-globulins in Landau–Kleffner syndrome. *Pediatr. Neurol.* **18**: 165–8.

Landau, W. M. & Kleffner, F. R. (1957). Syndrome of acquired aphasia with convulsive disorder in children. *Neurology* **7**: 523–30.

Lerman-Sagie, T., Statter, M. & Lerman, P. (1987). Low erythrocyte zinc content in acquired aphasia with convulsive disorder (the Landau Kleffner syndrome). *J. Child Neurol.* **2**: 28–30.

Lou, H. C., Brandt, S. & Bruhn, P. (1977a). Aphasia and epilepsy in childhood. *Acta Neurol Scand.* **56**: 46–54.

Lou, H. C., Brandt, S. & Bruhn, P. (1977b). Progressive aphasia and epilepsy with a self-limited course. In *Epilepsy: the VIII International Symposium*, ed. J. K. Penry, pp. 295–303. New York: Raven Press.

Maccario, M., Hefferen, S. J., Kebusek, S. J., *et al.* (1982). Developmental dysphasia and electro-encephalographic abnormalities. *Dev. Med. Child. Neurol.* **24**: 141–55.

Mantovani, J. R. & Landau, W. M. (1980). Acquired aphasia with convulsive disorders: course and prognosis. *Neurology* **30**: 524–9.

Maquet, P., Hirsch, E., Metz-Lutz, M. N., *et al.* (1995). Regional cerebral glucose metabolism in children with deterioration of one or more cognitive functions and continuous spike-and-wave discharges during sleep. *Brain* **118**: 1492–520.

Maquet, P., Hirsch, E., Metz-Lutz, M. N., *et al.* (1999). PET studies of Landau–Kleffner syndrome and related disorders. In *Childhood Epilepsies and Brain Development*, ed. A. Nehlig, J. Motte, S. L. Moshe & P. Plouin, pp. 135–41. London: John Libbey & Co.

Marescaux, C., Hirsch, E., Finck, P., *et al.* (1990). Landau–Kleffner syndrome: a pharmacologic study of five cases. *Epilepsia* **31**: 768–77.

McKinney, W. & McGraw, D. A. (1974). An aphasic syndrome in children. *Can. Med. Assoc.* **110**: 637–9.

Metz-Lutz, M. N. & Massa, R. (1999). Cognitive and behavioral consequences of epilepsies in childhood. In *Childhood Epilepsies and Brain Development*, ed. A. Nehlig, J. Motte, S. L. Moshe & P. Plouin, pp. 123–34. London: John Libbey & Co.

Michalowicz, R., Jozwiak, S., Szwabowska-Orzeszko, E., *et al.* (1989). Zespol Landau–Kleffnera. *Wiad. Lek.* **42**: 256–9.

Mikati, M. A. & Saab, R. (2000). Successful use of intravenous imunoglobulin as initial mono-therapy in Landau–Kleffner syndrome. *Epilepsia* **41**: 880–86.

Ming, L., Xiao-ye, H., Jiong, Q., *et al.* (1996). Correlation between CSWS and aphasia in Landau–Kleffner syndrome: a study of three cases. *Brain Dev.* **18**: 197–200.

Morrell, F., Whisler, W. M., Smith, M. C., *et al.* (1995) Landau–Kleffner syndrome: treatment with subpial intracortical transection. *Brain* **118**: 1529–46.

Mouridsen, S. E. (1995). The Landau–Kleffner syndrome: a review. *Eur. Adolesc. Psychiatr.* **4**: 223–8.

Nakano, S., Okumo, T. & Mikawa, H. (1989). Landau–Kleffner syndrome: EEG topographic studies. *Brain Dev.* **11**: 43–60.

Nass, R., Gross, A., Wisoff, J. & Devinsky, O. (1999). Outcome of multiple subpial transactions for autistic epileptiform regression. *Pediatr. Neurol.* **21**: 464–70.

Nass, R., Heier, L. & Walker, R. (1993). Landau–Kleffner syndrome: temporal lobe tumor resection results in good outcome. *Pediatr. Neurol.* **9**: 303–5.

O'Donohoe, N. V. (1979). Learning disorders. In *Epilepsies of Childhood*, pp. 186–9. Boston, MA: Butterworth.

Otero, E., Cordova, S., Diaz, F., *et al.* (1989). Acquired epileptic aphasia due to neurocystericosis. *Epilepsia* **29**: 569–72.

O'Tuama, L. A., Urion, D. K., Janicek, M. J., *et al.* (1992). Regional cerebral perfusion in Landau–Kleffner syndrome and related childhood aphasias. *J. Nucl. Med.* **33**: 1758–6.

Pascual-Castroveiuo, I., Lopez-Martrin, V., Martinez-Bermejo, A., *et al.* (1992). Is cerebral arteritis the cause of the Landau–Kleffner syndrome: four cases in childhood with angiographic study. *Can. J. Neurol. Sci.* **19**: 45–52.

Pearce, P. S. & Darwish, H. (1984). Correlation between EEG and auditory percpetual measures in auditory agnosia. *Brain Lang.* **22**: 41–8.

Pearl, P. L., Carrazana, E. J. & Holmes, G. L. (2001). The Landau–Kleffner syndrome. *Epilepsy Reviews* **1**: 39–45.

Perniola, T., Margari, L., Buttiglione, M., *et al.* (1993). A case of Landau–Kleffner syndrome secondary to inflammatory demyelinating disease. *Epilepsia* **34**: 551–6.

Rapin, I. (1995). Autistic regression and disintegrative disorders: how important the role of epilepsy? *Semin. Pediatr. Neurol.* **2**: 278–85.

Rapin, I., Mattis, S., Rowan, A. J. & Golden, G. G. (1977). Verbal auditory agnosia and seizures in children. *Dev. Med. Child Neurol.* **19**: 192–207.

Ratmelli, G. P., Donati, F., Kaufmann, F., *et al.* (1998). Motor and cognitive profile during successful treatment in a case of continuous spike-waves during sleep. 3rd European Congress of Epileptology. *Epilepsia* **39** (suppl 2): 54.

Rintahaka, P. J., Chugani, H. T. & Sankar, R. (1995). Landau–Kleffner syndrome with continuous spikes and waves during slow-wave sleep. *J. Child Neurol.* **10**: 127–33.

Roger, J., Dravet, C., Bureau, M., Dreifuss, F. E., *et al.* (1985). *Epileptic Syndromes in Infancy, Childhood and Adolescence.* London: John Libbey Eurotext.

Roubertie, A., Touzery, A., Humbertclaude, V., *et al.* (1998). Continuous spikes and slow waves during sleep: neuropsychological aspects. 3rd European Congress of Epileptology. *Epilepsia* **39** (suppl 2): 19.

Roulet-Perez, E. (1995). Syndromes of acquired epileptic aphasia and epilepsy with continuous spike-waves discharges during sleep: models for prolonged cognitive impairment of epileptic origin. *Semin. Pediatr. Neurol.* **2**: 269–77.

Sat, L. & Dreifuss, F. (1973). Electroencephalographic findings in a patient with developmental expressive aphasia. *Neurology* **23**: 181–5.

Sawhney, I. M. S., Suresh, N., Dhand, U. K., *et al.* (1988). Acquired aphasia with epilepsy: Landau–Kleffner syndrome. *Epilepsia* **29**: 283–7.

Shields, D. (1995). Treatment modalities. Presented at the American Epilepsy Society Conference, Baltimore, MD, December 1995.

Shoumaker, R. D., Bennett, D. R., Bray, P. R., *et al.* (1974). Clinical and EEG manifestations of an unusual aphasic syndrome in children. *Neurology.* **24**: 10–16.

Siebelink, B. M., Bakker, D. J., Binnie, C. D., *et al.* (1988). Psychological effects of subclinical EEG discharges 2. General intelligence tests. *Epilepsy Res.* **2**: 117–21.

Sieratzki, J. S., Calvert, G. A., Brammer, M., *et al.* (2002). Accessibility of spoken, written and sign language in Landau–Kleffner syndrome: a linguistic and functional MRI study. *Epileptic Disord.* **3**: 79–89.

Solomon, G., Carson, D., Pavlakis, S., *et al.* (1991). Intracranial EEG monitoring in Landau–Kleffner syndrome associated with left temporal lobe astrocytoma. *Epilepsia* **32** (suppl 3): 56.

Solomon, G. E., Parson, D., Pavlakis, S., *et al.* (1993). Intracranial EEG monitoring in Landau–Kleffner syndrome associated with a left temporal lobe astrocytoma. *Epilepsia* **34**: 557–60.

Squires, K. C. & Hecox, K. E. (1983). Electrophysiological evaluation of higher level of auditory processing. *Semin. Hearing* **4**: 415–33.

Stein, L. K. & Curry, F. K. W. (1968). Childhood auditory agnosia. *J. Speech Hear. Disord.* **33**: 361–70.

Stores, G. (1990). Electroencephalographic parameters in assessing the cognitive function of children with epilepsy. *Epilepsia* **31**: 45–9.

Swarton, R. (1995). Laboratory evaluation. Presented at the American Epilepsy Society Conference, Baltimore, MD, December 1995.

Tassinari, C. A., Bureau, M., Dravet, C., *et al.* (1985). Epilepsy and continuous spikes and waves during slow sleep. In *Epileptic Syndromes in Infancy, Childhood and Adolescents*, ed. J. Roger, C. Dravet, M. Bereau, F. E. Dreifuss & P. Wolf, pp. 194–212. London: John Libbey Eurotext.

Tharpe, A. M., Johnson, G. D. & Glasscock, M. E. (1991). Diagnostic and management considerations of acquired epileptic aphasia or Landau–Kleffner syndrome. *Am. J. Otol.* **12**: 210–14.

Thysanura, C. A. (1998). Electrical status epilepticus in sleep. Presented at the Cleveland Clinic Conference, Cleveland, OH, June 1998.

Tuchman, R. F. & Rapin, I. (1997). Regression in pervasive developmental disorders: seizures and epileptiform electroencephalogram correlates. *Pediatrics* **2**: 670–77.

Van Dongen, H. R. & Loonen, M. C. B. (1977). Factors related to the prognosis of acquired aphasia in children. *Cortex* **13**: 131–6.

Volkmar, F. R. & Nelson, D. S. (1990). Seizure disorders in autism. *J. Am. Acad. Child Adolesc. Psychiatry* **29**: 127–9.

Wasterlain, C. G., Fujikawa, D. G., Penix L. & Sankar, R. (1993). Pathophysiologic mechanisms of brain damage from status epilepticus. *Epilepsia* **34**: 537–53.

Watters, G. B. (1974). The syndrome of acquired aphasic and convulsive disorder in children. *Can. Med. J.* **110**: 611–12.

White, H. & Sreenivasan, J. (1987). Epilepsy aphasia syndrome in children: an unusual presentation to psychiatry. *Can. J. Psychiatry* **32**: 599–601.

Wioland, N., Rudolf, G. & Metz-Lutz, M. N. (2001). Electrophysiological evidence of persisting unilateral-auditory cortex dysfunction in the late outcome of Landau and Kleffner syndrome. *Clin. Neurophysiol.* **112**: 319–23.

Worster-Drought, C. (1971). An unusual form of acquired aphasia in children. *Dev. Med. Child. Neurol.* **13**: 563–71.

Yamashita, S., Yamada, M. & Iwamoto, H. (2000). ESES syndrome with acquired aphaisa. Proceedings of the 32nd Congress of Japan Epilepsy Society. *Epilepsia* **41** (suppl 9): 71.

Yashima, Y., Endo, M., Yagiuchi, T., *et al.* (1987). Epilepsy–aphasia syndrome (word deafness) – course and prognosis over ten years. *Brain Dev.* **9**: 166.

Yasuhara, A., Yoshida, H., Hatanaka, T., *et al.* (1991). Epilepsy with continuous spike-waves during slow sleep and its treatment. *Epilepsia* **31**: 59–62.

Zovan, N. & Choyakh, F. (1977). Es potentiaels evoques auditifs precoces, de latoence moyenne et tardifs dans un cas d'aphasic acquise-epilepsie (syndrome de Landau–Kleffner). *Rev. Laryngol. Otol. Rhinol. (Bord)* **40**: 299–308.

7

Other epilepsy language syndromes

In addition to the acquired aphasia with epilepsy syndromes, there are other syndromes in which the loss or non-development of language skills, along with the emergence of epilepsy, may be prominent.

Perisylvian-opercular syndromes

The perisylvian syndromes consist of a congenital type and an acquired type, both presenting with pseudobulbar palsy and epilepsy. Language remains intact, but speech is inhibited.

Congenital perisylvian syndrome

The congenital bilateral perisylvian (opercular) syndrome presents with a developmental pseudobulbar palsy with epilepsy and mild to moderate mental retardation. Often, other congenital defects are found. Imaging studies reveal bilateral perisylvian migration abnormalities (Kuzniecky *et al.*, 1989; Kuzniecky *et al.*, 1991a; Kuzniecky *et al.*, 1991b; Kuzniecky *et al.*, 1993a; Kuzniecky *et al.*, 1993b; Kuzniecky *et al.*, 1994).

Clinical

The syndrome becomes apparent in infancy or early childhood as dissociation between automatic and voluntary movements of the mouth and face. Characteristic of this syndrome is that severe voluntary oromotor problems are noted, with preserved non-voluntary emotional movements. The child demonstrates developmental delays (60%) and mild to moderate mental retardation (50–80%). Dysarthria or, in severe cases, mutism with preserved comprehension is seen.

Seizures are usually seen (87–90%), often beginning at age eight to 12 months. Some patients (20%) have a history of infantile spasms in the first few months of life. Generalized seizures are common (80%). Absence seizures may be seen. Head drops and atonic and tonic seizures occur often (70%). Partial epilepsy may also be noted (9%). A mixed seizure disorder is seen in about half the patients (40–60%). The seizures are stable but frequent in 55%. Nearly one-third (30%) have infrequent seizures or seizures that are controlled by therapy (Kuzniecky *et al.*, 1989; Kuzniecky *et al.*, 1991a; Kuzniecky *et al.*, 1991b; Kuzniecky *et al.*, 1993a; Kuzniecky *et al.*, 1993b; Kuzniecky *et al.*, 1994).

Examination

All patients present with the congenital pseudobulbar palsy manifest as perioral signs, speech and swallowing difficulties, and dysarthria. Oropharyngeal dysfunction and dysarthria are seen in all. Other findings include poor palate function (40%), impaired tongue movements, an exaggerated jaw jerk, and a preserved gag reflex. The child may be floppy, with hypotonia (30%) or other motor deficits (25%). Limb malformations with arthrogryposis may be found (30%). Associated neurological problems include mental retardation and pyramidal signs, such as spasticity and accentuated tendon reflexes (Kuzniecky *et al.*, 1989; Kuzniecky *et al.*, 1991a; Kuzniecky *et al.*, 1991b; Kuzniecky *et al.*, 1993a; Kuzniecky *et al.*, 1993b; Kuzniecky *et al.*, 1994).

Diagnosis

Electroencephalogram

EEG abnormalities and seizures, if present, present interictally with generalized bilateral slow spike-wave discharges and multifocal epileptic discharges, involving especially the central-temporal parietal regions. The background activity may be slowed (50%). Ictal records usually show generalized or bilateral synchronous fast spike-wave discharges or a low-voltage recruiting pattern (30%). Occasionally, bilateral central-temporal discharges are seen. Children without seizures may have a normal EEG.

Neuroradiology

Despite the classic clinical features of a combination of congenital pseudobulbar facial, swallowing, and chewing weakness, with intractable epilepsy and mental retardation, the diagnosis is usually made retrospectively after an MRI has been obtained (Belousova *et al.*, 1998).

Bilateral perisylvian imaging abnormalities are the cardinal feature. CT and MRI scans show symmetrical bilateral perisylvian abnormalities with increased cortical thickness. The MRI best demonstrates the thickened insular cortex with small gyri, a widely open Sylvian fissure (secondary to the abnormal opercularization), and a dysplasia of the posterior frontal cortex. Polymicrogyri tend to be around the Sylvian fissure, especially the posterior portion. Irregularity of the cortical white-matter junction is characteristic of the associated polymicrogyria, although in some patients the cortical white-matter junction may appear smooth. Extension of the perisylvian cortical abnormalities is variable. Enlarged ventricles are often present.

Bilateral involvement is a poor prognosticator associated with developmental delays and motor dysfunction.

Cause

The syndrome is caused by a bilateral structural defect in the anterior opercular area, usually a bilateral perisylvian opercular cortical polymicrogyria dysplasia. Acquired bilateral opercular destructive lesions have also been described. Other causes that have been considered include congenital cytomegalovirus infection, in utero ischemia, and chromosomal mutations, although cytogenic studies have shown no abnormalities (Kuzniecky *et al.*, 1989; Kuzniecky *et al.*, 1991a; Kuzniecky *et al.*, 1991b; Kuzniecky *et al.*, 1993a; Kuzniecky *et al.*, 1993b; Kuzniecky *et al.*, 1994).

Treatment

Treatment is variable. Often, the child is on multiple anticonvulsants (67%). If the seizures are intractable, surgery may be helpful. A corpus callosotomy, either anterior or complete, is the most common approach when the epilepsy is severe to intractable (Kuzniecky *et al.*, 1989; Kuzniecky *et al.*, 1991a; Kuzniecky *et al.*, 1991b; Kuzniecky *et al.*, 1993a; Kuzniecky *et al.*, 1993b; Kuzniecky *et al.*, 1994).

Acquired epileptiform opercular syndrome

With acquired epileptiform opercular syndrome, there is a combined persistent drooling, oral apraxia, and a peculiar unawareness of the presence of food in the mouth (oral sensory agnosia). Infrequent seizures develop in most children. The course fluctuates over several years (Roulet *et al.*, 1989; Shafrir & Prensky, 1995).

Clinical

The children mostly girls, are often preschoolers. They may be developmentally slowed but respond well to special help. No pre-existing neurologic abnormality has been noted. The child develops recurrent prolonged episodes of severe oral apraxia, dysarthria, and drooling, similar to the congenital opercular syndrome of children. Each episode lasts weeks to months, and is associated with exacerbation of epileptiform activity on the EEG. The episodes may have an insidious onset of drooling and an inability to blow bubbles or drink through a straw. Eating then becomes slowed, as chewing and swallowing may become disorganized. The child is otherwise alert, active, responsive, and able to follow commands involving other body parts. There is a gradual decrease in speech output, poor pronunciation, and loss of previously achieved vocabulary. Some clumsiness becomes apparent.

Within a year, infrequent, brief, partial seizures associated with a centrotemporal spike-wave discharge may emerge, with occasional generalization. The seizures may manifest as a blank stare, eyelid fluttering, and blinking observed in the daytime, and can be confirmed by EEG. Quivering or twitching of the left angle of the mouth and tongue lasting up to hours when awake may be noted (Roulet *et al.*, 1989; Shafrir & Prensky, 1995).

Course

The symptoms wax and wane as the course evolves to one of relapses and remissions, fluctuating over several years. Each active episode may last weeks to months, evolving in a characteristic manner, beginning with the inability to protrude the tongue and subsequent worsening of the oral motor function. During the active EEG times, the drooling worsens, with retention of food and without chewing efforts lasting up to hours. Speech output decreases to occasional single words, yet comprehension appears normal. During relapses, a mild ataxia may be noted without any signs of other dysfunctions. Between the spells, expressive language improves but the oromotor deficits persist. In recovery, no language problems of word or sound substitutions, echolalia, or palilalia are noted (Roulet *et al.*, 1989; Shafrir & Prensky, 1995).

Examination

The examination is normal except for continuous drooling and a mild developmental delay. The oral examination shows an oral apraxia but normal oral reflexes. Involuntary emotional movements of the face are apparent (Roulet *et al.*, 1989; Shafrir & Prensky, 1995).

Diagnosis

The EEG and neuroradiology confirm the diagnosis. The fluctuating course is atypical for a structural lesion, and no lesion is found (Roulet *et al.*, 1989; Shafrir & Prensky, 1995).

Electroencephalography

A basic EEG shows spike-wave discharges over the centrotemporal areas with variable spread, including occasional runs of a generalized 2.5 to five per second spike-wave activity. Status epilepticus during slow-wave sleep has been recorded. The EEG improves markedly when clinical symptoms subside, but with the return of the symptoms the EEG again reveals a marked increase in voltage and field of the temporal spike, the appearance of generalized spike or polyspike and slow-wave discharges occasionally associated with atypical absence seizures, as well as ESES. The EEG abnormalities correlate with the severity of the neural deficits, yet the neurologic problems are not felt to be ictal manifestations.

Video-EEG studies show generalized spike-wave discharges maximal over the involved temporal area. In the daytime, these are associated with blank stare and eyelid fluttering. The oral movements do not correlate with the discharges. At night, the near-continuous spike-wave discharges are not associated with any movements.

Neuroimaging

The MRI is normal initially but later may show a mild diffuse atrophy. An FDG-PET shows a hypometabolism area in the mesiotemporal area and patchy mild hypometabolism in both frontal lobes, with later studies showing slight worsening of the regional hypometabolism.

Other tests

Evoked responses, EMG, and nerve conduction testing are normal, as are tests for metabolic, infectious, and inflammatory causes. A barium swallow shows only incoordinated oral components of swallowing.

Neuropsychologic testing

Psychological testing reveals a marked impairment of expressive language, with relative strengths in arithmetic, riddles, and reading decoding.

Cause

This syndrome may share a similar mechanism with Landau–Kleffner syndrome, representing a neurological disorder in which long-standing electrical dysfunction of perisylvian neurons causes bilateral neurological dysfunction. This may be caused by disruption of normal connections or by an excessive inhibitory reaction to the epileptiform discharges (Engel & Wilson, 1986).

Therapy

Various antiepileptic drugs have been tried without significant response. A response is seen when felbamate or clonazepam is added. Some children appear to benefit from a combination of anticonvulsants and a ketogenic diet. Some children may require oral surgery to help with the drooling, resulting in transient improvement. This does not help the chewing and swallowing component. Tube feeding may be needed (Roulet et al., 1989; Shafrir & Prensky, 1995).

Infectious and immunologic speech regression

Post-encephalitis language disorders

Younger children appear more vulnerable to enteroviral illnesses such as the Western equine virus. With neonatal enteroviral encephalitis, an increased amount of language and speech deficits are seen as sequelae. Children with enterovirus infections in the first year of life may be found to have definite sequelae, including seizures, small heads, depressed intelligence, and delayed language development. No clinical symptoms, signs, or laboratory findings in the acute encephalitic state have proven helpful in prognosticating the outcome, except for the presence of seizures in the acute state. The infection appears to affect the nervous system at an important stage of cerebral development at the time of the injury. The more immature the nervous system, the greater the impairment (Sells *et al.*, 1975).

Protracted partial complex status syndrome

This is an extremely rare and frustrating disorder occurring in both children and adults. The condition presents with acute mixed, recurring, drug-resistant seizures associated with deteriorating intelligence, an emerging aphasia, and evolving major behavioral problems, often psychotic. The attack is prolonged, usually with eventual remission, although rarely there may be recurrence. This can be considered to be a symptomatic regionalized partial seizure syndrome, but commonly it is referred to as a protracted epileptiform encephalopathy (Mikati *et al.*, 1985).

Clinical presentation

This syndrome presents with four stages: (1) a deterioration phase, (2) an obtundation phase, (3) an improvement phase, and (4) a normalization phase. The very few children reported usually experienced the onset in mid childhood.

Deteriorative phase

The patient experiences an acute progressive confusion, deterioration of language abilities, and emergence of frustration behaviors over a few weeks. A mixed seizure disorder, usually including complex partial seizures, emerge. Adversive and focal tonic–clonic seizures may be noted. A marked psychosis, including hallucinations, agitation, aggression, echoing what is heard, labored efforts to talk, and delusions of grandeur may be noted. Gastrointestinal upsets and transient high blood pressure may occur. Occasionally, choreoathetoid and other extrapyramidal as well as pyramidal symptoms may be noted.

Obtundation phase

The patient then experiences a deterioration of consciousness, interrupted by periods of alertness and responsiveness over several months. A varying expressive aphasia with marked frustrations emerges. Spoken efforts may be jumbled together with some relevance to external stimuli. There may a refusal to eat and erratic sleep cycles. The seizures may decrease, although apneic episodes may be noted.

Improvement phase

The patient then begins to become increasingly alert and establish improved sleep habits over the next few months. Behavior problems re-emerge, including aggressive tendencies.

Recovery or relapse phase

Over the next few months, normalization usually occurs as seizures cease, the EEG normalizes, and both intelligence and behavior recover. The recovery may be incomplete. Rarely, there is a recurrence (recycling), with further regression and less recovery.

Subtypes

There are various types of this syndrome. Some patients present with aphasia associated with bilateral temporal-occipital EEG discharges, severe for about a month, then followed by a gradual recovery. Others present with altered consciousness with confusion and seizures, including prominent automatisms, adversive movements, and focal clonic movements associated with bilateral continuous seizure activities. This persists for weeks, to be followed by a gradual recovery.

The childhood form presents with an altered consciousness with confusion, aphasia, mixed seizures (including automatisms, partial complex seizures, adversive seizures, and focal clonic seizures), a florid psychosis, and vegetative symptoms. The course is prolonged over months. At the end, recovery is usual but not necessary complete. A recurrence within the year may leave the child essentially mute and demented, with drug-resistant multifocal seizures.

Considerations

Those dealing with the child often think of schizophrenic or other major psychoses, a central nervous system (CNS) degenerative or infectious disorder, or confusional migraines, although a minor or complex partial status should also be considered.

Examination

When first seen, the patient may present with uncontrollable behavior or depressed consciousness, aphasia, and often subtle pyramidal and extrapyramidal signs.

Diagnostics

In desperation to find a diagnosis, many tests are performed but little is found. The EEG shows abnormal discharges unilateral or bilaterally, but usually from the temporal, frontal, or posterior (occipital) areas. Runs of up to ten-second-long high slow discharges are seen, which become more rhythmic and slower. Between these discharges, the background activity is slow. Other studies include a

CSF examination, immunologic and virologic studies, a toxo-metabolic work-up, a CT or MRI scan, and isotopic scans, all of which are usually normal.

Cause

The etiology is not known. This is a very rare condition, of which little is known. One child case presented at a time when two other children from the same region presented with an encephalitis-like picture following an upper respiratory infection, suggesting a possible infectious cause, but studies did not confirm the cause.

Course

This syndrome often occurs in young adults. It is seen rarely in children or older adults. The course is prolonged (months), usually ending with full recovery. Rarely, the problem may recur, producing further regression, or it may end with only partial recovery of functions.

Outlook

The outlook is usually good with full recovery in adults, but the prognosis is less good in children, especially if recurrent attacks are noted. In some cases, there is limited to little recovery and the patient remains severely handicapped. The language, learning processing, and emotional and behavioral problems seen acutely may persist if the patient does not recover after the acute stage.

Treatment

The condition is resistant to anticonvulsive and psychiatric medication, including barbiturate coma induction, although occasionally there may be a patient who responds somewhat to one of these approaches. The seizure is not thought to be amenable to surgery. The family needs much support and the patient, especially if they do not recover, needs intensive rehabilitation.

Rasmussen's syndrome

In 1958, Rasmussen and colleagues described children with a rare disorder beginning in the first decade of life after infancy (Rasmussen et al., 1958; Aguilar & Rasmussen, 1960). These children showed an insidious onset and a gradual progression of unilateral brain dysfunction, with intractable focal seizures, hemiparesis, and ultimate dementia (McNamara, 1995). This entity is now known as Rasmussen's syndrome.

Rasmussen's syndrome is a specific progressive disease affecting primarily one hemisphere, accompanied by intractable epilepsy and leading to a slowly progressive hemispheric dysfunction and mental impairment, with a progressive atrophy of the affected hemisphere. Characteristic is the emergence of Kojewnikow's syndrome of epilepsia partialis continuans, especially the childhood form. The diagnosis is confirmed by pathologic findings of perivascular lymphocytic cuffing, microglial nodules, and microglial proliferation (So & Andermann, 1997).

Clinical

The disorder usually begins in childhood between the ages of one and 15 years. The rare adult-onset cases tend to be bilateral and to have more localized epileptogenic activity in the temporal and occipital areas (So & Andermann, 1997). Some patients have a history of an infectious episode of some sort at or shortly before the onset of seizures. The infection itself is not particularly impressive (Piatt et al., 1988).

Seizures

The seizures usually began before age ten and persist, being resistant to anticonvulsant therapy. Progressive partial focal seizures, with or without secondary generalization, emerge. Simple partial motor seizures are seen in all patients, with some patients also developing complex partial seizures. In some (20%), the onset may be an episode of status epilepticus. Most exhibit more than one seizure pattern. The seizures are frequent in many patients (67%), occurring at least daily. The simple motor seizures often degenerate into epilepsia partialis continua, if not already present at the onset; these can last hours to years. The seizures usually come from one hemisphere, with contralateral corresponding focal epileptiform activity. Independent seizures from either hemisphere may develop with disease progression (So & Andermann, 1997; Piatt et al., 1988).

Unilateral progressive cerebral damage

A spastic hemiparesis ipsilateral to the focal seizures develops gradually over three months to ten years, usually in a smoldering manner, although occasionally abrupt deficits may occur. Hemiatrophy of the involved side may become evident, particularly in cases of early onset. The motor deficit eventually leads to loss of voluntary hand function. The ability to walk is not lost. There is often a deterioration of intellectual function and speech and language skills, as well as other neurologic deficits (Rasmussen et al., 1958). Mild to severe mental retardation usually emerges (85%). Other cortical deficits may emerge, including progressive hemianopsia, cortical sensory loss, and progressive dysphasia, in descending order (So & Andermann, 1997; Piatt et al., 1988). Behavior disorders may also be seen (Piatt et al., 1988).

Course

There is a three-stage clinical course. Stage I is from the time of seizure onset to the time of development of the hemiparesis, lasting from three months to ten years. Stage II is the period of active neurologic deterioration subsequent to the appearance of the hemiparesis, lasting from two months to ten years. The patient may become aphasic and hemiplegic, with developmental arrest or regression. Psychological deficits and behavior disorders are apparent (Capovilla *et al.*, 1997). Seizures continue to intensify during this time. In stage III, the patient plateaus and the seizures may lessen in severity.

Examination

Initially at the seizure onset, the examination may be normal. Later, an emerging spastic hemiparesis with unilateral atrophy and ipsilateral functional deficits become apparent, including ipsilateral loss of sensation, loss of contralateral vision, a receptive or expressive aphasia (if the dominant hemisphere is involved), and memory problems.

Diagnostics

The clinical, electrical, and MRI features are diagnostic for Rasmussen's syndrome from the onset of the disease. Early signs include stereotyped focal seizures associated with contralateral EEG focal slow activity and with contralateral MRI focal abnormalities. If the patient is not operated on early, the frequency of seizures increases progressively. Intractability is established within months of onset (Granata *et al.*, 2000).

Electroencephalography

Nearly all patients show low-voltage polymorphic slow waves in the affected hemisphere, with more localized epileptiform waveforms amid the gradually spreading involved area of slow-wave abnormality. The persistent focal slow or epileptic EEG activity appears in all cases between one day and four months after the onset of the seizures. Bilateral independent discharges may be found in one-third of patients. Even when bilateral, asymmetry is usually present sufficiently to permit lateralization to one hemisphere (90%). Occasional bilaterally synchronous spike-wave complexes are seen (45%) (Rasmussen *et al.*, 1958; Granata *et al.*, 2000).

Recorded seizures tend to be poorly localized, and the correlation between the ictal EEG and clinical signs is often poor, especially in epilespia partialis continua. Independent seizures can be recorded from each hemisphere in a few patients. The EEG abnormalities are progressive, both in the degree of severity and the topography (So & Andermann, 1997).

Serial studies show that the initial simple partial seizures are associated with the intermittent variable slow activities, at which point the CT and MRI are normal. As the seizure pattern develops, localized hypoperfusion in the focal slowing area appears on the SPECT. The seizures may recur as multifocal seizure sites. The MRI then begins to show focal mild atrophy. At the onset of the epilepsia partialis continua, there may be contralateral appearance of central spikes and marked continuous slowing, with occasional independent vertex spikes associated with the appearance of mild hemiparesis (Capovilla *et al.*, 1997).

Radiology

Neuroimaging confirms the diagnosis. CT can demonstrate a progressive lateralized cerebral atrophy with localized or lateralized functional abnormalities, while MRI can reveal focal abnormalities within the first month. White-matter hyperintensification with signal enlargement of the Sylvian fissure and lateral ventricular atrophy involving the frontal and parietal areas, as well as some atrophy of the caudate head, may be seen (Granata *et al.*, 2000). Patches of increased protein density may be seen in the cortex and sometimes in the white mater before the appearance of the atrophy. Bilateral signal abnormalities may be seen.

Metabolic functional studies, as with PET and SPECT, may show lateralized focal abnormalities of glucose metabolism at the site of the seizure focus before the atrophy. Lateralized regional hypoperfusion may be seen interictally, whereas hyperperfusion correlates with the ictal state. Proton magnetic resonance spectroscopy shows reduced *N*-acetyl-L-aspartate concentration in the diseased hemisphere and sometimes elevated lactate levels in patients presenting with epilepsia partialis continuans (Piatt *et al.*, 1988; So & Andermann, 1997).

Other tests

Occasionally, the spinal fluid may reveal an excess of inflammatory cells or protein evaluations, but this does not parallel the clinical activity. Viral studies have been unrewarding. Occasional CSF oligoclonal banding and elevated immunoglobulin G (IgG) findings have been noted. Antibodies to type 3 glutamate receptor (GluR3) have been demonstrated, but no consistent abnormalities have been seen in blood tests (Rasmussen *et al.*, 1958; Capovilla *et al.*, 1997; Piatt *et al.*, 1988).

Neuropsychologic studies

Psychological studies often reveal global impairments in mental functions. Functional problems in patients with a unilateral disease are often diffuse or bilateral. Neuropsychological testing demonstrates bilateral deficits in 60–70% (So & Andermann, 1997).

Epidemiology

This is a relatively uncommon condition, occurring worldwide without any seasonal or epidemic pattern and seemingly non-familial (So & Andermann, 1997).

Pathology

The common pathologic findings are of perivascular lymphocytic cuffing (7%), microglial nodules in the cortex, and to a lesser degree in the white matter, and neuronal loss, originally thought to be suggestive of a chronic viral infection (Rasmussen *et al.*, 1958; McNamara, 1995). Astrogliosis associated with neuronal loss is a common non-specific finding in epilepsy, but the microglial inflammatory infiltrate is not usual (Piatt *et al.*, 1988). Occasionally, some spongy degeneration and some more destructive areas with little if any inflammatory reaction may be found. In more rapidly advancing cases, more intensive inflammatory changes may be noted, especially with the epilepsia partialis continua. Re-biopsy of the involved area appears to show an advancing pathologic front (Yacubian *et al.*, 1999).

Outlook

The course of this syndrome is relentless, and efforts to control the seizures or to overcome hypothesized suspect causes are not very effective.

Cause

The etiology of Rasmussen's encephalitis has been postulated to be a chronic or slow focal virus infection (Rasmussen *et al.*, 1958; Aguilar & Rasmussen, 1960), an immune reaction following an acute viral infection, or a focal immune reaction (Pardo *et al.*, 2000). The exact cause and mechanism is not known. It is speculated that the syndrome may be an autoimmune disorder involving antibodies bound to nerve cells that are potentially damaging to the brain. A nerve protein, GluR3, has been studied. Active immune T-cells toxic to the nerve cells have been found in the inflammatory brain biopsies from Rasmussen's patients. There may be a history of a minor infection or head injury, but the exact trigger of an abnormal reaction remains unknown.

Treatment

Medical treatment, including antiepileptic drugs and other pharmacological therapies, as well as corticosteroids and gamma globulins, are of very little value in Rasmussen's encephalitis, but they can delay the need for radical surgery that is inevitable in most cases (Capovilla *et al.*, 1997). The seizures, and particularly the epilepsia partialis continuans, appear resistant to antiepileptic therapy (So & Andermann, 1997). A ketogenic diet has also been tried.

Steroids, antiviral agents (such as aciclovir, ganciclovir, and zidovudine), interferon, plasmaphoresis exchange (to remove the GluR3 antibodies) (Capovilla *et al.*, 1997), immunoglobulins, and immunosuppressive agents (intravenous cyclophosphamide) have all been tried separately or in combination. Seizures and motor function may respond more than intellectual function (Knight *et al.*, 1999), but the response is often only transient. With steroids and immunoglobulins, behavior problems and psychoses as well as fluid retention have occurred. Sooner or later, after several months, the patient relapses and continues to deteriorate (So & Andermann, 1997). In a single case, immunoglobulin immunoadsorption was effective, preventing the need for surgery (Fusco *et al.*, 2000).

Neurosurgical approaches

Surgery, especially if conservative, often provides only a pause in the progression, to be followed later by a reactivation. There has been debate over the extent of surgical removal that is necessary to halt the disease and yet preserve functions, especially if language is involved. When motor, sensory, and language functions are preserved at least partially, there may be reluctance to be more vigorous in the surgical removal, but this results in a markedly reduced chance for lasting seizure control (So & Andermann, 1997). A hemispherectomy, although sacrificing some functions, often may lead to markedly better control and, in a majority, alleviation of seizures. Even language abilities are recovered to a degree beyond the usual expectations.

Cortical excision may modestly reduce the seizure frequency but does not halt the disease progression or neurologic deterioration. Any benefits are temporary (Aguilar & Rasmussen, 1960). It serves essentially as a diagnostic biopsy and little more (So & Andermann, 1997). If not already present, a dysarthria may emerge even after the excision (Piatt *et al.*, 1988).

A hemidecorticectomy may provide respite, with relief and recovery of language functions. After a year, however, the resistant seizures will return and language will regress. Reinvestigation may reveal residual overlooked tissue, which, if removed, may lead to seizure control and language recovery. Residual epileptic tissue may inhibit recruitment of the right hemisphere for language functions (Boatman *et al.*, 1999).

An early hemispherectomy is followed by complete seizure remission, stabilization of the neurologic deterioration, and general improvement in functioning, as it may halt the disease process (Piatt *et al.*, 1988; So & Andermann, 1997). Children achieve epilepsy and motor skill benefits from either an anatomically total or a subtotal functional hemispherectomy (Hecker *et al.*, 1991; Tenembaum *et al.*, 1999). A hemispherectomy provides improved (86%) to complete (60–75%) seizure control. General cognitive functions improve due to removal or disconnection of the diseased interfering hemisphere, and only a few patients show any decline. Residual defects include spastic hemiplegia (but improved gait) and visual neglect to the opposite side, in which the patient ignores items on that side. Most children make appropriate cognitive gains (So & Andermann, 1997; Knight *et al.*, 1999). Recovery of language processes appears to be related to the age of onset and duration of the illness. In the preschool years, children improve significantly. In childhood, if the hemispherectomy includes the language area, an amazing degree of recovery may ensue, especially if the surgery is performed within a year or so after onset. Even in adolescence, useful recovery can be obtained with intense remediation.

In this disorder, there is an acquired aphasia, but speech can develop in the other hemisphere, unlike in Landau–Kleffner syndrome, in which both sides are involved. Children operated on have hypometabolism of the non-resected pre-frontal cortex, but this is not seen after hemispherectomy. Postoperative prefrontal hypometabolism and persistent developmental delays may persist if the patient is operated on years after the seizure onset (Caplan *et al.*, 1993; So & Andermann, 1997).

REFERENCES

Aguilar, J. M. & Rasmussen, J. (1960). Role of encephalitis in pathogenesis of epilepsy. *Arch. Neurol.* **2**: 663–76.

Belousova, E., Perminov, V., Baev, A., *et al.* (1998). Congenital bilateral perisylvian syndrome. 3rd European Congress of Epileptology. *Epilepsia* **39** (suppl 2): 54.

Boatman, D., Stephenson, D., Vining, E., *et al.* (1999). Left mesial temporal lobe dysfunction can interfere with right sided language function. *Epilepsia* **40** (suppl 7): 45–6.

Caplan, R., Surtiss, S., Chugani, H. T., *et al.* (1993). Thought processing, language, glucose metabolic patterns and pathology in hemispherectomy patients with Rasmussen's encephalitis. *Epilepsia* **34** (suppl 6): 101.

Capovilla, G., Paladin, F. & Bernadina, B. D. (1997). Rasmussen's syndrome: longitudinal EEG study from the first seizure to epilepsia partialis continua. *Epilepsia* **38**: 483–8.

Engel, J. & Wilson, C. L. (1986). Evidence for enhanced synaptic inhibition in epilepsy. In *Neurotransmitters, Seizures and Epilepsy*, ed. G. Nistico, pp. 1–13. New York: Raven Press.

Fusco, L., Granata, T., Gobbi, G., *et al.* (2000). The role of medical treatment in Rasmussen's encephalitis. *Epilepsia* **41** (suppl 7): 129.

Granata T, Fusco L, Gobbi G., *et al.* (2000). Early clinical and instrumental findings of Rasmussen's encephalitis. *Epilepsia* **41** (suppl 7): 114.

Hecker, A., Guekos-Thoni, U., Egli, M., *et al.* (1991). Hemispherectomy for Rasmussen Syndrome. 19th International Epilepsy Congress. *Epilepsia* **32** (suppl 1): 18.

Knight, E. S., Oxbury, J. M., Oxbury, S. M., *et al.* (1999). Long term cognitive development following treatment of Rasmussen's encephalitis. *Epilepsia* **40** (suppl 7): 48.

Kuzniecky, R., Andermann, F. & Guerrini, R. (1991a). Congenital bilateral perisylvian ayndrome: a new recognizable entity. 19th International Epilepsy Congress. *Epilepsia* **32** (suppl 1): 16.

Kuzniecky, R., Andermann, R., Guerrini, R., *et al.* (1991b). Electrographic findings in the congenital bilateral perisylvian syndrome. *Epilepsia* **32** (suppl 3): 51.

Kuzniecky, R., Andermann, F. & Guerrini, R. (1993b). Congenital bilateral perisylvian syndrome: study of 31 patients. The congential bilateral perisylvian syndrome multicenter collaborative study. *Lancet* **341**: 608–12.

Kuzniecky, R., Anderman, F., Guerrini, R., *et al.* (1994). The epileptic spectrum in the congenital bilateral perisylvian syndrome. *Neurology* **44**: 379–85.

Kuzniecky, R., Andermann, F., Tampieri, D., *et al.* (1989). Bilateral central macrogyria; epilepsy, pseudobulbar palsy and mental retardation – a recognizable neuronal migration disorder. *Ann. Neurol.* **25**: 547–54.

Kuzniecky, T., Mutto, S., King, D., *et al.* (1993a). Magnetic resonance imaging in childhood intractable partial epilepsy: pathologic correlations. *Neurology* **43**: 681–7.

McNamara, J. O. (1995). Autoimmunity and Lennox. Presented at the American Epilepsy Society Conference, Baltimore, MD, December 1995.

Mikati, M. A., Lee, W. L. & DeLong, G. R. (1985). Protracted epileptiform encephalopathy: an unusual form of partial complex status epilepticus. *Epilepsia* **26**: 563–71.

Pardo, C. A., Irani, D., Vining, E. P., *et al.* (2000). The immunopathology of Rasmussen's syndrome: chemokines and chemokine-receptors response. *Epilepsia* **41** (suppl 7): 82.

Piatt, J. H., Hwang, P. A., Armstrong, D. C., *et al.* (1988). Chronic focal encephalitis (Rasmussen syndrome): six cases. *Epilepsia* **29**: 268–79.

Rasmussen, T., Olszewski J. & Lloyd-Smith, D. (1958). Focal seizures due to chronic localized encpehalitiies. *Neurology* **8**: 435–45.

Roulet, E., Deonna, T. & Despland, P. A. (1989). Prolonged intermittent drooling and oromotor apraxia in benign childhood epilepsy with centrotemporal spikes. *Epilepsia* **30**: 564–8.

Sells, C. J., Carpenter, R. L. & Ray, C. G. (1975). Sequelae of central nervous system enterovirus infections. *N. Engl. J. Med.* **293**: 1–4.

Shafrir, Y. & Prensky, A. L. (1995). Acquired epileptiform opercular syndrome: a second case report, review of the literature, and comparison to the Landau Kleffner syndrome. *Epilepsia* **36**: 1050–57.

So, N. S. & Andermann, F. (1997). Rasmussen's syndrome. In *Epilepsy: A Comprehensive Textbook*, ed. J. Engel & T. A. Pedley, pp. 2379–88. Philadelphia: Lippincott-Raven.

Tenembaum, S., Soprano, A. M., Pomata, H., *et al.* (1999). Epilepsy and neuropsychological outcome after surgery in children with Rasmussen's encephalitis. 23rd International Epilepsy Congress. *Epilepsia* **40** (suppl 2): 85.

Yacubian, E. M., Rosemberg, S., Jorge, C. I., *et al.* (1999). Pathological variability in a series of 17 patients with Rasmussen's syndrome. 23rd International Epilepsy Congress. *Epilepsia* **40** (suppl 2): 57–8.

8

Seizure-management effects

Hippocrates warned, "What is one man's pleasure is another man's poison." This can be applied to antiepileptic drugs. What helps one patient may do nothing for a second patient and may produce undesirable side effects in a third patient.

Antiepileptic drug helps and hindrances

Pharmacologic principles

An antiepileptic drug does not affect only a specific brain site and a specific function. Rather, it affects the entire brain and many functions. Some basic principles help in understanding these effects.

Some seizures are due to excessive discharges of parts of the brain, as with partial seizures. Some seizures are due to bursts of inhibition from deeper portions of the brain, as with absence, myoclonic, and atonic seizures. With focal discharge, enlargement of the discharge area and the spread to involve distant sites are important.

Inhibiting excessive excitation and vice versa

Anticonvulsants act by inhibiting excess discharges, by provoking excessive inhibition, or by stopping the discharge spread. The actions of the brain are mediated by neurotransmitters. There are inhibitory neurotransmitters and excitatory neurotransmitters. Antiepileptic drugs tend to mimic the neurotransmitters, block the neurotransmitter actions, facilitate the production of neurotransmitters or inhibit the breakdown and removal of them.

Stopping the focus, enlargement, and spread

Antiepileptic action may be to inhibit a focus from firing, to limit the focus from becoming large enough to produce a seizure, or to limit the spread from the focus to other parts of the brain. If the area of discharge increases in size or strength of firing, it may involve adjacent or sometimes distant sites, sufficient to overcome the natural inhibition of the nervous system, and a seizure event thus occurs. Even if a seizure does not occur, the enlarged discharge area, or the response of the adjacent brain to inhibit the discharge, may impair functions within the involved area. Drugs that inhibit discharging cells may also inhibit related cognitive and language functions.

Drugs affect more than just seizure discharges

If the discharging focus inhibits or distorts a cognitive, linguistic, or behavior signal traveling the involved neural pathway, the antiepileptic drugs that inhibit the focus may improve the related brain functions. Drugs that inhibit only the enlargement of the focus are less apt to benefit the associated dysfunctions. Drugs that primarily prevent the spread may have little benefit to the function in that area.

The antiepileptic medication effect targets specific neurotransmitters or neurons, not brain regions. The effect of the drug affects the entire brain, wherever the neurotransmitter or neuronal targets are located, not just at the seizure focus. Consequently, the drug can affect other related functions.

Drugs that inhibit undesired excessive brain discharges tend to also inhibit desired brain functions, such as alertness, rate of thinking, and language flow. Drugs that augment brain activity to overcome the inhibition of seizures produced by bursts of excessive inhibitory activity tend not to impair alertness, cognition, or language activities but occasionally they can remove inhibitions from unwanted activities, i.e. behaviors.

Older versus newer drugs

The antiepileptic drugs discovered in the early twentieth century dominated the medication control attempts of epilepsy throughout that century. These drugs are based on the original barbiturate structure. They tend to be inhibitory drugs, causing sedation and slowed functions. This effect extends beyond the brain, calming down excessive reactions in other organs. The barbiturates and their derivatives produce both good effects and side effects in the central nervous system and in other organs. The established antiepileptic drugs are so similar in structure, i.e. of a barbiturate background, that if more than one or two are prescribed together the drugs are more apt to augment adverse aspects than to improve seizure control. Thus, the rule of thumb was one drug usually, two drugs seldom, three drugs rarely, and four or more drugs never. Newer drugs that are novel in design are less apt to be additive in side effects.

Neurotransmitters are messenger agents promoting or inhibiting cell activities, depending on the type of neurotransmitter endings. These neurotransmitter agents also facilitate language, learning processes, and emotions. The newly designed antiepileptic drugs are often targeted to specific neurotransmitter systems involved in seizure production, and thus can be selected in additive combinations without being additive in side effects. However, these new drugs may also alter the neural functions subserved by the transmitter(s), both cognitive and behavioral. The newer drugs, being designed to mimic neurotransmitters, are more limited in action to the CNS, where both desired and undesired effects are seen. The side effects appear to affect primarily brain function. Thus, researchers learned to begin at lower dosages and make increases slowly to avoid the initial sensitivity by allowing the brain chemistry to adjust to the new drugs.

Inhibition versus excitation

The inhibitory antiepileptic drugs, like the barbiturates, inhibit the excess discharges of the partial seizures but also increase the inhibition of the inhibitory minor seizures. A side effect of such drugs may therefore be precipitation or augmentation of absences, atonic drops, and myoclonic jerks. Drugs that stimulate the brain may overcome the inhibition of minor epilepsy types of seizures but may bring out partial and generalized tonic–clonic seizures. The newer drugs are less apt to fit into the categories of inhibition versus stimulation.

Often, neurotransmitters are described as inhibitory or excitatory, but a neurotransmitter that acts as an inhibitory neurotransmitter in the temporal lobe and limbic system may act as an excitatory neurotransmitter in the frontal lobe. Neurotransmitters in the immature brain of a young infant may have one effect, but as the brain matures it may have the opposite effect. Furthermore, an active seizure site may change in its relationships to inhibitory and excitatory input circuits. If the area is damaged, cells may be lost and the remaining inhibitory input circuits may grow instead on to other inhibitory cells, resulting in the inhibition of inhibition, i.e. the creation of excitatory activity. Repeated seizures may lead to loss of effectiveness and even to paradoxical effects of selected drugs.

Rational polypharmacy

Chosen and used properly, antiepileptic drugs are apt to improve seizure control but not necessarily improve other disturbances so frequently found to be a part of the epilepsy syndrome, i.e. the learning struggles, the language disturbances, and the emotional aspects. The drugs neither find the individual a job nor help with socialization. Used improperly, anticonvulsants do not produce good seizure control and are more likely to aggravate cognition, emotion, or language problems and thus, directly or indirectly through frustration, increase the seizure frequency.

Rational drug use, especially when more than one antiepileptic drug is required, means choosing those that do not duplicate action and side effects, that complement actions, and, in consideration of a specific patient, do not bring out potential functional weaknesses. In the behavioral realm, this includes choosing an epileptic agent or drug combinations so as to enhance both seizure control and benefit related emotional side effects.

Antiepileptic drug effects on speech and language

Henry & Browne (1987) reviewed the antiepileptic drug effects on speech and language for the St Francis Epilepsy Center Conference. Anticonvulsants can affect speech and language. At a high dose, or in patients especially sensitive to the drug, the speech may be slowed, slurred, or hesitant, and the patient's overall thinking processing, including the processing of language, may be impaired. Auditory memory may be impaired. Pre-existing language-processing problems can be worsened. The use of multiple anticonvulsants or combinations of anticonvulsants with other drugs affecting the brain, such as tranquilizers, antidepressants, stimulants, etc., is more apt to produce the same problems as strong doses of a single medication. Polytherapy (the use of multiple drugs) may lessen rather than improve seizure control in some patients.

Anticonvulsant drugs rarely improve speech or language problems, unless underlying epileptiform activity interferes with the language process. Even in the latter case, improvement is often incomplete and occurs only in some patients. When a child has a seizure disorder and a speech or language problem, the child needs appropriate anticonvulsant medications selected and monitored carefully, along with speech and language therapy for the speech or language problems.

No medication is without potential side effects. The ideal drug controls the problem for which it is taken and produces no unwanted side effects, but there is no such drug. If the child presents with slowed language or mental processing, or with the appearance of slowed, slurred, unclear speech, the cause may be missed seizures or excessive anticonvulsant drug blood levels. A seizure cause will clear. The anticonvulsant intoxication will remain until the dose is changed if it is a long-acting drug, or may clear over hours but recur daily if it is a rapidly acting drug. If there is no obvious seizure by history, anticonvulsant blood levels should be checked, preferably at the time of day that the problem occurs.

Parents and teachers tend to blame problems in learning, behavior, or language on the medications rather than on the epilepsy itself or the handling of the epileptic child. Drug levels can be checked to avoid overdosages. A more careful evaluation of the problem may reveal that it is not the medication but rather the seizure disorder, and reactions to it, that is the problem.

Drugs for major seizures

Drugs that are used most often to treat partial seizures and generalized tonic–clonic seizures include the barbiturates, the hydantoins, carbamazepine, and valproate, which is a broad-spectrum drug.

Barbiturates

The barbiturates include phenobarbital, mephobarbital, metharbital, and a related drug, primidone. Mephobarbital and metharbital were touted as avoiding the behavioral side effects of the barbiturates, but only because the levels proved not to be sustained at an adequate dosage. Barbiturates can impair verbal learning and depress auditory processing, especially auditory discrimination and auditory memory (especially sequential memory), and impair language comprehension and verbal expression. These effects are seen at higher therapeutic levels. A reduction of spontaneous speech efforts and speech slurring may be noted. If a focal seizure discharge interferes with speech or language, occasionally phenobarbital may help to overcome this. Otherwise, there are no direct benefits with speech and language problems.

Hydantoins

The hydantoins consist of phenytoin and the older drugs ethotoin and mephenytoin, which are no longer used. Rarely, phenytoin has been claimed to benefit children with speech or language problems who have a temporal lobe epileptiform EEG. There is no report of any significant language or speech problems nor benefits noted with phenytoin at therapeutic levels, although one patient with aphasia presenting with the utterance of nonsensical "words" was noted that cleared when the patient was switched to phenobarbital. If phenytoin levels are slightly high or if the patient is especially sensitive to the drug, slowed and slurred speech, often with a slowed speaking rate, is seen as an early symptom of intoxication. Phenytoin may impair auditory memory.

Carbamazepine

Carbamazepine, in both regular and long-acting forms, is the only drug in this group. A new, related drug, oxcarbamazepine, may offer similar benefits with fewer side effects. Carbamazepine may speed up speech and improve vocabulary. Some patients are more talkative when on carbamazepine. One child with chronic speech articulation and language-processing problems normalized abruptly when started on carbamazepine for bitemporal complex partial epilepsy. No speech or language impairments have been noted with carbamazepine. Periods of slurred speech may occur if the drug levels get high, especially if the patient takes the medicine on an empty stomach. Neither carbamazepine monotherapy nor carbamazepine in combination with vigabatrin alter P300 potentials (Mervaala *et al.*, 1993).

Valproate

Valproate is a useful drug for nearly all types of seizures. It may improve a child's ability to communicate. Impairments in speaking have been noted with the use of this drug. Slurred speech has been a problem with stronger doses. When used in combination with other drugs, the protein-binding potential of valproate may drive more of the unbound form of other protein-binding drugs into the brain, resulting in signs of intoxication (slurred speech, memory problems, etc.) despite normal drug levels on testing. Some children have been said to display "speaking ability damage," with retardation of speech, slowed motor behavior, and slurring of speech, the latter associated with ataxia and nystagmus, thus suggesting intoxication.

Rarely, valproate may induce hearing, motor, and cognitive impairments. In several studies, 25–42% of individuals, following complaints, were found to have worsening of hearing. Often, this was associated with motor and cognitive impairment. Worsening was documented in those with prior audiograms (Karageorgiou *et al.*, 1991; Morales *et al.*, 1992). After discontinuing the medication, 91% of patients improve. Three patterns of impairment are seen: low-frequency changes only when a severe high-frequency deficit is present, high-frequency changes when a mild low-frequency deficit is present, and both high- and low-frequency changes (Armon *et al.*, 1991). Valproate and ethosuximide significantly prolong auditory conduction velocity, as shown by brainstem auditory evoked testing (Morales *et al.*, 1992). At supratherapeutic serum valproate levels, the III–IV interpeak latency is prolonged, suggesting that valproate influences brainstem conduction (Karageorgiou *et al.*, 1991).

Drugs for minor seizures

Minor seizure medications are used for minor seizures such as absence stares, atonic drops, akinetic pauses, and myoclonic drops. Such medications include the succinimides, the benzodiazepines, the diones (which are no longer used), and valproate.

Benzodiazepines

This group includes diazepam, clonazepam, nitrazepam, and lorazepam, and a similar drug, clorazepate. These drugs may all render a child more talkative but are apt to make the speech slurred and difficult to understand. Sometimes it is difficult to hear what the child is saying due to the very soft speech. The spoken efforts may appear to be blocked, and sentences and phrases may be incomplete. This is seen when such drugs are used at high therapeutic doses or if the child is especially sensitive to the drugs. Diazepam has been associated with slurring of speech with a dysarthria. The saliva accumulation accentuates articulation problems.

With clonazepam, speech problems include a "thick tongue." The child's speech may be slurred. Swallowing difficulties are a major difficulty. Some children may have problems in handling an excess of saliva. Slurring of speech, an increase in spoken efforts but with difficulties in being understood are seen, along with blocking or incompleteness of sentences and phrases (Browne, 1970; Gottschalk *et al.*, 1972; Gottschalk, 1977; Wilson *et al.*, 1983).

Clobazam has been associated with an aphasia in which the patient spoke nonsensical words with a monotone pattern lacking any emphasis. When the drug was discontinued, the aphasia cleared up. Clorazepate has also been linked with a tendency towards slurred speech.

Diones

The diones consist of trimethadione and paramethadione. These are now used infrequently, although they have not been associated with any specific speech or language problems.

Succinimides

The succinimides consist of ethosuximide methsuximide, and phensuximide; the latter two are no longer commonly used. These drugs are relatively free of language-impairment potentials. Ethosuximide has been reported to improve verbal learning. Speech disturbances have been suggested, but no specific problems have been identified and no other family members exhibited speech or language difficulties.

New anticonvulsants

In the past decade, a number of new drugs that differ markedly from the older established anticonvulsants have emerged. These are available for partial seizures, especially complex partial and secondarily generalized seizures, but some of these new drugs have shown the potential for widespread actions on many seizure types. The new drugs have been designed to mimic neurotransmitters that carry messages between cells in the brain.

Felbamate is a drug for partial epilepsies and Lennox–Gastaut syndrome. Potentially, it may offer a broader spectrum of activity. However, some individuals cannot tolerate the drug, developing either aplastic anemia or hepatitis, leading to a marked reduction in the use of this very effective antiepileptic drug. There are no specific language impairments. Some individuals may do better in speech, because felbamate has a brightening rather than a sedative effect. One retarded child brightened up and began to talk when placed on the drug.

Gabapentin was originally designed to help with nerve pain but it was found to be effective for partial seizures. It is safe and thus useful for elderly patients, who have problems tolerating medications. At high dosages, speech may be slurred, but otherwise there are no specific speech and language problems noted.

Lamotrigine is another new drug released for partial epilepsies but with the potential to be another broad-spectrum antiepileptic medication. If given to a patient already on valproate, lamotrigine must be initiated at a lower dosage and increased very slowly to avoid rashes. In retarded patients, lamotrigine may produce improvements in alertness, mobility, speech, and independence in 65%. Rarely, speech disorders and dysarthria have been reported.

Levetiracetam has not been associated with any specific speech or language disorders, although experience with this drug is somewhat limited.

Losigamone, a drug that is still in trial, has been reported to produce dysarthria in a few patients.

Sulthiame has produced drooling, which can affect articulation.

Tiagabine may produce speech difficulties if the dose is built up too rapidly or to too high a level. Thus, the medication is begun at a low dosage and increased slowly. A very small percentage of patients on this drug may experience speech problems, such as dysarthria, or language problems (0.2–0.4%).

Oxcarbamazepine is related to carbamazepine, but it is metabolized in the body by a different pathway, avoiding the toxic by-products that carbamazepine may produce. Speech and language problems have been reported at higher doses.

Topiramate is a newer, potent anticonvulsant with numerous methods of action in the brain. It has been released for partial and primarily generalized seizures, but it may prove to be very broad spectrum in its potential as it exhibits multiple types of antiepileptic activity. As it is a potent antiepileptic drug, it is also at high risk to produce other brain effects, many of which are undesirable. If it is started at too strong a dose or increased too rapidly, the patient may become drowsy and confused, with problems in thinking, especially if the patient had a prior history of problems in thinking or in behavior. Language problems may be significant, with speech hesitancy and word-finding (memory) difficulties. This sensitivity is seen especially in the first few months of use. Therefore, the rule of thumb in prescribing this medication is to start low and increase slow. Even after the initial extrasensitivity of the first few months has subsided, there may be problems in speech and language, with aphasia, dysnomia (word-finding disturbances), and hesitancy (1–11%). Such problems, although usually transient, may recur with increasing dosages. These patients have retrieval problems for semantic information. Problems in initiating speech may be noted.

Impairment of language as a side effect of the sulfa-containing antiepileptic drugs (zonisamide and topiramate) is different from the side effects of other anticonvulsants. This suggests that these drugs may interfere with the chemistry in language neurocircuitry. Nearly 4% of patients placed on topiramate complain of language-only deficits, such as anomia, impaired verbal expression, other language problems, and impaired cognition. Retarded patients with limited vocabulary become mute but more alert (Ojemann *et al.*, 1999).

Vigabatrin was a very effective drug in patients with complex partial seizures and with West's syndrome, but soon after release it was found to produce peripheral vision loss. It was withdrawn from the market. Some patients experienced memory problems, word-finding difficulties, and word-substitution problems when on the drug.

Zonisamide is another new drug for complex partial seizures that potentially may help with myoclonic seizures. Memory difficulties and slowness of thought may impair speaking efforts in a few patients. Zonisamide produces anomia (12%) and dysnomia (12%). In a trial of the drug a lower verbal IQ score was seen with a trend for poorer performance IQ in half the patients on high-dose zonisamide (Ojemann *et al.*, 1999). Communication difficulties may be seen (Mandelbaum *et al.*, 2001).

Seizure surgery and speech and language functions

Gates (1999) reviewed surgical options at an American Epilepsy Society pre-conference on the vagal nerve stimulator. Seizure surgery candidates are evaluated to determine the laterality and focality of the seizure discharge.

Temporal lobectomy

Children with seizures not responding to tolerated antiepileptic mediations used appropriately, and especially those who may be developing language or learning problems, may be considered for a temporal lobectomy not only for seizure control but also to avoid the adverse effects on functioning and socialization. Early surgery may avoid the risk of language and memory decline and take advantage of the young brain's plasticity to allow greater recovery of functions.

Preoperative work-up

The dominant temporal lobe is more limited in the amount of brain tissue that can be resected. Speech needs to be localized and other speech areas (lateral-temporal, suprafrontal) located. The speech area is not always where it is supposed to be. Reorganization of language function after focal brain injury shows that contra-hemisphere contributions can emerge, even in adulthood. There is a risk of post-operative aphasia even in right temporal lobectomy (Speer *et al.*, 2001).

Although the side of the seizures is a key predictor of language change, the age of onset may also be important, since later onset increases the risks for postoperative language deficits. Women have more language sites, with less lateralization and more symmetric verbal memory and hippocampal volume correlations (Loring *et al.*, 1988; Langfiitt & Rausch, 1996; Trenerry *et al.*, 1995). A greater risk of decline is associated with higher performance level (Chelune *et al.*, 1991). Removal of damaged cortex improves comprehension and general fluency (Saykin *et al.*, 1995; Hermann & Wyler, 1988; Davies *et al.*, 1995; Loring *et al.*, 1988).

Hemisphere dominance for language should be assessed before approaching any temporal surgery, in light of the variability of lateralization and localization found (Devinsky *et al.*, 2000). There are a variety of approaches used in determining the lateralization and localization of language in individuals, including handedness and family history, neuropsychological results, especially naming, the Wada test, regional cerebral activation of blood flow (PET, functional magnetic resonance imaging (fMRI)), and electrocorticography (EcoG). Newer, less invasive methods of assessing language laterality and localization such as fMRI and transcranial magnetic activity are being researched. Each new technique shows biases.

Intracarotid amytal (Wada) testing

The Wada test, in which a fast-acting barbiturate is injected into the arteries carrying blood to the brain, one side at a time is most useful. This results in half of the brain being anesthetized briefly. During this time, specific psychologic and language tests are performed to see which skills are lost when one side of the brain is put to sleep.

The pediatric intracarotid amobarbital procedure can clarify the hemispheric language dominance in most verbal, school-age, preadolescent children with at least borderline intelligence and in many children with mental retardation. In children, the testing requires extra pretest teaching and emotional preparation. Memory retention scores tend to be lower in children than in adults and thus must be interpreted cautiously, especially in children who are retarded (Szabo & Wyllie, 1993; Williams & Rausch, 1991). Most of the children who fail the test are less than 12 years of age, with left language dominance and left-sided lesions (Szabo & Wyllie, 1993; Williams & Rausch, 1991). This testing has been performed in children with fairly good responses, especially after eight years of age. In patients undergoing temporal lobectomy after neuropsychological testing and amytal testing but no cortical stimulation mapping, those with a left dominant temporal lobe epilepsy showed no significant loss of language functions and actually gained in many parameters after a conservative resection (Davies *et al.*, 1995).

Functional imagery

Hemispheric dominance for language can be assessed by fMRI, a non-invasive technique for demonstrating cerebral activation associated with language tasks, which correlates well with the WADA test. The results may influence further diagnostic work-up and should be performed before other invasive diagnostic procedures, as occasionally the fMRI unexpectedly reveals right-hemispheric language dominance, influencing further presurgical diagnostic assessment (Speer *et al.*, 2001).

Cortical mapping

Cortical mapping of language functions in patients before a standard temporal lobotomy or lateral resections may reduce the incidence of postoperative language impairments, such as anomia. Mapping of eloquent cortex may be done by electrocorticography before surgery and also as part of the surgical approach. Atypical large cortical representations or multiple sites of language, such as those involving the inferior or anterior temporal cortex, are seen in patients with lower IQ, fewer years of education, poorer verbal memory, reduced confrontation naming, and reduced verbal fluency (Devinsky *et al.*, 2000; Loring & Meador, 2001).

Surgical approaches

The extent of temporal neocortical resection varies. Resection of the superior temporal gyrus may be done (Loring *et al.*, 1988). The goal of functional surgery is to remove or destroy cellular centers or to interrupt neural pathways of seizure spread. The most common seizure surgery is the removal of all or, more often, part of the temporal lobe for control of complex partial seizures resistant to medical therapy. The major concern is that the surgery should not remove any vital language center. To optimize the results, as much hippocampus as possible should be resected. The risk of taking more of the hippocampus posteriorly is damage to vital arteries, so these vessels need to be left intact. Memories already stored are not affected because the storage is more diffuse throughout the brain.

Results

About 70–80% of patients can be rendered seizure-free. About 90% show significant improvement, but 7% do not improve.

The temporal lobe is involved intimately with higher-level perceptual processing of sounds. A number of studies have focused on identifying possible postoperative changes in hearing function. Many have evaluated dichotic listening. In some patients, contralateral ear deficits are combined with improved postoperative discrimination in ipsilateral ears. These studies suggest that very little, if any, improvement in central auditory functioning is expected following temporal lobe surgery. Some report markedly improved skills in dichotic digit tests and P300 event-related potentials. Some children may show slight improvement in central auditory processing, but others show minimal improvement. Severe discrimination deficits found in the ear contralateral to the diseased hemisphere may be ameliorated following surgery. Testing, utilizing the SCAN test for central auditory processing in children, dichotic digit tests, duration pattern tests, and the P300 event-related potential test performed immediately postoperatively and one year later in children, reveal postoperative improvements in some patients but no changes or poorer postoperative performance in others. Temporal lobotomies, while controlling seizures, may not always improve auditory processing (Cranford *et al.*, 1996).

Postoperative complications

The complication rate is no higher than 1%. Conservative surgery on the dominant (i.e. language-related) temporal lobe of severely handicapped seizure patients may result in an anomia for the names of people and things more than for verbs. Risks for anomia appear greater in patients with no identifiable early risk factors for epilepsy. Other language-related memory problems might occur, especially in the first few months after the surgery. Fluency is not affected. Some patients experience aphasic symptoms that improve or normalize over time with dominant temporal lobe surgery. This is not seen in non-dominant temporal lobe patients, who instead may have problems in remembering things they have seen. Postoperative language declines are greater in patients who do not have a classical syndrome of mesial temporal lobe epilepsy, i.e. early onset age and hippocampal sclerosis (Milner, 1975; Loring et al., 1988). Both left and right temporal lobectomy patients show variable decreases in episodic verbal memory, but those with a right temporal lobectomy show no language decreases and may show improvement instead (Davies et al., 1995).

Postoperatively, children, particularly those with a left temporal focus, may show a reduced language performance (Lendt et al., 1999). Children and adolescents younger than 17 years do not appear at any unusual risk of postoperative verbal impairment. Up to 10% may experience a decline in verbal intelligence skills, although 9% experience significant improvement in verbal functioning. Risks for decline include the age at which surgery is undertaken and the presence of structural lesions other than mesial temporal sclerosis (Loring & Meador, 2001).

Neocortical resections

Gates (1999) found that the majority of refractory partial epilepsies of childhood onset are extratemporal, i.e. from some part of the brain other than the temporal lobe. If a heterotopia or focal dysplasia is found, surgery can be considered. In lesional partial epilepsy, both the lesion and the epileptic halo must be mapped out. Neocortical non-lesional surgery is less successful and more risky than temporal lobectomy. Multiple subpial transections may be considered, especially in areas involving vital functions.

Corpus callosum sectioning

In patients with seizures resistant to medication who are not candidates for resection of a seizure site, a corpus callosotomy may be considered to prevent the spread of the discharge, especially if the seizures are traumatic to the patient. This is not curative, but it may lessen both the frequency and severity of seizures. Candidates for this approach include those who have multifocal seizures that do not respond well to antiepileptic medications, with multifocal to generalized cerebral damage, and in whom the seizures are physically traumatic to the individual. A corpus callosum sectioning allows about 71% of patients to have a significant and valuable reduction in seizure frequency and/or intensity, but none become seizure-free (Rayport et al., 1991).

Expressive language deficits after a callosotomy have been reported in patients with mixed cerebral dominance (Crone et al., 1992). Occasional side effects include disturbances of language production, with continued mutism and impairment of attention and memory. This is most apt to occur in patients with mixed dominance and multifocal cerebral damage that undergo a two-stage approach. There is a marked decrease in spontaneous speech, repetition is intact, and paraphasic errors are rare. The individual improves with time but continues to show a lengthy verbal response latency and short phrase length. When speech is elicited, its rate can be excessive rather than slow or labored. No deficit in receptive language function is observed. The deficit occurs only after the second stage, sectioning of the posterior portion. This is not seen in individuals with right-sided dominance (Rayport *et al.*, 1984). Following an 80% callosal section study, no patients had any long-term language deficit for they seemed able to compensate and recover their skills (Crone *et al.*, 1992).

There may also be appearance of non-dominant hemispheric dysphasia due to a mixed dominance. The left-hand and left-hemisphere dominance may contribute to a dysgraphia, as may the right-hand, right-hemisphere dominance. There may be a residual mutism. Alexia without agraphia may be seen in patients with a poorly dominant hemisphere with occipital damage and a splenium section.

The possible etiologies may include underlying problems with the non-dominant hemisphere that is damaged and thus dysfunction that is compensated by the corpus callosum with the influence from the dominant hemisphere. Surgical injury to the neighboring structures may originate from traction. A single-stage commissurotomy may lead to this. Prior seizure activity and drugs may have masked the emergence of a dysfunction. Serial lesions cause fewer defects than a single, larger lesion.

Subpial transections

The concept of multiple subpial transactions (MSTs) for control of medically intractable seizures in language, memory, and sensory motor cortex is based on the concept of horizontal epileptic discharges and vertical functional organization of the cerebral cortex (Dogali *et al.*, 1992). MSTs do not disrupt behaviors but interfere with neuronal synchronization (Fried, 1999). The MST disconnects horizontal connections to decrease seizure propagation, preserving columnar functional organization (Loring *et al.*, 1988). This is a surgical procedure designed to eliminate the capacity of cortical cells to generate epileptiform discharge without interfering substantially with normal function (Morell *et al.*, 1992). This has been performed in Broca's and Wernicke's areas (Loring & Meador, 2001).

This approach is developed especially for those with Landau–Kleffner acquired aphasia with epilepsy syndrome (Loring & Meador, 2001). It also has been used in epilepsia partialis continuans, for focal or motor sensory seizures, as well as for focal cortical dysplasias, heterotopias, and Rasmussen's syndrome. MSTs have been used with sagittal-cortical transactions on both sides of the brain to suppress propagation to the ipsilateral but not contralateral focus or in the focus itself.

Following surgery, one-third of patients recover completely; the remainder improve dramatically and are able to speak in sentences, but they still require special language training programs (Morell *et al.*, 1992). An acute anomia and paraphasia without significant language impairment is seen afterwards (Devinsky *et al.*, 1993). This may be mild in nearly half the patients. There may be moderate dysnomia in about 22%, with partial recovery over time. Patients are able to return to school or work (Loring & Meador, 2001).

Patients who undergo routine neurosurgery encroaching on primary language areas may experience greater language declines. If surgery is planned near a primary language region, mapping may help to reduce but will not totally avoid the risks. MSTs may be performed on such language regions. This approach is generally tolerated better in motor regions than in language regions. In language areas, there may be a 90% or more reduction in seizure frequency, but a significant dysnomia is seen in 69% half a year after surgery. MST is associated with poorer postoperative naming, verbal fluency, and oral reading compared with patients who undergo a standard anterior temporal lobectomy, especially at about six months postoperatively (Loring & Meador, 2001).

Hemidecortication and hemispherectomy

Hemispherectomies, as used in patients with Rasmussen's syndrome and with some developmental unilateral brain malformations, result in a spastic hemiparesis and loss of related other contralateral sensory, visual, and motor functions, including language if the dominant hemisphere is involved. A surprising amount of recovery ensues, including language, as the other hemisphere takes over. This is seen especially when the surgery is performed in a younger child.

Infants in whom a severely damaged brain half is removed (hemidecortication) show resultant language deficits to be far less than in an adult, although these children tend to have a lowered overall IQ. It would seem that in the remaining normal brain tissue, language and non-verbal abilities compete for the limited number of remaining intact nerve cells. In predicting language after hemispherectomy, the integrity of the non-resected hemisphere seems to be a reliable index that integrates and accounts for a number of variables mentioned previously in the literature (De Bode *et al.*, 2000).

Vagal stimulation

Gates (1999), Ben-Manachem (1999), and Frost (1999) reviewed their experiences for the American Epilepsy Society pre-conference on vagal nerve stimulation. Vagal nerve stimulation (VNS) is mainly an option for non-surgical candidates, offering chances of a significant reduction in seizure frequency by 25–30%, and in some up to 50%, over the ensuing year (Fried, 1999). Partial seizures are helped the most, but generalized tonic–clonic attacks and atypical absences as well as the atonic and tonic attacks of Lennox–Gastaut syndrome may benefit. Seizures are shorter, with a fast recovery and less tendency toward clustering. Improvements in alertness, verbal skills, memory, mood, and school performance emerge at three months and are even better at 15 months. Total control is attained rarely. The approach is effective, safe, and reversible.

The implantation of the vagal nerve on the side may lead to hoarseness and swallowing difficulties if excessive traction is placed on the recurrent laryngeal nerve, causing a paralysis. Occasionally, patients may complain of throat pain or cough. The stimulus itself may produce voice alterations (hoarseness or tremulousness) in up to 13% of patients. Other symptoms noted, especially when the stimulator emits an electrical charge, include a gagging sensation, cough, hoarseness, coughing when swallowing, or exertional shortness of breath. Rarely, the voice may change in pitch during the firing of the stimulus. Adverse effects are apt to affect speech rather than produce any language problems. Precipitation or perhaps an exacerbation of psychosis has been reported in one patient.

Special diets

There have been no special problems affecting speech or language with children who are on special diets for seizure control. Low blood sugar, especially in the morning time when beginning the ketogenic diet, may impair functioning, but this has been avoided by monitoring and by initiating the diet slowly. Several children with intractable seizures and multiple episodes of status, when placed on a ketogenic diet, have gradually lost their language; they had previously had normal speech development. The interictal EEGs showed multifocal spikes in sleep. The children tend to develop autistic behaviors. The seizures, however, are controlled on the ketogenic diet (Shafrir, 1999).

REFERENCES

Armon, C., Paul, R. G., Miller, P., *et al.* (1991). Valproate induced hearing impairment: active ascertainment in an epilepsy clinic population and result of therapeutic intervention. *Epilepsia* **32** (suppl 3): 8.

Ben-Manachem, E. (1999). History and theories of action. Presented at the American Epilepsy Society Conference, Orlando, FL, 1999.

Browne, T. R. (1970). Drug therapy, clonzepam. *N. Engl. J. Med.* **299**: 212–15.

Chelune, G. J., Naugle, R. I. & Luders, H. (1991). Prediction of cognitive change as a function of preoperative ability status among temporal lobectomy patients seen at 6-month follow-up. *Neurology* **41**: 399–404.

Cranford, J. L., Kennalley, T., Svoboda, W., *et al.* (1996). Changes in central auditory rocessing following temporal lobotomies in children. *J. Am. Acad. Audiol.* **7**: 289–95.

Crone, N. E., Vining, E. P. G., Lesser, R. P., *et al.* (1992). A bilateral (mixed) language dominance: effects of corpus callosotomy. *Epilepsia* **33** (suppl 3): 27.

Davies, K. G., Maxwell, R. E., Beniak, T. E., *et al.* (1995). Language function after temporal lobectomy without stimulation mapping of cortical function. *Epilepsia* **36**: 130–46.

De Bode, S., Curtiss, S. & Methern, G. W. (2000). Hemispherectomy: integrity of the remaining hemisphere as a predictor of language outcome. *Epilepsia* **41** (suppl 7): 138.

Devinsky, O., Perrine, K., Hirsch, J., *et al.* (2000). Relation of cortical language distribution and cognitive functions in surgical epilepsy patients. *Epilepsia* **41**: 400–404.

Devinsky, O., Perrine, K. & Llinas, R. (1993). Anterior temporal language areas in patients with early onset of temporal lobe epilepsy. *Ann. Neurol.* **34**: 727–32.

Dogali, M., Devinsky, O., Luciano D., *et al.* (1992). Experiences with multiple subpial cortical transections for the control of intractable epilepsy in exquisite cortex. *Epilepsia* **33** (suppl 3): 100.

Fried, I. (1999). Non-resective strategies: stimulation and disconnection. Presented at the American Epilepsy Society Conference, Orlando, FL, 1999.

Frost, M. (1999). The epilepsy team approach to implantation. Presented at the American Epilepsy Society Conference, Orlando, FL, 1999.

Gates, J. (1999). Alternative to surgery if latter not possible. Presented at the American Epilepsy Society Conference, Orlando, FL, 1999.

Gottschalk, L. A. S. (1977). Effects of certain benzodiazepine derivatives on disorganization of thoughts as manifest in speech. *Curr. Ther. Res.* **21**: 192–206.

Gottschalk L. A., Elliot, H. W., Bates, D. E., *et al.* (1972). Content analysis of speech samples to determine effect of lorazepam on anxiety. *Clin. Pharmacol. Ther.* **13**: 323–8.

Henry, D. & Browne, M. (1987). Language and auditory processing deficits. Presented at the St Francis Epilepsy Symposium, Wichita, KS, 1987.

Hermann, B. & Wyler, A. (1988). Effects of anterior temporal lobectomy on language functions: a controlled study. *Ann. Neurol.* **23**: 585–8.

Hermann, B., Beghi, E., Besag, F. M. C., *et al.* (2001). Panel discussion 2. In *Epilepsia and Learning Disabilities*, ed. G. F. Ayala, M. Elia, C. M. Cornaggia & M. M. Trimble. *Epilepsia* **42**: 28.

Karageorgiou, C., Kontogianni, B. & Tagaris, G. (1991). Brainstem auditory evoked potentials in epileptics patients receiving long-term valproate monotherapy. 19th International Epilepsy Congress. *Epilepsia* **32** (suppl 1): 27.

Langfitt, J. T. & Rausch, R. (1996). Word-finding deficits persist after left anterior temporal lobectomy. *Arch. Neurol.* **53**: 72–6.

Lendt, M., Helmstaedtet, C. & Elger, C. E. (1999). Pre- and postoperative neuropsychological profiles in children and adolescents with temporal lobe epilepsy. *Epilepsia* **40**: 1543–50.

Loring, D. W. & Meador, K. J. (2001). Cognitive and behavior effects of epilepsy treatment. *Epilepsia* **42** (suppl 8): 24–32.

Loring, D. W., Meador, K. J., Martin, R. C. & Lee, G. P. (1988). Language deficits following unilateral temporal lobectomy. *J. Clin. Exp. Neuropsychol.* **11**: 41.

Mandelbaum, D. E., Kugler, S. L., Wenger, E. C., *et al.* (2001). Clinical experience with levetiracetam and Zonisamide in children with uncontrolled epilepsy. *Epilepsia* **42** (suppl 7): 183.

Mervaala, E., Kalviainen, R., Kjnononen, M., *et al.* (1993). Vigabatrin and carbamazepine monotherapy does not impair cognitive functions in event-related potentials. *Epilepsia* **34** (suppl 6): 95.

Milner, B. (1975). Psychological aspects of focal epilepsy and its neurosurgical management. In *Advances in Neurology*, ed. D. P., Purpura, J. R. Penry & R. D. Walter, Vol. 8. New York: Raven Press.

Morales, A., Verhulst, S., Faingold, C. L., *et al.* (1992). Absence epilepsy: brainstem auditory evoked responses (BAERs) before and during treatment. *Epilepsia* **33** (suppl 3): 63.

Morrell, F., Whisler, W. W., Smith, M. C., *et al.* (1992). Clinical outcome in Landau-Kleffner Syndrome treated by multiple subpial transection. *Epilepsia* **33** (suppl 3): 100.

Ojemann, L. M., Crawford, C. A., Dodrill, C. B., *et al.* (1999). Language disturbances as a side effect of Topiramate and Zonisamide therapy. *Epilepsia* **40** (suppl 7): 66.

Rayport, M., Ferguson, S. M. & Corrie, W. S. (1984). AES Society Proceedings. *Epilepsia* **25**: 5.

Rayport, M., Ferguson, S. M. & Schell, C. A. (1991). Long-term outcomes after corpus callosum section: neurosurgical, neurological, neuropsychiatric and neuropsychological aspects. *Epilepsia* **32** (suppl 3): 89.

Saykin, A. J., Stafiniak, P. & Robinson, L. J. (1995). Language before and after temporal lobectomy: specificity of acute changes and relation to early risk factors. *Epilepsia* **36**: 1071–7.

Shafrir, Y. (1999). Loss of speech in 2 patients with excellent seizure control on Ketogenic diet. *Epilepsia* **40** (suppl 7): 124.

Speer, J., Quiske, A., Altenmuller, D. M., *et al.* (2001). Unsuspected atypical hemisphere dominance for language as determined by fMRI. *Epilepsia* **42**: 957–9.

Szabo, A. & Wyllie, E. (1993). Intracarotid amobarbital testing for language and memory dominance in children. *Epilepsia* **34** (suppl 6): 31.

Trenerry, M. R., Westerveld, M. & Meador, K. (1995). MRI hippocampal volume and neuropsychology in epilepsy surgery. *Magn. Reson. Imaging* **13**: 1125–32.

Williams, J. & Rausch, H. R. (1991). Factors in children that predict memory performance on the intracarotid amobarbital procedure. *Epilepsia* **32** (suppl 3): 70.

Wilson, A., Petty, R., Perry, A. & Rose, F. C. (1983). Paroxysmal language disturbance in an epileptic treated with clobazam. *Neurology* **33**: 652–4.

9

Evaluation of speech and language problems

Much of learning and the day-to-day social interactions of life depend on communication. Subtle speech and language problems impair learning and inhibit social development. Discipline, explanations, and instructions are based largely on the spoken word.

Subtle seizure short-circuits may impair the epileptic child's functioning in many ways. Proper help depends on early recognition and confirmation of the problem, followed by appropriate, practical, remediative help. Children who have epilepsy are at risk of developing speech and language problems and should be evaluated at four levels, depending on their needs: (1) awareness and subsequent screening, (2) formal basic hearing and speech testing, (3) in-depth language-processing studies, as indicated, and (4) applied language arts, especially in practical situations, by both the therapist and others (parents, teachers, etc.). The main challenge is suspecting the problem and confirming that it exists (Bradford, 1980).

Too often, a physician tells the parents that a young child will probably grow out of the problem. This is not true. A child who has delayed speech or a deviation from normal that is significant enough to disturb the parents, frustrate the child, or be apparent to the teacher or physician should be referred for speech and language evaluation. Both relaxed testing and testing under stress is helpful, as stress can bring out deficits that may be overlooked in the usual, relaxed speech-testing situation.

Awareness and screening

Language problems in children with epilepsy occur frequently enough such that all children with epilepsy should be screened for possible speech and language problems. This is particularly true if the patient has complex partial seizures, especially if from the left hemisphere.

Talking with the child, the parents, and the school personnel can identify areas of possible problems. Some of the questions to be asked include:

1 Does the child seem to confuse similar words and sounds?
2 Does the child tend to misunderstand or confuse what others say?

3 Does the child get instructions confused?

4 Does the child seem forgetful, especially for things he or she has just been told?

5 Does the child get things he or she hears or says mixed up?

6 Does the child get parts of words or words within the sentence out of order?

7 Does the child have problems expressing their thoughts and ideas?

8 Does the child often feel misunderstood?

9 Does the child seem to never listen to important things that others say?

10 Does the child tend to forget names of people, places, or items that he or she should remember?

11 Does the child seem to struggle to say words at times and inconsistently stumble over familiar words?

12 Is the child able to pronounce words clearly?

13 Is the child's speech slow or slurred together?

14 Does the child stutter or stammer?

15 Was the child's speech and language development slowed?

16 Does the quality of the child's speech vary widely from day to day?

17 Can the child communicate adequately with others?

18 Is the child's speech and language a concern or frustration to the parents, to the child, or to those working with the child?

If any of these concerns appear and the child is known to have epilepsy, and especially if the child is on an anticonvulsant, referral to a speech and language pathology specialist is indicated. Although other things beyond speech and language disorders can produce such symptoms, the more symptoms that are noted, the greater is the need for the child to be evaluated by a speech pathologist.

In dealing with an epileptic child, a speech and language pathologist must be part of a team approach so that the results and recommendations of the testing can be integrated with the educational, parenting, and behavioral approaches developed to help the child.

Hearing evaluation

A proper speech and language evaluation begins with an evaluation of the child's hearing ability. Children with temporal lobe problems, especially involving the dominant temporal lobe, may have difficulties coping with noisy backgrounds. Testing should include assessment in both pure tone and speech recognition, as well as with a noisy background input.

The bright child with a hearing impairment may be able to get around a hearing test by reading lips, or, if the tester obscures their face behind a book or clipboard, by seeing the reflection of the tester's face in a mirror, window, or picture reflection. Watching the child's eyes in response may hint that such is occurring. A skilled tester may also be able to trick the child by mouthing one word while saying another, to see whether the child responds to the spoken word or the mouthed word.

The administration of valproate has been associated with hearing loss. This has been confirmed by audiometry (Karageorgiou *et al.*, 1991; Morales *et al.*, 1992). This can be a low-frequency deficit, a high-frequency deficit, or both (Armon *et al.*, 1991). Stopping the drug results in improvements in many children.

Noise-background testing

Another significant difficulty experienced by some individuals with seizures from the dominant temporal lobe is distinguishing sounds in a noisy environment. The individual may pass a routine audiometry test in the silence of the sound chamber and may respond normally during brainstem auditory evoked and P300 cognitive evoked testing, yet they may still have problems in a noisy setting. Therefore, part of the testing should include testing the individual's abilities in a noisy background. This should be performed with routine audiometry and cognitive evoked potential testing.

Auditory evoked potentials

If a child passes the routine audiometric testing but still does not seem to hear, then a brainstem auditory evoked response test is desirable. A series of tones given to the ears is recorded from the brain in a series of waves that denote the passage of the signal from the ear to auditory centers in the brain. By measuring the resulting waves, the examiner can determine whether there are any blocks or delays in the transmission of the sound signals to the receiving areas of the brain. Brainstem auditory evoked potential testing shows slowing of auditory conduction with valproate and ethosuximide (Morales *et al.*, 1992). At high dosage levels, valproate is especially apt to slow the brainstem conduction (Karageorgiou *et al.*, 1991).

Cognitive evoked potentials

For those children who pass the above hearing tests yet still do not seem to hear, and for those suspected of having a central deafness (as with epileptic children with an acquired agnosia or aphasia with epilepsy syndrome), the P300 cognitive testing approach may be desirable. The response to periodic changes in pitch to the incoming signals, if abnormal, may help to indicate that the child who has been misdiagnosed as retarded or autistic is actually a child with a central language-processing problem. Individuals with seizures coming from the temporal lobe may have difficulties in distinguishing these different stimuli normally. The difference between the two signals must be widened for them to discriminate the differences, showing that they have problems. Decreased and delayed responses have been reported with chronic seizures, with complex partial seizures, and with some antiepileptic drugs.

Auditory event-related potentials, especially the P300, are said to reflect a general cognitive functioning (Mervaala *et al.*, 1993). The responses are influenced by ongoing initial cognitive activity, possibly related to activation of the hippocampal formation and amygdala. A delayed P300 has been associated with disturbances of cognitive processing and may relate to the language processing, including memory problems and intolerance to noisy situations seen especially in patients with epilepsy of the dominant temporal lobe (Syrigou-Papavasiliou *et al.*, 1985).

The cognitive deficit of the P300 abnormalities found is the result of the epilepsy itself, not the antiepileptic drug changes. Delays and depressed responses of P300 response are not significant with all generalized seizures but are noted with generalized tonic–clonic seizures (even after the first seizure) and most prominent with complex partial seizures, even before medication. This is seen more often with left temporal EEG discharges early in the seizure course (Haan & Schulz, 1991; Aktekin *et al.*, 1999).

Medications do not appear to be responsible for the P300 abnormalities in epileptic patients because this latency was also increased in patients not yet on medication (Haan & Schulz, 1991). The mean P300 latencies are longer than normal in patients with newly diagnosed epilepsy (Aktekin *et al.*, 1999). In untreated patients, N1 responses are normal, but P300 latencies may be prolonged and partial P300 amplitudes enhanced, preceded by attenuation of the response, suggesting subtle attention deficits early in epilepsy. Patients with chronic epilepsy have prolonged P300 latencies (Mervaala *et al.*, 1993). No changes are seen with the addition of antiepileptic therapy, although adverse effects may be associated with prolonged therapy (Haan & Schulz, 1991; Aktekin *et al.*, 1999). Addition of antiepileptic medication, such as carbamazepine or vigabatrin, does not produce the defect (Syrigou-Papavasiliou *et al.*, 1985).

Speech and language assessment

If problems are suspected, especially in epileptic children at special risk for language impairments, a referral to a speech pathologist should be pursued. The pathologist should be knowledgeable and experienced in working with children, especially handicapped children. The examiner should also be alert for and able to recognize subtle seizures that may interfere with listening and responses.

Language tests are tools to help the evaluator understand the child, the child's problems, and the child's needs in the way of help, including the approaches that the child will probably respond to best. There are nearly as many tests as there are testers. Each test is somewhat different in what it tests. Each test is only an aid to help the evaluator, and each is only as good as the tester. Only those tests that will help the examiner arrive at the answers needed to develop help for the child should be used.

The evaluator needs information on the medical condition of the child and the drugs the child is on, particularly the current blood levels of any antiepileptic drugs in use. Also important are the results of any psychologic testing results (if done) and the description of academic and emotional problems, including a description of what situations brings out the problems. This will help in selecting the most appropriate test for the child.

Areas of testing

General language development approaches measure three areas, speech, language functions, and language processing. Speech quality assessment includes the accuracy of pronunciation (articulation), the smoothness of the flow (fluency), and the tone, inflections, and the general quality of the voice. Receptive and expressive language functions as well as the use of expressive language, including vocabulary abilities, grammar, etc., need to be interpreted. Language functions during informal sessions, such as informal play sessions, may yield much information. Both formally and informally, any differences in the child's performance in a relaxed situation versus a stressful situation is important to observe, for stress tends to bring out errors. In addition, the therapist should observe the structure and movements of the lips, tongue, palate, and throat in speech efforts, looking for an oromotor apraxia.

The home and school environment of the child should be considered. Children have been referred because of pronunciation and grammar problems, which, in retrospect, mirrored those of the parent or teacher.

In the epileptic child, special attention should be paid to evaluating short-term and long-term memory for what is heard. Epileptic children may not perform significantly lower on many tests of communication skills, but they may be quite poor in language usage. A child may have had demands met with relatively little use for language. The parents may need to be more alert and react more to non-verbal demands.

Observations

Observations of the patient during the evaluation are most important. Some tests may precipitate emotional and behavior reactions, which need to be addressed in remediation. Rarely, a test may precipitate a seizure, which, if confirmed (retesting with an ongoing EEG is desirable), may suggest alternate pathways in seizure management, such as conditioning behavioral approaches. Some children can overcome weak areas by using "crutches," i.e. techniques to get around the problem. If the technique is useful now and will continue to be useful in the future, then both the evaluator and the patient have gained; if the technique used now in simpler tasks is likely to be impeding in the future in more complex tasks, such as by slowing down or confusing performance efforts, then the approach should be altered or substituted by a better one.

More intensive testing of language processing

Auditory processing problems are more common than suspected in epileptic children. These problems interfere with learning. The abilities to associate what is heard with other facts may be reduced, although memory both for what is just heard and for things learned in the past may be impaired. Both short-term and long-term auditory memory are learning processes that are especially vulnerable to the effects of partial seizures and most especially those involving the temporal lobes, particularly the left temporal lobe. This may not show up on routine speech testing and should be looked at more intensively.

Based on the observations and the results of the initial testing, and in full consideration of the problems experienced by the child and the risks associated with the seizure disorder, more comprehensive evolution into specific areas may be required. Several types of testing may be considered, including tests that evaluate any prior tested area in more depth, tests that evaluate language processing, and tests that look into applied language, as with conversation, listening, and reading. Comparative testing in vulnerable situations (noise, stress), and carefully observing the child's reactions and performance in such environments, may be most useful.

Such testing can be run both in a regular, rather sterile testing situation with a very supportive tester (unlike classroom demands), and in special situations in which many children with epilepsy may have problems. Performance of a concomitant EEG may be of great value in such situations, to see whether the situation accentuates the seizure tendencies. Such situations may include the utilization of a stressful testing approach and performance in both a quiet and a noisy background. A background of people speaking may be more stressful than white noise.

By using questions such as "Are you sure?" or "What was that?", the evaluator can create self-doubts and anxiety in the client. Facial expressions and body language can be potent in producing the same effects during testing. Such stresses may bring out the language deficits and may even precipitate seizures. This information is most valuable in developing an immediate remediative approach. It can lead to recommendations for changes in the environment, the use of relaxation and stress management therapy, and other help (timeout, etc.) when the child begins to become stressed until the child can be gradually conditioned to cope with the normal stresses of life. It may be that the approaches rather than the medications need to be changed. In a series of children with left temporal lobe epilepsy, tested utilizing the Porch Index of Communicative Abilities for Children, the testing was divided into two phases with a special approach. At a certain point, the examiner introduced stress into the testing situation by giving the appearance of a doubtful reaction and by statements causing the child to feel stressed. The child's performance often deteriorated markedly from normal to frankly aphasic. This did not happen with children without seizures. Often, this response to stress correlated with experiences within the classroom and at home.

This information may help to differentiate whether a child can perform in the optimum state of a quiet one-on-one testing situation but in a more realistic noisy classroom and/or if the child is under stress, performance may falter and fail. If the latter is the case, then the environment (classroom noise) and the approaches (non-stressful management until the child can be taught to handle the stress better) may be an important part of the remediation. Children, especially those with a dominant temporal lobe seizure, who display excessive activity and deficient attention, occasionally with an increased seizure frequency, in a noisy classroom setting may be found to deteriorate in test performance when stress is added. One boy who demonstrated such performance deterioration improved markedly when he was placed in a quieter classroom setting until he could gradually be trained to handle the noisier environment.

Neurodiagnostics

If a child experiences a rather sudden or progressive change or loss of language, then the evaluation should include a wake and sleep EEG, with special attention being paid to the temporal lobe areas for possible seizure discharges or localized slowing that might suggest a seizure or other underlying neurologic problem causing the speech and language changes.

If the history indicates a regression of language, the child may require an all-night EEG to exclude the possibility of nocturnal activations of spike-wave status in sleep seen with some of the language regression syndromes. Such children usually require an all-night sleep recording to document the disorder. In hospital, evaluation with video-EEG telemetry to properly evaluate the sleep state may be supplemented with a bedside speech and language evaluation while being monitored, which may be helpful in noting any relationships between the seizure discharges and the language abnormalities.

MRI is indicated especially for resistant partial seizures, for complex partial seizures, and for those seizures associated with speech and language regression. P300 auditory evoked potential testing may be helpful in studying the language regression with epilepsy syndromes, as may a SPECT or PET scan.

Applying the test results

The therapist takes the information gathered and translates it into a statement answering specific questions. What are the child's needs? The answer to this is obtained through the history and observations. How have these needs been demonstrated and confirmed? The answer to this is derived from the testing results. What help does the child need to improve function? How can they get that help?

To do this effectively, the therapist must sit down and review the results and observations in view of the specific questions that are likely to be asked by concerned patients, teachers, and physicians. How does the problem relate to the medical problems and the medications being taken? How does the problem affect the child's self-image, social communication attempts, responses to discipline, following of directions, basic learning, and both emotional development and behavior? What can be done about problem areas beyond speech and language performance, to include learning, social interactions, and related emotional areas? How does stress affect the language problem? This leads to the development of a comprehensive remediative approach.

The final approach should be clear to the parents, the medical personnel, and the school staff, i.e. not written in linguistic specialty jargon understandable only to another speech therapist. With this information, the speech therapy consultant can work with other members of the school or preschool team and the parents (and counselors if involved) to develop a rounded program for home and school use.

REFERENCES

Aktekin, B., Ozkaynak, S., Oguz, Y., *et al.* (1999) Short term effects of antiepileptic drugs on P300 in patients with epilepsy. 23rd International Epilepsy Congress. *Epilepsia* **40** (suppl 2): 124.

Armon, C., Paul, R. G., Miller, P., *et al.* (1991). Valproate induced hearing impairment: active ascertainment in an epilepsy clinic population and result of therapeutic intervention. *Epilepsia* **32** (suppl 3): 8.

Bradford, L. J. (1980). Understanding and assessing communicative disorders in children. *J. Dev. Behav. Pediatr.* **1**: 89–95.

Haan, J. & Schulz, G. A. (1991). Cognitive evoked potentials in complex partial and generalized epilepsies. 19th International Epilepsy Congress. *Epilepsia* **32** (suppl 1): 117.

Karageorgiou, C., Kontogianni, B. & Tagaris G. (1991). Brainstem auditory evoked potentials in epileptics patients receiving long-term valproate monotherapy. 19th International Epilepsy Congress. *Epilepsia* **32** (suppl 1): 27.

Mervaala, E., Kalviainen, R., Kjnononen, M., *et al.* (1993). Vigabatrin and carbamazepine monotherapy does not impair cognitive functions in event-related potentials. *Epilepsia* **34** (suppl 6): 95.

Morales, A., Verhulst, S., Faingold, C. L., *et al.* (1992). Absence epilepsy: brainstem auditory evoked responses (BAERs) before and during treatment. *Epilepsia* **33** (suppl 3): 63.

Syrigou-Papavasiliou, A., LeWitt, P. A., Green, V., *et al.* (1985). P300 and temporal lobe epilepsy. *Epilepsia* **26**: 528.

10

Management of speech and language problems in epilepsy

Speech and language therapy can be divided into three types: speech therapy (usually articulation therapy), one-on-one language therapy, and language therapy as part of a team approach

The stress of speech therapy

Some children with epilepsy may find therapy stressful, possibly even triggering seizures. The tendency is for speech therapy to be canceled until the seizures can be controlled. Without the stress, the child may regain control, only for seizures to break through again when the child returns to speech therapy. In such cases, the therapist needs to know about the seizures and how to handle them. A low-key initiation with stress-helps may overcome the stress. If small seizures do occur, the therapist may let the child rest and then resume, always in a relaxed manner. A combined speech and behavioral approach works best.

Special speech and language therapy approaches

Therapy is aimed at trying to overcome identified problems. Initially, this may be individualized, one-on-one therapy with the child, but eventually it may move on to group therapy in which the therapist works with a group of children with similar problems. The next stage is to continue the therapy in the regular classroom (or a preschool program) via the teacher with the therapist serving as consultant to the teacher.

Help at home

The parent and family need to be involved in the therapy, incorporating it into their interactions at home. Hopefully, the family may be able to model proper speech as well as interact appropriately with the child in therapy. The family should be included in some of the speech therapy sessions and drawn into active participation. The therapist should sit down at regular intervals to provide updated information on the progress and goals. Homework to carry on therapy approaches should be given to the family. There may be times at which the parents need individual counseling sessions. Much of discipline and parenting is based on communication. The family may need to adapt their parenting techniques to the child's communication difficulties.

The parents may be able to reinforce the child's proper responses by repeating back good or near-correct efforts. If a child is struggling to perform but is making progress, the parent should wait patiently and not jump in with the correct statement or affirmation; however, waiting too long is frustrating to the child and to the parent. The skilled therapist needs to explain and show the parents how long to wait, when to intervene, and how to help. It requires both art and skill between the parents and the therapist to time things correctly.

Much of discipline is dependent on verbal instructions. The therapist may need to review the disciplinary approaches and teaching techniques at school and at home, moderating the approaches to fit the child's abilities. Less talk and more demonstration is desirable. Rather than a lengthy lecture on what should be done, the therapist should provide written lists of things to be done. Problems in discipline may be due to misunderstandings and forgetting, rather than disobedience; the problem, therefore, may be the discipliner and not the person being disciplined. A simple short phrase when the child is attending is far more useful than a lengthy lecture, especially with language-impaired children.

Classroom approaches to learning and language problems

Children with problems related to speech and/or language may exhibit problems in the classroom. These may include attention deficits, auditory deficits, conceptual deficits, and coordination deficits. Henry & Browne (1987), in their review of speech and language problems in children with epilepsy for the St Francis Epilepsy Conference, provided guidelines for working with language impaired children.

Attention

A child with a disability may be inattentive, especially when surrounded by stimuli. The child with a left temporal seizure disorder may seem inattentive and overly active in a noisy setting, although a few are more attentive in such an environment. Such children are easily distracted by noise and activity. They cannot sit still. They appear to be upset easily by psychological distress such as hunger and by physical distress. Children seem to daydream and may lose their train of thought midstream. The child with a left temporal lobe seizure may get stuck on part of an assignment and never get through, whereas the child with a right temporal disturbance may rush through assignments, making careless errors.

The teacher should place the child where there are few distractions and where they can easily assimilate the information being presented, such as in front of the room and away from the windows or any sources of noise. The student's desk should be clear of unnecessary items. The teacher should accentuate material that the child is meant to be attending to, call on the child to gain a higher attention, and ask the child to take notes on relative materials.

If environmental noise is a problem, a similar desensitization program can be established. The initial placement is in a relatively noise-free environment, monitoring the child's reactions and performance to any noisy intrusions. Gradually, the child needs to be desensitized to a noisy environment, working towards more normal situations. There may be times when the child is allowed or encouraged to have a timeout period to escape from the pressures of the surrounding noise when signs and symptoms of intolerance begin to emerge. The world is noisy and the child needs to be trained to tolerate it, not to escape it.

Auditory comprehension

Students with auditory defects may seem to not accurately hear stimuli or to not satisfactorily process information that they do hear. This can be broken down into three categories. Some children have difficulty in giving written and/or verbal responses to oral instructions. Some children may have difficulty detecting, perceiving, and comprehending that which they hear. Some children have trouble remembering what they have just heard (short-term memory) or what they heard in the past (long-term memory), or both.

These children may appear too attentive, straining to "see" what is being said. They confuse similar sounding words, such as pin/pen, all/oil, map/nap, etc. They frequently ask for repetition when instructions are oral, and they prefer tasks that require little or no listening.

The teacher should maximize visual instruction and use visual aids such as blackboards, written outlines, maps, graphs, charts, and pictures. Oral instructions should be repeated, but written instructions should be given when possible. The child should sit in the front or the middle of the room, close to the teacher. (However, such seating is often considered a place of punishment, the where unruly students are put, so involving the patient as a helper to the teacher may help to overcome the stigma of the placement.) Simple verbal instructions should be used, and the child should be encouraged to seek clarification of instructions. The teacher should check that the student has understood the instructions.

Conceptualization deficits

Children with conceptual deficits may have difficulties or be unable to classify and categorize experiences. Such children tend to think and comprehend concretely rather than abstractly. They may exhibit one or more of a group of behaviors. Some cannot think of words to explain common relationships and seem to "beat around the bush" when trying to explain. Other children, in spoken and written language, are unable to use concepts involving time, feelings, and emotional reactions. Others may have difficulty making inferences, drawing conclusions, and seeing patterns, trends and generalizations. Some cannot easily determine similarities and differences, or make relationships and apply them to various situations. Some lack an abstract vocabulary.

The teacher, in discussing abstract concepts, should offer as many examples as possible. In class discussions, the students should be encouraged to respond and accept their responses in developing abstract concepts. The teacher may consider restricting the questions in written work so that they are more concrete, not necessarily for the whole class but for the particular individual.

Organizational deficits

Some students are disorganized and may appear to be at loose ends. They may display one or more of the following characteristics: misplacing or forgetting items, messy work habits, incorrect sequencing of thoughts, arrival at class unprepared, and giving disorganized responses but never arriving at the point.

The teacher should check the student's note-taking in class to make sure that the necessary information is correctly written and underlined, etc. The student should keep a separate notebook for each class. They should write down all assignments on a separate notepad, checking them off as they are completed. The lecture or discussion may be outlined and presented to the student before class. The student should be encouraged to work at a modest pace and to check all work before handing it in.

Verbal expressive deficits

Children with verbal expressive deficits may have trouble putting thoughts into words. They may be slow to answer questions orally. Responses, whether oral or written, may be unclear, improperly sequenced, or otherwise disorganized.

The teacher should call on students when they raise their hands. Tactfully, the teacher may assist the student who seems to stumble. The teacher may try to call on the student by surprise. The student may know the answer but be unable to verbalize a response adequately. The teacher may help by giving questions that require only a yes/no response or only simple responses, gradually building up the in response complexity, as the child is able to handle the task.

General classroom management

Henry & Browne (1987), referring to a handout originated by Peddicord of the Children's Hearing Clinic of the University of Arizona, explained how such approaches can be adapted to children with epileptic and language-processing problems. Children with auditory processing deficits typically demonstrate one or more problems, such as poor auditory attending skills, deficits in discriminating important versus unimportant stimuli in noisy backgrounds, limitations in auditory memory and recall, and delays in receptive auditory language development. Certain approaches can help such children in the classroom.

Classroom placement

A self-contained, structured environment is more effective than an open, unstructured teaching environment for children with auditory deficits.

Look and listen

Children function better when they can both look and listen. Preferential seating should be a major consideration for them.

Classroom seating

The child should be assigned a seat away from hallways or street noises and close to the teacher so they can better utilize hearing and visual cues. If audiometry shows that one ear functions far better than the other, the child should be seated so as to favor the best ear.

Gain attention

Always get the child's attention before giving directions or instructions, such as by calling the child's name or by touching them gently. The first few words that are spoken should not bear important information, for those words are only the "attention-getters." Once attention is gained, then the important message can be communicated.

Check comprehension

Ask the child questions related to the subject and be certain that the child is following and understanding the discussion.

Rephrase and restate

Encourage the child to indicate when they do not understand what has been said. Rephrase the question or statement, since certain words contain sounds or blends that are not discriminated easily. Sometimes, by substituting words and simplifying the grammar, the intended meaning may be conveyed more readily.

Use brief instructions

Keep instructions relatively short. The child with problems with a limited auditory memory span may lose out otherwise. Similarly, at home the parents should be guided to state things simply and to avoid long lectures.

Pre-tutor the child

Ask the child to read ahead on the subject to be discussed in the class so they become familiar with new vocabulary and concepts and thus are prepared to follow and participate in the classroom. The parents can help with this.

List key vocabulary

List key vocabulary on the blackboard, then try to build the discussion around this.

Use visual aids

Visual aids help the child to use relative strengths in visual processing to augment language-processing weaknesses. Sometimes, a parent may feel that the child understands when actually the child reads body language and guesses at the desired response.

Give individual help

Whenever possible, provide individual help to fill in gaps in language and understanding stemming from the child's auditory disability.

Create a quiet study area

Provide an individual studio area relatively free from auditory and visual distractions to improve the child's ability to discriminate from conflicting stimuli.

Involve resource personnel

Inform resource personnel of planned vocabulary and language topics to be covered in the classroom so that pre-tutoring can supplement classroom activities during individual therapy. At home, the television, radio, and music players should be switched off at times of study.

Write instructions

Children with auditory processing problems may not follow verbal instructions accurately. Write assignments on the board so they can copy them in a notebook. Use a buddy system by giving the classroom the responsibility to be certain the child is aware of the assignments made during the day.

Encourage participation

Encourage participation in expressive language activities, such as reading, conversation, story-telling, and creative dramatics. Parents can help with this.

Monitor efforts

Children with impaired auditory functions become fatigued more readily than other children and thus may not attend because of the continuous strain from efforts to keep up and compete in the classroom. Provide short, intensive periods of instruction, with breaks during which the child can move around.

Inform parents

Provide the parents with consistent input so that they can understand the child's successes and difficulties, as well as meet the need for supplementary tutoring outside of school. The methods of working successfully with the child at school can and should be incorporated into home approaches.

Evaluate the progress

Do not assume that the program is working. Evaluate the child's progress on a systematic schedule. It is far better to modify a program than to wait until a child has encountered yet another frustration and failure.

Henry & Browne (1987), referring to another handout of Peddicord from the Children's Hearing Clinic of the University of Arizona, quote a mnemonic, 'SPEECH,' to guide those working with auditory impaired children: State the topic to be discussed. Pace the conversation at a moderate speech with occasional pauses to permit comprehension. Enunciate clearly without exaggerated lip movements, facing the child. Enthusiastically communicate, using body language and natural gestures. Check comprehension before changing topics.

The environment

If a child, especially with dominant complex partial epilepsy, is found to be distractable in a noisy environment, and particularly if this is validated by specific audiologic testing, then the mere removal of the child from the noisy setting may do much to improve attention and learning while reducing unwanted behaviors and also even seizure activities. Some children may use acting-out behavior to escape the cacophony of the classroom. They can escape by being sent to the principle's office or to the hall in timeout. However, the world is noisy: the removal should be the first step, but then the child should be desensitized gradually to tolerate the noisy background. Success is the eventual return to the classroom, at which time the child has been trained to tolerate the noise.

Other aspects

The epilepsy, the language, and the emotions are all tied together in one individual. Stress one aspect of this triad and all go out of balance. It is most important to observe any relationships between language functioning, seizure occurrence, and behavioral reactions. If such is seen, which is common, it is most important to determine which initiates the other and to address the trigger in the therapy. The emotional state of the patient is most important and is a vital component of speech and language therapy, both in prevention and in remediation of the therapy. However, in counseling, the counselor often falls back on talk therapy, which may aggravate the patient. Sometimes, the behavioral therapist must be trained to work with the language impairment before they begin to work with the patient. It is difficult to segregate and compartmentalize therapies, for they should all be blended together in one common approach to the patient.

Speech therapy should be constructed to meet the needs of real-life situations, not the special situation of a one-on-one therapy room or specialized classroom. All working with the child and not just the therapy sessions should practice therapy.

REFERENCE

Henry, D. & Browne, M. (1987). Language and auditory processing deficits. Presented at the St Francis Epilepsy Symposium, Wichita, KS, 1987.

11

Behavior consequences

A child with epilepsy complicated by language problems may develop frustration behaviors, especially if the language struggles are overlooked. An adolescent with complex partial seizures experienced problems in understanding what her parents told her to do as well as struggles to learn what she had been taught in school. She felt misunderstood. Her seizures remained uncontrolled. A full evaluation revealed language-processing weaknesses brought out by stress testing. Her major stresses were related to the misunderstandings and being misunderstood, which led to much anxiety. Combining language and counseling in stress management produced marked improvement in all areas, including the achievement of seizure control, without changing her medication.

The bridge between language, learning, and emotions

Behavior is influenced by the development of language function. In children, speech and language impairments are a risk factor underlying some psychiatric disorders (Beitman, 1985). Links between language delays and behavior are well known, leading to frustration, loss of self-esteem, educational failure, and lack of motivation, as well as impeded social and emotional relationships (Gordon, 1991). Children with speech disorders, especially boys (75%), tend to be referred for psychiatric assessment twice as early as children with other presenting symptoms (Chess & Rosenberg, 1974).

Children and adults with complex partial seizures, especially those involving the dominant temporal lobe, show a significantly increased incidence of language and emotional problems. It is logical to search for relationships between the types of emotional problems seen and the existence of language problems underlying these emotional states.

A child may present with an expressive aphasia and normal understanding. If a child has a developmental receptive aphasia, expressive aphasia is also often present as the ability to express one's self is dependent on a clear understanding of what others are saying. A child with a receptive aphasia usually presents with a global aphasia. Children with global language disturbances tend to be hyperactive and to have developmental problems. The more evidence of a receptive dysphasia, the more withdrawn the child can be, with impaired personal relationships and similarities to the autistic child (Caulfield *et al.*, 1989).

Social development and social interactions

Language is an essential tool for social behaviors. It is through language that the child interacts with the world around them. Through language, the child understands the feelings and desires of others. Through language, the child expresses emotions and feelings, learning to influence the behaviors of others. The subtler the language disorder, the more the child is at risk for incorrect diagnosis and inappropriate treatment. The disability may not be recognized, and the child may be blamed for a lack of cooperation , inattention, and inappropriate behavior (Gordon, 1991). Communication is the internalization of social modes and is used for self-regulation of behavior; it is the means of expressing emotions and feelings, and the mode of influencing the behavior of others.

Children with left frontal-temporal complex partial seizures may not show any obvious aphasic errors, but their language may be characterized by a reluctance to talk, a simplified language structure, and less spontaneous speech than other children of a similar age. As they get older, a tendency towards becoming an introvert emerges, especially in social interaction, suggesting an underlying problem of communication in social situations. Early, subtle language-processing problems may distort personality development.

Do disorders of communication lead to psychiatric disorders? Rarely, except with autistic behaviors, schizophrenia-like disorders, or elective mutism, is such an evolution evidenced clearly.

Circumlocutions

Anomia, the problem of recalling names of items and people, is more common in individuals with complex partial epilepsy, especially if the left brain half is involved. Adults with complex partial epilepsy can be most talkative but tend to talk around the subject. Those who display this trait most prominently have been found to have an anomia. The trait of talking around the topic may be more of a compensation trick than a true personality trait.

Domination

Some individuals who have problems in understanding what they hear may compensate by monopolizing the conversation so they do not have to listen. Thus, they avoid struggling to comprehend what is being said. This resembles what individuals with hearing deficits and some individuals with "recovered autism" have been noted to do.

Personality traits

Certain personality traits resembling an obsessive-compulsive personality style (introversion, writing overly detailed notes, giving lengthy detailed explanations to the physician in fear of leaving out some important fact) may be more common in people with a left-sided seizure disorder. These traits could relate to an insecure language-processing skill. If an individual is "burned" again and again in social interactions because of misunderstandings due to an underlying aphasic tendency, they tend to withdraw from future social actions and become a loner, even to the point as to be classified as having a "schizoid personality."

Anxiety

Anxiety is another common finding in individuals with seizures, especially complex partial seizures. The misunderstandings of subtle aphasias may lead to excessive anxiety, which impedes seizure control.

Psychosis lateralization

Major psychotic disorders differ depending on whether the seizure comes from the left or the right brain side. Left-sided seizures are more apt to be associated with thought disorders, which may be language-related. Such problems include schizophrenia and paranoia. Childhood autism is associated with an increased incidence of seizures emerging as the child grows up. More than expected, the site of the seizure tends to be the left temporal lobe area, i.e. the language area of the brain. A major obstacle to be overcome in autism, if the child is ever to fit into society, is the language barrier. If this can be overcome, the behavioral characteristics of the autistic child who has successfully matriculated into adulthood is quite similar to the abnormal personality traits seen in some individuals with left-sided complex partial seizures. Charles Barlow, in a lecture at the University of Chicago School of Medicine, described it as: "The temporal lobe appears to be the bridge between psychiatry and neurology, and at any one moment in time no one is certain which direction on that bridge the patient is headed." Language is at one end of that bridge.

Presenting problems in children

Children seen for psychiatric problems have been studied, comparing those with speech and language difficulties with those who have no such problems (Cantwell *et al.*, 1980; Cantwell *et al.*, 1981). Slightly more than half (53%) of children with developmental speech and language problems develop significant behavior problems. The incidence of psychiatric diagnoses in children with developmental or acquired speech and language disorders is four to five times greater than expected. Of these, about 15% have multiple diagnoses. Boys (73%) are affected more commonly. The speech and language problems may be developmental or acquired.

Behavior diagnosis

The most common diagnosis is of a behavior disorder in 26%, including ADHD (15%), oppositional behavior (7%), and conduct disorder (4%). Pervasive developmental disorders, i.e. infantile autism, were found in 1%. Other problems found included emotional disorders (18%), avoidant disorders (8%), separation anxiety disorders (2%), anxiety disorder (2%), adjustment disorders (5%), and chronic depressive disorder (2%). Also noted in a miscellaneous group (7%) were academic underachievement, parent–child problems, interpersonal problems, and a schizoid disorder. Unspecified interpersonal disorders were seen in 5%. Mental retardation is found in about 4% (Cantwell *et al.*, 1980; Cantwell *et al.*, 1981).

Speech versus language impact

A mixed speech and language problem places the child more at risk for behavior problems than those who have only speech problems. The incidence of psychiatric problems is much greater in those with speech and language problems (87%) than in those with only speech problems (13%).

Speech and language problems associated with psychiatric difficulties to children include comprehension difficulties (62%) and processing problems (56%). Children with difficulties in expressive language also have behavior problems (75%). The milder speech and language problems, including expressive language and articulation-disabled children, are often not recognized as such and thus are more apt to cause difficulties than those with more severe presentations. Children with more severe speech and language problems often are not seen for their psychiatric problems as the focus is on the language. Other influential factors include a depressed verbal IQ found in 89% of the psychiatrically ill group.

Children with epilepsy are even more apt to have such problems overlooked, especially if the problems are variable. The speech and language problem may be thought of as part of the epilepsy. This leads to the attitude that if the epilepsy is controlled, then the problem will be cured. Rarely is this true for children with seizures. Indeed, the chances are more that the anticonvulsants may harm rather than help speech and language.

Frustration of language that is lost or not developed

Dealing with the frustration of lost language, or with language that is never gained normally, or with language skills that vary from day to day has a major impact on social development and functioning. The consequences of such speech and language difficulties are usually behavioral disturbances that eventually become more handicapping than the cause. This is seen in elderly patients after a stroke and similarly in children who experience developmental speech and language problems. However, therapy is aimed at the stroke in the elderly and at the language disturbance in the child, with the frustration behaviors often overlooked. In a few children, the behavior disturbance is so marked that it draws therapeutic attention, leading to psychiatric intervention, but too often without any search to find out why the behavior has emerged. The child is labeled "autistic," "attention deficit/hyperactive," "angry," "depressed," or "withdrawn;" the label is treated but the cause is never found for lack of search.

Post-stroke acquired aphasia emotions

Elderly people suffering an acquired aphasia from a stroke exhibit marked behavior changes. Those with a receptive aphasia often cannot stay on task; they are described as flighty and fidgety, and they cannot sit still. Those with an expressive aphasia, which prevents them from expressing their thoughts, either tend to withdraw or may exhibit explosive tempers and much anger. Children exhibit similar reactions to a developmental receptive or expressive aphasia.

The language problem: the emotional risks

Although Alajouanine & Lhermitte (1965) first noted behavior problems appearing in children with receptive and expressive language problems, the awareness of the relationships of speech and language problems and behaviors in children became most apparent through the work of Cantwell and colleagues (Cantwell *et al.*, 1980; Cantwell *et al.*, 1981).

Receptive stresses

Children with receptive language problems interfering with understanding often tend to be wordy but to substitute sounds and words, sometimes inventing new words. They talk around an idea with active use of clichés and stock phrases. At times, they tend to echo. They tend to be wordy, talking much but not saying much. Few substantive words a used. If severe, the receptive problems appear as disordered and confused comprehension, and the child may retreat to being silent, rely on jargon, or echo back what was said. They struggle to understand, and language tends to cause more confusion than clarification to them. Behaviors ascribed to such children by various authors are of attention problems often with hyperactivity, and uninhibited or negativistic behaviors, often with temper tantrums. Perseverative behaviors are noted. The children are described as confused and may appear dull. They are usually non-social and tended to be fearful of new situations, strange places, and strangers. They may seem easily agitated. Socially, they tend to be superficial and uninvolved, often with poor social skills. Their mothers tend to be overprotective. Such children often tend to become loners.

An expressive aphasia may be an isolated occurrence, but a developmental receptive aphasia is usually associated with a secondary expressive language aphasia, for the child often has faulty input upon which to develop expressive skills Children with global language disorders tend to be hyperactive with developmental problems, unlike those with expressive speech disorders.

Autistic

The more evidence of a receptive dysphasia, the more withdrawn a child can appear, with resultant impaired personal relationships and behaviors similar to autistic children with autism. This often leads to the misdiagnosis of autism without any investigation of the possibility of a receptive aphasia. To make the diagnosis of autism, one must first exclude the existence of a developmental aphasia. One prominent theory of autism is that it is a severe receptive-associative impairment involving primarily, but not exclusively, language. The more evidence for a receptive dysphasia, the more withdrawn a child may be, with impaired personal relationships and behaviors similar to those of an autistic child.

Psychotic

Receptive language-impaired children tend to be disorganized and agitated in unstructured verbal situations, with poor comprehension. This may be misinterpreted as psychotic behaviors.

Inattentive and distractable

There is a particular link between language disorders and attention deficit disorders, which appears to relate to the constitution and temperament of the child. An overly reactive child may react with hyperactivity.

In summary, the behavior problems seen with a receptive language problem such as a receptive aphasia include attention and activity problems, autistic-like behaviors, agitation (situational), problems with social interactions (usually superficial) and withdrawal, and developmental delays in general.

Expressive frustrations

The discrepancy between adequate cognition and inadequate verbal expression provides fertile soil for misunderstandings and a faulty interaction with the environment (Caulfield *et al.*, 1989). A good environment seems to minimize defense maneuvers. A number of stresses affecting the child are due to frustration related to the difficulties of not being able to communicate except through actions and gestures. The response depends on the child's temperament. The frustrated child will react with tantrums. The reactive child reacts with hyperactivity. A child who is aware of the disability and who is being teased often develops defensive behaviors, which may appear bizarre withdrawn, disorganized, angry, or retarded (Gordon, 1991).

Children with expressive aphasias usually talk little, with slow, struggling, effortful speech. Their efforts may lack the normal prosody that conveys emotional speech. Words are few and may be limited to substantive nouns, action verbs, and a few significant modifiers. There may be few words but with much meaning. Grammar is poor. The children often seem to be aware of their errors. Severely affected children may be limited to monosyllable or double-syllable words or even to grunts and snorts. In general, these children are reduced to a struggle to express their ideas.

A discrepancy between cognition and inadequate verbal expression leads to misunderstandings and faulty interactions with the environment. Emotional accompaniments are prominent but different from those in children with a receptive aphasia. When the child has difficulty trying to communicate thoughts, often only frustration emerges. Such children often seem frustrated and perplexed yet very attentive. Discrepancies between cognition and inadequate verbal expression lead to misunderstandings and thus faulty interactions with others in the environment. Emotional affects tend to be extreme. A good environment minimizes such defensive maneuvers but does not overcome the frustrations of not being able to communicate.

Shy and retiring
Parents and teachers may describe the child as quiet, friendly, shy, or even fearful, responding to but not initiating social interactions. The child may be reluctant to use their limited language. Such children may be misdiagnosed as retarded.

Acting out anger
Children with expressive language problems may also be angry, with explosive reactions often noted, especially related to language-induced frustrations. The frustrated child may exhibit an explosive temper or a bizarre reaction. Problems with expression are more apt to lead to negative behaviors. Parents often perceive the children as difficult. However, the behavior itself is an expression of their frustration.

Overprotection
Maternal overprotection is prominent, with underdisciplining often noted. There is a higher level of negative behavior in children delayed in expressive language development. The parents see their child as shy, fearful, and reluctant to use what language they have.

Alternate communication
Behavior that may seem bizarre, angry, or withdrawn may be used as an alternative communication system. Behavior problems tend to serve as an alternative system, although few people pause to note this.

Diagnosis and management

Psychiatric disorders are diagnosed in about one-third of children with speech impairment and about two-thirds of children with both speech and language impairments (Cantwell *et al.*, 1980; Cantwell *et al.*, 1981). Similarly, problems in socialization with peers, a lack of special friends, and the presence of other problems as seen by the parents are increased when the speech impairment is complicated by language impairment.

Although many claim no relationships between psychiatric problems and speech-language problems in children complicated by other neurologic or familial dysfunctions, Rutter note that children with mental retardation and speech problems had six times the expected frequency of behavior problems (Cantwell *et al.*, 1981). Key family factors that may aggravate speech and language difficulties include family arguing, home stress, divorce, and alcoholism.

In children with epilepsy, influential factors include the seizure type and the medication being use. The variability of the seizure activity may tend to accentuate the struggle with language processing. Often, when the seizures are less controlled, the speech and language problems are worse. When the seizures become more prominent, the medication is increased, sometimes to excessive dosage or by using a number of medications, which tends to worsen the speech and language problems.

Diagnosis

The child will rarely "grow out of it," whether a speech or language delay or related behavior. Early intervention is required to avoid later problems. Whether the child is brought to a specialist because of the speech and language problem or because of the behavior, it is important to screen the child for both. Part of any speech and language evaluation should seek any relative behavior reactions or emotional difficulties in the child. Part of any behaviorist evaluation of a child should search for any delays or deviances in speech and language usage. If such is suggested by history, a full evaluation must be pursued; if problems are verified, the therapy should be a combined behavior–language therapy, not just one or the other. This also needs to be explained to the parents so that they can be involved in delivering the needed approaches at home as well as with the therapist and at school (Cantwell *et al.*, 1980; Cantwell *et al.*, 1981).

There is a strong link between language deficiencies and psychiatric disorders, especially for language disorders demonstrable only by special tests. The psychologist may be less aware of this link than a speech therapist. Affected children tend to be disorganized and agitated in unstructured verbal situations, with poor comprehension. Behavior may be misinterpreted as psychotic. If subsequent treatment is too verbally based, it is likely to be ineffective. If it is less language oriented, there is more chance of success (Gaultieri *et al.*, 1983). The type of language disorder needs to be identified before management can be organized. Watching the child at play may aid the differentiation of expressive language from those problems involving the structure of language processing (Gordon, 1991).

Whole-child therapy

More subtle language disorders are often misdiagnosed and thus treated improperly. The child is often blamed for a lack of cooperation, inattention, or abnormal behavior. Early recognition and therapy is highly important, not only to overcome the problems but to prevent the development of behavior difficulties. Early intervention prevents later problems. Young children with combined speech and language disorders who are at risk for psychiatric problems may benefit from early intervention in speech and language areas to prevent the development or persistence of psychiatric disorders (Cantwell *et al.*, 1981).

Bad behavior is the child's way of communicating a desire to escape a stressful situation. The behavior results in exclusion, which relieves the child, who feels rewarded, encouraging future resorting to similar approaches in the future. Then the teacher or therapist or parent, instead of listening to hear what the child is communicating by the behavior, acts only to reinforce the bad behavior by rewarding it.

Prognosis

Behavior problems born of language delays can persist, leading to increased introversion and withdrawal, as well as learning, social, and educational difficulties by late childhood (Richman *et al.*, 1983). Language behavior problems increase with time. Delayed speech in the toddler age may lead to increasing introversion and withdrawal by seven years of age in 50%; in early adolescence, learning, social, and educational difficulties emerge. Language disorders may lead to frustration, loss of self-esteem, educational failure, and a loss of motivation.

Later on, there is an impeded social and emotional relationship problems unless the home environment motivates communication. Teasing and rejection of the child because of the speech and language difficulties are adverse factors. Thus the evolution of a speech and language problem is one of the initial speech and language delays, followed by introversion, frustration, and giving up, with underachievement and ultimate relative school failure. Comprehensive remediation is the only way to avert this outcome.

REFERENCES

Alajouanine, T. & Lhermitte, F. (1965). Acquired aphasia in children. *Brain* **88**: 653–62.

Beitman, J. H. (1985). Speech and language impairment and psychiatric risk: toward a model of neurodevelopmental immaturity. *Psychiatr. Clin. North Am.* **8**: 721–36.

Cantwell, D. P., Baker, L. & Mattison, R. E. (1980). Psychiatric disorders in children with speech and language retardation. *Arch. Gen. Psychiatry* **37**: 423–6.

Cantwell, D. P., Baker, L. & Mattison, R. (1981). Prevalence, type and correlates of psychiatric diagnoses in 200 children with communication disorders. *J. Dev. Behav. Pediatr.* **2**: 131–5.

Caulfield, M. B., Fischel, J. E., DeBaryshe, B. D. *et al.* (1989). Behavioral correlates of developmental expressive language disorders. *J. Abnorm. Child Psychol.* **17**: 187–201.

Chess, S. & Rosenberg, M. (1974). Clinical differentiation among children with initial language complaints *J. Autism Child. Schizophr.* **4**: 99–109.

Gordon, N. (1991). The relationship between language and behavior. *Dev. Med. Child Neurol.* **33**: 86–9.

Gualtieri, C. T., Koriath, U., Van Bourgondien, M. *et al.* (1983). Language disorders in children referred for psychiatric services. *J. Am. Acad. Child Psychiatry* **22**: 165–77.

Richman, N., Stevenson, J. E. & Graham, P. J. (1983). The relationship between language development and behavior. In *Epidemiological Approaches in Child Psychiatry*, ed. M. W. Schmidt & H. Remschmidt. New York: Thieme-Stratton.

Part II

Learning problems

12

Learning challenges

Roughly half of children with epilepsy experience increased school difficulties due to retardation, intellectual decline, learning disabilities, and underachievement (Rutter *et al.*, 1970; Stores, 1978; Stores, 1987; Thompson, 1987; Aldenkamp *et al.*, 1990; Smith *et al.*, 2002). They falter and fail due to the affects of the seizures and seizure discharges, the seizure cause, and the medications (Aldenkamp, 1983; Reynolds, 1985; Wiberg *et al.*, 1987; Blennow *et al.*, 1990; Henricksen, 1990). Often, their difficulties are undiagnosed, misdiagnosed, or missed. Consequently, although the seizures may cease, the patient enters into the adult world unprepared and underemployed.

International experience

Over the past 50 years, numerous studies have been done in the USA and in Europe regarding the experiences of children with epilepsy in school. A representative sampling of the findings shows that needs exist.

Schooling

Problems of learning and behavior are over-represented in children with epilepsy. A majority (69%) of children with epilepsy attending ordinary schools have a below-average level of performance. Some (21%) show behavior disturbances (Holdsworth & Whitemore, 1974; Mellor & Lowint, 1977).

Teachers perceive children with epilepsy as having poor concentration and mental processing and to be less alert than their peers (Bennett-Levy & Stores, 1984). More than 50% of children with epilepsy are reported by their teachers as "just holding their own" in ordinary schools at a below-average level, whereas one-sixth fall behind seriously (Holdsworth & Whitemore, 1974).

Problems

Performance problems fall into four groups: retardation, declining intelligence, learning disabilities, and underachievement. Performance impairments are noted.

Retardation

A great variety of cognitive problems have been found in epileptic children (Trimble, 1990). Mental retardation normally presumes the existence of brain damage or a permanent dysfunction (Cornaggia & Gobbi, 2001). Impaired intelligence is seen in children whose seizures are associated with cerebral palsy or other brain disorders (Trimble, 1990).

Declining IQ

Even though a large number of children with epilepsy have school difficulties, only a minority show a loss of skills or a decreasing IQ. Children with an actual skill loss need to be evaluated for a specific cause and a remediative program planned (Cornaggia & Gobbi, 2001).

Learning disabilities

Learning disorders of epilepsy may be state-dependent, i.e. situationally related, or permanent. Situation-dependent learning disorders may evolve into permanent learning disabilities (Cornaggia & Gobbi, 2001). Academic problems arise from specific cognitive deficiencies rather than any generalized cognitive dysfunction. A wide variety of cognitive deficiencies have been found in children with epilepsy. These include impaired memory function and reduced attention span (Stores, 1973; Stores & Hart, 1976; Stores, 1981), difficulties in abstract reasoning (Long & Moore, 1979), reduced information processing efficiency (Fairwether & Hutt, 1969), auditory perception and language-processing problems, and problems of concentration (Fairwether & Hutt, 1969; Rugland, 1990).

Underachievement

About one-sixth of children with epilepsy with normal intelligence are under-achieving (Pazzaglia & Frank-Pazzaglia, 1976). Children with epilepsy show lower academic achievement scores relative to their IQ, with specific difficulties in arithmetic, spelling, reading, comprehension, and word recognition (Seidenberg *et al.*, 1986; Trimble, 1990). Children with epilepsy underachieve in school and even more in daily application of what they have learned. They have a higher rate of repeating grades and of special education placements (Bailet & Turk, 2000).

Performance

Children with epilepsy perform less well in verbal tests and show a higher than expected frequency of reading retardation. Many of these patients perform poorly in reasoning (Trimble, 1990). Speed of information processing, memory, vigilance alertness, sustained and focused attention, and motor fluency are important cognitive domains that are especially vulnerable to epileptic factors. Other areas of deficits are in language and problem solving, as well as perceptual and motor difficulties (Waxman & Geschwind, 1975; Dodrill, 1987; Brittain, 1980; Kupke & Lewis, 1985; Aldenkamp, 1987; Beaumont, 1987; Oxley & Stores, 1987; Aldenkamp *et al.*, 1990).

Behavior

Behavior and learning are often linked. Behavior changes may result from temporary or permanent cognitive deficits (Cornaggia & Gobbi, 2001). About 21% of children with epilepsy attending ordinary schools show behavior disturbances (Holdsworth & Whitemore, 1974). Behavior disturbances are found in 27% of children with epilepsy, with a rate of 15% in controls (Rutter *et al.*, 1970). Underachievement in school may be due to depressive reactions, the child's classmates' fears of seizures, or the hostility of the parents after a major seizure has occurred at school. Secondary psychological problems in epilepsy patients combined with the side effects of antiepileptic drugs may cause or increase learning problems (Henricksen, 1990).

Placement

Given a prevalence of epilepsy estimated as four to eight per 1000, most schools will have several pupils with epilepsy at any one time. It is important that the teacher is informed about the disorder and its management if they are to help in the assessment and remediation of children with epilepsy (Henricksen, 1990).

Dropout rate

Although the majority children with epilepsy attend ordinary schools, learning disabilities and school problems are frequent (Cavazutti, 1980; Ross & Tookey, 1988). Around 90–95% of children with epilepsy are in ordinary schools, but this drops to 67% by age 11 years and 58% by age 15 years (Verity & Ross, 1985; Henricksen, 1990). Children with epilepsy tend to drop out of school earlier. The dropout tendency relates somewhat to the sociological status and attitudes of the family (Suurmeijer *et al.*, 1978; Long & Moore, 1979; Aldenkamp *et al.*, 1990). By adolescence, only 33% of epileptic children are in the secondary school system, as compared with 68% of controls. This leads to occupational disadvantages and a higher unemployment rate (Rodin *et al.*, 1972; Thorbecke, 1987).

Special education services

About one-third of children with epilepsy receive some form of special education (Aldenkamp *et al.*, 1990). Around 30% of children with therapy-resistant epilepsies are receiving special education help as compared with 7% of non-epileptic children (Green & Hartlage, 1971; Holdsworth & Whitemore, 1974; Aldenkamp, 1983; Thompson, 1987; Ross & Tookey, 1988).

Functioning in society

Approximately 60% of epilepsy patients function well in society, 25% are somewhat incapacitated by psychosocial problems but integrated into society, and 15% need continuous care, not necessarily because of their epilepsy but for additional handicaps such as cerebral palsy, mental retardation, or psychiatric problems (Henricksen, 1990).

Federal Commission for the Control of Epilepsy and Its Consequences' findings

In 1975, the Federal Commission for the Control of Epilepsy and Its Consequences surveyed the status of the management of epilepsy in the USA (Commission for the Control of Epilepsy and Its Consequences, 1977–8). It was found that the seizures themselves are not as much a handicap as are the associated disabilities. The Commission summarized the overall needs for school children with epilepsy quite fully:

The child with epilepsy has a number of problems that interfere with the ability to learn. If undetected and uncorrected, those problems can present a severe handicap in later years, resulting in deficient education, inadequate job skills or qualifications, and severe social adjustment problems [Vol. I, Chapter 8, p. 87].

Intelligence

Forty-eight percent of individuals under active medical care for their epilepsy have intellectual disabilities and 54% have behavior problems ... The intelligence of individuals with epilepsy was average or above in 30 to 47%, borderline in 13 to 31%, mildly impaired in 6 to 19%, moderately retarded in 10.8 to 19% and severely defective in 10 to 22.8%. In school surveys, 25.8% were in special education and 7.4% were suspended. Those children with epilepsy only had little problem. Those children with epilepsy and related problems had difficulties [Vol. I, Chapter 3, p. 2].

Subtle intellectual impairments or mild learning disabilities present in over half of children with epilepsy can interfere with home and school adjustment. Psychological and psychometric evaluation therefore, should be included in the evaluation of children with epilepsy as well as adults [Vol. I, Chapter 4, p. 47].

School problems

Children who had epilepsy only had little problems in school. It was those who had related problems, either intellectual impairment or emotional problems, who had difficulty ... In public schools, if a child has epilepsy, he is likely to have other problems as well. He also may be mentally retarded, may have motor disorders, be emotionally disturbed, or have learning disabilities. These problems superimposed on epilepsy, greatly influence the child's learning [Vol. II, Part I, pp. 474–90].

Whitehouse (1971) noted: "Learning problems occur in 50% of epileptic children. The mildly affected patients with normal intelligence still have problems in learning but these are often unrecognized."

School problems are not necessarily due to seizures. In fact they afflict children whose seizures are controlled as well as those who continue to have them . . . The school problems were not necessarily due to the seizures. Such problems affected children whose seizures are controlled as well as those who continued to have seizures. The teacher's attitude was one serious problem. If the teacher did not understand epilepsy, if the teacher believed that the child was slow or feared that the child may have a seizure in class . . . Seizures may not be realized and the child branded as a "daydreamer" or inattentive if they were having absence seizures, or as difficult and unruly if they experienced psychomotor seizures. Sometimes parents also were in denial [Vol. I, Chapter 8, p. 87].

Learning problems in children with epilepsy are common and may stem from undiagnosed and subtle learning disabilities, from psychological and behavior problems that often accompany epilepsy, from mild or severe retardation or from under or over medication [Vol. I, Chapter 8, p. 8].

The child with epilepsy has a number of problems that interfere with the ability to learn. If undetected and uncorrected, those problems can present a severe handicap in later years, resulting in deficient education, inadequate adjustment problems [Vol. I, Chapter 8, pp. 83–98].

Placement

Yet the primary responsibility for providing the best possible education for handicapped children rests with the schools. If aware of their problems, schools can take a number of specific actions to help assure that handicapped children do indeed receive the education to which they are entitled [Vol. I, Chapter 8, pp. 83–98].

Although a sizable proportion of children with epilepsy were found to be in special education classes or in special schools, it was not possible to determine how many have been placed in those special situations because of the seizures and how many because of associated handicaps. For some children, such placement may not be suitable and may be used as a means of social ostracism . . . Since social ostracism is one of the major problems confronting children with epilepsy, it is important to contain these children in regular classroom situations, whenever possible. For some children such placement may not be suitable; however, there have never been systematic studies to determine under what conditions special placement may be advantageous for the child with epilepsy [Vol. I, Chapter 8, pp. 83–98].

Teachers believe children with epilepsy have twice as many problems ... such as lack of concentration, restlessness, and fidgeting ... as their classmates. The same problems that interfere with school performance also prevent employment of people with epilepsy ... Whether in a special or regular classroom situation though, the teacher must be alert to the special problems and needs of the child with epilepsy ... aware, for instance, that absence seizures can reduce learning time so that a child will require extra help ... and must work closely with parents, counselors, school psychologists, and the child to assure the best possible learning situation ... The informed teacher will realize that the child with epilepsy may also have learning disabilities and will provide the extra help needed [Vol. I, Chapter 8, pp. 83–98].

West Virginia experience, 1970–80

In the 1970s, the West Virginia University Medical Center's Pediatric Neurology program established a learning disability clinic. Sixty percent of the children referred were found to have a history of epilepsy. A number of the children were underachieving or failing in school because of unrecognized learning disabilities. Their difficulties were blamed on uncontrolled seizures or the medications. The developing of a more appropriate educational approach improved both learning achievement and seizure control.

Reviewing school evaluations and performance was considered a part of epilepsy management. In 15% of patients, the learning disability was predictable but not recognized in the first grade. Those with complex partial seizures were most apt to have learning disabilities. Those with generalized epilepsy syndromes did not tend to have as many learning problems unless their EEG demonstrated frequent EEG discharges or they had problems tolerating their anticonvulsants.

Problems of the complex partial epilepsy group were especially common in children with left temporal lobe epilepsy of early onset, who tended to present with problems of active seizures, language-processing problems, specific learning disabilities especially affecting memory, and situational emotional reactions. The EEGs tended towards bilateral activation with background slowing at the focus site. Those with primarily right-sided discharges had a different profile, with fewer memory problems, more prominent perceptual difficulties, and hasty, error-prone performance. Perceptual motor problems were common to all seizure types. Stress brought out dysfunctions in testing and in task-related school efforts. These children showed good responses to remedial help.

Some children with abnormal EEGs but with no epilepsy history were hospitalized on the general pediatric service for seizure observation for five days, but the nursing staff noted nothing to suggest seizures. Because of a history of learning difficulties in one child, the educational specialist was consulted. During testing, the specialist would note behaviors such as pauses in a child's pencil efforts, wandering off track, and then resuming the pencil efforts at drawing the line. The consultant wrote "absence seizure," and in her report she described both the symptoms and the effect on the academic performance along with recommendations on how the teacher could handle the spells. The child was successfully started on medication.

A number of the seizure patients had had seizure-related learning disabilities suspected by the parent or school but not confirmed by school testing. By selecting a test battery appropriate to the type of seizure disorder and the academic problems, the problems were documented sufficiently to develop, with the school, an appropriate placement and plan resulting in improvement in performance and in seizure frequency.

Relationships between school stresses, performance problems, and complex partial epilepsy were noted in some of the children with epilepsy, especially in those with language problems. Adding stress to portions of language testing frequently would cause the child's performance to deteriorate, occasionally precipitating both a blatant aphasia and an occasional seizure. For children with epilepsy who deteriorate with language stresses, behavior modification and stress management give a marked improvement in functioning.

With some children referred with grand mal epilepsy, the specialist questioned the diagnosis on the basis of the observed testing performance, error type, and personality manifestations, which led to the suspicion of a temporal lobe focus. In slightly more than two-thirds of this group, a subsequent EEG confirmed her suspicion of a focal rather than a generalized seizure onset. She generally was correct in suspecting the laterality of the focus.

Close monitoring of academic progress and behavior became a key element of seizure management in the clinic. At any sign of depressed or deteriorating achievement at the initial evaluation or thereafter, the school was contacted to develop an appropriate comprehensive evaluation covering overall intelligence (using a WISC IQ test), a testing of academic achievement levels, and a psycholinguistic battery after initial screening, all aiming towards a more appropriate educational meeting for the child's needs. The educational consultant would then monitor the progress of the child, working with the school.

Approach to learning problems

The approach to learning disabilities in epilepsy first concentrates on analyzing the different effects of the epileptic factors on cognitive function. The impact of seizure activity, localization of the epileptogenic foci, and the antiepileptic treatment of cognitive functioning should be evaluated (Aldenkamp et al., 1990).

REFERENCES

Aldenkamp, A. P. (1983). Epilepsy and learning behavior. In *Advances in Epileptology: The XIVth International Epilepsy Symposium*, ed. M. Parsonage, R. H. E. Grant, A. G. Craig & A. A. Ward, Jr, pp. 221–9. New York: Raven Press.

Aldenkamp, A. P. (1987). Learning disabilities in epilepsy. In *Education and Epilepsy 1987*, ed. A. P. Aldenkamp, W. C. J. Alpherts, H. Meinardi & G. Stores, pp. 21–38. Lisse: Swets & Zeitlinger.

Aldenkamp, A. P., Alpherts, W. C. J., Dekker, M. J. A., *et al.* (1990). Neuropsychological aspects of learning disabilities in epilepsy. *Epilepsia* **31** (suppl 4): 9–20.

Bailet, L. L. & Turk, W. R. (2000). The impact of childhood epilepsy on neurocognitive and behavioral performance. A prospective longitudinal study. *Epilepsia* **41**: 426–31.

Beaumont, M. (1987). *Epilepsy and Learning: Understanding the Learning Difficulties Experienced by Children with Epilepsy*. Melbourne: National Epilepsy Association of Australia.

Bennett-Levy, J. & Stores, G. (1984). The nature of cognitive dysfunction in schoolchildren with epilepsy. *Acta. Neurol. Scand.* **69** (suppl 99): 79–82.

Blennow, G., Heijbel, J., Sandstedt, P., *et al.* (1990). Discontinuation of antiepileptic drugs in children who have outgrown epilepsy: effects on cognitive function. *Epilepsia* **31** (suppl 4): 50–53.

Brittain, H. (1980). Epilepsy and intellectual functions. In *Epilepsy and Behavior*, eds. B. M. Kulig, H. Meiinardi & G. Stores, pp. 2–13. Lisse: Swets & Zeitlinger.

Cavazutti, G. B. (1980). Epidemiology of different types of epilepsy in school-age children of Modena, Italy. *Epilepsia* **21**: 57–62.

Commission for the Control of Epilepsy and Its Consequences (1977–8). *Plan for Nationwide Action on Epilepsy*. Bethesda, MD: National Institutes of Neurological and Communicative Disorders and Stroke.

Cornaggia, C. M. & Gobbi, G. (2001). Learning disability in epilepsy: definitions and classification. In *Epilepsy and Learning Disabilities*, ed. I. Ayala, G. F. M. Elia, C. M. Cornaggia & M. M. Trimble. *Epilepsia* **42**: 2–5.

Dodrill, C. B. (1987). Aspects of antiepileptic treatment in children. *Epilepsia* **29**: (suppl 3) 10–14.

Fairwether, H. & Hutt, S. J. (1969). Interrelationship of EEG activity and information processing on paced and self-paced tasks in epileptic children. *Electroencephalogr. Clin. Neurophysiol.* **27**: 701–10.

Green, J. B. & Hartlage, I. C. (1971). Comparative performance of epileptic and non-epileptic children and adolescents. *Dis. Nerv. System* **32**: 418–21.

Henricksen, O. (1990). Education and epilepsy: assessment and remediation. *Epilepsia* **31** (suppl 4): 21–5.

Holdsworth, H. & Whitemore, K. (1974). A study of children with epilepsy attending ordinary schools. l: their seizure patterns, progress and behaviors in school. *Dev. Med. Child Neurol.* **16**: 746–58.

Kupke, T. & Lewis, R. (1985). WAIS and neuropsychological tests, common and unique variance within an epileptic population. *J. Clin. Exp. Neuropsychol.* **7**: 353–66.

Long, C. G. & Moore, J. R. (1979). Parental expectations for their epileptic children. *J. Child Psychol. Psychiatry* **20**: 299–312.

Mellor, D. H. & Lowint, I. (1977). Study of intellectual function in children with epilepsy attending ordinary schools. In *Epilepsy: Eighth International Symposium*, ed. J. K. Penry, pp. 291–304. New York: Raven Press.

Oxley, J. & Stores, G. (eds.) (1987). *Epilepsy and Education*. London: Medical Tribune Group.

Pazzaglia, P. & Frank-Pazzaglia, I. (1976). Record in grade school of pupils with epilepsy: an epidemiological study. *Epilepsia* **17**: 361–6.

Reynolds, E. H. (1985). Antiepileptic drugs and psychopathology. In *The Psychopharmacology of Epilepsy*, ed. M. R. Trimble, pp. 49–65. Chichester, UK: John Wiley & Sons.

Rodin, E. A. Rennick, P., Dennerill, R., *et al.* (1972). Vocational and educational problems of epileptic patients. *Epilepsia* **13**: 149–60.

Ross, E. A. & Tookey, P. (1988). Educational needs and epilepsy in childhood. In *Epilepsy, Behavior and Cognitive Function*, ed. M. R. Trimble & E. M. Reynolds, pp. 87–97. Chichester, UK: John Wiley & Sons.

Rugland, A. L. (1990). Neuropsychological assessment of cognitive functioning in children with epilepsy. *Epilepsia* **31** (suppl 4): 41–44.

Rutter, M. Graham, P. & Yule, W. A. (1970). A neuropsychiatric study in childhood. *Clin. Dev. Med.* **3**: 237–55.

Seidenberg, M., Beck, N., Geisser, M., *et al.* (1986). Academic achievement of children with epilepsy. *Neurology* **26**: 753–9.

Smith, M. L., Elliott, I. M. & Lach, L. (2002). Cognitive skills in children with intractable epilepsy: comparison of surgical and nonsurgical candidates. *Epilepsia* **46**: 621–7.

Stores, G. (1973). Studies of attention and seizure disorders. *Dev. Med. Child Neurol.* **15**: 376–82.

Stores, G. (1978). Schoolchildren with epilepsy at risk for learning and behavior problems. *Dev. Med. Child Neurol.* **20**: 502–8.

Stores, G. (1981). Memory impairment in children with epilepsy. *Acta. Neurol. Scand.* **64** (suppl 89): 21–7.

Stores, G, (1987). Effects on learning of "subclinical" seizure discharges. In *Education and Epilepsy 1987*, ed. A. P. Aldenkamp, W. C. J. Alpherts, H. Meinardi & G. Stores, pp. 14–21. Lisse: Swets & Zeitlinger.

Stores, G. & Hart, J. (1976). Reading skills of children with generalized or focal epilepsy attending ordinary schools. *Dev. Med. Child Neurol.* **18**: 705–16.

Suurmeijer, T. P. B. M., van DAM, A. & Blijham, M. (1978). Socialization of the child with epilepsy and school achievement. In *Advances in Epileptology*, ed. H. Meinardi & A. J. Rowan, pp. 40–54. Lisse: Swets & Zeitlinger.

Thompson, P. J. (1987). Educational attainment in children and young people with epilepsy. In *Epilepsy and Education 1987*, ed. J. Oxley, G. Stores, pp. 15–24. London: Medical Tribune Group.

Thorbecke, R. (1987). Improving condition for the employment of people with epilepsy: environmental factors. In *Epilepsy and Employment*, ed. H. de Boer & J. Oxley, pp. 19–24. Heemstede: International Bureau for Epilepsy Publications.

Trimble, M. R. (1990). Antiepileptic drugs, cognitive function and behavior in children: evidence from recent studies. *Epilepsia* **34** (suppl 4): 30–34.

Verity, C. M. & Ross, E. M. (1985). Longitudinal studies of children's epilepsy. In *Pediatric Perspectives on Epilepsy*, ed. E. Ross & E. Reynolds, pp. 133–40. Chichester, UK: John Wiley & Sons.

Waxman, S. G. & Geschwind, N. (1975). The interictal behavior syndrome of temporal lobe epilepsy. *Arch. Gen. Psychiatry* **32**: 1580–86.

Whitehouse, D. (1971). Psychological and neurological correlates of seizure disorders. *Johns Hopkins Med. J.* **129**: 36–42.

Wiberg, M., Blennow, G. & Polski, B. (1987). Epilepsy in the adolescence. Implications for the development of the personality. *Epilepsia* **28**: 542–76.

13

The development of learning

The age of onset of the seizures is important as it may influence, inhibit, or impair cognitive processes developing at that time and thereafter. The clinical presentation of these effects relates to the seizure focus location but may be modified by the brain's ability to develop skills elsewhere.

Anatomy

The number of brain cells is estimated at more than 100 billion neurons. In utero, neurons develop at a rate of more than 250,000 per minute (Cowan, 1979). Each germinal neuron must not only migrate to its terminal destination, but also ultimately become connected to approximately 5000–15,000 other neurons (Cragg, 1975). Much of cell proliferation and migration is prenatal, while much of the development of axonal and dendritic connections is postnatal, alternating with pruning in spurts, with major cycles peaking in the toddler, in the prepubertal childhood period, and in early puberty. The left hemisphere cycles ahead of the right hemisphere by a year or two, which may relate to language dominance over non-language functions. The cycling varies somewhat in different parts of the brain (Thatcher, 1997). The timing of seizure insult sequelae may relate to the time of occurrence in the cycle.

Dendritic growth is the main avenue of learning development. The neurocircuity develops rapidly to be most complex at around two to three years of age. Thereafter, the cyclic pruning away of what is not used or needed occurs so that the circuitry is far less complex by adolescence. This tendency continues, although on a far less active status, for the remainder of a person's life. The adage "Use it or lose it!" applies aptly to the cognitive skills of an individual at any age.

As connections evolve and specialization sites emerge, functions lateralize. In the embryo, the left hemisphere appears destined for auditory-linguistic functions, while the right is destined for non-linguistic visual spatial performance processes. Even in left-handed people, verbal skills still tend to develop on the left or bilaterally, although language develops on the right in a few people. If the lateralization process is disrupted in infancy, often after a few months lag the skill begins to develop on the other side. This plasticity lessens gradually in childhood. By six to seven years, skills are largely lateralized. However, with therapy, even adolescents can regain a surprising amount of lost skills. With remediative approaches, some skills may be redeveloped well into adulthood.

An increase in the myelination of the nerve processes occurs especially in the first ten to 12 years of life. This is associated with changes at or within synapses as well as collateral growth of axons. New receptor cells grow to replace old or damaged ones. In some brain systems, there is use of different or less used neurocircuits that exist in excess. Brain development somewhat parallels myelination, which sweeps up the brainstem and from posterior to anterior throughout the cerebral hemispheres, the frontal lobes directing the process but also being the last to achieve the mature state by early adulthood. Language centers are fully myelinated by seven to nine years of age, and language skills mature similarly. The prefrontal-frontal lobe appears to direct other parts of the brain in development, with connections especially to the parietal and temporal areas. Learning changes from concrete thinking to abstraction abilities by adolescence. The adult brain is not completed until early adulthood. Even the adult continues to evolve in the style of learning well beyond adolescence.

Localization

Cerebral localization of function is an extremely complex phenomenon. The brain is not a mosaic of clearly delimited centers, each of which is responsible for a precise psychological function (Hecaen & Albert, 1978). There are centers related to specific types of learning, but these areas may serve more to coordinate scattered learning resources. Vision prime sites are in the occipital lobe, but as the sensation is passed forward it is noted, recognized, and then reacted to. Auditory receptive processes begin in the posterior area of the superior temporal gyrus. Short-term memory utilizes the mesial-temporal hippocampal areas of the brain. Key associations are made at the temporal-parietal juncture at the end of the Sylvian fissure, and the meanings of the input are understood. This is projected forward to the premotor areas for the mouth and face for speech or to the hand area immediately above for manual expression. The frontal lobe appears to coordinate this into an organized response. Language input is processed primarily in the dominant hemisphere (except for emotional and musical aspects of language), whereas visual motor functions are processed especially on the non-dominant side.

The hippocampus and adjacent area, so often involved in epilepsy, is a key site of learning. A most important functioning part of the hippocampus relates to memory problems. Hippocampal atrophy correlates with memory losses. There is temporal lobe heterogeneity in the control of verbal memory. Tasks with a high semantic content show greater involvement of the temporal neocortex (Fedio et al., 1993).

Cognitive development

Development of learning and intelligence is related to brain myelination. Within days after birth, the infant can discriminate between simple sets of numbered dots, rapidly recognizing three-dimensional items and discriminating visual size and shapes, followed closely by depth perception (Antell & Keating, 1983). The neonate prefers shapes most like a human face, especially those resembling the mother's face.

Infancy: sensorimotor stage

Infancy is a sensorimotor reactive stage of development. Within these first few years, through repetitive reflex movements with fortuitous behavioral reinforcements, certain movement patterns develop and become coordinated. The child learns to move in space, thus coming in contact with the environment in order to learn to manipulate this environment. Objects are recognized, manipulated, and then searched for. Finally, the child learns to plan purposeful movements for specific purposes, which is reinforced through the sensorimotor circuit. This is the age of the initial perceptual development, in which coordination (visual-motor) problems may arise. Disturbances at or before this time may result in perceptual-motor coordination problems, often with related emotional problems, including autism, hyperactivity, and personality trait difficulties, i.e. problems of dependence versus independence, socialization, and adjustability.

This is also the time of the emergence of early executive planning, with the child developing the basics of the awareness of the results of their actions and then the awareness that one can modify actions in accordance with what has been experienced. If this development is inhibited, exploration and intelligence itself appear stifled.

Toddlers: language stage

In the toddler age (two to five years), the main developmental task is language. The child has spent the majority of the latter part of infancy preparing for this. The toddler enters into the language stage as auditory processing develops into speech through the distinguishing of sounds, which are then related to objects and symbols. The child must get the sounds in the right order both in understanding and in production. One may note mispronunciations and other speech deviations, tangled speech, and grammar problems. Interferences at this stage include brain damage, hearing loss, emotional problems, epilepsy, and heredity. Related emotional reactions include agitation, hyperactivity, and autistic-like withdrawal, possibly including development of paranoid or schizoid personalities, controlling personalities, discipline problems, frustration reactions, and temper problems.

With epilepsy, in infancy and the toddler stage, a bilateral insult usually underlies any significant speech and language impairments resulting from the seizure process. With the language regression syndromes of epilepsy, the toddler must first have established the basics of the language before it can be lost. Thus, the onset of such syndromes occurs after this stage of development.

Early school age: perceptual maturation stage

In the early school age (four to seven years), following the maturation of language, perceptual recognition matures. The child begins to distinguish details and appearances as to presentations and differences, correlating these into vocal and manual (written, drawn, gestured) efforts in response. A child works rapidly on the recognition of similar symbols, even if they are dissimilar in formation or position in space. Children are overcoming problems of reversals during this period.

Distortions in these processes may manifest as dyslexia (reading) and dysgraphia (writing), and later as dysorthographia (spelling) and anarithmia or dyscalculia (math). Related activities affected include coordination in sports, housekeeping, manners, and music lessons. Emotional frustrations born of failures at this age include feelings of exclusion, rejection, and inadequacy; reactive responses include the child becoming apathetic, aggressive, discouraged, flight or fight patterns of attack, or giving up and running away. Delinquent behaviors or rigid-chaotic hyperactive symptoms may emerge. Problems of attention are noted, often with related problems of activity.

Later grade-school age: concrete operational stage

The grade-school child (age 7–12 years) continues to operate in a concrete operational stage of thinking. The child begins to apply recalled information in specific situations, developing conclusions, checking out ideas, and formulating new approaches. The concept of cause and result is developing. Basic social skills begin to emerge. Peers seem more important than parents.

Adolescent abstraction stage

By adolescence, the child enters into an abstract or more formal operational phase of learning. The teen is no longer on the presence of items being present and can develop logical approaches. The teen recapitulates the first five years of emotional development, with emphasis on gaining independence from the family. Thus, issues of independence versus dependence become important, as does the future.

Gender differences

In infancy, girls develop a month or so faster than boys. In childhood, there may be a difference of as much as a year. Non-verbal functions are more lateralized in males than in females (McGone, 1977). Children who attain puberty earlier show less lateralized skills. Their left and right hemispheres seem to share in more tasks. Since the female matures several years earlier than the male, the female brain may have less time to lateralize (Yule, 1980).

The intimately connected hemispheres of the female brain may communicate more rapidly and thus prove an advantage in integrating all the details and nuances in an intricate situation but may be less able to focus on a few relevant details. With less interference from the left hemisphere, a man might use his right hemisphere more precisely in deciphering a map or finding a three-dimensional object in a two-dimensional representation (Yule, 1980). A woman may tend to ask for directions, while a man may prefer to read a map.

Plasticity

Damaging brain insults, hereditary factors, or intermittent interruptions of seizure discharges distort or destroy the developing neurocircuity at any of these stages. This may lead to faulty learning development, resulting in a disturbance of intelligence and learning and academic problems. Severe insults may result in a developmental regression or loss. These sequelae often lead to the development of a reactive personality or behavioral problems.

Early and strategic insult to language zones in the left brain promotes a shifting of language functions to the right brain. Verbal functions remain relatively intact but visuospatial skills are impaired, a "crowding" hypothesis accounting for this compromise. In patients with early left lesions, language receives higher developmental priority and transfers to the intact right hemisphere, while visuospatial functions are assigned to the damaged left brain. Thus, with identical twins, if one experiences a left hemisphere stroke at birth resulting in a right hemiplegia, the child's language impairment is far less than expected, but the child, through developmental plasticity, may have only a verbal learning weakness but associated with a non-dominant perceptual problem. This is seen in about 30% of individuals with a right hemiplegic cerebral palsy. Patients with right language dominance and late injury do not show these adjustments. If the genetically coded language hemisphere is injured early, laterality may be reversed and crowding of verbal and visuospatial functions in one hemisphere is unlikely.

Studies of learning deficits in children do not support the idea that early injury may lead to a complete shift of function to the opposite side. Selective memory or attention losses in children with cortical or subcortical epilepsy indicate that the deficits may emerge several years after the onset of the epilepsy (Fedio & Mirsky, 1969). If there is a switch of hemispheric dominance due to early brain damage in epileptic individuals, this may affect cognitive skills. For normal development of cognitive skills, both hemispheres must function properly (Van der Vlugt & Bakker, 1980).

With epilepsy due to a major destructive brain lesion, the cognitive relationships are not what would be expected normally. It is possible to identify accurately such complex partial seizure patients with unilateral cerebral dysfunction even though the group does not show laterality confirmed by neurosurgery or postmortem evidence (Dennerll, 1964). Observed cognitive deficits may depend primarily on the electrical activity of the epileptic focus. The focus does not always coincide with the topographic localization of the atrophic lesion (Ladavas *et al.*, 1979). There may be a lack of any unilaterality of the EEG discharge, leading to difficulties relating a psychologic deficit to a presumed dominant hemisphere (Quadfasel & Pruyser, 1955).

Laterality

There is a continuum in handedness that results in an ordering of hemispheric specialization, from strong lateralization with right-handedness with no familial left-handedness, to weak (atypical or bilateral) hemispheric specialization in left-handed subjects with a familial left-handedness (Piazza, 1980). About the same percentage of left-handedness is seen in the non-epileptic population with learning disabilities and in the epileptic population. The normal learning-disabled population has nearly twice as many left-handed individuals. The incidence of left-handedness is increased in the left temporal lobe group and decreased significantly in the right temporal lobe group.

Left hemisphere

The dominant (left) hemisphere utilizes analytic approaches whereas the non-dominant right hemisphere favors non-language functions, including spatial concepts and "gestalt" recognition (Blakemore *et al.*, 1966; Stores, 1981; Brittain, 1981). Lesions in the dominant hemisphere are more likely to be associated with performance difficulties, especially in verbal and mathematical spheres (Dreifuss, 1983), often resulting in severe, obvious language dysfunctions in older children (Berrant *et al.*, 1980).

Early and late childhood left-hemisphere lesions significantly lower both verbal and performance scores. There are definite verbal/performance differences between children with right temporal lobe epilepsy and those with left temporal lobe epilepsy (Fedio & Mirsky, 1969). In children with left-sided epileptic lesions, there are deficits in learning, sequencing, and memorization of verbal materials, whereas those with a focus on the right side show subtler deficits in tests of non-verbal memory. There is little deficit of learning in children with generalized epilepsy (Hecaen, 1976; Kim *et al.*, 1988).

The left hemisphere may be a major repository for motor learning (Geschwind, 1976). As tasks become more complex, speed and accuracy deteriorate, which may affect the speed of decision-making in situations of increased complexity. This does not seem to be determined by the language deficit or etiology of the condition (Dee, 1973).

In the first year after the diagnosis of an epileptic condition, no significant hemispheric differences are apparent (Ladavas *et al.*, 1979). Unlike patients with epileptic foci in the right hemisphere, impaired performance for patients with a left hemispheric focus may increase over time (Berrant *et al.*, 1980). Epileptic patients with lateralized left hemisphere EEG abnormalities show greater losses with age in performance on several cognitive measures as compared with right hemisphere lateralized abnormality patients (Seidenberg *et al.*, 1981; Beaumanoir *et al.*, 1985).

Frontal and temporal abnormalities with left-sided lesions are more impairing than lesions in other sites (Dreifuss, 1983). Poor performance on the intelligence subtests in the absence of any significant psychiatric thought disorder is generally associated with prefrontal lobe dysfunction (Golden & Berg, 1983).

Right hemisphere

Disruption to right-hemispheric processes is not always clinically obvious (Berrant *et al.*, 1980). The right hemisphere has some motor learning skills, although perhaps not to the extent of the left hemisphere (Geschwind, 1976). The right hemisphere advantage is more of a manipulative skill that appears as a consequence of the earlier emergence of language in the left hemisphere. Perceptual skills may suffer if a lesion involves the non-dominant hemisphere (Stores, 1976).

Learning problems

Some children struggle to learn because one or more of the stages of learning is significantly below their overall intelligence. This is a learning disability if it inhibits academic performance in reading, writing, math, spelling, etc. Some children struggle because their overall intelligence is three standard deviations below the average; this is retardation. Both are learning problems. It is reasonable to assume that some children may be retarded but have specific learning disabilities relative to their overall intellectual level.

There are confusions between various specialties in term usage. Dyslexia, i.e. disturbed, distorted reading efforts, may be seen due to a variety of learning disabilities. There are as many as 20 types of dyslexia. People speak of a perceptual motor problem or a visual-motor problem, but these are the same type of handicap. There are a variety of approaches to reading, including phonetic and sight recognition. Some languages are more phonetically based and some involve more sight recognition.

The most efficient way of reading is to be able to combine both methods. Spelling problems are called dysorthographia. In discussing math problems, one talks of a dyscalculia or an anarithmia; there are as many as 70 potential types of math problems. Math is particularly difficult as it involves three symbol systems, namely numerical, operational, and alphabetical symbols. It also involves spatial relationships (as with math columns), memory (for multiplication tables), and reading skills (for story problems) at the basic levels. Higher math skills involve abstract spatial concepts and relationships, which tend to favor boys' thought processing, although at lower levels girls tend to do better in basic math computation. It is no wonder that the parent, after being shuffled around from expert to expert (teacher, special educator, occupational/physical therapist, psychologist, neurologist), ends up uttering, "I don't know what any of you are talking about. All I know is that my child can't read."

Mental retardation

Mental retardation is intelligence three standard deviations or more below average. Severe mental retardation is usually due to some brain defect or damage, whereas mild retardation may be idiopathic and possibly familial. Some children do not score low enough to be classified as retarded but do not score not high enough to be normal. They are overwhelmed in regular classes but they become bored when placed in classes for retarded children. They tend to learn little and become unprepared for life. Frequently, they drop out of school early.

Mental retardation is most often seen in children whose first seizures were preceded by neurologic abnormalities or with generalized catastrophic seizure syndromes of early childhood, including infantile spasms and some myoclonic and atonic mixed syndromes. For other seizure types, there is no strong correlation between early age of onset and mental retardation. The IQ in this age group equals that of controls (Lesser *et al.*, 1986). No differences in IQ are seen between right and left temporal lobe foci (Camfield *et al.*, 1984).

Deteriorating intelligence

Some children in early grades of school are of higher intelligence levels, but their IQ declines as they progress through school. The cause needs to be determined. Overlooked seizures, misused medications, or nocturnal seizures may contribute. Overlooked learning disabilities may also cause a deterioration of test performance over the years. A discouraged child who has given up trying may drop as many as 20–30 points due to the emotional state. An intellectual decline may also be artificial if dissimilar tests are used or when changing from a pediatric IQ test to an adult IQ test in adolescence. For the most part, there is no real change in the intelligence of many children with epilepsy. Intellectual regression in epileptic children is most often correlated with toxic doses of anticonvulsant drugs, polypharmacy, and early age of seizure onset (Bourgeois *et al.*, 1983).

Intelligence styles and problem areas

The importance of differentiating the types as well as stages of learning and of related learning disabilities has been emphasized (Kirk & Kirk, 1971). Such problems pertain to various areas of the brain, although these skills appear more widespread than are the speech centers.

Learning styles

Many individuals, although tending to favor one or other style of learning, tend to learn by both auditory and visual approaches to learning. Some children are predominantly auditory learners, learning best by listening and talking. They may favor the auditory approach because of a weak visual-motor learning channel. They would rather listen than read, and they prefer to talk than to write. Other children are essentially visual learners, which may be a result of an underlying auditory processing defect. They would rather read or look at pictures or, even better, go on a field trip or try something out rather than listen. Those who show these preferences to an extreme may be learning-disabled.

Learning disabilities

Learning disabilities indicate that the child is significantly outside of the normal range for their age and overall intellectual level and that the deviation interferes with various academic skills, such as reading, writing, spelling, math, understanding, and expression. Such problems are not due to a lack of prior training or to environmental factors. There are as many definitions of learning disabilities as there are learning disabilities.

In children with epilepsy, the risks for learning disabilities, often subtle, may be found in half of the group, especially in those with partial epilepsy. The child most at risk is the child, especially a boy, who develops partial seizures, especially involving the frontal-temporal brain area, before age six years, with seizures that are not controlled easily with medications, especially if on phenytoin monotherapy. In the child epilepsy population, the gender ratio is 60% (in the epilepsy population) to 83% (in the general learning-disabled population) male. However, any and all children with epilepsy are at risk and need to be monitored for such problems (Svoboda, 1979).

Auditory channel disorders

Some children experience learning disabilities involving one or more of the stages of auditory learning. Often, such children also have a visual perceptual difficulty if the problem is of early onset.

Perception and discrimination

The child may not hear the differences between similar sounds or words such as "cat" and "catch." They may have problems understanding what others say. Their difficulties may be reflected in their own speech, with mispronunciations and struggles with phonetic approaches in reading. Such children may have more trouble in a noisy background, and they may appear fidgety, inattentive, or withdrawn.

Memory

Children with poor auditory memory skills may twist and get written and spoken numbers and letters in the wrong order. Phonics abilities are poor. The child does not learn easily by rote memory and needs many repetitions. Such children may grasp the idea but not the order of a series, sometimes repeating the concepts but not able to repeat the words. They may have difficulties in learning and recalling useful names, numbers, rhymes, addresses, the alphabet, counting, and, later on, math. Such a child does not remember facts or instructions given. The child's speech is often delayed, mispronounced, twisted, or out of order. Such children read primarily by sight recognition but may confuse similar words, often resorting to guesses. Grammar may be poor.

Reception

Children with problems in understanding the meanings of spoken words exhibit an inability to understand fully what they have been told or instructed to do. The child hears but appears to struggle in trying to retain useful information and therefore prefers to see rather than to hear information. Such children respond best to visual cues. The child may appear inattentive and hyperactive and often is a loner, although occasionally such children may try to be the leader so they do not have to listen to what others say. Often, such children do not get along well with peers and seem hurt easily. They may withdraw and even seem autistic. When they do try to communicate, it is more by gestures and demonstrations than with meaningful words.

Association

Children with problems in auditory associations may have difficulties relating what they hear with other bits of information in order to understand relationships and develop meaningful responses. They have difficulties in attaching meanings and relationships to words and sounds. They may struggle in finding alternative solutions. They may not understand the relationships of ideas and objects. They do not easily grasp the ideas of stories, outlines, and humor. They tend to do foolish things, not learning from past experiences. This may carry over into discipline, in that they often fail to relate what they have been told to do or not to do in similar experiences in the past.

Expression

The child has problems in communicating in speech with reasonable fluency, often struggling with hesitations and stuttering when trying to express ideas. Such children may appear shy or dull. They can express themselves better by pantomime or writing, and they often rely on gesture and demonstration. They talk little or else they may display an excessive irrelevant chatter with little substance. Verbal responses are limited. The child's mother or other family member may do much of the talking. These children may become so frustrated that they withdraw in tears or may explode in anger and frustration.

Visual-motor disorders

Some children have disabilities in one or more of the visual-motor learning processes, independent of any auditory learning disabilities.

Perception and discrimination

Perception and the discrimination of key details are complex. Various groups of problems may be seen. Some children may have trouble discriminating key details from a busy picture or page. They have trouble in noting visual cues in reading, often confusing similar letters or words. They may display struggles with reading and spelling, with reversals, adding or omitting letters and words. They may forget visual cues in word recognition. They may confuse similarly shaped letters and words such as "h" and "n" or "horse" and "house." They may omit details in drawing. They may be poor at tidying their rooms as they overlook things.

Some children cannot recognize and differentiate symbols, shapes, and items when presented in differing positions, sizes, or appearances. They may struggle in recognizing figures, letters, numbers, and words. They tend to have difficulties with letters and recall. They may confuse words and letters of similar appearance.

Some children have difficulties in spatial arrangement. They are known for reversals and confusions of letters and words that differ only in direction, such as "b" and "d," or "b" and "p," or "6" and "9," or "was" and "saw." These children struggle in reading and in writing. Rotations, reversals, transpositions, and mirroring are prominent. Writing seems sloppy. Their drawings are sterile and disorganized. They are often confused in left–right concepts and in directions. They may get lost in a building easily. They tend to be uncoordinated. They may also struggle in math with difficulties in carrying and borrowing and even in staying within columns. Fractions are overwhelming.

Memory

Some children cannot recall what they have previously seen correctly. Such children may display poor reading abilities, with difficulties in sight recognition approaches. They do better in phonetic approaches. They tend to vocalize what they read so they can hear themselves and thus understand. They may lose their place easily. Reversals and getting things out of order are common. They may struggle to copy items, especially items from the chalkboard to paper.

Reception

Some children do far better in understanding what others say than in recognizing visual cues. They tend to be inattentive and often do not use visual cues. Their workbook performance is slow. They do far better if items are explained to them and they do not have to rely on written instructions. Diagrammatical instructions are overwhelming.

Association

Children with visual association difficulties have trouble relating visual concepts. They struggle to classify and categorize items. They have difficulties in finding alternative solutions to problems. They have trouble attaching meanings and relationship to visual stimuli. They often fail to see and use visual cues appropriately, or they may dwell on the cues and fail to see the whole picture. They are not good at craftwork or puzzles. They cannot derive a story or outline from a picture or cartoon and often do not understand them.

Expression

Children with manual expression problems have difficulties in imitating and expressing ideas through gestures. They prefer to speak rather than to write or draw. Their drawings are often crude, with dislocated parts. Their penmanship is often poor, irregular, and malaligned. They often avoid arts and crafts. They are poor in charades, dramatizations, and pantomime. They often have fine motor coordination problems. They tend to be self-conscious.

Auditory-visual integration problems

Some children have problems in integrating sensations. They may have problems in attaching a phonetic sound to a letter. Often, they have problems in integrating sensory feedback to motor acts, and thus may be uncoordinated and clumsy.

Learning levels

Some children are imbalanced in their levels of learning. Some comprehend well but perform poorly; others may do just the opposite, performing fairly well but without adequate understanding of what they have just done.

Age effect

Many of these skills are developed in early to mid childhood. The four-year-old may display numerous reversals and perceptual problems normally, but this is a disability if it is still present by eight years of age. The teenager tends to be fairly set in their ways and often, if learning problems are untreated, by adolescence the emotional frustration surpasses the underlying learning problems. Usually one helps the teen to use whatever strengths are present and to develop alternative approaches in areas of excessive weakness, as applied especially to future vocational needs and life skills.

Home problems

Learning problems are not limited to school. They also affect home life. The child who has problems in auditory understanding may not understand when told to do something. The child with association problems may not be able to associate past discipline to present situations. The child with perceptual problems may be sloppy at the table and seem superficial in tidying their bedroom. Children with memory problems may not remember to do the things they have been told to do.

REFERENCES

Antell, S. E. & Keating, D. P. (1983). Perception of numerical invariance in neonates. *Child Dev.* **54**: 696–701

Beaumanoir, A., Potolicchio, S. R. & Nahory, J. R. (1985). The importance of telemetric recording in the study of neuropsychological function in epileptics. *Electroencephalogr. Clin. Neurophysiol.* **43**: 542–50.

Berrant, S., Boll, T. J. & Giordani, B. (1980). Hemispheric site of epileptogenic focus: Cognitive, perceptual and psychosocial implications for children and adults. In *Advances in Epileptology XIth Epilepsy International Symposium*, ed. R. Ganger, F. Angeleri & J. K. Penry, pp. 185–90. New York: Raven Press.

Blakemore, C. B., Ettlinger, G. & Falconer, M. A. (1966). Cognitive abilities in relation to the frequency of seizures and neuropathology of the temporal lobes in man. *J. Neurol. Neurosurg. Psychiatry* **29**: 268–72.

Bourgeois, B. F. D., Presky, A. I., Palkes, H. S., *et al.* (1983). Intelligence in epilepsy, a prospective study in children. *Ann. Neurol.* **14**: 438–44.

Brittain, H. (1981). Epilepsy and intellectual functions. In *Epilepsy and Behavior '79*, ed. B. M. Kulig, H. Meinardi & G. Stores, pp. 2–12. Lisse: Swets & Zeitlinger.

Camfield, P. R., Gates, R., Ronen, G., *et al.* (1984). Comparison of cognitive ability, personality profile and school success in epileptic children with pure right versus left temporal lobe EEG foci. *Ann. Neurol.* **15**: 122–6.

Cowan, M. W. (1979). The developing brain. In *The Brain*, pp. 65–79. San Francisco: W. H. Freeman.

Cragg, B. G. (1975). The development of synapses in the visual system of the cat. *J. Comp. Neurol.* **160**: 147–66.

Dee, H. L. & Van Allen, M. W. (1973). Speed of decision making processes in patients with unilateral disease. *Arch. Neurol.* **28**: 163–6.

Dennerll, R. D. (1964). Prediction of unilateral brain dysfunction using Wechsler test scores. *J. Consult. Psychol.* **289**: 278–84.

Dreifuss, F. E. (1983). *Pediatric Epileptology.* Boston: John Wright PSG.

Fedio, P. & Mirsky, A. F. (1969). Selective intellectual deficit in children with temporal lobe or centrencephalic epilepsy. *Neuropsychologia* **7**: 287–300.

Fedio, P., August, A., Sato, S., *et al.* (1993). Left and right brain stimulation and reversed laterality of language and spatial functions: fixed specialization versus transfer of functions. *Epilepsia* **34** (suppl 6): 703.

Geschwind, N. (1976). The apraxias: neural mechanisms of disorders of learned movements. *Am. Sci.* **53**: 188–95.

Golden, C. J. & Berg, C. J. (1983). Interpretation of the Luria–Nebraska battery by item interpretation: intellectual processes. *Clin. Neuropsychol.* **5**: 23–8.

Hecaen, H. (1976). Acquired aphasia in children and the ontogenesis of hemispheric function specialization. *Brain Lang.* **3**: 114–34.

Hecaen, H. & Albert, M. L. (1978). *Human Neuropsychology.* New York: John Wiley & Sons.

Kim, Y., Royer, F., Bontele, C., *et al.* (1988). Temporal sequencing of verbal and nonverbal materials: The effects of laterality of lesion. *Cortex* **16**: 135–43.

Kirk, S. & Kirk, W. (1971). *Psycholinguistic Learning Disabilities: Diagnosis and Remediation.* Urbana, IL: University of Illinois Press.

Ladavas, E., Umnila, C. & Provincialli, I. (1979). Hemispheric dependent cognitive performance in epileptic patients. *Epilepsia* **20**: 493–502.

Lesser, R. P., Luders, H., Wylie, E., *et al.* (1986). Mental deterioration in epilepsy. *Epilepsia* **27** (suppl 2): 105–23.

McGone, J. (1977). Sex differences in the cerebral organization of verbal functions in patients with unilateral brain lesions. *Brain* **1000**: 775–93.

Piazza, D. M. (1980). The influence of sex and handedness in the hemispheric specialization of verbal and nonverbal tasks. *Neuropsychologia* **18**: 163–76.

Quadfasel, A. F. & Pruyser, P. W. (1955). Cognitive deficits in patients with psychomotor epilepsy. *Epilespia* **4**: 80–90.

Seidenberg, M., O'Leary, D. S., Berent, S., *et al.* (1981). Changes in seizure frequency and test–retest scores on the Wechsler Adult Intelligence Scale. *Epilespia* **22**: 75–83.

Stores, G. (1976). The investigation and management of school children with epilepsy. *Publ. Health (London)* **90**: 171–7.

Stores, G. (1981). Problems of learning and behavior in children with epilepsy. In *Epilepsy and Psychiatry*, ed. E. H. Reynolds & M. R. Trimble, pp. 33–48. New York: Churchill Livingstone.

Svoboda, W. B. (1979). Epilepsy and learning problems. In *Learning about Epilepsy*, pp. 185–200. Baltimore, MD: University Park Press.

Thatcher, R. W. (1997). Human frontal lobe development. In *Development of the Prefrontal Cortex*, ed. N. A. Krasnegor, G. R. Lyon & P. S. Goldman-Rakic, pp. 85–115. Baltimore, MD: Paul H. Brookes.

Van der Vlugt, H. & Bakker, D. (1980). Lateralization of brain function in persons with epilepsy. In *Epilepsy and Behavior '79*, ed. B. M. Kulig, H. Meinardi & G. Stores, pp. 30–35. Lisse: Swets & Zeitlinger.

Yule, W. (1980). Educational achievement. In *Epilepsy and Behavior '79*, ed. B. M. Kulig, H. Meinardi & G. Stores, pp. 152–8. Lisse: Swets & Zietlinger.

14

Learning difficulties

Up to 50% of children with epilepsy have learning difficulties (Rutter *et al.*, 1970; Holdsworth & Whitmore, 1974; Whitehouse, 1976; Stores, 1978; Stores, 1987; Thompson, 1987), with up to 30% at risk of developing serious learning problems (Aldenkamp, 1991). The main problems are mental retardation, intellectual decline, learning disabilities, and underachievement. The seizure type and etiology, age of onset, frequency, severity, duration, and effects of seizure therapy modify the academic presentations. Some problems are potentially reversible, but others are permanent (Cornaggia & Gobbi, 2001).

Around 50% of children with epilepsy have some school difficulties, but less than 1% attend special epilepsy schools (Cornaggia & Gobbi, 2001). Around 30% of children with therapy-resistant epilepsies receive special education help (Green & Hartlage, 1971; Holdsworth & Whitmore, 1974; Aldenkamp, 1983; Thompson, 1987; Ross & Tookey, 1988). Children with epilepsy tend to drop out of school earlier. By adolescence, only 33% of epileptic children are in the secondary school system (Rodin *et al.*, 1972; Thorbecke, 1987). The dropout tendency relates somewhat to the sociological status and attitudes of the family (Suurmeijer *et al.*, 1978; Long & Moore, 1979; Aldenkamp *et al.*, 1990). This leads to occupational disadvantages and a higher unemployment rate (Rodin *et al.*, 1972; Thorbecke, 1987).

Learning problem confusion

A specific cognitive functional impairment is a reduction in the capacity of the child to learn. This is a learning disability, which is different to mental retardation and intellectual deterioration. In some countries such as the UK, the term "learning disability" is used to define both mental retardation and learning disorders. However, the usual definition of a learning disability includes a significant disturbance in academic achievement or daily living activities that require reading, mathematics, or writing skills. As applied, a child with mental retardation has a depressed IQ, whereas a child with a learning disorder has a normal IQ (Cornaggia & Gobbi, 2001).

Epilepsy may cause a learning disability coinciding with the cortical area involved in the seizure focus without causing mental retardation. When this occurs before the acquisition of the learning ability, this may lead to a depressed intellectual performance. Those children who appear to be mentally retarded may improve completely if this specific cognitive dysfunction is adequately treated early (Cornaggia & Gobbi, 2001).

Intelligence and retardation

The distribution of intelligence in children with epilepsy is skewed towards a lower range, but it can vary widely from year to year in an individual (Tarter, 1972; Holmes, 1987). In childhood epilepsy, intelligence has been found to be below average in up to 57%, with only 9% showing an IQ above 110 (Whitehouse, 1971).

Retardation means that the intellectual average is three standard deviations below normal (Seidenberg et al., 1985). In the general population, 1–2% of people are retarded. Around 20–29% of people with epilepsy are mentally retarded (Pazzaglia & Frank-Pazzaglia, 1976; Besag, 1995). About 15% may fall in the moderate to severe retardation range. Retardation with seizures is seen slightly more often in males than females (Richardson et al., 1981).

Epilepsy in the retarded population

Epilepsy is more common (25%) in the retarded population, the incidence being inversely proportional to the intellectual level (Richardson et al., 1981). The incidence of underlying brain damage or maldevelopment as a cause for both is also inversely proportional to the intellectual level in the more retarded population (Corbett, 1981). With mild retardation, only 3–6% have epilepsy (Browne & Reynolds, 1981). With severe retardation, 31% have seizures but only 18% are having active treatment (Kaufman & Katz-Garris, 1974).

Seizure type

Children with absence seizures do the best, with an average IQ in the range 106–13 (Collins & Lennox, 1946; Zimmerman et al., 1984), yet 34% of children score in the borderline range and 15% are retarded (Cheminal et al., 1998). Children with partial seizures show higher intelligence than those with generalized tonic–clonic seizures. Children with mixed seizures have significantly lower IQs (Lennox & Lennox, 1960; Fedio & Mirsky, 1969; Brittain, 1980). Some of the seizure syndromes of infancy and early childhood, especially those associated with distinctly abnormal EEG patterns (burst-suppression, hypsarrhythmia, slow spike-wave discharges), often are associated with marked intellectual impairments.

Modifiers

A tendency towards lower intelligence scores is seen in younger epileptic children and in those who have adverse perinatal factors, early onset of epilepsy, symptomatic epilepsy, non-familial epilepsy, a mixed seizure disorders with multiple seizure types, a greater seizure frequency, or a higher lifetime total number of seizures (Mellor and Lowit, 1977; Browne & Reynolds, 1981; Seidenberg *et al.*, 1985). Children younger than ten years at the time of seizure onset gain skills more slowly than those with an age of onset greater than ten years (Neyes *et al.*, 1999).

Cause

The combination of neurologic deficits and seizures contributes to the lower IQ, but children with idiopathic epilepsy also show some cognitive problems (Mellor & Lowit, 1977). The intelligence of children with idiopathic epilepsy is in the average range but with a tendency to cluster toward the lower end, especially in performance areas, with scores slightly lower than their sibs. Factors contributing to lower IQ scores are early age of onset, longer duration, persistence of seizures, and anticonvulsant effects (Rodin *et al.*, 1986).

Children with symptomatic epilepsies and those with mixed and multifocal seizures have significantly lower IQ scores than those with idiopathic seizures, especially with familial idiopathic epilepsy (Halstead, 1957; Tarter, 1972; Klove & Matthews, 1974; Brittain, 1980; Bourgeouis *et al.*, 1983; Cornaggia & Gobbi, 2001). Children with frank brain damage (such as cerebral palsy or other brain disorders), inborn errors of metabolism, and neurocutaneous disorders are most apt to be impaired (Corbett, 1981; Trimble, 1990).

Age of onset

There is no correlation between early age of onset and mental retardation, except in those with neurological abnormalities preceding the first seizures and those with early childhood seizure syndromes including infantile spasms (Sillanpaa, 1973; Lesser *et al.*, 1986).

Frequency and duration

Seizure frequency or duration, especially with signs of underlying acquired brain damage, relate to a lower intelligence (Halstead, 1957; Browne *et al.*, 1981). The highest incidence of mental retardation (57%) is seen in children with very frequent seizures (Keith *et al.*, 1955). In a study, only 45% of students who had an accumulative total of more than 1000 seizures were considered mentally normal (Keating, 1960).

Intellectual variability

The wide fluctuations in IQ performance seen in children with epilepsy on retesting may relate to changes in seizure control and Reynolds (Browne *et al.*, 1981; Bargemeister, 1962; Seidenberg *et al.*, 1981; Trimble, 1990). IQ is not the sole criterion of intelligence, since emotional disorders, slowness of mental reactions, lack of concentration, and shortened memory span may impair the performance on testing, leading to incorrect estimates (Sillanpaa, 1973).

Intellectual decline

Although it is now felt that epilepsy does not usually lead to an intellectual decline (Cornaggia & Gobbi, 2001), in some patients epileptic deterioration does occur (Brittain, 1980; Corbett, 1981; Rodin, 1968; Waxman & Geschwind, 1975). This may relate to repeated seizures or to overmedication (Onuma, 2000).

Over the years, a small but significant intellectual decline occurs in some individuals, even when seizures are controlled (Aldenkamp et al., 1990). More often, seizures in remission are associated with stability or improvement of intellect. Patients with partial seizures followed for a decade showed only subtle losses, if any, in intellectual functions. In most children with epilepsy, intelligence remains stable (Holmes et al., 1998). However a small but significant group shows a progressive intellectual decline over time (Holmes, 1987). A drop in academic performance may be seen in the first year following the seizure onset (McNelis et al., 2000). A greater than ten-point IQ drop may occur in 11% of patients; over a longer period, 20% experience a fall of at least 12 IQ points on serial testing. This is thought to be related to seizure control, seizure frequency, drug intoxication, and polypharmacy (Bourgeouis et al., 1983; Palkes et al., 1982). Non-convulsive status is seen more often in patients who actually lost skills (Besag et al., 1991).

Causes and modifiers

IQ deterioration in children may relate to a high initial seizure frequency, a poorer response to anticonvulsant therapy, a more disturbed family environment, or an excess of focal seizures, often secondarily generalizing (Browne & Reynolds, 1981). Brighter individuals appear more prone to intellectual decline (Tarter, 1972).

Seizure type

Major seizures are more associated with deterioration than are minor seizures, with the exception of the minor motor group (Tarter, 1972). The majority of cases of intellectual deterioration are seen in children with more severe epileptic syndromes (O'Donohoe, 1979). Declines in intelligence functions, memory, and behavior have been reported with repeated seizures. Animal and human studies suggest that uncontrolled seizures lead to nerve cell losses that parallel the deterioration of cognitive functions and emotions (Svoboda, 1979).

Cause

Declines are more apt to be seen in children with symptomatic epilepsy (Tarter, 1972; Sillanpaa, 1973; Bourgeouis et al., 1983). In children with idiopathic epilepsy, deterioration is found in only 9.8%, whereas in symptomatic epilepsies, deterioration is found in 26–37%, especially in those with abnormal neurologic findings (Tarter, 1972; Pond, 1974; Brittain, 1980). Deteriorating intelligence in epileptic individuals may suggest an active lesion (Milner, 1975).

Age of onset

Significant declines are seen most often in children with seizures of early onset, even if the seizures are protracted (Tarter, 1972; Diaz *et al.*, 1977; Bourgeouis *et al.*, 1983; Vargha-Kahdem, 2001). Recurrent seizures during early development may cause long-term deleterious effects for reasons that are unknown (Holmes *et al.*, 1999).

Seizure frequency

Seizures may lead to a decrease in intelligence if they are frequent, prolonged, or severe (Collins, 1951; Reitan, 1974; Dodrill, 1976; Reynolds, 1981). The role of seizure frequency in intellectual decline has been questioned (Tenny, 1955; Chaudhry & Pond, 1961; Stores, 1976b; Besag *et al.*, 1991).

Duration

Recurrent seizures may result in long-term detrimental changes in the developmental brain (Holmes *et al.*, 1999). Intellectual deterioration, especially in memory, appears to be related to the duration of the epilepsy (Tarter, 1972).

Severity

Lessening of intelligence may relate more to the severity than to the type of seizure (Tarter, 1972). Seizures interfere not only with neuronal development through the destruction of neurons by hypoxia, but also with the growth of nerve fibers and possibly RNA production in the brain (Ounsted *et al.*, 1966).

Status epilepticus

Following epileptic status in children, developmental deterioration is seen in 34%; 36% go on to develop epilepsy. About 79% of these children will have been abnormal before the status. Non-idiopathic, non-febrile status is a strong predictor for sequelae (Wirrell & Barnard, 1999). A drop in IQ of nearly 20 points may follow an episode of spike-wave stupor (Moe, 1971; Ballenger *et al.*, 1983).

Drug effects

A loss of mental ability in children may be associated with high-dosage medication, polypharmacy, or, rarely, low folate levels (Trimble *et al.*, 1980; Bourgeouis *et al.*, 1983; Thompson, 1983).

Diagnosis

When faced with intellectual deterioration, the underlying cause of the seizure disorder, the seizure frequency, and the medications in use, especially the potential of intoxication, must be reviewed (Prensky *et al.*, 1971). An active investigation is necessary until a cause is found (Cornaggia & Gobbi, 2001). If no identifiable cause is found, overnight EEG monitoring in children may reveal frequent EEG abnormalities, such as spike-wave discharges (Besag *et al.*, 1991).

Learning disabilities

Many children with epilepsy exhibit a higher incidence of learning disabilities associated with their seizure disorder, creating difficulties in academic achievement. This is especially apparent in their first years of schooling (Ives, 1970; Gerson *et al.*, 1972; Whitehouse, 1976; Wunsche *et al.*, 1977; Morgan & Groh, 1980). Children with epilepsy resemble other children with learning disabilities, except the former exhibit more difficulties in the speed of performance (Aldenkamp, 1991).

Laterality of the seizure focus

Learning disabilities related to the laterality of the focus tend to be seen with partial seizures rather than with generalized seizures; with absence seizures, memory abilities are lower than with controls (Cheminal *et al.*, 1998).

The left hemisphere is usually dominant for language processing as well as functions including analysis, details notation, ordering of items, time notation, and the process of calculation in math. Verbal skills include not only speech but also memory, reasoning, verbal learning, and related verbalized emotions. The right hemisphere relates to the processing of non-verbal skills, including the recognition and remembering of geometric shapes, spatial arrangements and relationships, directions, right–left differentiation, and a sense of time. The right hemisphere helps people remember time and spatial patterns, such as melodies, face, shapes, and forms (Svoboda, 1979).

Etiology

Epileptiform foci may alter dominant hemispheric processing of language, which can lead to a neuropsychological disorder such as learning disabilities (Riva *et al.*, 1991). The P300 "cognitive peak" is altered in about half of patients with epilepsy, often with dominance shifts to the other side. An MRI lesion renders a hemisphere unlikely to become language-dominant. A less severe focal MRI lesion, such as hippocampal atrophy, may be associated with both functional dominance and the P300 dominance to shift contralaterally (Kanazawa *et al.*, 2000). The right brain is capable not only of language comprehension but also of completely substituting for the left hemisphere, even its expressive capacity (Sidtis *et al.*, 1981; Piccirilli *et al.*, 1988).

Partial seizures

Lateralized interictal discharges may be related to functional hemisphere specialization, even if no brain lesions are detectable (Muszkat *et al.*, 1991). The epileptogenic focus, acting like a lesion focus, can alter the cerebral mechanisms underlying cognitive activity (Piccirilli *et al.*, 1988). The pattern of functional cerebral representation in focal epileptic patients depends on the focus site, as shown in individuals with untreated benign, focal, lesionless epilepsy. Interictal PET demonstrates an area of cerebral hypometabolism superimposed with the EEG focus (Engel *et al.*, 1982).

Frontal lobe seizure foci

Individuals with a frontal epileptiform focus, especially right frontal disturbances, may have difficulties with organization, planning, and independent work efforts, especially those tasks that depend on developing one answer as a base to the next step. A left frontal disturbance is more apt to disturb the smooth flow of spontaneous speech (Svoboda, 1979).

Left temporal lobe foci

Left temporal lobe seizures occur more frequently and often have an earlier age of onset than right temporal lobe seizures. Children with complex partial epilepsy exhibit language-based learning disabilities resembling the non-epileptic population with specific learning disabilities without any depression of intellect (Breier *et al.*, 1999). They may be depressed in immediate memory and verbal attentiveness (Muszkat *et al.*, 1991).

Children with left temporal lobe epilepsy tend toward problems in immediate memory and verbal attention (Muszkat *et al.*, 1991), including verbal and to a lesser degree visual spatial memory, as well as problems in concept formation. The mild impairment of visual spatial memory may relate to difficulties in using verbal mediation strategies as a means of facilitating learning and recall of non-verbal material (Battaglia, 1998). Weaknesses in information, digit span, and arithmetic subtests are seen (Muszkat *et al.*, 1991). Memory problems may be noted in understanding and remembering, in remembering words and names, math tables, rhymes, prayers, addresses, and phone numbers. Sometimes, what is recalled may be a similar but incorrect word, and this confusion will show up in understanding, speech, or written efforts (Svoboda, 1979).

In school, problems in reading and later in spelling may be noted. Phonetic approaches, such as blending sounds together into words, may be difficult. Such children often have problems sounding out words. They may confuse similar sounds or words. Sometimes, the child gets the sounds or the letters in the wrong order. These problems carry over to speech and spelling as well as to reading. Basic spelling rules may be of little help as they too may be forgotten. An early hint of potential reading difficulties in school would be delayed or distorted development of speech and language, which may be seen with later difficulties in phonic approaches to reading. Boys seem to be more at risk than girls (Svoboda, 1979).

Math problems emerge by third grade or earlier. Children may confuse or not recognize operations, such as addition, subtraction, multiplication, or division. They may subtract larger numbers from smaller numbers. They may carry over the last number of the problem as the answer (this mistake is a form of perseveration). They may write numbers literally; for example, when told to write 164, they may write 100, 60, and 4. They often place the comma place markings incorrectly in numbers of four or more digits (Svoboda, 1979).

Children with temporal lobe epilepsy and dysembryoplastic neuroepithelia tumors are prone to significant learning disabilities that do not respond to surgical excision of the tumors, suggesting that it is the severe continuing epilepsy, not the tumor, that impairs intelligence (Knight *et al.*, 1998).

Right temporal lobe foci

Children with right temporal lobe epilepsy may show a significantly poorer performance on visual spatial performance, visual spatial memory, and non-verbal attention (Muszkat *et al.*, 1991; Battaglia, 1998; Cornaggia & Gobbi, 2001). IQ performance tests are lower, with problems in block design, object assembly, and coding (Muszkat *et al.*, 1991).

Children with right-sided seizures seem less prone to overt disturbances. They are more apt to develop perceptual problems in recognizing what they see or non-language patterns that they hear, such as remembering and recognizing shapes, patterns, and forms. Such problems are often referred to as visuospatial difficulties, visual/motor problems, or perceptual (motor) problems. The children tend to have problems recognizing letters, numbers, and familiar words. In reading or writing, they may reverse, invert, or twist the letters around in their mind. In spelling, they may add or omit letters, or sometimes double or even triple up a letter. Difficulties in copying from the board may be noted. Writing tends to be very sloppy, with blotches and extra markings. Letters may vary in size, shape, form, and tilt. Spacing is erratic, with little attention paid to the paper lines. Letters may be fused together, or the child may devise new letters. Significant math details may be overlooked or confused, such as the operation signs or math columns. Problems also occur with borrowing and carrying in maths (Svoboda, 1979).

Such perceptual problems often result in clumsiness and a poor sense of left–right, directions, and time, as well as problems in table manners (spilling), sports (clumsy), housekeeping (overlooks obvious items), and in learning to sight-read music. Children may have problems recognizing social cues on other people's faces, resulting in disturbed social relationships. In reacting to their difficulties, they may become quite rigid and adherent to set schedules, going to pieces when the unexpected happens (Svoboda, 1979).

Bitemporal lobe foci

Early age of onset of seizures (before five years of age) involving both temporal lobes increases the risks for both auditory and visual-motor processing deficits and thus a lower intelligence. This is often manifest as more severe memory difficulties, inattentiveness, and distractibility, with incomplete work efforts. Anoxia, hypoglycemia, brain edema, or ischemia to the immature brain may produce bilateral damage sufficient to cause seizures and marked memory disturbances. The child may not be able to remember something long enough to learn it. Without past memories to rely on, the child may seem to be severely retarded. In adults, bilateral temporal lobe removal produces a severe memory problem, but intelligence and speech remain intact as the individual has a prior stored knowledge base (Svoboda, 1979).

Benign Rolandic epilepsy

The epileptiform focus itself can determine language laterality. A benign Rolandic mid-temporal central spike may be unilateral or bilateral-independent in presentation. Benign Rolandic epilepsy may influence language lateralization, even before treatment, as seen in children with normal intelligence and no demonstrable structural lesion. A right-hemispheric focus relates to the expected left language lateralization. A left unilateral focus shows a different pattern of functional representation, suggesting involvement of the right hemisphere in language mechanisms. This results in significantly poorer performance in tasks testing higher verbal and visual motor functions (Piccirilli *et al.*, 1988).

Underachievement

Underachievement in relation to the IQ has long been recognized in children with epilepsy (Rutter *et al.*, 1970; Stores & Hart, 1976; Baird *et al.*, 1980; Ford *et al.*, 1983). Children with epilepsy make less academic progress than expected for their IQ, age, and grade level (Seidenberg *et al.*, 1985; Seidenberg *et al.*, 1986), with much performance scatter seen (Halstead, 1957). Of those with normal IQs (58%), most have learning difficulties with an indifferent performance in class (Ounsted *et al.*, 1966; Holdsworth & Whitmore, 1974; O'Donohoe, 1979). In regular classrooms, 15.6% of children with epilepsy and normal intelligence fall behind significantly (Wilkus & Dodrill, 1976; Pazzaglia & Frank-Pazzaglia, 1976; Baird *et al.*, 1980;

Holdsworth & Whitmore, 1974). Often, these children are not pushed to meet their potential. They may be promoted socially or else placed according to their actual functioning.

Academic effects

Children with epilepsy underachieve especially in arithmetic, but also in spelling, reading, comprehension, and word recognition (Seidenberg et al., 1985; Seidenberg et al., 1986). Although they are placed appropriately per grade, the Wide Range Achievement Test shows such children to be about one year behind in reading vocabulary recognition and one year and eight months behind in math (Green & Hartlage, 1971). The strongest risk factors to academic performance are the age of the child, age of seizure onset, lifetime total seizure frequency, and presence of multiple seizures (especially absence and tonic–clonic) (Seidenberg et al., 1985; Seidenberg et al., 1986).

Contributing factors

Seizure type

Children with partial seizures do better than those with mixed generalized seizures. Children with generalized tonic–clonic seizures, especially if complicated by absence attacks, have more achievement problems (Sillanpaa, 1973; Seidenberg et al., 1985; Seidenberg et al., 1986). Children with complex partial epilepsy, despite having normal IQ, are often low in academic achievement, with poor school performance (Ounsted et al., 1966).

Missed and subclinical seizures

Subclinical spike-wave bursts may interfere with registration, storage, and recall of information, leading to underachievement (Baird et al., 1980). Children with absence attacks with active interictal epileptic discharges have more problems than those with normal interictal EEGs (Cheminal et al., 1998). In children who exhibit a fluctuating concentration, marked insecurity, and widely variable school performance, subclinical seizures are found in 25%, which were often missed absence attacks.

Cause

Children with symptomatic epilepsy are more apt to underachieve than those with idiopathic seizures (Sillanpaa, 1973), yet even the epileptic discharges cause problems.

Gender

With epilepsy, a significantly higher proportion of boys than girls experience educational difficulties (Barlow, 1978). Boys have more problems in spelling, arithmetic, and reading comprehension. Girls show a developmental advantage for the acquisition of specific cognitive skills of verbal reasoning, language skills, and pattern matching that relates to reading acquisition, and this carries over to children with epilepsy. Girls generally do better than boys in language-related academic areas, such as reading and spelling, rather than academic performance in general. Girls are similar to boys or perhaps perform below boys in higher arithmetic and in some types of reading (Seidenberg et al., 1985; Seidenberg et al., 1986).

Onset age

Underachievement is more common in children with early-onset seizures, especially in the first year of life and especially if brain damage is present. Otherwise, the older the child, the further behind is their performance (Seidenberg et al., 1985; Seidenberg et al., 1986).

Frequency

Underachievement is seen in children with at least overall average intelligence and good seizure control (Stores, 1976b; Porter et al., 1973; Rutter et al., 1970; Holdsworth & Whitmore, 1974).

Antiepileptic medication

Although most often blamed for school problems by teachers and many parents, neither antiepileptic medications nor the number of medications taken seem to be a significant predictor variable for academic functioning (Seidenberg et al., 1985; Seidenberg et al., 1986).

Behavior aspects

Underachievement in academic subjects is associated with behavior disturbances, especially conduct disorders (Green & Hartlage, 1971; Rutter, 1977). Children with epilepsy are at special risk for developing complications behaviors (20%), often as a result of learning underachievement, although the behavior may then accentuate the learning difficulties (Holdsworth & Whitmore, 1974; Stores, 1976a; O'Donohoe, 1979). About half of misbehaving children are referred for psychologic testing, especially those with major seizures, inattentiveness, or behavior problems (Wilkus & Dodrill, 1976; Holdsworth & Whitmore, 1974).

Anxiety

Underachievement may be due to the anxiety about having a seizure in school distracting a child from learning (Henricksen, 1990). Underachievement may arise because of anxiety or stress at an earlier critical learning skill development period. Parents and teachers often expect less of the epileptic child academically and in concentration (Rutter, 1977). A few parents will expect more of their child than they themselves produced academically. Children with epilepsy may be performing appropriately for their skills and intelligence, yet 38% may be described as not working productively and thus making lower than average grades.

Motivation

Underachievement may be related to temperamental influences, anxiety, past stresses at a critical period, lack of motivation, avoidance of learning (often due to prior failures), or undetected cognitive dysfunctions (Rutter, 1977). About 10% underachieve despite average or above-average intelligence and potentials. The children can and do learn, but they seem to lack the motivation and independent work habits required to meet promotional requirements. Some even seem to escape learning activities by acting out behaviors, illness complaints, or not doing their work or handing in assignments. Some are never prepared (Gerson *et al.*, 1972). Epileptic children tend to develop skills more to satisfy personal needs and to avoid any behaviors required in conforming to the demands of peers and superiors.

Attention problems

Attention problems are seen in underachieving children. Underachievers are often misdiagnosed as having ADHD. About 42% of children with epilepsy are described as inattentive. There is no relationship to the seizure type, seizure frequency, drug effects, basic intelligence, or the gender of the child. The possibility of a relationship of the attention to subclinical seizure discharges has been raised (O'Donohoe, 1979; Baird *et al.*, 1980).

Absenteeism

Usually, seizures are not a reason to miss school or to be sent home from school. A low rate of absenteeism is often reported (Rutter, 1970; Holdsworth & Whitmore, 1974), yet the absenteeism rate may be twice that of non-epileptic students (Ross & West, 1978).

Other problems

Children with epilepsy are also often handicapped by slowness of thinking, a lack of concentration, memory problems, and coordination difficulties (Halstead, 1957; Stores, 1976b), as well as speech and language problems, motor developmental difficulties, sensory deficits, and growth problems.

REFERENCES

Aldenkamp, A. P. (1983). Epilepsy and learning behavior. In *Advances in Epileptology: The XIVth International Epilepsy Symposium*, ed. M. Parsonage, R. H. E. Grant, A. G. Craig & A. A. Ward, Jr, pp. 221–9. New York: Raven Press.

Aldenkamp, A. P. (1991). Learning disabilities in epilepsy. 19th International Epilepsy Congress, Rio De Janeiro, Brazil. *Epilepsia* **32** (suppl 1): 25.

Aldenkamp, A. P., Alpherts, W. C. J., Dekker, M. J. A. & Overweg, J. (1990). Neuropsychological aspects of learning disabilities in epilepsy. *Epilepsia* **31** (suppl 4): 9–20.

Baird, H. W., John, E. R., Ahn., H. & Maisel, E. (1980). Neurometric evaluation of epileptic children who do well and poorly in school. *Electreoncephalogr. Clin. Neurophysiol.* **48**: 684–93.

Ballenger, C. E., King, D. W. & Gallagher, B. B. (1983). Partial complex status epilepticus. *Neurology* **33**: 1545–52.

Bargemeister, B. B. (1962). Epilepsy. In *Psychological Techniques in Neurologic Diagnosis*, pp. 62–90. New York: Hoeber Medical Books.

Barlow, C. F. (1978). Risk factors of infancy and childhood: interrelationship of seizure disorders and mental retardation. In *Mental Retardation and Related Disorders*, pp. 68–75. Philadelphia: FA Davis.

Battaglia, F. M. (1998). Neuropsychological aspects of TLE in children. 3rd European Congress of Epileptology. *Epilepsia* **39** (suppl 2): 70.

Besag, F. M. C. (1995). Epilepsy, learning and behavior in childhood. *Epilepsia* **36** (suppl 10): 58–63.

Besag, F. M. C., Fowler, M. & Pool, F. (1991). Cognitive deterioration in children with epilepsy. 19th International Epilepsy Congress. *Epilepsia* **32** (suppl 1): 15.

Bourgeouis, B. F. D., Prensky, A. L., Pales, H. S., Talent, B. K. & Busch, S. G. (1983). Intelligence in epilepsy: a prospective study in children. *Ann. Neurol.* **14**: 438–44.

Breier, J. I., Clark, A., Cass, J., Wheless, J. W. & Constantinou, J. E. C. (1999). Profiles of cognitive performance in TLE patients with and without learning disability. *Epilepsia* **40** (suppl 7): 47–8.

Brittain, H. (1980). Epilepsy and intellectual functions. In *Epilepsy and Behavior '79*, ed. B. M. Kulig, H. Meinardi & G. Stores, pp. 2–12. Lisse: Swets & Zeitlinger.

Browne, S. W. & Reynolds, E. H. (1981). Cognitive impairments in epileptic patients. In *Epilepsy and Psychiatry*, eds. E. H. Reynolds & M. R. Trimble, pp. 147–63. New York: Churchill Livingstone.

Chaudhry, M. R. & Pond, D. A. (1961). Mental deterioration in epileptic children. *J. Neurol. Neurosurg. Psychiatry* **24**: 213–20.

Cheminal, R., Laurayre, P., Quisquempois, J. M., *et al.* (1998). Neuropsychological abnormalities in absence epilepsy. 3rd European Congress of Epileptology. *Epilepsia* **39** (suppl 2): 120.

Collins, A. L. (1951). Epileptic intelligence. *J. Consult. Psychol.* **15**: 392–9.

Collins, A. L. & Lennox, W. G. (1946). Intelligence of 300 private epileptic patients. *Res. Publ. Assoc. Nerv. Ment. Dis.* **26**: 586–97.

Corbett, J. (1981). Epilepsy and mental retardation. In *Epilepsy and Psychiatry*, ed. E. H. Reynolds & M. R. Trimble, pp. 138–145. New York: Churchill Livingstone.

Cornaggia, C. M. & Gobbi, G. (2001). Learning disability in epilepsy: definitions and classification. In *Epilepsia and Learning Disabilities*, ed. G. F. Ayala, M. Elia, C. M. Cornaggia & M. M. Trimble. *Epilepsia* **42**: 2–5.

Diaz, J., Shain, R. J. & Bailey, B. G. (1977). Phenobarbital induced brain growth retardation in artificially reared rat pups. *Biol. Neonate* **32**: 77–82.

Dodrill, C. B. (1976). Neuropsychology. In *Textbook of Epilepsy*, ed. J. Laidlaw & A. Richens, Vol. II, pp. 282–91. London: Churchill Livingstone.

Engel, J., Brown, W. J., Kuhl, D. E., *et al.* (1982). Pathology findings underlying focal temporal lobe hypometabolism in partial epilepsy. *Ann. Neurol.* **12**: 512–28.

Fedio, P. O. & Mirsky, A. F. (1969). Selective intellectual deficits in children with temporal lobe or centrencephalic epilepsy. *J. Neuropsychol.* **7**: 287–300.

Ford, C. A., Gibson, P. & Dreifuss, F. E. (1983). Psychological considerations in childhood epilepsy. In *Pediatric Epileptology*, ed. F. Dreifuss, pp. 277–95. Boston: John Wright PSG.

Gerson, I. M., Barnes, T. C., Mannino, A., Fanning, J. M. & Burns, J. J. (1972). EEG of children with various learning problems. *Dis. Nerv. Syst.* **33**: 170–77.

Green, J. B. & Hartlage, L. C. (1971). Comparative performance of epileptic and non-epileptic children and adolescents. *Dis. Nerv. Syst.* **32**: 418–21.

Halstead, H. (1957). Abilities and behavior of epileptic children. *J. Ment. Sci.* **103**: 28–47.

Henricksen, O. (1990). Education and epilepsy: assessment and remediation. *Epilepsia* **31** (suppl 4): 21–5.

Holdsworth, L. & Whitmore, K. (1974). A study of children with epilepsy attending ordinary schools. *Dev. Med. Child Neurol.* **16**: 746–58.

Holmes, G. L. (1987). *Psychosocial Factors in Childhood Epilepsy*, pp. 112–24. Philadelphia: W. B. Saunders.

Holmes, M. D., Dodrill, C. B., Wilkus, R. J., Ojemann, L. M. & Ojemann, G. A. (1998). Is partial epilepsy progressive? Ten year follow-up of EEG and neuropsychological changes in adults with partial seizures. *Epilepsia* **39**: 189–93.

Holmes, G. L., Sarkisian, M., Ben-Ari, Y. & Chevassus-Au-Louis, N. (1999). Effects of recurrent seizures in the developing brain. In *Childhood Epilepsies and Brain Development*, ed. A. Nehlig, J. Motte, S. L. Moshe & P. Plouin, pp. 263–76. London: John Libbey & Co.

Ives, L. A. (1970). Learning difficulties in children with epilepsy. *Br. J. Disord. Commun.* **5**: 77–84.

Kanazawa, O., Yoshino, M., Sasagawa, M., *et al.* (2000). VIQ-PIQ discrepancies in partial epilepsy on the relation to lateralities of focal MRI lesions, P3 peaks and focal spikes. Proceedings of the 32nd Congress of Japan Epilepsy Society. *Epilepsia* **41** (suppl 9): 64.

Kaufman, K. R. & Katz-Garris, L. (1974). Epilepsy mental retardation and anticonvulsant therapy. *Am. J. Ment. Defic.* **84**: 256–9.

Keating, L. E. (1960). A review of the literature on the relationship of epilepsy and intelligence in school children. *J. Ment. Sci.* **15**: 1042–59.

Keith, H. M., Ewert, J. C., Green, M. W., *et al.* (1955). Mental status of children with convulsive disorders. *Neurology* **5**: 419–25.

Klove, H. & Matthews, C. G. (1974). Neuropsychological studies of patients with epilepsy. In *Clinical Neuropsychology: Current Status and Applications*, ed. R. M. Reitan & L. A. Davidson, pp. 237–67. New York: John Wiley & Sons.

Knight, E. S., Oxbury, J. M., Middleton, J. A. & Oxbury, S. M. (1998). Cognitive function after temporal lobe epilepsy surgery (TLES) for dysembryoplastic neuroepithelial tumor (DNET) in children aged <6years. 3rd European Congress of Epileptology. *Epilepsia* **39** (suppl 2): 119.

Lennox, W. G. & Lennox, M. E (1960). *Epilepsy and Related Disorders*. London: Churchill Livingstone.

Lesser, R. P., Luders, H., Wyllie, E., Dinner, D. S. & Morris, H. H. (1986). Mental deterioration in epilepsy. *Epilepsia* **27** (suppl 2): 105–23.

Long, C. G. & Moore, J. R. (1979). Parental expectations for their epileptic children. *J. Child Psychol. Psychiatry* **20**: 299–312.

McNelis, A. M., Austin, J. K., Dunn, D. W., Rose, D. & Creasy, K. (2000). Academic achievement in children with new-onset seizures. *Epilepsia* **41** (suppl 7): 238.

Mellor, D. H. & Lowit, I. (1977). A study of intellectual function in children with epilepsy attending ordinary schools. In *Epilepsy: Eighth International Symposium*, ed. J. K. Penry, pp. 291–4. New York: Raven Press.

Milner, B. (1975). Psychological aspects of focal epilepsy and its neurosurgical management. *Adv. Neurol.* **8**: 299–321.

Moe, P. (1971). Spike wave stupor. *Am. J. Dis. Child* **121**: 307–13.

Morgan, A. M. B. & Groh, C. (1980). Visual perceptual deficits in young children with epilepsy. In *Epilepsy and Behavior '79*, ed. B. M. Kulig, H. Meinardi & G. Stores, pp. 169–71. Lisse: Swets & Zeitlinger.

Muszkat, M., Ggorz-Reinhard, A. M., Masuko, A., *et al.* (1991). Neuropsychological performance in children with partial, non-lesional epilepsy. 19th International Epilepsy Congress. *Epilepsia* **32** (suppl 1): 24.

Neyes, L. G. J., Aldenkamp, A. P. & Meinardi, H. M. (1999). Prospective follow-up of intellectual development in children with recent onset of epilepsy. *Epilepsy Res.* **34**: 85–90.

O'Donohoe, N. V. (1979). Mental handicap and epilepsy. In *Epilepsies of Childhood*, pp. 143–6. London: Butterworth.

Onuma, T. (2000). Classification of psychiatric symptoms in patients with epilepsy. Proceedings of the 32nd Congress of Japan Epilepsy Society. *Epilepsia* **41** (suppl 9): 43–8.

Ounsted, C., Lindsay, J. & Normal, R. (1966). Biological factors in temporal lobe epilepsy: intelligence. In *Clinics in Developmental Medicine*, pp. 62–71. London: Heinemann.

Palkes, H. S., Prensky, A. L., Bourgeois, B. F. D., Talent, B. K. & Busch, S. G. (1982). Intelligence of epileptic children: a prospective study. *Ann. Neurol.* **12**: 2–6.

Pazzaglia, P. & Frank-Pazzaglia, I. (1976). Record in grade school of pupils with epilepsy: an epidemiological study. *Epilepsia* **17**: 361–6.

Piccirilli, M., D'Alessandro, P., Tiacci, C. & Ferroni, A. (1988). Language lateralization in children with benign partial epilepsy. *Epilepsia* **29**: 19–25.

Pond, D. A. (1974). Epilepsy and personality disorders. In *Handbook of Clinical Neurology*, ed. P. Vinken and G. Bruyn, Vol. 15, pp. 576–92. New York: Elsevier.

Porter, R. J., Penry, J. K. & Dreifuss, F. E. (1973). Responsiveness at the onset of spike-wave bursts. *Electroencephalogr. Clin. Neurophysiol.* **34**: 239–45.

Prensky, A. L., DeVivo, D. C. & Palkes, H. (1971). Severe bradykinesia as a manifestation of toxicity to antiepileptic medications. *J. Pediatr.* **78**: 700–704.

Reitan, R. M. (1974). Psychological testing of epileptic patients. In *Handbook of Clinical Neurology*, ed. P. J. Vinken & G. W. Bruyn, Vol. 15, pp. 559–75. New York: Elsevier.

Reynolds, E. H. (1981). The management of seizures associated with psychological disorders. In *Epilepsy and Psychiatry*, ed. E. H. Reynolds & M. R. Trimble, pp. 322–36. New York: Churchill Livingstone.

Richardson, E. A., Killer, H., Katz, M. & McLaren, J. (1981). A functional classification of seizures and its distribution in a mentally retarded population. *Am. J. Ment. Def.* **85**: 457–66.

Riva, D., Zorzi, C., Devoti, M. & Pantaleoni, C. (1991). Hemispheric prevalence on dichotic verbal tasks in children with functional epilepsy. 19th International Epilepsy Congress. *Epilepsia* **32** (suppl 1): 15.

Rodin, E. A. (1968). *The Prognosis of Patients with Epilepsy*. Springfield, IL: Charles C. Thomas.

Rodin, E. A., Rennick, P., Dennerill, R. & Yin, Y. (1972). Vocational and educational problems of epileptic patients. *Epilepsia* **13**: 149–60.

Rodin, E. A., Schmaltz, S. & Twirty, G. (1986). Intellectual functions of patients with childhood-onset epilepsy, *Dev. Med. Child Neurol.* **28**: 25–33.

Ross, E. A. & Tookey, P. (1988). Educational needs and epilepsy in childhood. In *Epilepsy, Behavior and Cognitve Function*, ed. M. R. Trimble & E. M. Reynolds, pp. 87–97. Chichester, UK: John Wiley & Sons.

Ross, E. A. & West, P. B. (1978). Achievement and problems of British eleven year olds with epilepsy. In *Advances in Epileptology, Psychology, Pharmacotherapy and New Diagnostic Approaches*, ed. H. Meinardi & A. J. Rowan. Lisse: Swets & Zeitlinger.

Rutter, M. (1977). Brain-damage syndromes: I Childhood: Concepts and findings. *J. Child Psychol. Psychiatr.* **18**: 1–21.

Rutter, M., Graham, P. & Yule, W. (1970). A neuropsychiatric study in childhood. In *Clinics in Developmental Medicine*, pp. 237–55. London: Spastics Society and Heinemann.

Seidenberg, M., Beck, N., Geisser, M., *et al.* (1985). Academic achievement of children with epilepsy. *Epilepsia* **26**: 540.

Seidenberg, M., Beck, N., Geisser, M., *et al.* (1986). Academic achievement of children with epilepsy. *Epilepsia* **27**: 753–9.

Seidenberg, M., O'Leary, D. S., Berent, S. & Bell, T. (1981). Changes in seizure frequency and test-retest scores on the Wechsler Adult Intelligence Scale. *Epilepsia* **22**: 75–83.

Sidtis, J. J., Volpe, B. T., Wilson, D. N., Rayport, M. & Gazzaniga, M. S. (1981). Variability in right hemisphere language function after callosal section: evidence for a continuum of generative capacity. *J. Neurosci.* **1**: 323–31.

Sillanpaa, M. (1973). Medico-social prognosis of children with epilepsy. *Acta. Paediatr. Scand. Suppl.* **237**: 6–114.

Stores, G. (1976a). Behavioural effects of anti-epileptic drugs. *Dev. Med. Child Neurol.* **17**: 647–58.

Stores, G. (1976b). The investigation and management of school children with epilepsy. *Publ. Health, London* **90**: 171–7.

Stores, G. (1978). Schoolchildren with epilepsy at risk for learning and behavior problems. *Dev. Med. Child Neurol.* **20**: 502–8.

Stores, G. (1987). Effects on learning of "subclinical" seizure discharges. In *Education and Epilepsy 1987*, ed. A. P. Aldenkamp, W. C. J. Alpherts, H. Meinardi & G. Stores, pp. 14–21. Lisse: Swets & Zeitlinger.

Stores, G. & Hart, J. (1976). Reading skills of children with generalized and focal epilepsy attending ordinary school. *Dev. Med. Child Neurol.* **18**: 705–16.

Suurmeijer, T. P. B. M., van DAM, A. & Blijham, M. (1978). Socialization of the child with epilepsy and school achievement. In *Advances in Epileptology*, ed. H. Meinardi & A. J. Rowan, pp. 40–54. Lisse: Swets & Zeitlinger.

Svoboda, W. B. (1979). Epilepsy and Learning Problems. In *Learning About Epilepsy*, pp. 186–200. Baltimore, MD: University Park Press.

Tarter, R. E. (1972). Intellectual and adaptive functioning in epilepsy. *Dis. Nerv. Syst.* **33**: 763–70.

Tenny, J. W. (1955). Epileptic children I Detroit's special school program, a study. *Exceptional Children* **21**: 162–7.

Thompson, P. J. (1983). Phenytoin and psychosocial development. In *Antiepileptic Drug Therapy in Pediatrics*, P. Morselli, C. E. Pippinger & J. K. Penry, pp. 193–200. New York: Raven Press.

Thompson, P. J. (1987). Educational attainment in children and young people with epilepsy. In *Epilepsy and Education 1987*, ed. J. Oxley & G. Stores, pp. 15–24, London: Medical Tribune Group.

Thorbecke, R. (1987). Improving condition for the employment of people with epilepsy: environmental factor. In *Epilepsy and Employment*, ed. H. de Boer & J. Oxley, pp. 19–24. Heemstede: International Bureau for Epilepsy Publications.

Trimble, M. R. (1990). Antiepileptic drugs, cognitive function and behavior in children: evidence from recent studies. *Epilepsia* **31** (suppl 4): 30–35.

Trimble, M. R., Thompson, P. J. & Huppert, F. (1980). Anticonvulsant drugs and cognitive abilities. In *Advances in Epileptology: XIth Epilepsy International Symposium*, ed. R. Canger, F. Angeleri & J. K. Penry, pp. 199–204. New York: Raven Press.

Vargha-Kahdem, F. (2001). Generalized versus selective cognitive impairments resulting from brain damage sustained in childhood. In *Epilepsia and Learning Disabilities*, ed. G. F. Ayala, M. Elia, C. M. Cornaggia & M. R. Trimble. *Epilepsia* **42**: 37–40.

Waxman, S. G. & Geschwind, N. (1975). The interictal behavior syndrome of temporal lobe epilepsy. *Arch. Gen. Psychiatry* **32**: 1580–86.

Whitehouse, D. (1971). Psychological and neurological correlates of seizure disorders. *Johns Hopkins Med. J.* **129**: 36–42.

Whitehouse, D. (1976). Behavior and learning problems in epileptic children. *Behav. Neuropsychiatry* **7**: 23–9.

Wilkus, R. J. & Dodrill, C. B. (1976). Neuropsychological correlates of the electroencephalogram in epileptics. I. Topographic distribution and average rate of epileptiform activity. *Epilepsia* **17**: 89–100.

Wirrell, E. & Barnard, C. (1999). Status epilepticus in children: developmental deterioration and exacerbation of epilepsy. 23rd International Epilepsy Congress. *Epilepsia* **40** (suppl 2): 69.

Wunsche, W., Todt, H., Gamnitzer, B. & Lorenz, K. (1977). Untersuchung der Schullestungen bei kindern mit cerebralen anfeallsleiden. *Arztl. Jungendkunde* **68**: 305–19.

Zimmerman, F. T., Burgmeister, B. & Putnam, T. (1984). The ceiling effect of glutamic acid upon intelligence in children and adolescents. *Am. J. Psychiatry* **104**: 593.

15

Learning problems with seizure types

Seizures may excite, distort, inhibit, or alter cognitive efforts when they are prolonged, are continuous, occur in a series, or even when they occur singly (Meador, 2002). Discharges may disrupt processing, thus interfering with attention, learning processing, or storage or retrieval of information. Discharges may disrupt consolidation processes of encoding, storage, and retrieval. Seizures are more deleterious to cognition if they are due to underlying brain damage. Brain damage may reduce the capability of the brain to react adaptively. The developing brain may compensate through plasticity. Damage to the mature brain may result in cognitive loss. Anticonvulsants may change neural functioning, affecting learning processes. Frequent sleep discharges may directly or indirectly disrupt brain functioning and, in the young child, brain development (Aldenkamp et al., 1990; Binnie et al., 1990; Blennow et al., 1990; Dam, 1990). Resultant cognitive impairments may be minimal to severe and progressive, depending on the seizure type, cause, and epileptic syndrome (Dam, 1990).

Epilepsy, of any type and at any age, may exist in benign and not so benign forms. Simple absence seizures are far less impairing than minor motor or atypical absence syndromes, especially in early syndromes (Farwell et al., 1984). Children with generalized seizures may have problems with intelligence and attention (Rennick et al., 1969; Wilkus & Dodrill, 1976), whereas children with partial seizures may have problems with learning disabilities, including perception and memory (Fedio & Mirsky, 1969; Stores, 1971). Even minor seizures and subclinical seizure activity may be damaging to neurons, which parallels the emergence of cognitive functions (Farwell et al., 1985a; Dam, 1990).

Generalized seizures

Generalized seizures include generalized tonic–clonic attacks, the absence seizure group, and the related minor motor (atonic, myoclonic) group, commonly thought to be of subcortical-cortical orgin, involving the thalamus, and related closely to the central reticular networking of the upper brainstem and thalamus as well as the frontal cortex (Lansdell & Mirsky, 1964).

Intelligence and learning

In simple idiopathic epilepsies, intelligence is slightly lower than that of the normal population (Fedio & Mirsky, 1969). Symptomatic epilepsy or the resistant syndromes of early childhood may be associated with cognitive deficits (Mirsky *et al.*, 1960; Giordani *et al.*, 1985; Binnie *et al.*, 1990). Increased seizure frequency, repeated seizures, or status can cause brain damage, resulting in a poorer performance, possibly due to loss of neurons (Farwell *et al.*, 1985a; Giordani *et al.*, 1985; Dam, 1990). Widespread hippocampal neuron loss follows multiple seizures or a long duration of epilepsy (Mirsky *et al.*, 1960; Margerison & Corsellis, 1966; Rausch *et al.*, 1978; Mourritzen, 1982; Babb *et al.*, 1984; Dam, 1990).

Awareness and attention

Generalized seizures are associated with depressed attentivity and alertness related to the seizure frequency, the antiepileptic drugs, and the developmental age of the child (Reitan, 1974; Binnie *et al.*, 1990; Rausch *et al.*, 1978). Vigilance is impaired both during and between attacks, even when the EEG is normal (Fedio & Mirsky, 1969; Stores, 1971). Vigilance, like the generalized discharges themselves, may involve the thalamic nuclei or the central-reticular brainstem areas. Vigilance may relate more to the background slowing on the EEG than to the actual epileptiform discharges (Mirsky *et al.*, 1960).

Generalized epilepsy is not a single epilepsy entity. Separate subcortical mechanisms may exist in the regulation of cortical activity and consciousness, functioning independently of each other. Attention problems may be due to a persistent disturbance of central-subcortical structures. A complex arrangement of different mechanisms appears to underlie various disturbances subdividing the generalized epilepsies. The finding of defects in attention and general activation in generalized epilepsies is an effect of the non-specific dysfunctioning of the thalamic system itself (Waxman & Geschwind, 1975; Stores, 1978; Ladavas *et al.*, 1979; Brittain, 1980; Kertesz, 1983; Mellanby *et al.*, 1984; Mungas *et al.*, 1985; Binnie *et al.*, 1987; Renier, 1987; Binnie, 1988; Aldenkamp *et al.*, 1990).

Perceptual-motor processing

Children with generalized epilepsy are often impaired in visual perception (Stores, 1971), including visuospatial organization and sequencing (Giordani *et al.*, 1985) and organizational abilities (Tarter, 1971), which can affect visual learning (Klove & Matthews, 1974). Rapid recognition may be impaired (except with myoclonic epilepsy), possibly due to attention problems (Brittain, 1980). Perseverative errors are prominent. Perceptual motor processes may relate to the integrity of the reticular activating system (Fedio & Mirsky, 1969).

Memory

Children with a generalized seizure disorder have no obvious memory defects (Fedio & Mirsky, 1969; Stores, 1971). There may be problems with visual sequential memory related to attention and perception problems.

Academics

Children with generalized epilepsies, including subclinical seizure discharges, show a wide range of reading skills (Stores & Hart, 1976). Those with idiopathic seizures often perform satisfactorily (Dreifuss, 1983). Awareness deficits do not appear to impair the acquisition of reading skills (Stores & Hart, 1976). Over time, no deleterious effects, and even some improvements, are seen in those on antiepileptic medications (Mandelbaum *et al.*, 1993).

Testing

Psychological test scores in general, and especially with absence attacks, may be widely variable, perhaps related to subclinical epileptiform activity (Lansdell & Mirsky, 1964; Stores, 1980). Brief generalized discharges slow performance, whereas longer discharges, especially spike-wave discharges, lead to errors. Prolonged spike discharges are associated with impaired complex cognition but not necessarily any impairment in the performance of simple tasks (Reitan, 1974).

Generalized tonic–clonic (GTC) epilepsy

Tonic–clonic attacks have significant adverse effects on overall learning (Dodrill, 1978; Dodrill, 1986; Klove & Matthews, 1974; Brittain, 1980; Seidenberg *et al.*, 1981; Aldenkamp *et al.*, 1990; Rennick *et al.*, 1969). If the source of the seizures is subcortical, there may not be homologous tissue available to mediate recovery from the original insult (O'Leary *et al.*, 1981).

Intelligence and learning

GTC seizures, especially symptomatic ones, tend to lower intelligence (Matthews & Klove, 1967; Whitehouse, 1971). Those with GTC upon awakening or GTC plus absence attacks (Brittain, 1980; Halstead, 1957) perform better than those with GTC in sleep (Sillanpaa, 1973). In children, intelligence tends to be lower with early onset, greater frequency, or longer duration of seizures (Sillanpaa, 1973; Dikmen *et al.*, 1977; Hall & Marshall, 1980; O'Leary *et al.*, 1981). The deleterious effects of early-onset seizures, as well as early initiation of antiepileptic drugs, to a child's developing brain may lower both simple and complex functioning (O'Leary *et al.*, 1981). However, many (80%) young infants with GTC seizures develop normally and become free of seizures (Matsumoto *et al.*, 1983).

Awareness and attention

Children with GTC, especially beginning before age five years, may be impaired in tasks requiring the repetition of simple motor acts, as well as in attention and concentration (O'Leary et al., 1981).

Perceptual-motor skills

Children may have problems in visual perceptual skills, eye–motor coordination, and occasionally in form-constancy. Some problems are reported in visuospatial orientation and sequencing abilities (Giordani et al., 1985).

Memory

Children, especially those with early onset of GTC before five years of age, may be impaired in tasks requiring memory and complex problem solving (O'Leary et al., 1981), with weaknesses of visual sequential memories and both rote and remote memory (Lewinski, 1947).

Absence epilepsies

Children with absence attacks may have learning difficulties due to problems of attention and memory (Cheminal et al., 1998).

Intelligence and learning

Intelligence and school performance are minimally impaired in absence seizures, especially in simple forms, although in some (36%) children the IQ may be below average (Dodrill, 1976; Dikmen, 1980; Gerber et al., 1983; Keating, 1960; Hermann et al., 1980). Children with mixed absence and GTC seizures may need special education (39%) (Benninger et al., 1983). Of children with atypical absences, 36% are of below-average intelligence, up to 34% are of borderline intelligence, and 15% are mentally retarded, especially with slow discharge rates (Browne et al., 1974). Absences in young brain-damaged children often coexist with other minor seizures, such as akinetic, myoclonic, and tonic attacks, commonly associated with lower IQs (Whitehouse, 1976; Brown & Reynolds, 1981).

Intellectual performance is more disturbed in children with active interictal epileptiform discharges on the EEG (Benninger et al., 1983; Cheminal et al., 1998). Any association with frequency is debatable (Halstead, 1957; Sillanpaa, 1973; Brittain, 1980). Unrecognized or subclinical absence discharges may dramatically inhibit learning and testing, resulting in depressed scores (Sillanpaa, 1973; Browne et al., 1974; Besag, 2001), especially in complex tasks, such as copying complicated figures, searching tasks, and word fluency, but not in motor control, vigilance, or memory areas.

Awareness and alertness

Attentiveness, especially sustained attention (Hertoft, 1963; Ounsted et al., 1963; Loiseau et al., 1983; Dam, 1990), may be impaired, particularly in younger children, perhaps due in part to frequent subclinical seizures (Ives, 1970).

Reaction and response time

Reactivity as related to seizure bursts varies between individuals (Halgren, 1982). Impairments may be seen with bursts that last longer than three seconds (Mirsky & Van Buren, 1965; Geller & Geller, 1970; Browne et al., 1974). A seizure of less than five to ten seconds is often overlooked. Responses to auditory stimuli are normal one second before the discharge but reduced at the onset, especially at 0.5–1.5 seconds after the onset. Recovery is rapid after the discharge ceases, although by 0.5 second only 20% have recovered (Barlow, 1978).

Reaction time may be prolonged (65%), especially in more complex tasks (Schwab, 1941; Kooi & Hovey, 1957; Tizard & Margerison, 1963; Logan & Freeman 1969; Chastrain et al., 1970; Porter et al., 1973; Wechsler, 1973; Browne et al., 1974; Binnie, 1980). There appear to be differences between typical and atypical absence seizures (Stores, 1971). There may be a second or so of improved reactivity just before the burst, but this is lost with the burst. Recovery is prolonged, with a gradual recovery during and after the attack. Such problems present without overt seizures as transient cognitive impairments (Sengoku et al., 1990), even when no EEG disturbance is noted, suggest a persistent disturbance of subcortical mechanisms (Stores, 1973; O'Donohoe, 1979).

Perceptual motor problems

Absences bursts affect visual-motor performance. A paroxysm lasting for more than three seconds results in errors emerging one to two seconds after the spike-wave activity begins, with recovery about one to two seconds before the cessation of the spike-wave burst (Goode et al., 1970). A majority of children (60%) show visuomotor processing impairments, including in spatial perception, perceptual memory, and time perception. Drawings may be simple, crude, and distorted. Efforts may be perseverated. Auditory processes may remain intact, and some children may respond during a seizure (Freman et al., 1973).

Memory

In children with absence epilepsy, both antegrade and retrograde memory tends to be depressed during an attack (Jus & Jus, 1962; Cheminal et al., 1998). Impairments of short-term memory are seen with discharges (Hutt & Fairweather, 1975). The degree of impairment varies from total recall to total amnesia. The memory impairment may begin four seconds before the discharge or not until up to a few seconds into the attack. There may be amnesia for events for a few seconds afterwards (Barlow, 1978; Freman *et al.*, 1973). Memory between attacks remains relatively intact.

Academics

The frequency of the attacks of absence seizures appears to have no real relationship to reading skills (Stores & Hart, 1976).

Task state effects

Both concentration and monotony facilitate absence seizure occurrence. Absences may occur in the anxiety of a task situation, such as with a test or a potential failure situation, as well as during periods of inattention, such as with boring activities (Lindsay *et al.*, 1979; Stores, 1980). EEGs may be more synchronized during various mental tasks that demand attention and fine motor skills, such as mental arithmetic or automatized visual motor tasks (Schlack, 1980).

Minor motor seizures

Children with myoclonic seizures, especially older children, often have other generalized seizure types. Sometimes, a brief stare may precede a myoclonic jerk (Livingston, 1974). Minor seizures and subclinical activity may damage the neurons in certain circumstances (Farwell *et al.*, 1984; Farwell *et al.*, 1985a; Dam, 1990). The etiologies may have known adverse effects on learning in addition to the seizures.

Intelligence and learning

Individuals with minor motor seizures tend toward lowered intelligence, especially in verbal processing (Davies-Eyesneck, 1952). Patients with juvenile myoclonic epilepsy usually have normal IQs, whereas patients with infantile spasms have a poor cognitive prognosis (Hermann *et al.*, 1980). Cortical spikes associated with myoclonic jerks do not appear to alter cognition (Fenwick, 1981).

Alertness and attention

Myoclonic seizures do not seem to be associated with attention deficits (Stores, 1971).

Effort effects

Concentration may precipitate myoclonic jerks, as in tasks of sustained attention and concentration, especially in individuals of normal intelligence. Discharges can be triggered by complex written or mental math computation. Tension or anxiety regarding the results appears to increase this seizure tendency (Foerster, 1977).

Myoclonic–atonic epilepsy

Some children with associated atonic and absence seizures and a slow spike-wave EEG may be handicapped in learning, with language skills and social abilities being most vulnerable. Many of these children may be normal before the onset, but 72% will be retarded later.

Akinetic myoclonic epilepsy

Mental retardation is common, with 27% of children being of borderline intelligence and 53% being mentally retarded. The retardation is often severe to profound in half the retarded group. Personality disorders are seen in 33% in the retarded group but in only 6% of the non-retarded group. One year after the last seizure, 35% of patients are retarded and 8% have a behavior problem.

Progressive myoclonic epilepsies

Individuals with progressive myoclonic epilepsy may develop severe dyslexia without concomitant aphasia, although a prior history of speech and language delays may be obtained. There may be reading problems, including problems with reading italicised words. Reading is performed with irregularly stressed word sounding. Comprehension is mediated by a symbol–sound conversion in the absence of a direct semantic route. This language disorder with subsequent surface dyslexia may be the first symptom of progressive myoclonic epilepsy (Piras *et al.*, 1991).

Lafora body myoclonic progressive epilepsy

The intelligence of the child with this disorder tends to be slightly lower than average. At entry into school, the child appears normal. After a few years, at around age ten years, school difficulties begin to appear soon after the first symptoms of the syndrome. Progress in school is impaired at times when the child is subjected to special attention or feels mentally stressed. The child tends to drop out of school due to difficulties in mobility. Some years after the onset of the disorder, speech becomes dysarthric; in later stages, the speech is slow, incoherent, and difficult to understand. Sometimes, speech clears when the patient is in a sauna or is febrile. Apathy and rapid dementia have been reported occasionally. A progressive dementia often emerges (Koskiniemi *et al.*, 1974).

Non-Lafora myoclonic progressive epilepsy

Mild mental deterioration and psychiatric symptoms develop very slowly despite severe handicaps from the myoclonus, often resulting in poor penmanship for years. The IQ may fall by about ten points. Digit span and arithmetic tests are most affected. Tests of similarities, information, and comprehension are least affected.

Speech is slow and dysarthric and finally becomes unintelligible (Koskiniemi, 1974).

Juvenile myoclonic epilepsy (JME)

Patients with JME are usually of normal intelligence (Hermann *et al.*, 1980). JME episodes are often precipitated by higher mental activity in handiwork (42%), writing (28.9%), thinking (13.2%), mental calculation (7.9%), and drawing (2.6%). Triggers may be confirmed in testing, included writing (68.4%), spatial constructions (63.2%), written calculation (55.3%), mental calculation (79%), and reading aloud or silently (5.3%), and not just by sleep deprivation and awakenings (Matsuoka, 2001).

Focal atonic

Children with onset of atonic seizures may show an inability to maintain school grades, with hyperactive behavior and clumsiness or ataxia, despite having normal intelligence. In slow-wake sleep, continuous generalized slow-spike and wave discharges may be seen. The patients demonstrate ictal bilateral or contralateral spike-wave discharges. Localized hypoperfusion in the parietal region is seen by ictal SPECT, suggesting that these are partial seizures (Fukushima *et al.*, 2001).

Syndromes

The relationship between epileptic syndromes and intellectual ability depends on multiple factors, including the etiology, especially the presence of a brain lesion (which can also cause psychological deficiencies), age of onset, type, frequency, and location of the seizure (Dam, 1990).

Febrile convulsions

Early reports suggesting risks for retardation (41%) or neurodevelopmental delays (28%) following the onset of febrile seizures have not been confirmed (Aicardi, 1988). No reading problems are noted (Commission for the Control of Epilepsy and Its Consequences, 1977; Wallace, 1976; Wallace & Cull, 1979). Most children (80–90%) with simple febrile seizures are mentally and physically normal (Commission for the Control of Epilepsy and Its Consequences, 1977; Matsumoto *et al.*, 1983). Children are at risk for developmental delays with complex febrile seizures if the child had discernible neurologic abnormalities before the onset (22%), if the seizure is early in the susceptible period, or if it is focal, prolonged, or repetitive in the first day of the illness (Ouelette, 1974; Commission for the Control of Epilepsy and Its Consequences, 1977; Wallace & Cull, 1979). Otherwise, early academic performance, attention, and behavior are not affected, even if the child is treated with phenobarbital (Gururaj, 1980; Rintahaka *et al.*, 1993; Chang *et al.*, 2000).

Infantile spasms

Infantile spasms feature the emergence of myoclonic spasms and a deterioration of developmental skills in infancy, with an EEG characterized as hypsarrhythmic. When the spasms start, development ceases and often regresses. Infantile spasms appear to be initiated in the upper brainstem with cortical involvement. Focal discharges may also be seen. The cortex may lack normal inhibitory activity in subcortical structures. Some children who are found to have diffuse malformations exhibit abnormal psychometric development before the onset of seizures (Dulac *et al.*, 1999).

When the hypsarrhythmic EEG emerges, neurologic function deteriorates. The continuous slow-wave activity may interfere with cognitive function. The occurrence of paroxysmal electrical discharge in the cortical area undergoing rapid maturation is known to prevent fine-tuning of the synaptic network important for cognitive development. The psychomotor outcome relates to the location and number of brain lesions and the later outcome of the epilepsy (Dulac *et al.*, 1999).

The long-term prognosis in children with infantile spasms is poor, with mental and neurologic development being affected in over 80% of symptomatic cases and in more than half of the cryptogenic forms (Glaze *et al.*, 1988; Cavazzuti *et al.*, 1984; Dam, 1990). Retardation to some degree is apparent in most children (84.9%–96%), varying from mild to severe, with many patients being severely retarded (Livingston, 1974; Sillanpaa, 1973). Children with idiopathic West syndrome may have a normal IQ, and many (about two-thirds) have no cognitive impairment, but almost all have emotional or adoptive behavior problems (Rener-Primec *et al.*, 1999). In the symptomatic group, only 5% develop normally (Glaze *et al.*, 1988; Cavazzuti *et al.*, 1984; Dam, 1990). In 83% of those treated with ACTH and in 89% of those not treated, mental retardation is observed (Kurokawa *et al.*, 1980).

A better outcome for mental and behavioral functions is seen in males lacking any family history of seizures, with prior normal development, and with no preexisting brain damage, who develop the idiopathic form of onset after one year without episodes of early status. A lower frequency and severity of attacks in children otherwise neurologically normal is also more favorable, as are brief, symmetrical spasms that are rapidly controlled or outgrown (Sillanpaa, 1973; Chevrie & Aicardi, 1978; Matsumoto *et al.*, 1981; Koo & Hwang, 1992). If a cortical lesion as an initiating focus is found, surgery may markedly improve the outlook. The outcome is often apparent within a few months of the onset (Sillanpaa, 1973).

Cognitive impairments can range from selective cognitive disorders to major mental retardation with autistic behaviors; the latter is seen especially with diffuse malformations or destructive brain lesions, with ictal discharges associated with reduced cortical blood flow. Specific cognitive deficits develop in patients with focal epileptogenic involvement, such as visuomotor problems, with occipital-parietal focal epileptic involvement and speech delays seen with temporal parietal involvement, especially if these precede or appear simultaneous with the spasms (Matsumoto *et al.*, 1981; Dulac *et al.*, 1999).

Lennox–Gastaut syndrome

This syndrome presents in childhood with a mixed seizure disorder (atypical absence, atonic/myoclonic, and especially tonic attacks). It is often fairly resistant to anticonvulsants. It usually has a slow spike-wave generalized EEG picture and mental retardation. This is an age-dependent syndrome, most common in childhood but also seen in infancy and in adolescence (Dravet, 1999).

These children often are not as retarded as those with infantile spasms, but they have more severe behavior problems. Mental retardation is observed in 99% of patients with onset in infancy and in 84% of those with onset thereafter (Kurokawa *et al.*, 1980), especially if they first had infantile spasms. At the time of the seizure onset, 30% are retarded; when the seizure activity lessens toward the end of the Lennox–Gastaut period, 92–98% are retarded.

Good prognostic factors include later onset in childhood, previously normal development, an idiopathic form, EEG showing a better developed background, and no focal abnormalities. Nearly half (42%) of those children not retarded before the onset a not retarded afterwards. The idiopathic form without retardation before the onset shows only a slightly higher incidence of recovery from seizures and normal intelligence in follow-up. Regardless of the type of treatment, late-onset seizures are more apt to cease spontaneously than those that begin in the first two years of life (Blume *et al.*, 1973).

Poor prognostic indicators include early onset, symptomatic nature (especially following West's syndrome), frequent seizures, prolonged periods of aggravation, recurrent status epilepticus, persistence of slow EEG background activity, association with focal abnormalities, and diffuse slow-spike wave activity on the EEG (Beaumanoir, 1985; Dam, 1990). Of those children who are abnormal before the onset, many (73%) are abnormal in follow-up (Fremion *et al.*, 1980). The earlier the onset of the syndrome, the greater is the degree of retardation (Barlow, 1978). In the third decade of life, the typical slow spike-wave picture fades and focal temporal lobe abnormalities may emerge. Despite the retardation, the main problem is with behavior.

Neonatal seizures

Neonatal seizures are often symptomatic of some underlying insult. The infant brain recovers better than the adult brain. However, there is a special vulnerability of parts of the infant brain. Early seizures may inhibit brain growth and development, with less DNA, RNA, protein, and cholesterol accumulation. Neonatal seizures reduce the number of cells in the brain cortex and also reduce cell size. Delayed developmental milestones are seen. With early seizures, there is less myelin accumulation, reduced synaptic protein, and possibly reduced cell dendritic connections (Wasterlain *et al.*, 1999). Aberrant networks established by recurrent seizures increase brain vulnerability to future injury. Thus, neonatal seizures alter the brain in a maladaptive manner (Stores, 1990). Anticonvulsant drugs (phenobarbital, phenytoin, possibly carbamazepine and valproate) at therapeutic levels may inhibit brain cellular, especially cerebellar, growth in the immature brain.

The mortality of neonatal seizures is 23%, and long-term sequelae occur in 29–35%. Abnormal neurologic signs in the first year of life, before the onset of seizures, may be an important prognostic indicator of intellectual disability later in life (Barlow, 1978; Ellenberg *et al.*, 1984; Dam, 1990). With modernization of neonatal seizure recognition and care, the mortality rate has decreased but sequelae have increased, with the percentage of normal development fairly consistent at 53% (Ericksson & Zetterstrom, 1979).

Reflex epilepsies

Reflex epilepsy are those attacks triggered by a repetitive stimulus, such as flashing lights, colors, video games, or even voice timbre, music, or intensive cognitive tasks. Apart from the well-known phenomenon of sensitivity to flashing lights, other precipitating factors include emotional stress at home or at school, boredom or overconcentration, and physical fatigue (Stores, 1976). Occasionally, children with photogenic epilepsy may show compulsive neurotic trends, with a tendency to precipitate seizures in a manipulative fashion (Mosovich, 1974). No significant correlations with any academic problems are seen, except for disturbances created by seizures precipitated by an academic activity.

In reflex epilepsy, 80% or more of the seizures may be precipitated by a specific stimulus or event. Idiopathic generalized reflex epilepsies seem to depend on the activation of higher mental activities in one of two forms: (1) seizures induced by thinking and spatial tasks, and (2) seizures induced by writing, written calculations, or drawing that requires action-programming activity. Reflex epilepsies induced by thinking and clinical tasks are often generalized and may involve decision-making, as seen with calculations, card and board games, and spatial tasks but not with writing efforts. Seizures precipitating mental activities are almost exclusively related to idiopathic generalized epilepsies and often occur with myoclonic seizures such as JME. Neuropsychological tasks of reading, speaking, and writing, written arithmetic calculation, mental arithmetic calculation, and spatial construction may provoke epileptic discharges in 7.9% of patients. Tasks that require the use of hands (writing (68.4%), written calculations (55.3%), and spatial constructions (64.2%)) provoke the most discharges. Neuropsychologic testing provokes myoclonic seizures in 84.2%, generalized tonic–clonic seizures in 60.5%, absences in 50%, secondary generalized tonic–clonic seizures in 5.3%, simple partial seizures in 2.6%, and complex partial seizures in 2.6% (Matsuoka, 2001).

Reading epilepsy, an infrequent form of epilepsy, is considered a form of myoclonic epilepsy triggered by a group of sensory stimuli on a hyperexcitable cortical focus. Several factors may contribute to the seizure production, including the visual pattern, proprioceptive impulses from the jaw and ocular muscles, and attention to reading. Reading in a loud voice or writing, speaking, or whispering may contribute. Others have considered this to be a communicative disorder with the seizure provoked by superior cognitive functions. Reading efforts may lead to a generalized seizure proceeded by brief jaw movements, occurring only while reading. This may be of adolescent onset (Mesri & Pagano, 1987).

The EEG may show predominantly left-hemisphere discharges, with the EEG discharge preceded by brief jaw movements in some patients. Paroxysmal discharges may occur when an interpretative component of what is being read is present. The absence of discharge during observation of comic strips with meaning but without reading, as well as reading of an announcement or in math calculation, suggests a cognitive component (Mesri & Pagano, 1987).

Existence of a primary reception of writing (reading or characters) involves the occipital cortex. Intervention of association areas whose functions would be in the connections between the primary receiving area and those areas processing and providing meaning to the input material is involved (Mesri & Pagano, 1987).

Partial epilepsies

Children with partial seizures do better than those with generalized seizures but still display problems in learning (Wilkus & Dodrill, 1976). It is important to establish the location and extent of any underlying lesion, as this may indicate the sort of specific learning disability to expect and lead to more appropriate management (Stores, 1987; Henricksen, 1990). The epileptogenic focus may alter cerebral mechanisms underlying cognitive activity. Frequent partial seizures are associated with reduced verbal IQ and academic failure (Ounsted et al., 1966; Binnie et al., 1990).

Intelligence and learning

Partial seizures impact on the overall intelligence less than generalized seizures, but children with partial veizures present more often with learning disabilities (Whitehouse, 1976). The location of the partial seizure focus and electrical discharges relate to specific types of learning disability (Milner, 1968b; Wolf, 1979; Bradford, 1980; Brittain, 1980). Children with partial secondarily generalized seizures perform the poorest (Giordani *et al.*, 1983). The pattern of functional cerebral representation in focal epileptic patients depends on the focus site, as shown in individuals with untreated benign focal non-lesion epilepsy (Milner, 1954; Rausch *et al.*, 1978). Learning deficits tend to be lateralization specific, i.e. dominant hemisphere for verbal materials and non-dominant for non-verbal materials. Verbal deficits, particularly for meaningful material, are seen with the language-dominant hemisphere discharges (Milner, 1954; Fedio & Mirsky, 1969; Binnie *et al.*, 1990). Children with left unilateral cerebral injury tend to show verbal impairments (Fedio & Mirsky, 1969), especially if the child is right-handed (Reitan, 1974), although through plasticity language functions may be salvaged by being transferred to the non-dominant hemisphere. Performance is significantly poorer on tasks of higher verbal and visual-motor functions (Piccirilli *et al.*, 1988). In children, the right brain is capable not only of language comprehension but also of completely substituting for the left hemisphere, even its expressive capacity (Sidtis *et al.*, 1981; Piccirilli *et al.*, 1988). Impairments on tests using visual spatial material are seen with non-dominant hemisphere disturbances (Milner, 1954; Fedio & Mirsky, 1969; Binnie *et al.*, 1990).

Attention

Attention problems are more common with generalized seizures than with partial seizures (Rennick *et al.*, 1969), although they may be seen with partial seizures. Such attention problems are often associated with specific cognitive dysfunctions (Giordani *et al.*, 1983). Children with partial seizures have more problems in school than would be expected for their intelligence (Whitehouse, 1976). Significant differences in all perceptual tasks may be seen with a focus along the superior posterior temporal region (Boatman *et al.*, 1992). Persistent focal discharges are associated with impaired reactivity (Fenwick, 1981).

Memory

Although memory difficulties have been attributed mostly to bilateral lesions in the hippocampus, severe-type specific memory problems may be caused by unilateral impairment of specific structures outside the hippocampal-limbic circuitry (Aldenkamp *et al.*, 1990), both within the temporal lobe and in the frontal-prefrontal area (Kertesz, 1983).

Academics

Naming and reading follow the expected lateralization of language processes to the left and spatial functions to the right hemisphere. Inhibition during language tasks is significantly greater on the left and activity occurs significantly earlier on the left during language tasks. The reverse is seen during spatial tasks, with the right side being more affected (Schwartz *et al.*, 1992). Reading, memory, and visuomotor tasks are better in children with controlled focal seizures (Mandelbaum *et al.*, 1993).

Simple partial epilepsies

Simple focal seizures are not associated with prominent cognitive problems. Epileptogenic damage to either lobe causes deficits in visual spatial abilities (Read, 1981). Right posterior brain lesions produce impairment of tasks involving perceptual complex materials (Sherwin & Efron, 1980). A slight diminution of copying abilities and problems in recall are also noted. Any memory problems found may be secondary to a postictal effect of the seizure spread.

Benign partial epilepsies

Benign focal epilepsy is characterized by infrequent idiopathic partial seizures, if any, which are self-remitting and not thought to be associated with any neuropsychological or neurologic deficits (Gulgonen *et al.*, 2000). The interictal EEG shows frequent discharges that may disturb specific cognitive processes, such as reading, counting, grammar, and spelling (Metz-Lutz *et al.*, 1999).

Benign epilepsy centro-temporal (Rolandic) of childhood (BECT)

BECTs were once thought to be free of any learning impairments (Heijbel & Behman, 1975; Loiseau *et al.*, 1983; Lerman, 1985), but significant impairments in performance IQ, auditory and visual memory (immediate and delayed), and visual spatial abilities (Gerber *et al.*, 1983; Croona *et al.*, 1998), as well as in coordination, have been noted (Berges *et al.*, 1968). Attention and concentration problems, often with hyperactivity, have been found (Croona *et al.*, 1998; Turkdogan *et al.*, 1999). These may emerge about six months after the onset. Clinical or subclinical epileptogenic activity in the central region might be related causally to dominant-hemisphere dysfunction. Cognitive and behavioral problems can precede the development of epileptic activity and clinical seizures, or vice versa (Turkdogan *et al.*, 1999).

The epileptiform focus itself can determine laterality (Piccirilli *et al.*, 1988; Dam, 1990). Children with a predominantly left-sided discharge may show depressed digital retention test scores (Beaumanoir *et al.*, 1964), with a lower verbal intelligence (Turkdogan *et al.*, 1999). In patients with a focus on the left side, hemispheric dominance may be atypical, with the right-hemisphere assuming responsibility for language processing, even without any lesion being present. Children with a right-hemispheric focus show the expected left language lateralization. Children with predominantly right-sided discharges may display visuomotor impairments (Beaumanoir *et al.*, 1964; Gerber *et al.*, 1983), but the verbal/non-verbal balance is not altered (Heijbel & Behman, 1975). Right-sided or bilateral discharges impair attention (Piccirilli *et al.*, 1994).

Benign occipital epilepsy of childhood (BOEC)

Children with occipital paroxysms may have subtle cognitive defects, especially those with continuous spikes and waves during slow sleep, as seen in BOEC and idiopathic photosensitive occipital lobe epilepsy. Flickering lights and photosensitive patterns may produce seizures (Gulgonen *et al.*, 2000). Bioccipital discharges in epileptic children are associated with problems in visual processing, including perception and discrimination, and in attention (Berges *et al.*, 1968; Reitan, 1974). Auditory and visual memory and mental arithmetic may be impaired (Gulgonen *et al.*, 2000).

Benign partial sensory evoked spikes

Children with sensory evoked parietal spikes show no changes on computerized test performance, suggesting no impairment of information processing efficiency (Morales *et al.*, 1993).

Gelastic seizures

In gelastic seizures with hypothalamic harmatomas, the dysplasia is intrinsically epileptogenic (Berkovic *et al.*, 1997). In younger children, an intellectual regression and severe behavior problems are probably related to the strategic posture of this malformation, with the spread of epileptic discharges by hypothalamic-amygdalar connections (Deonna, 1999).

Complex partial seizures (CPEs)

CPEs, more than simple partial epilepsy, has adverse effects on learning (Dodrill, 1978; Dodrill, 1986; Klove & Matthews, 1974; Brittain, 1980; Seidenberg *et al.*, 1981; Aldenkamp *et al.*, 1990), even when a lesion is not radiologically apparent (Stores, 1987). The effect in children is widespread. A generalized reduction of total cerebral tissue, especially white matter, corresponding to this extends beyond the temporal lobe (Herman *et al.*, 2002). CPEs are commonly thought of as originating from the temporal lobe but they may also be of frontal origin. Both areas often involve the limbic system.

Frontal lobe epilepsy

More is known about the cognitive and behavioral deficits of temporal lobe epilepsy than of frontal lobe epilepsy (Swartz *et al.*, 1993). Children with a frontal epileptogenic focus may not show severe deficits, but they do have a variety of impairments of frontal functions.

Intelligence and learning

Intellectual functioning is relatively normal (Riga *et al.*, 1998). A subgroup of CPE patients exhibit a language-based learning disability that is not due to reduced intellect (Breier *et al.*, 1999).

Attention and awareness

Frontal disturbances, especially involving the prefrontal cortex, may impair attention (Kertesz, 1983; Mellanby *et al.*, 1984). More impulsive responses may be seen.

Planning and organization

Patients with frontal lobe lesions appear unable to implant a plan of action, even though the plan may be detailed in language form. Dorsolateral frontal lobe lesions interfere with the developing of a plan of action in sorting tasks (Zimmerman *et al.*, 1951). Difficulties in continuous self-paced tasks that rely on learning from experiences and difficulties with mazes are seen. Patients with a right frontal problem have difficult in sorting. Those with a left frontal focus seem to recover better after surgery (Milner, 1975).

Reaction time

Reaction times are increased in patients with frontal lobe epilepsy (Swartz *et al.*, 1993).

Memory

Frontal lesions, especially those especially involving the prefrontal cortex, show more impairment of memory, especially recent task memory (Ladavas *et al.*, 1979; Kertesz, 1983; Mellanby *et al.*, 1984). Memory problems attributed to bilateral lesions in the hippocampus may be caused by unilateral impairment of specific structures outside the hippocampal-limbic circuitry (Mellanby *et al.*, 1984; Aldenkamp *et al.*, 1990). Patients with left frontal epileptic foci appear significantly impaired in long-term memory (Riga *et al.*, 1998).

Academics

The transient impairments of numerical and verbal skills following intracarotid injection of sodium amobarbital in neurosurgical patients may be due to perfusion of parts of the frontal lobe of the injected dominant side over and above the perfused temporal lobe (Serafetinides, 1969).

Temporal lobe/complex partial epilepsy

The temporal lobe is closely integrated with the frontal lobe, especially in shared limbic structures. Executive functions may be transiently impaired post-temporal lobectomy, whereas problem solving and both verbal and non-verbal fluency may improve.

Intelligence and learning

Complex partial seizures, especially those of early onset, are more apt to be associated with a channel depression and related learning disabilities than to an overall depressed intelligence (Browne & Reynolds, 1981).

The intelligence of children with CPE is only slightly reduced as compared with children with generalized seizures (Bray, 1962; Ounsted et al., 1966). The seizures may have significant adverse effects on specific learning areas, especially verbal processing, even in idiopathic forms of anterior temporal lobe epilepsy (Dodrill, 1978; Dodrill, 1986; Klove & Matthews, 1974; Brittain, 1980; Seidenberg et al., 1981; Browne & Reynolds, 1981; Stores, 1987; Aldenkamp et al., 1990). Long-term refractory temporal lobe epilepsy is associated with a progressive cognitive decline and increasing hippocampal damage unrelated to the age of onset, education, seizure frequency, interictal discharges, or antiepileptic drugs in use. Interictal discharges may produce transient cognitive impairments (Jokeit & Ebner, 1999; Meador, 2002). Evoked potential testing shows the P300 to be delayed and lower in amplitude, suggestive of a disturbance of cognitive processing (Syrigou-Papavasiliou et al., 1985).

The type of cognitive processing deficit depends on the laterality of dominance as well as the laterality of the seizure focus. In younger children with temporal lobe epilepsy, the dominant lobe is not necessarily the left, for plasticity may have shifted cognitive skills. The side of the epileptic focus alters the processing of verbal information, but in different ways depending on the side of the focus (Stores & Hart, 1976; Camfield et al., 1984; Rugland, 1990).

Dominant CPE occurs more often and earlier than non-dominant foci, but it is often misdiagnosed as generalized epilepsy. The child who has a left temporal lobe seizure disorder that begins before six years of age is at risk for auditory channel learning disabilities, such as impairments of verbal learning skills pertaining to retention and learning of verbal materials, word-finding skills (Quadfasal & Pruyser, 1955; Hermann et al., 1980), and serial information processing. Naming difficulties are more common (Waxman & Geschwind, 1975; Stores, 1978; Ladavas et al., 1979; Brittain, 1980; Kertesz, 1983; Mellanby et al., 1984; Mungas et al., 1985; Binnie et al., 1987; Renier, 1987; Binnie, 1988; Aldenkamp et al., 1990). Such children often do poorly on verbal comprehension, communication, and vocabulary (Fedio & Mirsky, 1969). Aphasic traits, including the impairment of verbal reasoning, may be detected (Reitan, 1974). Such individuals may make unusual interpretations of what they think others say, which affects interpersonal relationships adversely. Left temporal lobe epileptics are poorest in verbal dichotic stimuli, whereas right temporal lobe epileptics are less deviant, although they are still depressed to subnormal (McIntyre *et al.*, 1976).

Verbal skill breakdown with dominant temporal seizures is due not to an initial encoding disability but to a breakdown in information processing after it is recognized. False recognition errors are noted, probably due to a problem in storage or retrieval processing. This affects verbal memory and categorization regardless of whether the material is visual or auditory (Risberg & Ingvar, 1973; Rausch, 1981). Children may have some difficulties in comprehension, but they tend to have more difficulties in information and vocabulary, which is the reverse of adults (Fedio & Mirsky, 1969; Novelly, 1982). In older children, deductive reasoning seems to be impaired. Imagery is not utilized as a mnemonic aid (Read, 1981). A more reflective cognitive style may be noted (McIntyre *et al.*, 1976).

Intelligence is less apt to be disturbed with right temporal lobe epilepsy as compared with those with a left dominant focus (Meyer & Falconer, 1960). Lesions of the non-dominant anterior temporal lobe may produce some auditory learning deficits. Diminished auditory processing of verbal materials may relate directly to the proximity of a focus in one primary receptive and associative area but affecting both sides. It may be that the deficit of the right CPE does not have a direct effect, but rather the effect is to disrupt other intact functional systems, although this is not apparent (Cavazzuti *et al.*, 1984). Children with right-sided CPE show more performance impairments than verbal intelligence impairments. Problems in non-verbal performance and memory tasks, such as temporal and visual-spatial patterns and relationships, as well as in visual-spatial perception, relationships, and sequencing are seen (Reitan, 1974; Fedio & Mirsky, 1969). Other problems include perceptual motor disabilities and poor memory for non-verbal materials. Problem-solving, design fluency, and verbal fluency problems may be noted. Perseverations may be seen postoperatively (Fedio & Mirsky, 1969; Stores, 1971).

Awareness and attention

Temporal lobe patients do not have significant attention deficits, although some children appear distractable to environmental stimuli (Fedio & Mirsky, 1969; Mirsky *et al.*, 1960; Rausch *et al.*, 1978). Children with a left CPE may be inattentive, and boys in particular may be hyperactive, especially in a noisy setting (Stores, 1978). Children with right temporal seizures may not pay sustained attention to any visual details; when they get older, they may tend to rush through items, their impulsivity tending to be branded as hyperactivity.

Perceptual-motor processing

Involvement of the non-dominant right temporal lobe affects non-verbal perceptive abilities of perceptive discrimination (Barlow, 1978) and understanding of temporal and spatial patterns and relationships (Rennick *et al.*, 1969; McDaniel & McDaniel, 1976). This includes perceptual recognition, spatial relationships, directed attention (Waxman & Geschwind, 1975; Stores, 1978; Ladavas *et al.*, 1979; Brittain, 1980; Kertesz, 1983; Mellanby *et al.*, 1984; Mungas *et al.*, 1985; Binnie *et al.*, 1987; Renier, 1987; Binnie, 1988; Aldenkamp *et al.*, 1990), and related visual memory for non-verbal items (Stores, 1971). Children may have trouble in discriminating simple shapes, especially in figure-background retrieval (Fedio & Mirsky, 1969). Mazes are a challenge (Milner, 1968a). These perceptual problems may relate to extension of the seizure discharge into the right parietal lobe (Read, 1981).

Perceptual recognition and detailed visual analysis of unfamiliar stimuli, figures, and facies may be noted (Milner, 1968a). Right temporal lobe epileptic individuals are faster, although more impulsive, especially in spatial organization tasks, with a resulting increased number of errors. This is more prominent in older children. Individuals with left temporal lobe epilepsy are slower in responding in matching figures, with a more reflective cognitive style (McIntyre *et al.*, 1976). Such problems may affect coordination, as in copying and recall (Fedio & Mirsky, 1969). Some individuals can perform simple motor acts but not complicated ones, with reduced coordination noted. This is seen in 16% of individuals with temporal lobe epilepsy, especially in girls (85%), and is unrelated to any temporal lobe pathology. This may depress both full-scale and performance IQ performance.

Reaction time

Delayed reaction time appears to be due to both a reduction of motor speed and impairment of other cognitive processes, as related to epileptic factors (Zheng *et al.*, 2000).

Memory

Memory deficits are seen as an inevitable consequence of temporal lobe dysfunction (Glowinski, 1973; Hutt & Gilbert, 1980; Stores, 1981; Loiseau *et al.*, 1982; Binnie *et al.*, 1990). The patient complains but appears able to perform daily activities, revealing little on clinical examination or screening (Mayeux *et al.*, 1980). Specific testing variably shows generalized memory impairments and selective memory deficits (Mirsky *et al.*, 1960; Denman & Wanamaker, 1983). The laterality of the epileptic lesion relates to the type of memory deficit seen. The left temporal lobe specializes in the learning and retention of verbal information. The right temporal lobe pertains to visual-spatial and non-verbal material.

Dominant (left) temporal lobe seizure patients may be impaired in verbal learning (Stores, 1978), with deficits in verbal short-term memory, serial information processing, complex verbal processing, and delayed recall. The short-term memory problem is one especially of encoding and consolidation, without major laterality differences noted (Zimmerman *et al.*, 1951). Such patients remember less and forget more rapidly but complain the least (Barlow, 1978; Delaney *et al.*, 1980; Hendriks *et al.*, 1998). Dominant temporal lobe patients show more impairment for long-term memory tasks (Ladavas *et al.*, 1979). Naming problems are more prevalent with left posterior EEG abnormalities (Waxman & Geschwind, 1975; Stores, 1978; Ladavas *et al.*, 1979; Brittain, 1980; Delaney *et al.*, 1980; Kertesz, 1983; Mellanby *et al.*, 1984; Mungas *et al.*, 1985; Binnie *et al.*, 1987; Renier, 1987; Binnie, 1988; Aldenkamp *et al.*, 1990). Tasks such as memorizing poetry and recalling in a noisy situation may be difficult (Fedio & Mirsky, 1969). The basic problem is an impairment in the use of categories in memory retrieval (Snyder & Blaxton, 1992). Both circumlocution and circumstantiality may compensate for the anomia, a common disability (Mayeux *et al.*, 1980). There may be a mild impairment on visual-spatial memory in left temporal lobe epilepsy patients, which may be related to difficulties in using verbal mediation strategies as a means of facilitating their learning and recall of non-verbal material (Battaglia, 1998). Children have to try more times to learn, with a poorer recall noted for verbal material (Fedio & Mirsky, 1969; Brown & Reynolds, 1981). Impairment of verbal reasoning and learning functions are also noted (Rennick *et al.*, 1969).

People with right CPE show less depression of delayed verbal memory scores than those with left CPE (Rausch *et al.*, 1978), although patients with right temporal lobe epilepsy complain significantly more about their memory functioning in daily life (Hendriks *et al.*, 1998). When a defect of immediate recall of the right temporal lobe is found, it suggests that the lesion in either temporal lobe may decrease auditory processing capabilities (Cazvazzuti *et al.*, 1984) or, through plasticity, transfer may have occurred. Significant impairments of non-verbal visual memory are seen in right CPE patients (Delaney *et al.*, 1980; Brown & Reynolds, 1981), especially in visual-spatial and perceptual motor tasks (Stores, 1971). There appears to be a greater deficit of storage of non-verbal information than of retrieval (Giovagnoli *et al.*, 1995).

Defects include problems in remembering designs, faces, and figures (Milner, 1975), seen with mesial damage, which especially affects delayed memory skills (Zimmerman *et al.*, 1951). Children have significantly poorer performance on non-verbal tasks, such as visual-spatial memory and non-verbal attention (Fedio & Mirsky, 1969; Brown & Reynolds, 1981; Battaglia, 1998), and prove to be more disrupted for spatial long-term memory tasks (Ladavas *et al.*, 1979). In copying efforts, they often forget much and leave out portions, especially after a brief delay (Brown & Reynolds, 1981). Children with temporal lobe epilepsy have problems with visual sequential memory, especially if the right temporal lobe is involved, thus getting items out of order. Some problems in visual memory and closure as well as picture relationships may be seen after a right temporal lobectomy (Rennick *et al.*, 1969; Giovagnoli *et al.*, 1995).

Older children and adults with right CPE may have problems in recognizing melodic changes and familiar tunes (Milner, 1968a; Fedio & Mirsky, 1969).

Such memory impairments, found even in idiopathic forms of anterior temporal lobe epilepsy (Browne & Reynolds 1981; Stores, 1987), appear to be related to a general impairment of verbal functioning, which itself may be depressed. Non-verbal memories and perceptual motor processes are less impaired (Quadfasel & Pruyser, 1955). Most often, this relates to a naming disturbance, i.e. an anomia (Denman & Wanamaker, 1983), resulting from an epileptic focus in the inferior left temporal lobe. This resembles a word-selection anomia (Mayeux *et al.*, 1980). Improvements in some but not all patients may follow a temporal lobectomy (Powell *et al.*, 1975).

Temporal lobe dysfunction, by affecting several mechanisms of the verbal memory system, is at risk for developing memory problems by its impact on several mechanisms in the verbal memory system (Aldenkamp *et al.*, 1990). The hippocampus may function more as a network of systems, and therefore to excise any part may break down the chain of action (Kortenkamp, 1996). The hippocampus and adjacent temporal regions are critical in learning for the maintenance of time-limited memory storages or retrieval. Delayed recall of learned material can occur without the participation of the mesiotemporal structures (Giovagnoli *et al.*, 1995). Mesial damage affects delayed memory skills (Zimmerman *et al.*, 1951). Verbal and non-verbal tasks problems have been correlated to hippocampal neuronal loss from the left and right sides, respectively, especially the site of the loss in late adolescence and adults microscopically. Patients with left hippocampal sclerosis do more poorly than those with right hippocampal sclerosis on both immediate and delayed prose recall (Baxendale *et al.*, 1998). Prolonged or repeated refractory temporal lobe epilepsy leads to progressive cognitive decline and hippocampal damage.

Removal of an atrophic left hippocampus is associated with the best verbal skill recovery. Removal of normal hippocampus results in the greatest loss of skills (Kortenkamp, 1996). Postoperative declines are more apt to be seen on the left. Any frontal area declines occurr within the first year after surgery.

Patients with bilateral anterior temporal ictal foci are more likely to have memory deficits involving the verbal and visual domains, suggesting bilateral hippocampal dysfunction (Mirsky *et al.*, 1960; Rausch *et al.*, 1978; Morrell, 1980; Prevey *et al.*, 1988), especially auditory sequential memory problems (Baratz & Mesulam, 1982). Patients with independent bilateral temporal foci have a lower mental cognition than patients with unilateral foci (Mirsky *et al.*, 1960). After bilateral destruction of the medial parts of the temporal lobes, there is no impairment of attention and no loss of preoperative acquired skills or intelligence, but there is a loss of the transition from short-term to long-term memory (Milner & Scoville, 1968; Milner, 1968b).

Academics

Patients with complex partial seizures have more learning difficulties (Stores, 1987). Seizure frequency, seizure intractability, and use of phenytoin may influence learning adversely in temporal lobe epilepsy (Reynolds, 1985; Rodin *et al.*, 1986; Andrews *et al.*, 1986; Trimble, 1988; Aldenkamp *et al.*, 1990). Children with left temporal epilepsy often present with verbal channel difficulties, which may be subtle enough to be overlooked, although the presence of speech and language problems may be a clue (Stores *et al.*, 1978; Stores & Piran, 1978; Stores, 1980). Memory problems may produce difficulties in basic reading processes by impairing the development of stable word recollection (Reynolds, 1985). Such children have difficulties learning new word lists (Brown & Reynolds, 1981). Boys with persistent left temporal foci often have impaired reading skills and accuracy, with phonetic difficulties, especially if they are on phenytoin (Stores, 1978). Boys with a non-dominant temporal focus fail in practical performance (Stores & Hart, 1976; Stores, 1978; Camfield *et al.*, 1984; Rugland, 1990; Henricksen, 1990).

Spelling and especially math are often more difficult for these children. Arithmetic tests in individuals with seizure onset before age six years show that those with shorter duration do better than those with longer duration of CPE (Oxbury *et al.*, 1998). Children with a non-dominant temporal focus are much less apt to have difficulties with reading and math, but they may still be impeded early in school by their perceptual problems affecting reading and writing and later math. Other school concerns include absenteeism and behavior problems. Children with persistent generalized subclinical EEG seizures are often felt to be overachieving.

Multifocal seizure disorders

The presence of multifocal seizure foci is related to certain types of cognitive and psychiatric complications. Such patients are often depressed in intelligence, and the cognitive profile may be more irregular, depending on the locations of the foci.

REFERENCES

Aicardi, J. (1988). Epileptic syndromes in childhood. *Epilepsia* **29** (suppl 3) 1–5.

Aldenkamp, A. P., Alpherts, W. C. J., Dekker, M. J. A., *et al.* (1990). Neuropsychological aspects of learning disabilities in epilepsy. *Epilepsia* **31** (suppl 4): 9–20.

Andrews, D. G., Bullen, J. G., Tomlinson, L., *et al.* (1986). A comparative study of the cognitive effects of phenytoin and carbamazepine in new referrals with epilepsy. *Epilepsia* **27**: 128–34.

Babb, T. I., Jann Brown, W., Pretorius, J., *et al.* (1984). Temporal lobe volumetric cell densities in temporal lobe epilepsy. *Epilepsia* **25**: 729–40.

Baratz, R. & Mesulam, M.-M. (1982). Adult onset stuttering treated with anticonvulsants. *Arch. Neurol.* **38**: 132.

Barlow, C. F. (1978). Risk factors of infancy and childhood: interrelationship fo seizure disorders and mental retardation. In *Mental Retardation and Related Disorders*, pp. 68–75. Philadelphia: F. A. Davis.

Battaglia, F. M.(1998). Neuropsychological aspects of TLE in children. 3rd European Congress of Epileptology. *Epilepsia* **39** (suppl 2): 70.

Baxendale, S. A., van Paesschen, W., Thompson, P. J., *et al.* (1998). The relationship between quantitative MRI and neuropsychological functioning in temporal lobe epilepsy. *Epilepsia* **39**: 158–66.

Beaumnoir, A. (1985). The Landau–Kleffner syndrome. In *Epileptic Syndromes in Infancy, Childhood and Adolescence*, ed. J. Roger, C. Dravet, M. Bureau, F. E. Dreifuss & P. Wolf, pp. 181–91. London: John Libbey.

Beaumanoir, A., Baltis, T., Varfis, G., *et al.* (1964). Benign epilepsy of childhood with Rolandic spikes. *Epilepsia* **15**: 301–15.

Benninger, C. K. Lipinski, C. G. & Scheffner, D. (1983). Intellectual development, school and vocational success in patients suffering from absence epilepsy in childhood. Presented at the 15th Epilepsy International Symposium, Washington, DC.

Berges, J., Harrison, A., Lairy, G. C., *et al.* (1968). L'EEG del enfant dyspraxique. *Electroencephalogr. Clin. Neurophsyiol.* **25**: 208–20.

Berkovic, S. F., Kuzniecky, R. I. & Andermann, F. (1997). Human epileptogenesis and hypothalamic hamartomas: New lesions from an experiment of nature. *Epilepsia* **38**: 1–3.

Besag, F. C. (2001). Treatment of state-dependent learning disabilities. In *Epilepsia and Learning Disabilities*, ed. G. F. Ayala, M. Elia, C. M. Cornaggia & M. R. Trimble. *Epilepsia* **42**: 46–9.

Binnie, C. D. (1980). Deterioration of transitory cognitive impairments during epileptiform EEG discharges; problems in clinical practice. In *Epilepsy and Behavior '79*, ed. B. R. Kulig, H. Meinardi & G. Stores, pp. 91–7. Lisse: Swets & Zeitlinger.

Binnie, C. D. (1988). Seizures, EEG discharges and cognition. In *Epilepsy, Behaivor and Cognitive Function*, ed. M. R. Trimble & E. H. Reynolds, pp. 45–51. London: John Wiley & Sons.

Binnie, C. D., Channon, S. & Marston, D. (1990). Learning disabilities in epilepsy: Neurophysiological aspects. *Epilepsia* **31** (suppl 4): 2–8.

Binnie, C. D., Kasteleijn-Nolst Trenite, D. G. A., Smit, A. M., *et al.* (1987). Interactions of epileptiform EEG discharges and cognition. *Epilepsy Res.* **1**: 239–45.

Blennow, G., Heijbel, J., Sandstedt, P., *et al.* (1990). Discontinuation of antiepileptics. *Epilepsia* **31** (suppl 4): 50–53.

Blume, W. T., David, R. B. & Gomez, M. R. (1973). Generalized sharp and slow wave complexes associated clinical features and long-term follow-up. *Brain* **98**: 289–308.

Boatman, D. F., Cronse, N. E., Lesser, R. P., *et al.* (1992). The localization of speech perception processes using direct cortical electrical interference and electrocorticography. *Epilepsia* **33** (suppl 3): 119–20.

Bradford, L. J. (1980). Understanding and assessing communicative disorders in children. *Dev. Behav. Pediatr.* **1**: 89–95.

Bray, P. F. (1962). Temporal lobe syndromes in children. *Pediatrics* **70**: 517–38.

Breier, J. I., Clark, A., Cass, J., *et al.* (1999). Profiles of cognitive performance in TLE patients with and without learning disability. *Epilepsia* **40** (suppl 7): 47–8.

Brittain, H. (1980). Epilepsy and intellectual functions. In *Epilepsy and Behavior*, ed. B. M. Kulig, H. Meiinardi & G. Stores, pp. 2–13. Lisse: Swets & Zeitlinger.

Brown, W. S. & Reynolds, E. H. (1981). Cognitive impairments in epileptic patients. In *Epilepsy and Psychiatry*, ed. E. H. Reynolds & M. R. Trimble, pp. 147–63. New York: Churchill Livingstone.

Browne, T. R., Penry, S. K., Porter, R., *et al.* (1974). Responsiveness before, during and after spike-wave paroxysms. *Neurology* **24**: 659–65.

Camfield, P. R., Gates, R., Ronen, G., *et al.* (1984). Comparison of cognitive ability, personality profile and school success in epileptic children with pure right versus left temporal lobe EEG foci. *Ann. Neurol.* **15**: 122–6.

Cavazzuti, G. B., Ferrari, P. & Lalla, M. (1984). Follow-up study of 482 cases with convulsive disorders in the first year of life. *Dev. Med. Child Neurol.* **26**: 425–37.

Chang, Y. C., Guo, N. W., Huang, C. C., *et al.* (2000). Neurocognitive attention and behavior outcome of school age children with a history of febrile convulsions. A population study. *Epilepsia* **41**: 412–20.

Chastrain, G. E., Lettsich, E., Miller, L. H., *et al.* (1970). Pattern sensitive epilepsy: part 2. Clinical changes, tests of responsiveness and motor output, alterations of evoked potentials and therapeutic measures. *Epilepsia* **11**: 151–62.

Cheminal, R., Laurayre, P., Quisquempois, J. M., *et al.* (1998). Neuropsychological abnormalities in absence epilepsy. 3rd European Congress of Epileptology. *Epilepsia* **39** (suppl 2): 120.

Chevrie, J. J. & Aicardi, J. (1978). Convulsive disorders in the first year of life: neurological and mental outcome and mortality. *Epilepsia* **19**: 47–67.

Commission for the Control of Epilepsy and Its Consequences. (1977). Prevention related to febrile convulsions. In *Plan for Nationwide Action on Epilepsy*, Vol. IIIB, pp. 256–68. Bethesda, MD: National Institutes of Neurological and Communicative Disorders and Stroke.

Croona, C., Kihlgren, M., Lundberg, S., *et al.* (1998). Neuropsychologic findings in children with benign childhood epilepsy with centrotemporal spikes. 3rd European Congress of Epileptology. *Epilepsia* **39** (suppl 2): 18.

Dam, M. (1990). Children with epilepsy: the effect of seizures, syndromes and etiological factors on cognitive functioning. *Epilepsia* **31** (suppl 4): 26–9.

Davies-Eyesneck, M. (1952). Cognitive factors in epilepsy. *J. Neurol. Neurosurg. Psychiatry* **15**: 39–44.

Delaney, R. C., Rosen, A. J., Mattson, R. H., *et al.* (1980). Memory function in focal epilepsy; a comparison of non-surgical unilateral temporal lobe and frontal lobe samples. *Cortex* **6**: 103–17.

Denman, S. B. & Wanamaker, B. B. (1983). Neuropsychological memory scale in temporal lobe epileptic patients. *Epilepsia* **24**: 258.

Deonna, T. (1999). Developmental consequences of epilepsies in infancies. In *Childhood Epilepsies and Brain Development*, ed. A. Nehlig, J. Motte, S. L. Moshe & P. Plouin, pp. 113–22. London: John Libbey & Co.

Dikmen, S. (1980). Neuropsychological aspects of epilepsy. In *A Multidisciplinary Handbook of Epilepsy*, ed. B. P. Hermann, pp. 236–73. Springfield, IL: Chas. C. Thomas.

Dikmen, S., Matthews, C. G. & Harley, J. P. (1975). The effect of early versus late onset of major motor epilepsy upon cognitive-intellectual performance. *Epilepsia* **16**: 73–81.

Dikmen, S., Matthews, C. G. & Harley, J. P. (1977). Effects of early versus late onset of major motor epilepsy on cognitive-intellectual performance: further considerations. *Epilepsia* **18**: 31–6.

Dodrill, C. B. (1976). Neuropsychology. In *Textbook of Epilepsy*, ed. J. Laidlow & A. Reichens, Vol. II, pp. 282–91. London: Churchill Livingstone.

Dodrill, C. B. (1978). A neuropsychological battery for epilepsy. *Epilepsia* **19**: 611–23.

Dodrill, C. B. (1986). Correlates of generalized tonic–clonic seizures with intellectual, neuropsychological, emotional and social functioning in patients with epilepsy. *Epilepsia* **27**: 399–411.

Dravet, C. (1999). The Lennox–Gastaut syndrome: from baby to adolescent. In *Childhood Epilepsies and Brain Development*, ed. A. Nehlig, J. Motte, S. L. Moshe & P. Plouin, pp. 103–12 London: John Libbey & Co.

Dreifuss, F. (1983). *Pediatric Epileptology*. Boston, MA: John Wright PSG.

Dulac, O., Chiron, C., Robain, OL., *et al.* (1999). Infantile spasms: a pathophysiological hypothesis. In *Childhood Epilepsies and Brain Development*, ed. A. Nehlig, J. Motte, S. L. Moshe & P. Plouin, pp. 93–102. London: John Libbey & Co.

Ellenberg, J. H., Hirtz, D. G. & Nelson, K. B. (1984). Age at onset of seizures in young children. *Ann. Neurol.* **15**: 127–34.

Ericksson, M. & Zetterstrom, R. (1979). Neonatal convulsions. *Acta Paediatr. Scand.* **68**: 807–11.

Fairweather, H. & Hutt, S. J. (1971). Some effects of performance variaibles upon generalized spike-wave activity. *Brain* **94**: 321–6.

Farwell, J. R., Dodrill, C. B., & Batzel, L. W. (1984). Neuropsychological function in children with epilepsy. *Epilepsia* **25**: 646.

Farwell, J. R., Dodrill, C. B. & Batzel, L. W. (1985a). Neuropsychological abilities of children with epilepsy. *Epilepsia* **26**: 395–400.

Farwell, J., Dodrill, C., Tempkins, N. & Wilkus, R. (1985b). Intellectual function in children with complex partial seizures. *Ann. Neurol.* **8**: 229–30.

Fedio, P. & Mirsky, A. F. (1969). Selective intellectual deficits in children with temporal lobe or centrencephalic epilepsy. *Neuropsychology* **7**: 287–300.

Fenwick, P. (1981). EEG studies. In *Epilepsy and Psychiatry*, ed. E. H. Reynolds & M. R. Trimble, pp. 242–53. New York: Churchill Livingstone.

Foerster, F. M. (1977). Epielspy evoked by higher cognitve functions: Decision making epilepsy. In *Reflex Epilepsy: Behavioral Therapy and Conditioned Reflexes*, pp. 124–34. Springfield, IL: Charles C. Thomas.

Freman, F. R., Douglas, E. F. O. & Penry, J. K. (1973). Environmental interaction and memory during petit mal (absence) seizures. *Pediatrics* **1**: 911–18.

Fremion, A., Emerson, R., Freeman, J. M., *et al.* (1980). Outcome of the Lennox Gastaut syndrome. *Ann. Neurol.* **8**: 229.

Fukushima, K., Kubota, H., Fujiwara, T., *et al.* (2001). Long-term follow-up of atypical benign partial epilepsy. Proceedings of the 33rd Congress of the Japan Epilepsy Society. *Epilepsia* **42** (suppl 6): 42–6.

Geller, M. & Geller, A. (1970). Brief amnestic effects of spike-wave discharges. *Neurology* **20**: 1089–95.

Gerber, M. J. Spindler, J., O'Rourke, C., *et al.* (1983). Anticonvulsant effects on cognitive functioning in children with epilepsy. Presented at the 15th Epilepsy International Symposium, Washington, DC.

Giordani, B., Berent, S., Sackellares, J. C., *et al.* (1983). Intelligence and academic achievement in patients with partial generalized and partial secondary generalized seizures. *Epilepsia* **24**: 258.

Giordani, B., Berent, S., Sackellares, J. C., *et al.* (1985). Intelligence test performance of patients with partial and generalized seizures. *Epilepsia* **26**: 37–42.

Giovagnoli, A. R., Casazza, M. & Gavanzini, G. (1995). Visual learning on a selective reminding procedure and delayed recall in patients with temporal lobe epilepsy. *Epilepsia* **36**: 704–11.

Glaze, D. G., Hrachovy, R. A., Frost, J. D., *et al.* (1988). Prospective study of outcome of infants with infantile spasms treated during controlled studies of ACTH and prednisone. *J. Pediatr.* **112**: 389–96.

Glowinski, H. (1973). Cogntive deficits in temporal lobe epilepsy. *J. Nerv. Ment. Dis.* **157**: 129–37.

Goode, D. J., Penry, J. K. & Dreifuss, F. E. (1970). Effect of paroxysmal spike-wave on continuous visual-motor performance. *Epilepsia* **11**: 241–54.

Gulgonen, S., Demirbilek, V., Kormaz, B., *et al.* (2000). Neuropsychological functions in idiopathic occipital lobe epilepsy. *Epilepsia* **41**: 405–11.

Gururaj, V. J. (1980). Febrile seizures, current concepts. *Clin. Pediatr.* **19**: 731–8.

Halgren, E. (1982). Psychological consequences of epilepsy. Presented at the 33rd Western Institute on Epilepsy Conference, Portland, OR.

Hall, J. H. & Marshall, P. C. (1980). Clonazepam therapy in reading epilepsy. *Neurology* **30**: 550–51.

Halstead, H. (1957). Abilities and behavior of epileptic children. *J. Ment. Sci.* **103**: 28–47.

Heijbel, J. & Behman, M. (1975). Benign epilepsy of children with centrotemporal EEG foci: Intelligence, behavior and school adjustment. *Epilepsia* **16**: 679–87.

Hendriks, M. P. H., Jacobs, S., Aldenkamp, A. P., *et al.* (1998). Memory complaints and the relation with memory functions in patients with partial seizures originating form the temporal or frontal lobes. 3rd European Congress of Epileptology. *Epilepsia* **39** (suppl 2): 120.

Henricksen, O. (1990). Education and epilepsy: assessment and remediation. *Epilepsia* **31** (suppl 4): 21–5.

Herman, B., Seidenberg, M., Bell, B., *et al.* (2002). The neurodevelopmental impact of childhood-onset temporal lobe epilepsy on brain structure and function. *Epilepsia* **43**: 1062–71.

Hermann, B. P., Schwartz, M. S., Karnes, W. E. & Vahdat, P. (1980). Psychopathology in epilepsy: relationship to seizure type and age of onset. *Epilepsia* **21**: 15–23.

Hertoft, P. (1963). The clinical, electroencephalographic and social prognosis in petit mal epilepsy. *Epilepsia* **4**: 298–314.

Hutt, S. J. & Fairweather, H. (1975). Information processing during two types of EEG activity. *Electroencephalogr. Clin. Neurophysiol.* **39**: 43–51.

Hutt, S. J. & Gilbert, S. (1980). Effects of evoked spikewave discharges upon short-term memory in patients with epilepsy. *Cortex* **16**: 445–57.

Ives, L. A. (1969). Learning difficulties in children with epilepsy. *Br. J. Dis. Commun.* **405**: 177–84.

Ives, L. A. (1970). Learning difficulties in children with epilepsy. *Br. J. Dis. Commun.* **5**: 77–84.

Jokeit, H. & Ebner, A. (1999). Long term effects of refractory temporal lobe epilepsy on cognitive abilities: a cross sectional study. *J. Neurol. Neurosurg. Psychiatry* **76**: 44–50.

Jus, A. & Jus, K. (1962). Retrograde amnesia in petit mal. *Arch. Gen. Psychiatry* **6**: 116–71.

Keating, L. E. (1960). A review of the literature on the relatinship of epilepsy and intelligence in school children. *J. Ment. Sci.* **105**: 1042–59.

Kertesz, A. (1983). *Localization in Neuropsychology.* New York: Academic Press.

Kimura, D. (1963). Right temporal-lobe damage. *Arch. Neurol.* **8**: 265–71.

Klove, H. & Matthews, C. G. (1974). Neuropsycholgoical studies of patients with epilepsy. In *Clincial Neuropsychology: Current Status and Applications*, ed. R. M. Reitan & L. A. Davidson, pp. 237–66. Washington, DC: VH Winston & Sons.

Koo, B. & Hwang, P. A. (1992). Developmental assessment of patients with cryptogenic and symptomatic infantile spasms. *Epilepsia* **33** (suppl 3): 5.

Kooi, K. A. & Hovey, H. B. (1957). Alternations in mental functions and paroxysmal cerebral activity. *Arch. Neurol. Psychiatry* **1978**: 264–71.

Kortenkamp, S. R. (1996). Neuropsychological correlates of subfield-specific hippocampal pathology. Presented at the American Epilepsy Society Conference, San Francisco, CA.

Koskiniemi, M. (1974). Psycholgocial findings in progressive myoclonic epilepsy without Lafora bodies. *Epilepsia* **15**: 537–45.

Koskiniemi, M., Donner, M., Majouri, H., Haltia, M. & Norio, R. (1974). Progressive myoclonus epilepsy. *Acta Neurol. Scand.* **50**: 307–32.

Kurokawa, T., Goya, N., Fukuyama, Y., *et al.* (1980). West syndrome and Lennox Gastaut syndrome: a survey of natural history. *Pediatrics* **65**: 81–8.

Ladavas, E. Umnila, C. & Provincialli, I. (1979). Hemisphere dependent cognitve performance in epileptic patients. *Epilepsia* **20**: 493–502.

Lansdell, H. & Mirsky, A. F. (1964). Attention in focal and centrencephalic epilepsy. *Exp. Neurol.* **9**: 463–9.

Lerman, P. (1985). Benign partial epilepsy with centro-temporal spikes. In *Epileptic Syndromes in Infancy, Childhood and Adolescence*, ed. J. Roger, C. Dravet, M. Bureau, F. E. Dreifuss & P. Wolf, pp. 150–59. London: John Libbey.

Lewinsky, R. J. (1953). The psychometric pattern. III: epilepsy. *Am. J. Orthopsychiatry* **17**: 714–21.

Lindsay, J., Ounsted, C. & Richards, P. (1979). Long-term outcome in children with temproal lobe seizures. No 1: social outcome and childhood factors. *Dev. Med. Child Neurol.* **21**: 285–98.

Livingston, S. (1974). Diagnosis and treatment of childhoodmyoclonic seizures. *Pediatrics* **53**: 542–6.

Logan, W. J. & Freeman, J. M. (1969). Pseudo-degenerative disease due to diphenylhydantoin intoxication. *Arch. Neurol.* **21**: 631–7.

Loiseau, P., Pestre, M., Dartigues, J. F., *et al.* (1983). Long-term prognosis in two forms of childhood epilepsy: typical absence seizures and epilepsy with rolandic (centrotemporal) EEG foci. *Ann. Neurol.* **13**: 642–8.

Loiseau, P., Signoret, J. L., Strube, E., *et al.* (1982). Nouveaux procedes d'appereciation des troubles de la memoire chez les epileptiques. *Rev. Neurol.* **183**: 387–400.

Mandelbaum, D. E., Burack, G. D. & Daswani, A. A. (1993). Effects of seizure type and education on psychological functioning in epileptic children. *Epilepsia* **34** (suppl 6): 72.

Margerison, J. H. & Corsellis, J. A. N. (1966). Epilepsy and the temporal lobes. *Brain* **89**: 499–530.

Matsumoto, A., Watanabe, K., Negoro, T., *et al.* (1981). Long-term prognosis after infantile spasms: a statistical study of prognostic factors in 200 cases. *Dev. Med. Child Neurol.* **23**: 51–65.

Matsumoto, A., Watanabe, K., Siguura, M., *et al.* (1983). Long-term prognosis of convulsive disorders in the first year of life: mental and physical development and seizure persistence. *Epilepsia* **24**: 321–9.

Matsuoka, H., Okuma, T., Oemo, T. & Saiato, H. (1986). Impairment of parietal cortical functions associated with episodic prolonged spike-and-wave discharge. *Epilepsia* **27**: 432–6.

Matsuoka, H. (2001). Neuropsychology of epilepsy. Proceedings of the 33rd Congress of the Japan Epilepsy Society. *Epilepsia* **42** (suppl 6): 42–6.

Matthews, C. G. & Klove, H. (1967). Differential pscyholgoical perfromacnes in major motor, psychomotor, and mixed seizure classifcation of known and unknown etiology. *Epilepsia* **8**: 117–28.

Mayeux, R., Brandt, J., Rosen, J., *et al.* (1980). Interictal memory and language impairment in temporal lobe epilepsy. *Neurology* **30**: 109–25.

McDaniel, J. W. & McDaniel, M. L. (1976). Visual and auditory cognitive processing affected by epilepsy. *PDM* **7**: 38–42.

McIntyre, M. B. P., Pritchard, P. B., III & Lombroso, C. T. (1976). Left and right temporal epileptics: a controlled inspecctiuon of some psychological differences. *Epilepsia* **17**: 377–86.

Meador, K. J. (2002). Cognitive outcomes and predictive factors in epilepsy. *Neurology* **58** (suppl 5): 21–8.

Mellanby, J., Hawkins, C. & Wilks, I. (1984). The relationship between seizures and amnesia in experimental epilepsy. *Acta Neurol. Scand.* **99**: 119–24.

Mellor, D. H. & Lowint, I. (1977). Study of intellectual function in children with epilepsy attending ordinary schools. In *Epilepsy: Eighth International Symposium*, ed. J. K. Penry, pp. 291–4. New York: Raven Press.

Mesri, J. C. & Pagano, M. A. (1987). Reading epilepsy. *Epilepsia* **28**: 301–4.

Metz-Lutz, M. N. & Massa, R. (1999). Cognitive and behavioral consequences of epilepsies in childhood. In *Childhood Epilespies and Brain Development*, ed. A. Nehlig, J. Motte, S. L. Moshe & P. Plouin, pp. 123–34. London: John Libbey & Co.

Meyer, V. & Falconer, M. A. (1960). Patterns of cognitive test performance as functions of the lateral localization of cerebral abnormalities in the temporal lobe. *J. Ment. Sci.* **103**: 758–72.

Milner, B. (1954). Intellectual function of the temporal lobe. *Psychol. Bull.* **51**: 42–62.

Milner, B. (1968a). Visual recognition and recall after right temporal-lobe excision in man. *Neuropsychology* **6**: 191–209.

Milner, B. (1968b). Disorders of memory after brain lesions in man. *Neuropsychology* **6**: 175–9.

Milner, B. (1975). Psychological aspects of focal epilepsy and its neurosurgical management. In *Advances in Epilepsy: Neurosurgical Management of Epilepsies*, ed. D. P. Purpura, J. R. Penry, & R. D. Walter, Vol. 8, pp. 299–321. New York: Raven Press.

Milner, B. & Scoville, W. B. (1968). Loss of recent memory after bilateral hippocampal lesions. *J. Neurol. Neurosurg. Psychiatry* **20**: 11–21.

Mirsky, A. F. & Van Buren, J. M. (1965). On the nature of the "absence" in centrencephalic epilepsy: a study of some behavioral, electroencephalographic and autonomic factors. *Electroencephalogr. Clin. Neurophysiol.* **18**: 334–8.

Mirsky, A. F., Primac, D. W., Marsan, C. A., *et al.* (1960). A comparison of the psychological test performance of patients with focal and nonfocal epilepsy. *Dev. Exp. Neurol.* **2**: 75–89.

Morales, A., Kelly, D. P., Shaw, S. R., *et al.* (1993). Information processing during focal evoked electroencephalographic epileptiform activity. *Epilepsia* **34** (suppl 6): 45.

Morrell, F. (1980). Memory loss as a Todd's paralysis. *Epilepsia* **21**: 185.

Mosovich, A. (1974). The significance of epileptic seizures in infancy and childhood. *S. Afr. Med. J.* **48**: 750–52.

Mouritzen, D. A. (1982). Hippocampal neuron loss in epilepsy and after experimental seizures. *Acta Neurol. Scand.* **66**: 601–42.

Mungas, D., Cindy, F., Walton, N., *et al.* (1985). Verbal learning differences in epileptic patients with left and right temporal lobe foci. *Epilepsia* **26**: 340–45.

Novelly, R. A. (1982). Minimal developmental dysphasia: constraints on specificity of expressive language with early onset left hemisphere epilepsy. *Epilespia* **23**: 430–39.

O'Donohoe, N. V. (1979). Mental handicap and epilepsy. In *Epilepsies of Childhood*, pp. 143–6. London: Butterworth.

O'Leary, D. S., Seidenberg, M., Berrent, S., *et al.* (1981). Effects of age of onset of tonic-clonic seizures on neuropsychological performance in children. *Epilepsia* **22**: 197–204.

Ouelette, E. M. (1974). The child who convulses with fever. *Pediatr. Clin. North Am.* **231**: 467–81.

Ounsted, C., Jutt, S. J. & Lee, D. (1963). The retrograde amnesia of petit mal. *Lancet* **1**: 163.

Ounsted, C., Lindsay, J. & Norman, R. (1966). Intelligence. In *Clinics in Developmental Medicine: Biological factors in Temporal Lobe Epilepsy*, pp. 62–71. London: Spastics Society and Heinemann.

Oxbury, S. M., Cambell, L., Baxendale, S. A., *et al.* (1998). Cognitive function in relation to duration of temporal lobe epilepsy (TLE) due to Ammon's Horn sclerosis. 3rd European Congress of Epileptology. *Epilepsia* **39** (suppl 2): 120.

Piccirilli, M. D., Alesandro, P., Sciarma, T., *et al.* (1994). Attention problems in epilepsy: possible significance of the epileptogenic focus. *Epilepsia* **35**: 1091–6.

Piccirilli, M., D'Allesandro, P., Tiacci, C. & Feronni, A. (1988). Language lateralization in children with benign partial epilepsy. *Epilepsia* **29**: 19–25.

Piras, M. R., Sechi, G. P., Mutani, R., *et al.* (1991). Developmental surface dyslexia in progressive myoclonic epilepsy. 19th International Epilepsy Congress. *Epilepsia* **32** (suppl 1): 25.

Porter, R. J., Penry, J. K. & Dreifuss, F. E. (1973). Responsiveness at the onset of spike-wave bursts. *Electroencephalogr. Clin. Neurophysiol.* **34**: 239–45.

Powell, G. E., Polkey, C. E. & McMillan, T. (1975). The new Maudsley series of temporal lobectomy. I: short-term cognitive effects. *Br. J. Clin. Psychol.* **24**: 109–24.

Prevey, M. L., Delaney, R. C. & Mattson, R. H. (1988). Test recall in temporal lobe seizure patients (a study of adaptive memory skills). *Cortex* **24**: 301–12.

Quadfasel, A. F. & Pruyser, P. W. (1955). Cognitive deficit in patients with psychomotor epilepsy. *Epilepsia* **4**: 80–90.

Rausch, R. (1981). Lateralization of temporal lobe dysfunction and verbal encoding. *Brain Lang.* **12**: 92–100.

Rausch, R., Lieb, U. P. & Crandall, P. A. S. (1978). Neuropsychologic correlates of depth spike activity in epileptic patients. *Arch. Neurol.* **35**: 699–705.

Read, D. E. (1981). Solving deductive reasoning problems after unilateral temporal lobectomy. *Brain Lang.* **12**: 116–27.

Reitan, R. S. (1974). Psychological testing of epileptici patients. In *Handbook of Clinical Neurology*, ed. P. J. Vinken & G. W. Bruyn, pp. 559–75. Amsterdam: North Holland.

Rener-Primec, Z. R., Tretnajak, V. G. & Kopac, S. (1999). Cognitive outcome in children with idiopathic form of West syndrome. 23rd International Epilepsy Congress. *Epilepsia* **40** (suppl 2): 163.

Renier, W. O. (1987). Restrictive factors in the education of children with epilepsy from a medical point of view. In *Education and Epilepsy 1987*, ed. A. P. Aldenkamp, W. C. J. H. Alpherts, H. Meinardi & G. Stores, pp. 3–14. Lisse: Swets & Zeitlinger.

Rennick, P. M. Perez-Borja, C. & Rodin, E. (1969). Transient mental deficits associated with recurrent prolonged epileptic clouded state. *Epilepsia* **10**: 397–405.

Reynolds, E. H. (1985). Antiepileptic drugs and psychopathology. In *The Psychopharmacology of Epilepsy*, ed. M. R. Trimble, pp. 49–65. Chichester, UK: John Wiley & Sons.

Riga, D., Saletti, V., Collino, L., *et al.* (1998). Neuropsychology of frontal epileptic activity. 3rd European Congress of Epileptology. *Epilepsia* **39** (suppl 2): 120.

Rintahaka, P. J., Anattila, S. & Ylitalo, V. (1993). Prognosis of children with first febrile convulsions before 12 months. *Epilepsia* **34** (suppl 6): 72.

Risberg, J. & Ingvar, D. H. (1973). Patterns of activation in the grey matter of the dominant hemisphere during memorizing and reasoning. *Brain* **96**: 737–56.

Rodin, E. A., Schmaltz, S. & Twitty, G. (1986). Intellectual functions of patients with childhood-onset epilepsy. *Dev. Med. Child Neurol.* **28**: 25–33.

Rugland, A. L. (1990). Neuropsychological assessment of cognitive functioning in children with epilepsy. *Epilepsia* **31** (suppl 4): 41–4.

Schlack, H. G. (1980). Changes of abnormal EEG patterns during mental tasks. *Epilepsia* **21**: 205.

Schwab, R. S. (1941). The influence of visual and auditory stimuli on the electroencephalographic tracing of petit mal. *Am. J. Psychiatry* **97**: 301–12.

Schwartz, T., Ojemann, G., Haglund, M., *et al.* (1992). Cerebral laterzazliation of neuronal activity during naming, reading and line matching. *Epilepsia* **33** (suppl 3): 120.

Seidenberg, M., O'Leary, D. S., Berent, S., *et al.* (1981). Changes in seizure frequency and test-retest scores on the Wechlser Adult Intelligence Scale. *Epilepsia* **22**: 75–83.

Sengoku, A., Kanazawa, O., Kawai, I., *et al.* (1990). Visual cognitive disturbance during spike-wave discharges. *Epilepsia* **31**: 47–50.

Serafetinides, E. A. (1969). Memory for words and memory for numbers. *J. Learn. Disabil.* **2**: 142–3.

Sherwin, I. & Efron, R. (1980). Temporal ordering deficits following anterior temporal lobectomy. *Brain Lang.* **11**: 195–203.

Sidtis, J. J., Volpe, B. T., Wilson, D. N., *et al.* (1981). Variability in right hemisphere language function after collosal section: evidence for a continuum of generative capacity. *J. Neurosci.* **1**: 323–31.

Sillanpaa, M. (1973). Medico-social prognosis of children with epilepsy: epidemiology study and analysis of 245 patients. *Acta Paediatr. Scand. Suppl.* **237**: 3–104.

Snyder, P. J. & Blaxton, T. (1992). Impaired semantic categorization in left temporal lobe epilepsy. *Epilepsia* **33** (suppl 3): 120.

Stores, G. (1971). Cognitive function in children with epilepsy. *Dev. Med. Child Neurol.* **13**: 390–93.

Stores, G. (1973). Studies of attention and seizure disorders. *Dev. Med. Child Neurol.* **17**: 647–58.

Stores, G. (1976). The investigation and management of school children with epilepsy. *Publ. Health, London* **9**: 171–7.

Stores, G. (1978). School-children with epilepsy at risk for learning and behavior problems. *Dev. Med. Child Neurol.* **20**: 502–8.

Stores, G. (1980). EEG studies in the behavioral assessment of people with epilepsy. In *Epilepsy and Behavior '79*, ed. E. M. Kulig, H. Meinardi & G. Stores, pp. 82–90. Lisse: Swets & Zeitlinger.

Stores, G. (1981). Memory impairment in children with epilepsy. *Acta Neurol. Scand.* **64** (suppl 89): 21–7.

Stores, G. (1987). Effects on learning of "subclinical" seizure discharges. In *Education and Epilepsy 1987*, ed. A. P. Aldenkamp, W. C. J. Alpherts, H. Meinardi & G. Stores, pp. 14–21. Lissee: Swets & Zeitlinger.

Stores, G. (1990). Electroencephalographic parameters in assessing the cognitive function of children with epilepsy. *Epilepsia* **31** (suppl 4): 45–9.

Stores G. & Hart, J. (1976). Reading skills of children with generalized or focal epilepsy attending ordinary school. *Dev. Med. Child Neurol.* **18**: 705–16.

Stores, G. & Piran, N. (1978). Dependency of different types in school children with epilepsy. *Psychol. Med.* **8**: 441.

Stores, G., Hart, J. & Piran, N. (1978). Inattentiveness in schoolchildren with epilepsy. *Epilepsia* **19**: 169–75.

Sullivan, E. G. & Gahagan, L. (1935). Intellgence of epileptic children. *Genet. Psychol. Monogr.* **17**: 314–74.

Swartz, B. E., Halgren, E., Daims, R., *et al.* (1993). Neurocognitive function in frontal lobe epilepsy. *Epilepsia* **34** (suppl 6): 33.

Syrigou-Papavasiliou, A., LeWitt, P. A., Green, V., *et al.* (1985). P300 and temporal lobe epilepsy. *Epilepsia* **26**: 528.

Tarter, R. E. (1971). Intellectual and adaptive functioning in epilepsy: a review of fifty years of research. *Dis. Nerv. Syst.* **33**: 763–70.

Tizard, B. & Margerison, J. H. (1963). Psychological functioning during wave-spike discharges. *Br. J. Soc. Clin. Psychol.* **3**: 6–15.

Trimble, M. R (1988). Anticonvulsant drugs: mood and cognitive unctions. In *Epilepsy, Behavior and Cognitive Function*, ed. M. R. Trimble & E. H. Reynolds, pp. 135–45. Chichester, UK: John Wiley & Sons.

Turkdogan, D., Zaimoglul, S., Yilmaz, Z., *et al.* (1999). Cognitive and behavioral characteristics in children with central spikes. 23rd International Epilepsy Congress. *Epilepsia* **40** (suppl 2): 230.

Wallace, S. J. (1976). Febrile fits. *Br. Med. J.* **1**: 333–4.

Wallace, S. J. & Cull, A. M. (1979). Long-term psychological outlook for children whose first fit occurs with fever. *Dev. Med. Child Neurol.* **21**: 28–40.

Wasterlain, C. G., Thompson, K. W., Kornblum, H., *et al.* (1999). Long-term effects of recurrent seizures on the developing brain. In *Childhood Epilepsies and Brain Development*, ed. A. Nehlig, J. Motte, S. L. Moshe & P. Plouin, pp. 237–65. London: John Libbey.

Waxman, S. G. & Geschwind, N. (1975). The interictal behavior syndrome of temporal lobe epilepsy. *Arch. Gen. Psychiatry* **32**: 1580–86.

Wechsler, A. F. (1973). The effect of organic brain disease on recall of emotionally charged versus neutral narrative texts. *Neurology* **23**: 130–35.

Whitehouse, D. (1971). Psychological and neurological correlates of seizures disorders. *Johns Hopkins Med. J.* **129**: 36–42.

Whitehouse, D. (1976). Behavior and learning problems in epileptic children. *Behav. Neuropsychiatry* **7**: 23–9.

Wilkus, R. J. & Dodrill, C. B (1976). Neuropsychological correlates of the electroencephalograph in epileptics: I. Topographic distribution and average rate of epileptiform activity. *Epilepsia* **17**: 89–100.

Wolf, S. M. (1979). Controversies in the treatment of febrile convulsions. *Neurology* **29**: 287–90.

Zheng, J., Okajima, H., Aikawa, H., *et al.* (2000). Delayed reaction time in patients with temporal lobe epilepsy. Proceedings of the 32nd Congress of Japan Epilepsy Society. *Epilepsia* **41** (suppl 9): 67.

Zimmerman, F. T. Burgemeister, B. B. & Putnam, T. J. (1951). Intellectual and emotional makeup of the epileptic. *Arch. Neurol. Psychiatry* **65**: 545–56.

16

Modifying factors

Epilepsy is not just one disease but rather a symptom of differing neurologic syndromes (Whitehouse, 1976), each of which is subject to multiple variables determining its final manifestation in a child. A combination of factors may determine the final presentation of epilepsy and its consequences. A combination of factors, such as epilepsy syndrome, etiology, presence of a lesion, onset age, frequency, duration, and location of brain involvement, may contribute to global or specific cognitive depression or deterioration (Dam, 1990).

Electroencephalograms

Generalized seizures with early burst suppression, hypsarrhythmia, or slow spike-wave appearance against a slowed background are usually associated with a significant degree of developmental delays and retardation. Slow spike-wave prolonged discharges in slow sleep are often associated with functional regression. A focal discharge on a slowed background, often associated with a symptomatic partial seizure, is at increased risk for specific learning problems. Multifocal spikes are usually associated with intellectual impairment and are often caused by an insult. Even so-called benign partial seizure discharges may not be so benign.

Idiopathic versus symptomatic epilepsy

From an etiologic viewpoint, there are two categories of epilepsy: symptomatic and idiopathic. New investigational methods are reducing the proportion of idiopathic cases (Collins & Lennox, 1947; Price *et al.*, 1948; Ounsted *et al.*, 1966; Rutter *et al.*, 1970; Dam, 1990). There is an intermittent term – cryptogenic epilepsy – used for patients with seizures that resemble a symptomatic form but for which no cause can be found, i.e. a presumed cause being undetected.

Idiopathic epilepsy

Up to 84% of patients in whom no cause for the seizures is found or suspected are mentally and physically normal (Collins & Lennox, 1947; Price *et al.*, 1948; Keating,

1960; Ounsted *et al.*, 1966; Tarter, 1971; Dikmen, 1980; Dam, 1990), especially if there is a family history of epilepsy (Klove & White, 1961; Rutter *et al.*, 1970). Those with idiopathic CPE are less impaired than those with symptomatic CPE or epileptic status (Ounsted *et al.*, 1966; Rennick *et al.*, 1969; Klove & Matthews, 1967; Matthews & Klove, 1967). However, with idiopathic epilepsy, there is a risk for general and specific psychologic impairments, especially if the onset is early in life (Keating, 1960; Klove & Matthews, 1966; Tarter, 1971; Klove, 1980). Such impairments may include a slightly lower intelligence, attention difficulties, memory problems (both auditory and visual), and academic underachievement (Gulgonen *et al.*, 2000).

Symptomatic epilepsy

Symptomatic epilepsy is more apt to be impairing than idiopathic epilepsies. Symptomatic generalized seizures are more apt to be associated with a depressed intelligence and attention problems, whereas partial seizures, especially if symptomatic, are more often associated with specific learning disabilities, including perception and memory problems (Collins & Lennox, 1947; Collins, 1951; Zimmerman *et al.*, 1951; Halstead, 1957; Ounsted *et al.*, 1966; Rennick *et al.*, 1969; Tarter, 1971; Waxman & Geschwind, 1973; Reitan, 1974, Klove & Matthews, 1974; Brittain, 1980; Klove, 1980; Brimer & Barudin, 1981; Bourgeois *et al.*, 1983; Meador, 2002; Henricksen, 1990). Brain damage or dysplasia alone may produce cognitive impairments, but if this is combined with epilepsy performance is even more disturbed (Dikmen & Reitan, 1978; Aldenkamp, 1983; Wiberg *et al.*, 1987; Dam, 1990). Learning difficulties in children with epilepsy may be caused by more localized brain damage or deformity. In many cases, seizures and electrographic findings are the only signs of pathology (Henricksen, 1990), although with demonstrable pathology the impairments are usually greater (Keith *et al.*, 1955; Binnie *et al.*, 1990).

In children, the commonest insults contributing to lowered intelligence include birth problems, generalized seizures before age one year, and head injuries (Dikmen & Reitan, 1978; Farwell *et al.*, 1980). Trivial head injuries may result in seizures later on, especially if there is a positive family history of seizures suggesting a genetic tendency (McLaurin, 1973). Although the cortical signs may be localized following a head injury, the psychological deficits may be more generalized (Dikmen & Reitan, 1978).

Impairment after an acute insult is usually greater than that following a relatively static insult. Early damage is usually bilateral, but the left hemisphere appears more vulnerable (Fitzhugh *et al.*, 1961). A more localized brain lesion is less impairing to intelligence than more widespread damage. Removal of a damaged hemisphere may depress the intelligence for a few months but the child recovers by one year. The presence of epileptogenic tissue disturbs functioning of other cortical areas (Milner, 1975).

Abnormalities on neurologic examination are often associated with impaired higher cortical functions (Rodin *et al.*, 1972; Dikmen *et al.*, 1975). Epilepsy is seen in 58% of individuals with cerebral palsy, often with intelligence depressed proportionally to the severity of the motor impairment (Rutter *et al.*, 1970; Mellor & Lowit, 1977).

Symptomatic temporal lobe epilepsy in childhood is often associated with lower intelligence and school problems (Matthews & Klove, 1967; Sillanpaa, 1973; Heijbel & Behman, 1975). The integrity of the anterior temporal lobe, in particular the subicular cortex, appears essential for many complex mental processes (Sherwin & Efron, 1980). Mesial temporal lobe structural damage may be associated with memory difficulties with recent recall without immediate memory disturbances. Localized anterior mesial temporal lesions are generally not associated with significant reduction in cognitive function (Tuxhorn *et al.*, 1998).

More common causes of childhood temporal lobe epilepsy are developmental etiologies, such as dysplasias or tumors, acquired insults or hippocampal sclerosis, and cryptogenic causes. Children with a malformation, dysplasia, or tumor etiology, who often develop seizures later in mid or late childhood, often display behavior problems without significant cognitive impairments (Knight *et al.*, 1998). Those with preceding insults (infection, hippocampal sclerosis, or head injury) often have seizures at the time of the insult and display developmental delays or intellectual disabilities. Those with cryptogenic etiology may have seizures at any time but they are less apt to show developmental delays or intellectual disturbances (Sztriha *et al.*, 2002).

Cognitive defects depend only on the electrical activity of the epileptic focus, for the epileptic focus does not always coincide with the topographic localization of the atrophic lesions. The latter can be considered to be unrelated to the former (Kurokawa *et al.*, 1980).

Location and laterality effects

Epileptic disturbances affect lateralized cognition functions more than pure lesions do (Dennerll, 1964). Auditory reception problems and memory difficulties are seen with left-sided discharges, whereas visual perception and associations may be weakened in right-sided discharges. Left-sided and bilateral discharges produce the greatest short-term memory problems. Clear-cut differences in immediate and short-term memory scores may not be apparent within a year of the diagnosis (Ladavas *et al.*, 1979).

Left-sided damage

Left hemisphere damage sustained during early childhood, especially before age four to five years, rarely produces any long-lasting aphasia, provided the homologous areas of the right hemisphere remain functional. There may be delays in the development of speech and language. Later, subtle deficits in the production or comprehension of higher aspects of language emerge, but these do not reflect difficulties in language per se but rather the limits established by a generalized reduction of intellectual abilities after hemispheric dysfunction. Verbal channel learning disabilities may be noted, especially auditory memory impairments (Vargha-Kahdem, 2001).

Extensive left hemisphere injury before age four to five years but after the onset of speech often results in initial aphasias symptoms, which generally resolve before hemispherectomy. Language production may even exceed comprehension ability. After age five to seven years, a mild version of the adult pattern of aphasia is seen, including speech arrest, transient mutism, anomia, and/or agrammaticism. These symptoms tend to be chronic. The patient may be able to communicate effectively through short phrases or sentences (Vargha-Kahdem, 2001).

Right-sided damage

Early right hemispheric acquired damage may result in a temporary interference with speech and language at the onset of a right hemisphere seizure disorder, but even extensive pathology of the hemisphere produces selective if any effects. Early insult damage after the acquisition of speech may be associated with some initial linguistic disturbances, such as slurring, disorganization, or irrelevant speech, but these resolve after hemispherectomy and the arrest of seizures, suggesting that the interference is from the spread of the seizures from the other side. Perceptual problems, including visual memory deficits, may be noted (Vargha-Kahdem, 2001).

Bitemporal damage

Bilateral medial temporal damage, such as with severe perinatal hypoxic-ischemic insults, may result in a severe memory problem seen in children as young as eight to ten years of age. There are marked impairments in recall and episodic memory for everyday events, but there is relatively preserved recognition and semantic memory, i.e. memory for facts. Such children are able to attend mainstream schools and to acquire average levels in intelligence language and literacy skills. However, the memory impairments show up in everyday tasks, such as remembering routes, appointments, messages, etc., leading to problems of independence in later life. Thus, the early insult damage really becomes manifest later on in life. The impairments are as severe with early onset as with later onset, suggesting that brain plasticity of early childhood does not help (Vargha-Kahdem, 2001).

Hemispheric damage

Children with hemispheric damage leading to hemispherectomy in childhood show a generalized pattern of cognitive impairment, with a dramatic loss of intellectual abilities, restricting both verbal and non-verbal functions. If a discrepancy between verbal and non-verbal abilities exists, it favors verbal abilities, suggesting that verbal functions tend to be rescued and non-verbal functions crowded out as a consequence of early hemispheric damage. This generalized impairment of all aspects of cognitive ability is independent of the laterality of the side involved. Early hemispherectomy can improve the outcome since it may minimize the chances of seizures producing further damage. Thus it can prevent chronic dysfunction in the remaining hemisphere, which may otherwise emerge early in life (Vargha-Kahdem, 2001).

Gender

Epileptic boys are found to be more at risk for poorer IQ scores, academic underachievement, inattentiveness, excessive activity, and poor sustained attention (Stores, 1981; Mellor & Lowit, 1977). Epileptic boys also have difficulties in real-life situations where a degree of persistence is required (Stores & Harts 1976).

Age of onset

Learning is more impaired with early onset of seizures and their treatment (Lennox *et al.*, 1946; Zimmerman *et al.*, 1951; Collins, 1951; Keith *et al.*, 1955; Rennick *et al.*, 1969; Tarter, 1971; Sillanpaa, 1973; Reitan, 1974; Klove & Matthews, 1974; Dodrill, 1975; Carson & Gilden, 1975; Brittain, 1980; Brown & Reynolds, 1981; Rausch, 1981; O'Leary *et al.*, 1981; Ford *et al.*, 1983; Tuxhorn *et al.*, 1998; Meador, 2002; Smith *et al.*, 2002). The effects appear more detrimental to the developing brain, especially with generalized seizures (Collins, 1951; Keith *et al.*, 1955; O'Leary *et al.*, 1981; O'Leary *et al.*, 1983; Rodin *et al.*, 1986; Holmes, 1987; Rugland, 1990b). This is particularly true if brain damage is found (Reitan, 1974; Dikmen & Matthews, 1977). Early seizures tend to occur in children with known neurologic abnormalities (Ellenberg *et al.*, 1984).

Early-age epilepsy inhibits cognition by interfering with brain development, inhibiting mitotic activity, affecting myelination, and reducing cell numbers and size (Renier, 1987). The insult occurs when the early structures of learning are being laid down (Ounsted *et al.*, 1966). Lower IQ scores are more common in the absence of a family history of epilepsy, especially in children with a mixed seizure pattern (Mellor & Lowit, 1977). The acquisition of verbal comprehension and factual knowledge is more impaired with earlier onset of epilepsy, especially with left-sided pathology (Oxbury *et al.*, 1998). Late onset in childhood of seizures correlates with higher IQ scores and less intellectual deterioration (Chaudry & Pond, 1961; Dikmen *et al.*, 1975; Bourgeois *et al.*, 1983).

Immature brains react differently than mature brains to seizures. The immature brain is especially vulnerable to seizure-induced neuronal death of specific neuronal populations. Different neuronal subpopulations are vulnerable at different ages (Wasterlain *et al.*, 1999). Seizures can modify, slow down, or accelerate a wide range of unique processes occurring during development that are essential for correction formation and wiring of brain circuitry, including mitotic activity, neuronal migration, neuritic arborization, synaptic formation, removal of redundant processes, and myelinization. This gives a poorer prognosis for cognitive development (Renier, 1987; Stores, 1990). These defects cannot be compensated for so well in later life (Aicardi, 1988).

Epileptic discharges in a vital emerging developmental area can be impairing. If epileptic activity is maximal at the time of normally occurring programmed development, then the consequences will be greater because the stabilization of connections for the consolidation of emerging cognitive functions cannot take place, possibly resulting in permanent structural changes. If epilepsy is unrecognized, persistent, or uncontrolled, then progressive, severe retardation may emerge over time. Seizures from buried areas, such as the cingulated, orbital-frontal, mesial-frontal, mesial-temporal area, may not be noticed. Complex partial seizures can easily escape diagnosis in younger children, as can frontal seizures (Deonna, 1999).

Early infancy onset

Very early infant seizures in the first two to three months of life result in a fairly high incidence of neurologic and intellectual deficits as well as seizure recurrence often associated with brain damage. Lower IQ scores are more common with non-familial seizures and in children with mixed seizure patterns (Mellor & Lowit, 1977). Mental and neurologic sequelae occur most often with seizure onset in the first six months. Such seizures are more often symptomatic or cryptogenic (Chevrie & Aicardi, 1978; Chevrie & Aicardi, 1979; Dikmen, 1980; Mellor & Lowit, 1977; Stores, 1981). The developmental prognosis for children with seizure onset and persistence before one year of life is poor with all seizure types, especially generalized seizures. Many of these children end up with below normal intelligence. Half of those with partial seizures achieve mental normality (Matsumoto *et al.*, 1983).

Preschool onset

Increased learning impairment is correlated inversely with the age of onset, with moderate to severe impairments seen in seizures before age five to seven years (Keith, *et al.*, 1955; Farwell *et al.*, 1984), and 27% being retarded (Sullivan & Gahagan, 1935; O'Leary *et al.*, 1981; Scarpa & Carassini, 1982). This is especially true if the child had preceding neurologic abnormalities, minor motor seizures, or infantile spasms (Bourgeouis *et al.*, 1983; Reitan, 1974). Children with onset of seizures before age five years perform significantly worse on verbal and performance IQ tests compared with children whose seizures begin later, regardless of whether the seizures are partial or generalized (O'Leary *et al.*, 1983). The performance of children with secondarily generalized seizures is worse than those with simple and complex partial seizures (O'Leary *et al.*, 1983; Collins, 1951; Keith *et al.*, 1955; Rodin *et al.*, 1986; Rugland, 1990b). Deficits are related somewhat to the focus location. The characteristics of interictal epileptiform discharges and maturation or disturbance of the EEG background determine the functional level of the child. EEG discharges during sleep can have deleterious effects on memory, language, cognitive functioning, and mood during the wake state (Renier, 1998).

School-age onset

Children with onset of seizures after five years of age typically display behavior problems more often than cognitive deficits (Hermann *et al.*, 1980). Late onset of protracted seizures causes less deterioration of intellectual ability than early onset. Children with onset of seizures before ten years of age show a 12% chance of deterioration; the later the onset of epilepsy is, the lesser the resulting impairment of abilities (Rennick *et al.*, 1969).

Frequency

The degree of seizure control may be a factor in cognitive outcome (Keith *et al.*, 1955; Glaser, 1967; Bagley, 1971; Sillanpaa, 1973; Dikmen & Matthews, 1977; Farwell *et al.*, 1980; Dam, 1990). An inverse proportionality may exist between the seizure frequency and intellectual level, especially with symptomatic epilepsy (Keating, 1960; Keith *et al.*, 1955; Scott *et al.*, 1967; Tarter, 1971; Whitehouse, 1971; Tarter, 1971; Holdsworth & Whitmore, 1974; Dikmen *et al.*, 1975; Seidenberg *et al.*, 1981; Camfield *et al.*, 1982; Dikmen, 1980; Brown & Reynolds, 1981). Many children having at least one seizure a month are slowed educationally and/or have disordered behavior (Holdsworth & Whitmore, 1974).

Memory may be less affected (Rausch, *et al.*, 1978). Seizure frequency and intractability relate to specific intellectual and memory impairments related to the side of the discharges (Powell *et al.*, 1975; Reynolds, 1985; Binnie *et al.*, 1990; Breier *et al.*, 1999). A consistent significant relationship exists between surface EEG recordings and performance. The amount of depth-spike activity correlates negatively with measures of intelligence. Patients with lateralized temporal lobe discharges tend to have higher memory scores relative to intelligence scores (Rausch *et al.*, 1978).

Repeated generalized tonic–clonic seizures over years, especially if associated with status, are associated with decreased functioning levels and intellectual performances, with mental dulling (Halstead, 1957; Wilkus & Dodrill, 1976; Camfield *et al.*, 1984; Dodrill, 1986). If the incidence of GTCs is less than a total of ten, then the incidence of retardation is 9%; when the incidence is greater than 1000, the incidence of retardation is 54%. There are no IQ differences with frequent absence attacks (Halstead, 1957; Dikmen, 1980). A similar trend with an even higher incidence of retardation is seen with frequent CPE. There is a reduced verbal IQ, memory problems, and academic failure, particularly if the seizures are symptomatic (Powell *et al.*, 1975; Rausch *et al.*, 1978; Dikmen, 1980; Ounsted *et al.*, 1966; Binnie *et al.*, 1990; Dam, 1990).

Children who have seizures in clusters, with seizure-free periods in between, have a higher intelligence and are better in certain academic skills (reading comprehension and arithmetic), suggesting that there may be a protective effect of more prolonged "rest" from seizures, allowing some recovery, that translates into higher functioning (Smith *et al.*, 2002).

Time of occurrence

Daytime seizures have direct effects on information possessing, i.e. alertness, short-term learning, and abstraction (Brittain, 1980; Dodrill, 1986; Renier, 1987). Postictal effects on learning may be overlooked and thus hard to accept (Aldenkamp *et al.*, 1990). Prolonged seizure discharges include non-convulsive status epilepticus during wakefulness and status epilepticus during slow-wave sleep, which may be associated with cognitive regression. Nocturnal seizures may have detrimental effects on language functions and memory (Renier, 1987). Some children with epilepsy might have a subtle disorder of arousal mechanisms in sleep, possibly associated with impaired daytime performance (Stores, 1990). Such sleep-related disturbances are associated with complaints of daytime lethargy and behavior disorders (Zaiwalla, 1989).

Duration

Deterioration of intellectual abilities appears to be associated with the duration of the disease (Farwell *et al.*, 1984; Rugland, 1990b; Smith *et al.*, 2002). After ten years of seizures, 24% of patients show signs of deterioration; after 25 years, 54% show some degree of deterioration (Tarter, 1971). People with symptomatic epilepsy may be the most prone to this effect (Dam, 1990). Prolonged epilepsy impairs neuropsychologic findings in long-term memory and short-term memory tasks (Ladavas *et al.*, 1979), but perhaps not in immediate recall (Macleod *et al.*, 1978).

The total number of seizures is related inversely to the IQ, except with absences. Frequent GTC over a long period of time leads to a deterioration of adaptive abilities and lowering of intelligence (Tarter, 1971; Dikmen, 1980). A lifetime number of tonic–clonic seizures above 100 shows worse functions. An increase in mental impairment and errors in language-related tasks is reported in those with longer duration of epilepsy, especially in people with GTC attacks (Tarter, 1971; Dikmen, 1980; Farwell *et al.*, 1984). Short- and long-term memory may also be affected (Koskiniemi *et al.*, 1974; Ladavas *et al.*, 1979). Cognitive dysfunction parallels a loss of brain neurons. Neuropathology studies of brains from epileptogenic patients with generalized seizures show a widespread loss of neurons in the hippocampus, which follows many generalized convulsions and a long duration of epilepsy (Margerison & Corsellis, 1966; Mouritzen, 1982; Babb *et al.*, 1984; Dam, 1990). Minor seizures and subclinical activity may damage the neurons in certain circumstances (Farwell *et al.*, 1985; Dam, 1990).

In children with CPE of onset before six years of age, problems are prominent, especially if the epilepsy has been present for more than ten years (Mirsky *et al.*, 1960). No IQ changes are seen (Farwell *et al.*, 1980), yet with left or bitemporal foci deficits in auditory short-term and sequential memory may be seen. Problems in arithmetic tests are noted. Attention problems may be seen. Hippocampal changes may occur with complex partial seizures (Farwell *et al.*, 1985; Dam, 1990). Longer duration of CPE in patients with Ammon's horn sclerosis is not associated with any decline in cognition (Oxbury *et al.*, 1998).

Intractability

Children with poorly controlled seizures are at high risk for learning, behavior, and emotional difficulties (Williams *et al.*, 1992). An intractable seizure disorder may lead to cognitive deterioration. Even a modest frequency of uncontrolled complex partial seizures over many years is associated with increased hippocampal atrophy and cognitive decline (O'Brien *et al.*, 1999; Jokeit & Ebner, 1999). With improved seizure control, there may be a slight rise in the IQ score, especially in performance scores (Brown & Reynolds, 1981; Seidenberg *et al.*, 1981).

Severity of attack

The severity of the attack, including the duration, intensity, degree of ictal involvement, and degree of postictal involvement, is important (Seidenberg *et al.*, 1981). Following a single seizure, recent memory depression is usually transient and may be limited to mere confusion, lasting up to 24 hours at most. A small defect in word fluency may be seen. With epileptic status or clustering, immediate memory is affected. Recent memory loss may be transient or permanent (Lindsay *et al.*, 1979). Permanent cerebral damage may occur from anoxia, lactic acidosis, and excessive action of neuro-excitatory neurotransmitters as a result of repetitive or prolonged seizures (Meador, 2002). When seizures are frequent or always in series, defects can be demonstrated by neuropathology examination (Dam, 1990).

Status

Status has a significant risk for mortality and morbidity in adults and very young children but much less so in older children. The effect of status is more deleterious than single seizures to intellectual functions (Dam, 1990; Dodrill, 1998). The outcome of status is worse among younger children if there are multifocal or generalized abnormalities. The younger child's brain is more vulnerable. Seizures are especially apt to be prolonged in children under 16 months of age (Chevrie & Aicardi, 1978; Sahin *et al.*, 2001). Resultant neuronal damage correlates with the duration of the seizure activity, and is proportional to the degree of severity, the severity and duration of the arterial hypotension, and the severity of the associated hypoglycemia, anoxia, lactic acidosis, and the effects of excessive excitatory neurotransmitters (Trieman, 2001). The parts of the brain most apt to be damaged are the hippocampus of the temporal lobe, the frontal and occipital lobes, the thalamus, and the Purkinje cells in the cerebellum (Stores, 1981).

Prolonged episodes of status may cause cognitive dysfunction, even in pediatric patients (DeLong & Heinz, 1997). About 34% of children show developmental deterioration and 36% develop epilepsy following status epilepticus. About 79% are abnormal before the status and 35% have no history of prior seizures. Risk factors for problems are a symptomatic, afebrile etiology (Wirrell & Barnard, 1999). Children over ten years of age in status have a far better outlook. Most children post-status continue to have seizures, and an ultimate seizure-free state is unlikely (unlike adults) (Sahin *et al.*, 2001).

Convulsive status

General convulsive status epilepticus may be followed by permanent cognitive deterioration, motor deterioration, and worsening of the epilepsy due to resultant cerebral damage (Binnie *et al.*, 1990).

Non-convulsive status

Non-convulsive status includes primarily absence status and complex partial status, although simple partial frontal, parietal, and occipital forms are also described (Ramsey, 1998). These cause children to perform with diminished responsiveness, as if they were retarded. Parents and teachers describe such children as "forgetful," "doing poorly at school," and "unresponsive," implying various degrees of cognitive and behavior disturbances (Stores, 1986; Stores, 1990). Problems in higher cortical functions, such as sustained attention, sequential planning, or various perceptual difficulties, e.g. spatial relationships, may be seen (Neidermeyer *et al.*, 1979; Nightengale & Welch, 1982; Matsuoka *et al.*, 1986). These problems resolve when recognized and treated. Chronic forms of non-convulsive status may lead to prolonged intellectual dysfunction (Binnie *et al.*, 1990).

Attitudes

Expectations are set to low, and the child is denied the usual encouragement to succeed (Stores, 1990). Teachers perceive epileptic children has having poor concentration and mental processing, as being less alert than their non-epileptic peers, and as being poor achievers, especially in math (Bennett-Levy & Stores, 1984).

Socioeconomic background

Epileptic children, especially boys, score lower than normal children, especially if the child comes from a lower socioeconomic environment (Mellor & Lowit, 1977). Early onset may lead to decreased school experience due to resultant absences from school (Dikmen *et al.*, 1975).

REFERENCES

Aicardi, J. (1988). Epileptic syndromes in childhood. *Epilepsia* **29** (suppl 3): 1–5.

Aldenkamp, A. P. (1983). Epilepsy and learning behavior. In *Advances in Epileptology, the XIVth Epilepsy International Symposium*, ed. M. Parsonage, R. H. E. Grant, A. G. Craig & A. A. Ward, Jr, pp. 221–8. New York: Raven Press.

Aldenkamp, A. P., Alpherts, W. C. J., Dekker, M. J. A., *et al.* (1990). Neuropsychological aspects of learning disabilities in epilepsy. *Epilepsia* **31** (suppl 4): 9–20.

Babb, T. I., Jann Brown, W., Pretorius, J., *et al.* (1984). Temporal lobe volumetric cell densities in temporal lobe epilepsy. *Epilepsia* **25**: 729–40.

Bagley, C. (1971). *The Social Psychology of the Child with Epilepsy*. London: Routledge and Kegan Paul.

Bennett-Levy, J. & Stores, G. (1984). The nature of cognitive dysfunction in schoolchildren with epilepsy. *Acta Neurol. Scand.* **69** (suppl 99): 79–82.

Binnie, C. D., Channon, S. & Marston, D. (1990). Learning disabilities in epilepsy: neurophysiological aspects. *Epilepsia* **31** (suppl 4): 2–8.

Bourgeois, B. F. D., Prensky, A. L., Palkes, H. S., *et al.* (1983). Intelligence in epeilspy: a prospective study in children. *Ann. Neurol.* **14**: 438–44.

Breier, J. I., Clark, A., Cass, J., *et al.* (1999). Profiles of cognitive performance in TLE patients with and without learning disability. *Epilepsia* **40** (suppl 7): 47–8

Brimer, R. W. & Barudin, S. L. (1981). Due process, right of education and the exceptional child: the road to equality in education. *Exceptional Peoples Quarterly* **39**: 197.

Brittain, H. (1980). Epilepsy and intellectual functions. In *Epilepsy and Behavior*, ed. B. M. Kulig & H. Meiinardi, pp. 2–13. Lisse: Swets & Zeitlinger.

Brown, W. S. & Reynolds, E. H. (1981). Cognitive impairments in epileptic patients. In *Epilepsy and Psychiatry*, ed. E. H. Reynolds & M. R. Trimble, pp. 147–63. New York: Churchill Livingstone.

Camfield, P. R., Gates, R., Ronen, G., *et al.* (1984). Comparison of cognitive ability, personality profile and school success in epileptic children with pure right versus left temporal lobe EEG foci. *Ann. Neurol.* **15**: 122–6.

Camfield, P. R., Ronen, G. N., Gates, R. D., *et al.* (1982). Temporal lobe peislpy in children: comparison of cognitive ability, personality profile and school success in children with pure right versus left EEG foci. *Ann. Neurol.* **12**: 206.

Carson, M. J. & Gilden, C. (1975). Treatment of minor motor seizures with clonazepam. *Dev. Med. Child. Neurol.* **17**: 306–10.

Chaudry, M. R. & Pond, D. (1961). Mental deterioration in epileptic children. *J. Neurol. Neurosurg. Psychiatry* **24**: 213–91.

Chevrie, J. J. & Aicardi, J. (1978). Convulsive disorders in the first year of life: neurological and mental outcome and mortality. *Epilepsia* **19**: 67–47.

Chevrie, J. J. & Aicardi, J. (1979). Convulsive disorders in the first year of life: persistence of epileptic seizures. *Epilepsia* **20**: 643–9.

Collins, A. L. (1951). Epileptic intelligence. *J. Consult. Psychol.* **15**: 393–9.

Collins, A. L. & Lennox, W. G. (1947). The intelligence of 300 private epileptic patients. *Res. Publ. Assoc. Res. Nerv. Ment. Dis.* **26**: 586–603.

Dam, M. (1990). Children with epilepsy: the effect of seizures, syndromes and etiological factors on cognitive functioning. *Epilepsia* **31** (suppl 4): 26–9.

DeLong, G. R. & Heinz, E. R. (1997). The clinical syndrome of early-life bilateral hippocampal sclerosis. *Ann. Neurol.* **42**: 11–17.

Dennerll, R. D. (1964). Cognitive deficits and lateral brain dysfunction in temporal lobe epilepsy. *Epilepsia* **5**: 177–91.

Deonna, T. (1999). Developmental consequences of epilepsies in infancies. In *Childhood Epilepsies and Brain Development*, ed. A. Nehlig, J. Motte, S. L. Moshe & P. Plouin, pp. 113–22. London: John Libbey.

Dikmen, S. (1980). Neuropsychological aspects of epilepsy. *In A Multidisciplinary Handbook of Epilepsy*, ed. B. P. Hermann, pp. 236–73. Springfield, IL: Chas. C. Thomas.

Dikmen, S., Matthews, C. G. & Harley J. P. (1975). The effect of early versus late onset of major motor epilepsy upon cognitive-intellectual performance. *Epilepsia* **16**: 73–81.

Dikmen, S. & Matthews, C. G. (1977). Effect of major motor seizure frequency upon cognitive-intellectual functions in adults. *Epilepsia* **18**: 21–9.

Dikmen, S. & Reitan, R. M. (1978). Neuropsychological performance in posttraumatic epilepsy. *Epilepsia* **19**: 177–83.

Dodrill, C. B. (1975). Diphenylhydantoin serum levels, toxicity and neuropsychological performance in patients with epilepsy. *Epilepsia* **15**: 593–600.

Dodrill, C. B. (1986). Correlates of generalized tonic-clonic seizures with intellectual, neuro-psychological, emotional and social functioning in patients with epilepsy. *Epilepsia* **27**: 399–411.

Dodrill C. B. (1998). The effects of seizures and various AEDs on cognition in cognitive organization of the brain. Presented at the American Epilepsy Society Conference, San Diego, CA.

Ellenberg, J. H., Hirtz, D. G. & Nelson, K. B. (1984). Age at onset of seizures in young children. *Ann. Neurol.* **15**: 127–34.

Farwell, J. R., Dodrill, C. B. & Batzel, L. W. (1984). Neuropsychological function in children with epilepsy. *Epilepsia* **25**: 646.

Farwell, J. R., Dodrill, B. B. & Batzel, L. W. (1985). Neuropsychological abilities of children with epilepsy. *Epilepsia* **26**: 395–400.

Farwell, J, Dodrill, C., Tempkins, N. & Wilkus, R. (1980). Intellectual function in children with complex partial seizures. *Ann. Neurol.* **8**: 229–30.

Fitzhugh, K. B., Fitzhugh, L. C. & Reitan, R. M. (1961). Psychological deficits in relation to acuteness of brain dysfunction. *J. Consult. Psychol.* **25**: 61–6.

Ford, C. A., Gibson, P. & Dreifuss, F. E. (1983). Psychosocial considerations childhood epilepsy. In *Pediatric Epileptology*, ed. F. Dreifuss, pp. 277–95. Boston, MA: John Wright PSG Inc.

Glaser, G. J. (1967). Limbic epilepsy in childhood. *J. Nerv. Ment. Dis.* **144**: 391–7.

Glowinski, H. (1973). Cognitive deficits in temporal lobe epilepsy. *J. Nerv. Ment. Dis.* **157**: 129–37.

Gulgonen, S., Demirbilek, V., Kormaz, B., *et al.* (2000). Neuropsychological functions in idiopathic occipital lobe epilepsy. *Epilepsia* **41**: 405–11.

Halstead, H. (1957). Abilities and behavior of epileptic children. *J. Ment. Sci.* **103**: 28–47.

Heijbel, J. & Behman, M. (1975). Benign epilepsy of children with centrotemporal EEG foci: intelligence, behavior and school adjustment. *Epilepsia* **16**: 679–87.

Henricksen, O. (1990). Education and epilepsy: assessment and remediation. *Epilepsia* **31** (suppl 4): 21–5.

Hermann, B. P., Schwartz, M. S., Karnes, W. E., *et al.* (1980). Psychopathology in epilepsy: relationship to seizure type and age of onset. *Epilepsia* **21**: 15–23.

Holdsworth, L. & Whitmore, K. (1974). A study of children with epilepsy attending ordinary schools, I: their seizure patterns, progress and behavior in schools. *Dev. Med. Child. Neurol.* **16**: 746–58.

Holmes, G. L. (2001). Pathogenesis of learning disabilities in epilepsy. In *Epilepsy and Learning Disabilities*, ed. G. F. Ayala, M. Elia, C. M. Cornaggia & M. M. Trimble. *Epilepsia* **42** (suppl 1): 13–18.

Jokeit, H. & Ebner, A. (1999). Long term effects of refractory temporal lobe epilepsy on cognitive abilities: a cross sectional study. *J. Neurol. Neurosurg. Psychiatry* **76**: 44–50.

Keating, L. E. (1960). A review of the literature on the relationship of epilepsy and intelligence in school children. *J. Ment. Sci.* **105**: 1042–59.

Keith, H. M., Ewert, J. C., Green, M. W. & Gage, R. P. (1955). Mental status of children with convulsive disorders. *Neurology* **5**: 287–92.

Klove, H. (1980). Neuropsychological consequences of epilepsy. *Epilepsia* **21**: 189–94.

Klove, H. & Matthews, C. G. (1967). Differential psychological performance in major motor, psychomotor and mixed seizure classification of known and unknown etiology. *Epilepsia* **8**: 117–28.

Klove, H. & Matthews, C. G. (1974). Neuropsycholgoical studies of patients with epilepsy. In *Clincial Neuropsychology: Current Status and Applications*, ed. R. M. Reitan & L. A. Davidson, pp. 237–66. Washington, DC: VH Winston & Sons.

Klove, H. & White, P. T. (1961). The relationships of degree of electroencephalographic abnormality to the distribution of Wechlser Bellevue scores. *Neurology* **13**: 423–30.

Knight, E. S., Oxbury, J. M., Middleton, J. A., *et al.* (1998). Cognitive function after temporal lobe epilepsy surgery (TLES) for dysembryoplastic neuroepithelial tumor (DNET) in children aged <6 years. 3rd European Congress of Epileptology. *Epilepsia* **39** (suppl 2): 119.

Koskiniemi, M., Donner, M., Majouri, H., *et al.* (1974). Progressive myoclonus epilepsy. *Acta Neurol. Scand.* **50**: 307–32.

Kurokawa, T., Goya N., Fukuyama, Y., *et al.* (1980). West syndrome and Lennox Gastaut syndrome: a survey of natural history. *Pediatrics* **65**: 81–8.

Ladavas, E., Umnila, C. & Provincialli, I. (1979). Hemisphere dependent cognitve performance in epileptic patients. *Epilepsia* **20**: 4939–502.

Lennox, W., McBride, M. & Potter, G. (1946). The higher education of epileptics. *Epilepsia* **3**: 182–97.

Lindsay, J., Ounsted, C. & Richards, P. (1979). Long-term outcome in children with temproal lobe seizures. No 1: social outcome and childhood factors. *Dev. Med. Child. Neurol.* **21**: 285–98.

Margerison, J. H. & Corsellis, J. A. N. (1966). Epilepsy and the temporal lobes. *Brain* **89**: 499–530.

Matsumoto, A., Watanabe, K., Siguura, M., *et al.* (1983). Long-term prognosis of convulsive disorders in the first year of life: mental and physical development and seizure persistence. *Epilepsia* **24**: 321–9.

Matsuoka, H., Okuma, T., Oemo, T., *et al.* (1986). Impairment of parietal cortical functions associated with episodic prolonged spike-and-wave discharge. *Epilepsia* **27**: 432–6.

Matthews, C. G. & Klove, H. (1967). Differential pscyholgoical perfromacnes in major motor, psychomotor, and mixed seizure classifcation of known and unknown etiology. *Epilepsia* **8**: 117–28.

McLaurin, R. L. (1973). Epilepsy and contact sports. *JAMA* **225**: 285–7.

Meador, K. J. (2002). Cognitive outcomes and predictive factors in epilepsy. *Neurology* **58** (suppl 5): 21–8.

Mellor, D. H. & Lowit, I. (1977). Study of intellectual function in children with epilepsy attending ordinary schools. In *Epilepsy: Eighth International Symposium*, ed. J. K. Penry, pp. 291–4. New York: Raven Press.

Milner, B. (1975). Psychological aspects of focal epilepsy and its neurosurgical management. In *Advances in Epilepsy*, ed. D. P. Purpura, J. R. Penry & R. D. Walter, Vol. 8, pp. 299–332. New York: Raven Press.

Mirsky, A. F., Primac, D. W., Marsan, C. A., *et al.* (1960). A comparison of the psychological test performance of patients with focal and nonfocal epilepsy. *Dev. Exp. Neurol.* **2**: 75–89.

Mouritzen, D. A. (1982). Hippocampal neuron loss in epilepsy and after experimental seizures. *Acta Neurol. Scand.* **66**: 601–42.

Neidermeyer, E., Fineyne, F., Riley, T., *et al.* (1979). Absence status (petit mal status) with focal characteristics. *Arch. Neurol.* **36**: 417–21.

Nightengale, S. & Welch, J. L. (1982). Psychometric assessment in absence status. *Arch. Neurol.* **39**: 516–19.

O'Brien, T. J., So, E. L., Meyer, F. B., *et al.* (1999). Progressive hippocampal atrophy in chronic intractable temporal lobe epilepsy. *Ann. Neurol.* **45**: 526–9.

O'Leary, D. S., Lovell, M. R., Sackellars, J. C., *et al.* (1983). Effects of age of onset of partial and generalized seizures on neuropsychological performance in children. *J. Nerve. Ment. Dis.* **171**: 624–9.

O'Leary, D. S., Seidenberg, M., Berrent, S., *et al.* (1981). Effects of age of onset of tonic-clonic seizures on neuropsychological performance in children. *Epilepsia* **22**: 197–204.

Ounsted, C., Lindsay, J. & Norman, R. (1966). Intelligence: biological factors in temporal lobe epilepsy. In *Clinics in Developmental Medicine*, Vol. 22, pp. 62–71 London: Heinemann.

Oxbury, S. M., Cambell, L., Baxendale, S. A., *et al.* (1998). Cognitive function in relation to duration of temporal lobe epilepsy (TLE) due to Ammon's horn sclerosis. 3rd European Congress of Epileptology. *Epilepsia* **39** (suppl 2): 120.

Powell, G. E., Polkey, C. E. & McMillan, T. (1975). The new Maudsley series of temporal lobectomy. I: short-term cognitive effects. *Br. J. Clin. Psychol.* **24**: 109–24.

Price, J. Kogan, K. L. & Tompkins, L. R. (1948). The prevalence and incidence of extramural epilepsy. In *Epilepsy: Psychiatric Aspects of Convulsive Disorders*, ed. P. M. Hoch & R. P. Knight, pp. 48–57. London: Heinemann.

Ramsey, E. (1998). Special populations. Cognitive concerns in adults and in the elderly. Presented at the American Epilepsy Society Conference, San Diego, CA.

Rausch, R. (1981). Lateralization of temporal lobe dysfunction and verbal encoding. *Brain Lang.* **12**: 92–100.

Rausch, R., Lieb, U. P. & Crandall, P. A. S. (1978). Neuropsychologic correlates of depth spike activity in epileptic patients. *Arch. Neurol.* **35**: 699–705.

Reitan R. S. (1974). Psychological testing of epileptic patients. In *Handbook of Neurology*, ed. O. Magnus & A. M. Lorentz, Vol. 15, pp. 559–75. Amsterdam: North Holland.

Renier, W. O. (1987). Restrictive factors in the education of children with epilepsy from a medical point of view. In *Education and Epilepsy 1987*, ed. A. P. Aldenkamp, W. C. J. Alpherts, H. Meinardi & G. Stores, pp. 3–14. Lisse: Swets & Zeitlinger.

Renier, W. O. (1998). Neuropsychological correlates of EEG changes in early childhood epilepsies. 3rd European Congress of Epileptology. *Epilepsia* **39** (suppl 2). 92.

Rennick, P. M., Perez-Borja, C. & Rodin, E. (1969). Transient mental deficits associated with recurrent prolonged epileptic clouded state. *Epilepsia* **10**: 397–405.

Reynolds, E. H. (1985). Antiepileptic drugs and psychopathology. In *The Psychopharmacology of Epilepsy*, ed. M. R. Trimble, pp. 49–65. Chichester, UK: John Wiley & Sons.

Rodin, E. A., Rennick, P., Dennerill, R., *et al.* (1972). Vocational and educational problems of epileptic patients. *Epilepsia* **13**: 149–60.

Rodin, E. A., Schmaltz, S. & Twitty, G. (1986). Intellectual functions of patients with childhood-onset epilepsy. *Dev. Med. Child Neurol.* **28**: 25–33.

Rugland, A. L. (1990a). Subclinical epileptogenic activity. In *Pediatric Epilepsy*, ed. M. Sillarpaa, S. I. Johnanessen, G. Blennow & M. Dam, pp. 217–23. London: Wrightson Biomedical.

Rugland, A. L. (1990b). Neuropsychological assessment of cognitive functioning in children with epilepsy. *Epilepsia* **31** (suppl 4): 41–4.

Rutter, M., Graham, P. & Yule, W. (1970). A neuropsychiatric study in childhood. *Clin. Dev. Med.* 35/36. London: Spastics Society & Heinemann.

Sahin, M., Menache, C. C., Holmes, G. L., *et al.* (2001) Outcomes of severe refractory status epilepticus in children. *Epilepsia* **42**: 1461–7.

Scarpa, P. & Carassini, B. (1982). Partial epilepsy in childhood; clinical and EEG study of 261 cases. *Epilepsia* **23**: 333–41.

Scott, D. F., Moffett, A., Matthews, A., *et al.* (1967). The effect of epileptic discharges on learning and memory in patients. *Epilepsia* **8**: 188–94.

Seidenberg, M., O'Leary, D. S. Berent, S., *et al.* (1981). Changes in seizure frequency and test-retest scores on the Wechlser Adult Intelligence Scale. *Epilepsia* **22**: 75–83.

Sherwin, I. & Efron, R. (1980). Temporal ordering deficits following anterior temporal lobectomy. *Brain Lang.* **11**: 195–203.

Sillanpaa, M. (1973). Medico-social prognosis of children with epilepsy: epidemiology study and analysis of 245 patients. *Acta Paediatr. Scand. Suppl.* **237**: 3–104.

Smith, M. L., Elliott, I. M. & Lach, L. (2002). Cognitve skills in children with intractable epilepsy: comaprison of sursgical and nonsurgical candidates. *Epilepsia* **46**: 621–7.

Stores, G. (1981). Problems of learning and behavior in children with epilepsy. In *Epilepsy and Psychiatry*, ed. E.H. Reynolds & M. R. Trimble, pp. 33–48. New York: Churchill Livingstone.

Stores, G. (1986). Nonconvulsive status epilepticus in children. In *Recent Advances in Epilepsy*, ed. T. A. Pedley & B. S. Meldrum, pp. 295–310. Edinburgh: Churchill Livingstone.

Stores, G. (1990). Electroencephalographic parameters in assessing the cognitive function of children with epilepsy. *Epilepsia* **31** (suppl 4): 45–9.

Stores, G. & Hart, J. (1976). Reading skills of children with generalized or focal epilepsy attending ordinary school. *Dev. Med. Child Neurol.* **18**: 705–16.

Sullivan, E. G. & Gahagan, L. (1935). Intelligence of epileptic children. *Genet. Psychol. Monogr.* **17**: 314–74.

Sztriha, L., Gururaj, A. K., Bener, A., *et al.* (2002). Temporal lobe epilepsy in children: Etiology in a cohort with new-onset seizures. *Epilepsia* **43**: 75–80.

Tarter, R. E. (1971). Intellectual and adaptive functioning in epilepsy: a review of fifty years of research. *Dis. Nerv. Syst.* **33**: 763–70.

Trieman, D. M. (2001). Status epilepticus. In *The Treatment of Epilepsy: Principles and Practice*, ed. E. Wyllie, pp. 681–97. Philadelphia: Lippincott Williams & Wilkins.

Tuxhorn, I., Pieper, T. & Moch, A. (1998). General cognitive function in children with temporal lobe epilepsy. 3rd European Congress of Epileptology. *Epilepsia* **39** (suppl 2): 129.

Vargha-Kahdem, F. (2001). Generalized versus selective cognitive impairments resulting from brain damage sustained in childhood. In *Epilepsia and Learning Disabilities*, ed. G. F. Ayala, M. Elia, C. M. Cornaggia & M. M. Trimble. *Epilepsia* **42**: 37–40.

Wasterlain, C. G., Thompson, K. W., Kornblum, H., *et al.* (1999). Long-term effects of recurrent seizures on the developing brain. In *Childhood Epilepsies and Brain Development*, ed. A. Nehlig, J. Motte, S. L. Moshe & P. Plouin, pp. 237–65. London: John Libbey.

Waxman, S. G. & Geschwind, N. (1973). The interictal behavior syndrome of temporal lobe epilepsy. *Arch. Gen. Psychiatry* **32**: 1580–86.

Whitehouse, D. (1971). Psychological and neurological correlates of seizure disorders. *Johns Hopkins Med. J.* **129**: 36–42.

Whitehouse, D. (1976). Behavior and learning problems in epileptic children. *Behav. Neuropsychiatry* **7**: 23–9.

Wiberg, M., Blennow, G. & Polski, B. (1987). Epilepsy in the adolescence. Implications for the development of the personality. *Epilepsia* **28**: 542–76.

Wilkus, R. J. & Dodrill, C. B. (1976). Neuropsychological correlates of the electroencephalograph in epileptics. I: topographic distribution and average rate of epileptiform activity. *Epilepsia* **17**: 89–100.

Williams, J., Sharp, G. B. & Griebel, M. I. (1992). Neuropsychological functioning in clinically referred children with epilepsy. *Epilepsia* **33** (suppl 3): 17.

Wirrell, E. & Barnard, C. (1999). Status epilepticus in children: developmental deterioration and exacerbation of epilepsy. 23rd International Epilepsy Congress. *Epilepsia* **40** (suppl 2): 69.

Zaiwalla, Z. (1989). Sleep abnormalities in children with epilepsy. *Electroencephalogr. Clin. Neurophysiol.* **72**: 29.

Zimmerman, F. T. Burgemeister, B.B. & Putnam, T. J. (1951). Intellectual and emotional makeup of the epileptic. *Arch. Neurol. Psychiatry* **65**: 545–56.

17

Transient cognitive impairments of epilepsy

Epilepsy may interfere with learning in at least six ways. Direct disruption of ongoing processing by epileptiform activity may interfere with the attending to, processing of, storing of, and retrieving incoming information, which may be task-specific. Discharges temporally distant from the learning experience may disrupt consolidation processes by which information is encoded, stored, and retrieved. Permanent damage to neural tissue reduces its ability to react adaptively to new information. In the developing brain, this may be compensated for by a degree of plasticity. In the mature brain, damage may produce cognitive loss. Antiepileptic drugs may alter neural functioning related to learning processes. Frequent chronic discharges occurring during sleep may result in direct or indirect disruption of brain functions (Binnie *et al.*, 1990). Subclinical epileptiform discharges in the EEG can adversely affect the child's performance (Henricksen, 1990). Subtle seizures are generally related to severe and global effects on cognitive functions, the most critical effects being on mentally demanding tasks (Aldenkamp *et al.*, 1998).

In simultaneous EEG recording and intellectual testing, unilateral left-sided epileptic adults often show no responses when a discharge is occurred during testing (Kooi & Hovey, 1956). When a child has active seizures and related learning problems emerge, it is easy to envision the seizure discharges short-circuiting vital learning pathways. However, children have infrequent seizures or even have their seizures controlled but still have the learning disabilities and are found to continue to have frequent epileptiform discharges on the EEG. Is there a relationship?

Important factors may include the degree of abnormality (Collins, 1951), the slowness of slow-spike wave and slow-wave discharges, and the background slowing (Tarter, 1971), even more than the focality of the discharge (Rodin *et al.*, 1972).

History

Observations from electroconvulsive shock therapy (ECT), electrocortical stimulation, and psychologic testing during EEG recording have contributed to the evolving concepts about transient cognitive impairments.

Electroconvulsive shock therapy

ECT produces an initial generalized paroxysm of electrical activity followed by depression of neural firing. The shock is not damaging, so changes must be due to the discharge itself (Duncan, 1949; McGaugh & Petrinovich, 1966). There is impairment of new learning immediately after ECT. The effect of unilateral ECT depends on the side stimulated. Verbal and auditory tasks are affected by dominant unilateral ECT, whereas non-verbal visual tasks are impaired by non-dominant unilateral ECT (Fink, 1979). Impairments of memory may last more than seven months after bilateral ECT (Squire *et al.*, 1981; Binnie *et al.*, 1990).

Electric brain stimulation

The effects of localized electrical brain stimulation resemble those of a temporary lesion or a focal seizure, with both excitatory and inhibitory responses. Deficits in memory and language follow responses to stimulation of particular neocortical sites (Ojemann, 1983). Memory problems follow deep bilateral limbic stimulation. Unimpaired perceptual discriminations during similar stimulation can still be made (Binnie *et al.*, 1990).

Simultaneous electroencephalographic intellectual testing

In simultaneous EEG intellectual testing, it is noted that impairments due to an epileptiform discharge may occur even when no clinical features are noted. Cognitive processes may be impaired or suspended during subclinical cortical epileptic activity (Aarts *et al.*, 1984). Choice reaction time delays are proportional to the discharge frequency and duration (Binnie, 2001).

Patients may fail to respond to a stimulus presented during generalized spike-wave discharges. Their reaction times are increased on paced tests (Kooi & Hovey, 1956). Absence attacks may delay answering (Stores, 1971). Cognitive dysfunction in children with absence epilepsy are not necessarily confined to spike-wave bursts but may occur between them (Mirsky, 1989; Stores, 1990). Reaction times are prolonged with generalized spike-wave discharges more than with brief spike-wave bursts, but more prolonged with brief spike-wave bursts than with frontal spike-wave bursts. Observable changes are seen only when the burst is more than three seconds in duration (Binnie, 2001).

Higher mental processes such as problem solving may be impaired during subclinical focal discharges. A deviant, delayed, or distorted response, if any, may occur if a burst comes between the seizure and the responses. With complex partial epilepsy, momentary verbal confusions may impede answers about half the time when a subclinical discharge occurs. Following the stimulus question, "don't know" responses, requests for repetitions of questions, "zero-quality" answers, or non-responses may be noted as related to discharges. Unilateral left-sided or bilateral discharges often relate to non-responses. Some patients may be able to respond despite the discharge (Kooi & Hovey, 1956).

Interictal epileptiform discharges may disrupt adaptive responses or may disrupt the function itself, relating to abnormal performances in specific tests (Tarter, 1971; Rausch *et al.*, 1978). This phenomenon may wear off (Kooi & Hovey, 1956).

Transient cognitive impairments

Discharges can be divided into clinical activity accompanied by observable symptoms and "subclinical" activity. Cognitive impairment occurs with interictal or subclinical discharges, both generalized and focal (Binnie *et al.*, 1987; Binnie, 1988; Binnie *et al.*, 1991; Stores, 1987). Individual epileptiform EEG discharges accompanied by a momentary disruption of adaptive cerebral function have been called transitory cognitive impairments (TCIs) (Schwab, 1939; Aarts *et al.*, 1984; Kasteleün-Nolst Trenite *et al.*, 1988; Binnie *et al.*, 1990). The concept is paradoxical, for a discharge causing a change in cognition is arguably not a subclinical event but an ictal event (Binnie, 2001).

TCIs are more than simple inattention. They are both material-specific and site-specific. Lateralized discharges are more likely to be accompanied by impairments of lateralized related psychological function. Left-sided discharges are often associated with errors in verbal tasks, while right-sided discharges are associated with visuospatial relationships. Specific tasks may activate or suppress focal discharges over those brain regions related to a specific cognitive activity. Lateralized discharges, whether spontaneous or induced by electrical brain stimulation, may be accompanied by an enhancement of functions located in the contralateral hemisphere. Short-term memory tests show impairment mainly when a discharge occurs during presentation of the material to be memorized but not during recall. Thus, TCIs may contribute to abnormal psychological test profiles (Binnie, 1999).

Clinical

When abnormal discharges are present in any part of the brain, cognitive functioning subserved by that area might be impaired temporarily. One cause of academic problems in children with epilepsy, especially in underachievers, may be ongoing subclinical EEG discharges (Kasteeijn-Nolste Trenite *et al.*, 1988; Siebelink *et al.*, 1988; Rugland, 1990a). Academic problems are seen as specific deficiencies rather than as generalized cognitive dysfunctions. Such difficulties may relate to disturbances in one of the various cognitive processes required for learning, such as perception, representation, sustained attention, strategy, or retrieval. Subclinical discharges decrease the capacity to process information with cognitive tasks (Tizard & Margerison, 1963a; Tizard & Margerison, 1963b; Hutt & Fairweather, 1975).

Significant correlation exists between the frequency of subclinical discharges and psychosocial difficulties, such as attention deficits, behavior disturbances, memory problems, language impairments, and dyslexia, and with cognitive impairments (Binnie *et al.*, 1987; Binnie, 1993; Binnie, 2001).

TCI occurs in up to 50% of patients during generalized or focal discharges. In children, these can lead to learning and academic problems. Generalized discharges disturb spatial tasks more readily, whereas verbal tasks are impaired only in one-third of occurrences. When spike-wave discharges occur within a few seconds preceding the presentation of a critical stimulus, both verbal and spatial task impairments have been noted. Discharges occurring during the stimulus presentation have the greatest effect on cognitive performance, suggesting that the stage of stimulus recognition is the most sensitive to discharges. Focal discharges have associated effects on spatial and verbal tasks (Aarts *et al.*, 1984; Binnie *et al.*, 1987; Kasteleijn Nolst-Trenite *et al.*, 1990). Even the benign focal epilepsies of childhood have been associated with TCIs and thus can cause learning deficits (Schwab, 1939).

Long-term video-electroencephalographic monitoring

The frequency of epileptic discharges, as well as manifest seizures, is influenced by the time of day, stress, activity, wakefulness, drowsiness or sleep, testing, and school activities. An ordinary 20-minute EEG recording does not necessarily give a representative picture of the situation. Long-term recordings, sometimes with video monitoring and telemetry, especially if combined with a computerized neuropsychological battery, make it possible to demonstrate the relationships between epileptic discharges and various activities, and to evaluate whether such discharges influence performance (Stores, 1987; Binnie, 1988). Functional testing is required because the amount of epileptic activity on a standard EEG, where the patient is lying down with their eyes closed, does not necessarily reflect the situation at school (Henricksen, 1990).

Video-EEG monitoring demonstrates that many short discharges are accompanied by subtle, previously unrecognized events. These may be especially difficult to detect if they fall within the patient's expected behavior repertoire. Even more subtle cognitive changes may not be recognizable by simple behavior observations but can be detected by relating changes in performance of continuous psychological tasks to epileptiform events during concurrent EEG monitoring (Aarts *et al.*, 1984; Rugland *et al.*, 1987).

In learning, information is rehearsed, elaborated, and associated through integration with previously stored knowledge, which extends over time beyond the initial processing. Interictal discharges may interfere with the consolidation process, as does ECT. Abnormalities of function in the intervals between the discharges can impair this further. The degree of generalization of a dysrhythmia may globally disrupt ongoing learning processes (Binnie *et al.*, 1990) and thus be more impacting than the actual epileptiform EEG abnormalities (Dodrill & Wilkus, 1978).

Epileptic discharges occurring in the intervals between overt seizures may be accompanied by subtle alterations in psychological or motor function. Some children without any history to suggest epilepsy may display difficulties in performing learning tasks. When an EEG is obtained, spike-wave discharges may emerge when concentration is required. Valoproate may help such children. Video-EEG studies can verify such cases (Binnie, 2001).

Modifiers

The extent of cognitive impairment during brief epileptiform bursts may vary with the number of spike components, the involvement of frontal-central regions (Mirsky, 1969), and especially the complexity of the task involving central cognitive processing (Aldenkamp *et al.*, 1990).

Generalized versus focal discharges

Performance suppresses discharges. Simple repetitive tasks may not be susceptible to TCIs. Tasks requiring concentration and persistence may be more vulnerable. In computer game testing synchronizing stimulus presentation to bursts, a subject performs twice as well when no discharge occurs as when discharges occur (Binnie, 2001). A variety of psychologic testing, including computerized games, have been utilized to evaluate patients with seizures, synchronizing the tests to epileptiform discharges, both focal and generalized (Aarts *et al.*, 1984).

Generalized spike-wave bursts

Subclinical generalized spike-wave discharges are often accompanied by TCIs, with simultaneous decline in cognitive functions (Schwab, 1939; Kooi & Hovey, 1957; Binnie, 1979). TCIs are brought out by difficult tasks and by generalized regular spike-wave bursts of duration greater than three seconds and also with even briefer discharges impairing more difficult task (Aarts *et al.*, 1984; Rugland *et al.*, 1987; Binnie *et al.*, 1990; Cornaggia & Gobbi, 2001). In children, pretest stress may increase the spike-wave discharge frequency, while post-test inactivation may decrease it. Individuals with pattern or photic sensitive generalized spike-wave discharges may show TCIs in tests such as object assembly (Brinciotti *et al.*, 1991).

Visuomotor tracking performance is impaired with bursts of more than three seconds in duration, but it is impaired only minimally with shorter discharges (Opp *et al.*, 1992). Reaction time responses are absent or delayed. The impact varies from patient to patient. In some children, even a 1% occurrence may reduce mental functions, although the patient may not be aware of this (Licht & Jacobsen, 1999). Verbal and particularly spatial functions may be disturbed with generalized discharges (Binnie, 2001).

The frequency of discharges is associated only slightly with seizure frequency, antiepileptic drug effects, or prognosis (Binnie, 2001). Testing is an alerting stimulation and thus tends to decrease discharge frequency unless the test is prolonged enough to become boring or unless it is performed when the child is under stress or is hypoglycemic. The discharge frequency relates to impairment occurrence. The surface EEG may reflect less than the depth EEG.

The content and complexity of the task being evaluated are significant. Simple tasks are less impacted than higher cortical functions. A child can easily complete a simple task during a burst of spike-wave discharges but will show increasing difficulty as the task becomes more demanding or the pace of work increases (Hutt *et al.*, 1977). Complex tasks involving central processing are more apt to be disrupted than those involving simple motor or sensory functions. Occurrence during the registration phase is the most disruptive (Mirsky & Van Buren, 1965).

Focal spikes

TCIs can produce both global inattention and specific memories impairments (Cornaggia & Gobbi, 2001). This is not simply a consequence of global inattention, since brief focal discharges exhibit some specificity (Binnie *et al.*, 1990). When abnormal discharges are present in any part of the brain, cognitive functioning subserved by that area might be impaired temporarily, producing restricted and specific deficits (Aarts *et al.*, 1984; Rugland *et al.*, 1987). A task may either suppress or activate the discharge. Activation may occur with certain tasks. Similar findings are seen regarding the type of deficit in relation to the side of discharge in 36% of children (Kasteleijn-Nolst Trenite *et al.*, 1990). In children with epilepsy, one cause of academic problems, especially in underachievers, may be ongoing subclinical EEG discharges (Kasteleijn-Nolste Trenite *et al.*, 1988; Siebelink *et al.*, 1988; Rugland, 1990a).

Focal spike-wave-induced cortical dysfunction may be clinically relevant for children with both frequent interictal discharges and cognitive problems. Focal interictal spikes in the posterior head regions transiently impair cortical processing, as manifested by delayed reaction times and increased non-perception and misperception of stimuli. Reactions time are prolonged significantly with large waves, regardless of the spike size. Reaction times are prolonged significantly only if the end of the slow wave overlaps the stimulus. The following slow wave (surround hyperpolarization) transiently disrupts aspects of cortical functioning in addition to whatever effect the spike itself may have (Shewmon & Erwin, 1988a; Shewmon & Erwin, 1988b). Tracking discharge rate doubles with focal discharges (Opp *et al.*, 1992).

Spiky EEG transients are not limited only to people with epilepsy (Binnie, 2001). The question is whether those individuals without any history of seizures who have learning problems and on EEG are found to have a spike discharge should be placed on medication? In some people, suppression of discharges by antiepileptic drugs has demonstrated improved psychological functioning (Binnie *et al.*, 1990).

Benign Rolandic spikes

Benign central-temporal epilepsy has been found to be associated with cognitive impairments, even in people without clinical seizures. Written efforts may tail off with the discharges. The error rate may increase. Educational problems are reported. Rarely, the performance of the opposite hemisphere is enhanced during the discharge. Those without seizures usually have only unilateral spikes. Problems found include phonological disorders, learning difficulties, attention problems, hyperactivity, and emotional instability. The verbal IQ may be depressed. Thus, both clinical and subclinical epileptiform activity in the central area may result in dominant hemispheric dysfunction. Such cognitive and behavioral problems can precede the development of epileptic activity and/or clinical seizures, or vice versa (Turkdogan *et al.*, 1999).

Laterality

Detected transient cognitive impairments produced by isolated focal spikes may affect performance in spatial or verbal tasks, depending on whether the discharge is right or left-sided, respectively (Aarts *et al.*, 1984; Rugland *et al.*, 1987). Lateralized discharges increase the reaction time when stimulus presentations or responses involve the affected hemisphere (Shewmon & Erwin, 1988; Binnie *et al.*, 1990). With spike-wave bursts, the effect is seen during the stimulus but not before the stimulus or after the response (Binnie, 2001).

Sometimes, unilateral discharges are associated with enhanced performance of tasks on the contralateral hemisphere (Regard *et al.*, 1985). Cognitive effects of deep brain stimulation show enhanced function of one hemisphere when the contralateral mesial temporal structures are stimulated (Binnie, 2001).

Left hemisphere

The left hemisphere is more verbal, especially in regard to the response (Binnie, 2001). Verbal functions are impacted by left-sided discharges, producing errors on verbal tasks (Aarts *et al.*, 1984; Binnie *et al.*, 1987; Binnie *et al.*, 1990; Dodrill, 1998; Binnie, 2001; Cornaggia & Gobbi, 2001). In a majority of patients, verbal functions are impaired regardless of which side the seizures emanate from (Binnie, 2001). When a left-sided discharge occurs, left hemisphere performance deteriorates but right hemisphere performance may be enhanced. Performance of a non-verbal task is not affected significantly by a discharge in either hemisphere (Regard *et al.*, 1985). The error rate increases if the stimulus is presented in the midst of the discharge. If the discharges occur within two seconds before the stimulus, the degree of disruption is greater (Binnie *et al.*, 1987; Aarts *et al.*, 1984). Increased concentration on a task results in a decrease in the rate of epileptiform discharges (Hutt *et al.*, 1977).

Right hemisphere

Subclinical discharges in either hemisphere were once thought to not interfere significantly with the performance of non-verbal tasks, but such problems in performance have now been reported (Regard *et al.*, 1985; Binnie *et al.*, 1990). Right hemispheric discharges are more apt to impair non-verbal functions, i.e. visual-spatial tasks, than verbal functions (Aarts *et al.*, 1984; Binnie *et al.*, 1987; Binnie *et al.*, 1990; Binnie, 2001; Cornaggia & Gobbi, 2001).

Frequency

There may be a relationship between the frequency of seizures or subclinical epileptiform discharges and impairments of learning and memory. The amount of such activity may be diminished in epileptic patients during testing (Scott *et al.*, 1967). Learning difficulties in general as well as specific learning disabilities are seen in children with epilepsy, especially those with frequent interictal discharges (Binnie *et al.*, 1990). Children perform most poorly and have the most difficulties at times of higher discharge rates. Increased task difficulties lead to a greater discharge rate and further transient cognitive disruptions (Siebelink *et al.*, 1988; Binnie, 2001).

Abnormal psychological profiles increase with an increase in the amount of interictal epileptiform activities, being greater in generalized than focal seizures. More specific materials are related to focal discharges. The frequency of discharges is associated only slightly with the seizure frequency (Binnie, 2001).

Discharges may be increased or reduced by non-specific cognitive activity or may be affected by specific stimuli as in reflex epilepsies. During various psychological tests, generalized discharges may be suppressed, but there may be focal activation of mesial-temporal discharges, with some showing a marked increase in discharges during memory tasks (Kooi & Hovey, 1956; Aarts *et al.*, 1984; Altafullah & Halgren, 1988). Focal discharges have been elicited or suppressed by cognitive tasks challenging the corresponding brain region (Binnie, 2001). Sometimes, unilateral discharges are associated with enhanced performance of tasks on the contralateral hemisphere (Regard *et al.*, 1985), including deep brain stimulation to the contralateral mesial-temporal structures (Binnie, 2001).

Duration

Impairing seizure discharges may be transient, brief, or prolonged. Observed cognitive deficits depend primarily on the electrical activity of the epileptic focus. The epileptic focus does not always coincide with the topographic localization of an atrophic lesion (Ladavas *et al.*, 1979).

Transient discharges

Very brief discharges of less than three seconds in duration are seen in interictal EEG of many patients and are commonly thought to have very little effect on psychological functions, which is largely true for generalized discharges. Perception and reaction time impairments are associated even with focal spikes of less than one to two seconds' duration, which appears to undermine the traditional distinction between interictal and ictal events by influencing the patient's responses (Shewmon & Erwin, 1988a; Shewmon & Erwin, 1988b; Stores, 1990). All epileptiform discharges may disturb functioning to some extent if the test batteries are sufficiently sensitive (Henricksen, 1990).

Brief bursts

TCIs are demonstrated most readily by difficult tasks and during generalized regular spike-wave bursts lasting more than three seconds (Goode *et al.*, 1970), but they can also be found during briefer and even focal discharges. Factors that influence clinical significance include the extent to which the discharges are bilaterally symmetrical, well organized, and comprised of spike or polyspike-wave complexes (Mirsky, 1969). The longer the duration, the greater the psychological effects (Stores, 1990).

Prolonged and epileptic status

The other extreme from transient discharges is continuous or near-continuous epileptic activity lasting hours, days, weeks, or longer without prominent motor manifestation, the so-called "non-convulsive status epilepticus." This may be overlooked and some affected children simply written off as unresponsive or cognitively depressed. Occasionally, an adolescent with this condition may be thought to be psychotic (Stores, 1986; Stores, 1990).

Performance effects

The significance of TCI accompanying subclinical EEG discharges for everyday functioning is uncertain, but there is experimental evidence that subclinical discharges may be accompanied by disruption of educational skills in children (Binnie *et al.*, 1990).

Intelligence and learning

Learning disorders may be a consequence of TCIs, associated with focal and/or generalized specific epileptiform EEG discharges (Schwab, 1939; Kooi & Hovey, 1956;

Binnie, 1979). Impaired learning may occur especially in tasks that are sensitive to the effects of subclinical discharges (Binnie et al., 1987; Binnie, 1988; Aldenkamp et al., 1990). Transient changes in cognition or motor function are difficult to recognize. Adverse effects of TCIs on performance of formal intelligence tests and on performance of educational tasks have been demonstrated (Siebelink et al., 1988; Binnie, 2001).

Attention and alertness

TCIs can produce global inattention. It is possible that some children diagnosed as having ADHD or autism may be affected by undiagnosed manifestations of epilepsy. Undiagnosed severe epileptic conditions, such as some frontal lobe epilepsies with subcontinuous specific EEG activity, including rapid activity lasting between one and 1.5 seconds, have been found to be associated with the onset of severe behavioral disturbances (sometimes with psychotic symptoms) and schizophrenia or autism-like syndromes in both children and adults (Cornaggia & Gobbi, 2001).

Perception

Generalized bursts during a given stimulus, even when less than one second in duration, impair perception. A very active right temporal-occipital focus may be related to a specific deficit in visual-spatial performance. With antiepileptic drug-induced seizure control and a 70% reduction in EEG spike activity, visuomotor skills recover (Cornaggia & Gobbi, 2001).

Reaction time

Subclinical discharges impair reaction time performance in 61% of patients performing simple and choice reaction time tests, even when some discharges last only one second. Patients are more impaired on more complex tests (Mirsky & Van Buren, 1965; Aarts et al., 1984; Binnie et al., 1990; Rugland, 1990a).

Memory

TCIs can produce problems in specific memory functions (Cornaggia & Gobbi, 2001). The acquisition phase of memory appears to be especially vulnerable if these discharges occur (Binnie et al., 1987), apparently because it prevents the consolidation of acquired information (Binnie, 1988; Stores, 1987).

Effect on test-taking

TCIs may account for the IQ testing variability in children with epilepsy (Bourgeois et al., 1983; Rodin et al., 1986). TCIs may be associated with increased errors during administration of a neuropsychological battery and resultant abnormal test profiles. This may relate to educational problems (Kasteleijn-Nolst Trenite et al., 1988).

More patients show a reduction (45%) than an increase (16%) in epileptogenic activity during testing. The testing increases concentration and reduces epileptogenic activity in some patients, but the stress may increase activity in others. Significant impairment of performance during the discharges is seen in 61% of children in tests of simple or choice reaction times or with more complex tests. With generalized discharges, 68% show impaired performance compared with 33% of patients with focal discharges. Even focal discharges of one second or less may be impairing (Mirsky & Van Buren, 1965; Aarts *et al.*, 1984; Binnie *et al.*, 1990; Rugland, 1990b).

Academics

Left-sided spikes are seen with reading disabilities (Stores & Hart, 1976; Camfield *et al.*, 1984; Rugland, 1990b). Subclinical discharges are also accompanied by an increased error rate on reading. Children read faster but less accurately when discharges occur, even when they are on medication. Drugs used to suppress the discharges result in an 80% improvement when the discharges are few. A 10% inverse response is seen when discharges occur more frequently. There is no evidence for hesitations in associations with errors, which might arouse suspicion that subtle seizures are occurring (Siebelink *et al.*, 1988; Binnie *et al.*, 1990).

Computerized neuropsychologic testing

Computerized neuropsychologic testing with simultaneous EEG recording may reveal the influence of epileptiform discharges on cognitive functions and help to evaluate the effects of antiepileptic drugs (Henricksen, 1990). It can be shown that subclinical epileptiform discharges in children may impair reaction time, choice time, verbal-spatial memory, and verbal and figurative problem solving, not necessarily relating to the discharge length. One is most apt to see abnormalities in reactions and responses if school problems are seen.

Specialized testing demonstrates that subclinical discharges impair performance in 61% of patients on simple and choice reaction time tests, even when some discharges last for only one second (Mirksy & Van Buren, 1965; Aarts *et al.*, 1984; Binnie *et al.*, 1990; Rugland, 1990b).

Information gained from specialized computerized neuropsychological testing, especially if it includes simultaneous EEG recording, can be shared with parents and teachers. Teachers thus learn the need for repeated instructions and the importance of checking whether the child has understood what is presented (Rugland, 1990a). Parents and teachers can see the effects of this testing approach, which may reveal the influence of epileptiform discharges on learning functions. This may help to monitor the effects of the antiepileptic drugs. In children with frequent epileptiform discharges but without clinical seizures, occasionally antiepileptic medication may have a limited effect on cognitive functioning, probably due to the child's intrinsic inattention (Henricksen, 1990).

Damaging subtle discharges

Frequent subtle seizures and the direct effects of interictal EEG epileptiform discharges (TCIs) may be an important factor causing learning disabilities. If the subclinical discharges are very frequent, they may amount to non-convulsive status epilepticus. If allowed to continue for along time, learning disorders may produce permanent learning disabilities (Cornaggia & Gobbi, 2001).

Therapy

Rugland (1993) reviewed the therapeutic considerations of children with subclinical discharges. The significance of TCIs accompanying subclinical EEG discharges for everyday functioning is uncertain. In some children, suppression of discharges by antiepileptic drugs has demonstrated improved psychological function.

In antiepileptic drug trials in reading impairments associated with TCIs, many children improved when medications produced significantly fewer discharges, but a few performed less well on medication. Valproate has been tested most commonly. Drug response time is less complex, but at higher drug levels the drug itself may impair verbal memory and spatial tasks. Correlating anticonvulsant blood levels to TCI occurrence and to performance may be useful in determining medication adjustments.

The definitely abnormal epileptiform EEG disturbance should be shown to correlate with a specific type of learning disturbance on testing, which correlates with an ongoing academic handicap, especially if clinical seizure activities are not shown. An appropriate drug, one least apt to produce academic side effects resembling the child's problem area, must then be prescribed. The adverse effects of antiepileptic treatment must be considered (Stores, 1990). The drug must be tolerated and shown to result in a definite significant improvement in the child's performance by objective verification, not just by first impressions. One endpoint may be aimed at obliteration of the EEG abnormality. If this cannot be shown within three months at an appropriate dosage, then the child should be withdrawn from the drug, watching for any possible deterioration of performance. If a drug does not objectively overcome the problem targeted, it should be stopped.

REFERENCES

Aarts, J. H. P., Binnie, C. D., Smit, A. M., *et al.* (1984). Selective cognitive impairment during focal and generalized epileptiform EEG activity. *Brain* **107**: 293–308.

Aldenkamp, A. P., Alpherts, W. C. J., Dekker, M. J. A., *et al.* (1990). Neuropsychological aspects of learning disabilities in epilepsy. *Epilepsia* **31** (suppl 4): 9–20.

Aldenkamp, A. P., Arenda, J. & Overweg-Plandsoen, W. C. G. (1998). Effects of subtle seizures and epileptiform EEG discharges on cognitive functions. 3rd European Congress of Epileptology, Warsaw, Poland. *Epilepsia* **39** (suppl 2): 99.

Altafullah, I. & Halgren, E. (1988). Focal medial temporal lobe spike-wave complexes evoked by a memory task. *Epilepsia* **29**: 8–14.

Binnie, C. D. (1979). Direction of transitory cognitive impairment during epileptiform EEG discharges: problems in clinical practice. In *Epilepsy and Behavior*, ed. B. M. Kuling, H. Meinardi & G. Stores, pp. 91–7. Lisse: Swets & Zeitlinger.

Binnie, C. D. (1988). Seizures, EEG discharges and cognition. In *Epilepsy, Behavior and Cognitive Function*, ed. M. R. Trimble & E. H. Reynolds, pp. 45–51. London: John Wiley & Sons.

Binnie, C. D. (1993). Significance and management of transitory cognitve impairment due to subclinical EEG discharges in children. *Brain Dev.* **15**: 23–30.

Binnie, C. D. (1999). Are interictal discharges subclinical? 23rd International Epilepsy Congress. *Epilepsia* **40** (suppl 2): 69.

Binnie, C. D. (2001). Cognitive performance, subtle seizures, and the EEG. In *Epilepsia and Learning Disabilities*, ed. G. F. Ayala, M. Elia, C. M. Cornaggia & M. M. Trimble. *Epilepsia* **42**: 16–18.

Binnie, C. D., Channon, S. & Marston, D. (1990). Learning disabilities in epilepsy: neurophysiological aspects. *Epilepsia* **31** (suppl 4): 2–8.

Binnie, C. D., Channon, S. & Marston, D. L. (1991). Behavioral correlates of interictal spikes. *Adv. Neurol.* **55**: 113–26.

Binnie, C. D., Kasteleijn-Nolst Trenite, D. G., Smit, A. M., *et al.* (1987). Interactions of epileptiform EEG discharges and cognition. *Epilepsy Res.* **1**: 239–45.

Bourgeois, B. F. D., Prensky, A. L., Palkes, H. S., *et al.* (1983). Intelligence in epeilspy: a prospective study in children. *Ann. Neurol.* **14**: 438–44.

Brinciotti, M., Matricardi, M., Paciello, F., *et al.* (1991). Subclinical spike-wave complexes and cognitive performance in epileptic children. 19th International Epilepsy Congress. *Epilepsia* **32** (suppl 1): 25.

Camfield, P. R., Gates, R., Ronen, G., *et al.* (1984). Comparison of cognitive ability, personality profile and school success in epileptic children with pure right versus left temporal lobe EEG foci. *Ann. Neurol.* **15**: 122–6.

Collins, A. L. (1951). Epileptic intelligen. *J. Consult. Psychol.* **15**: 393–9.

Cornaggia, C. M. & Gobbi, G. (2001). Learning disability in epilepsy: definitions and classification. In *Epilepsia and Learning Disabilities*, ed. G. F. Ayala, M. Elia, C. M. Cornaggia & M. M. Trimble. *Epilepsia* **42**: 2–5.

Dodrill, C. P. (1998). The effects of seizures and various ACDs on cognition in cognitive organization of the brain. Presented at the American Epilepsy Society Conference, San Diego, CA.

Dodrill, C. B. & Wilkus, R. J. (1978). Neuropsychological correlates of the electroencephalogram in epileptics. III: generalized non-epileptiform abnormalities. *Epilepsia* **19**: 453–62.

Duncan, C. P. (1949). The retroactive effect of electroshock on learning. *J. Comp. Physiol. Psychol.* **42**: 42–4.

Fink, M. (1979). Neuropsychology of ECT. In *Convulsive Therapy, Theory and Practice*, ed. M. Fink, pp. 107–29. New York: Raven Press.

Goode, D. J., Penry, J. K. & Dreifuss, F. E. (1970). Effect of paroxysmal spike-wave on continuous visual-motor performance. *Epilepsia* **11**: 241–54.

Henricksen, O. (1990). Education and epilepsy: assessment and remediation. *Epilepsia* **31** (suppl 4): 21–5.

Hutt, S. J. & Fairweather, H. (1975). Information processing during two types of EEG activity. *Electroencephalogr. Clin. Neurophysiol.* **39**: 43–51.

Hutt, S. J., Newton, J. & Fairweather, M. (1977). Choice reaction time and EEG activity in children with epilepsy. *Neuropsychologica* **156**: 257–67.

Kasteleijn-Nolst Trenite, D. G. A., Bakker, D. J., Binnie, C. D., *et al.* (1988). Psychological effects of sub-clinical epileptiform EEG discharges. I: scholastic skills. *Epilepsy Res.* **2**: 111–16.

Kasteleijn-Nolst Trenite, D. G. A., Smit, A. M., Velis, D. N., *et al.* (1990). On-line detection of transient neuropsychological disturbances during EEG discharges in children with epilepsy. *Dev. Med. Child Neurol.* **32**: 46–50.

Kooi, K. A. & Hovey, H. B. (1956). Alternations in mental functions and paroxysmal cerebral activity. *Arch. Neurol. Psychiatry* **78**: 264–71.

Ladavas, E., Umnila, C. & Provincialli, I. (1979). Hemisphere dependent cognitive performance in epileptic patients. *Epilepsia* **20**: 493–502.

Licht, E. A. & Jacobsen, R. H. (1999). Electrographic seizures and cognitive function: raising concerns for low frequency events. *Epilepsia* **40** (suppl 7): 59.

McGaugh, J. L. & Petrinovich, L. F. (1966). Neural consolidations and electroconvulsive shock re-examined. *Psychol. Rev.* **73**: 382–98.

Mirsky, A. F. (1969). Studies of paroxysmal EEG phenomena and background EEG in relation to impaired attention. In *Attention in Neurophysiology*, ed. C. R. Evans & T. B. Mulholland, pp. 310–22. London: Butterworth.

Mirsky, A. F. (1989). Information processing in petit mal epilepsy. In *Childhood Epilepsies: Neurophysiological, Psychosocial and Intervention Aspects*. ed. B. P. Hermann & M. Seidenberg, pp. 51–70. Chichester, UK: John Wiley & Sons.

Mirsky, A. F. & Van Buren, J. M. (1965). On the nature of the "absence" in centrencephalic epilepsy: a study of some behavioral, electroencephalographic and autonomic factors. *Electroencephalogr. Clin. Neurophysiol.* **18**: 334–8.

Ojemann, G. A. (1983). Brain organization for language from the perspective of electrical stimulation mapping. *Behav. Brain Sci.* **6**: 189–230.

Opp, J., Wenzel, D. & Brandl, U. (1992). Visuomotor coordination during focal and generalized EEG discharges. *Epilepsia* **33**: 836–40.

Rausch, R., Lieb, U. P. & Crandall, P. A. S. (1978). Neuropsychologic correlates of depth spike activity in epileptic patients. *Arch. Neurol.* **35**: 699–705.

Regard, M., Landis, T., Wieser, H. G., *et al.* (1985). Function inhibition and release: unilateral tachistoscopic performance and stereoelectroencephalographic activity in a case with left limbic status epilepticus. *Neuropsychologia* **23**: 575–81.

Rodin, E. A., Rennick, P., Dennerill, R. & Yin, Y. (1972). Vocational and educational problems of epileptic patients. *Epilepsia* **13**: 149–60.

Rodin, E. A., Schmaltz, S. & Twitty, G. (1986). Intellectual functions of patients with childhood-onset epilepsy. *Dev. Med. Child. Neurol.* **28**: 25–33.

Rugland, A. L. (1990a). Subclinical epileptogenic activity. In *Pediatric Epilepsy*, ed. M. Sillanpaa, S. I. Johananessen, G. Blennow & M. Dam, pp. 217–23. London: Wrightson Biomedical.

Rugland, A. L. (1990b). Neuropsychological assessment of cognitive functioning in children with epilepsy. *Epilepsia* **31** (suppl 4): 41–4.

Rugland, A. L. (1993). Subclinical discharges. Presented at the International Epilepsy Symposium, Oslo, Norway, July 1993.

Rugland, A. L., Bjaes, H., Henrickson, O., *et al.* (1987). The development of computerized tests as a routine procedure in clinical EEG practice for the evaluation of cognitive changes in patients with epilepsy. 17th Epilepsy International Congress 1987. *Epilepsia* **28** (suppl): 207.

Schwab, R. S. (1939). A method of measuring consciousness on petit mal epilepsy. *J. Nerv. Ment. Dis.* **89**: 690–91.

Scott, D. F., Moffett, A., Matthews, A., *et al.* (1967). The effect of epileptic discharges on learning and memory in patients. *Epilepsia* **8**: 188–94.

Shewmon, D. A. & Erwin, R. J. (1988a). The effect of focal interictal spikes on perception and reaction time. I: general considerations. *Electroencephalogr. Clin. Neurophysiol.* **69**: 319–37.

Shewmon, D. A. & Erwin, R. J. (1988b). The effect of focal interictal spikes on perception and reaction times. II: neuroanatomic specificity. *Electroencephalogr. Clin. Neurophysiol.* **69**: 338–52.

Siebelink, B. M., Bakker, D. J., Binnie, C. D., *et al.* (1988). Psychological effects of sub-clinical EEG discharges. 2: general intelligence tests. *Epilepsy Res.* **2**: 117–21.

Squire, L. R., Slater, P. C. & Miller, P. L. (1981). Retrograde amnesia and electroconvulsive therapy. *Arch. Gen. Psychiatry* **38**: 890–95.

Stores, G. (1971). Cognitive function in children with epilepsy. *Dev. Med. Child Neurol.* **13**: 390–93.

Stores, G. (1986). Nonconvulsive status epilepticus in children. In *Recent Advances in Epilepsy*, ed. T. A. Pedley & B. S. Meldrum, Vol. 3, pp. 295–310. Edinburgh: Churchill Livingstone.

Stores, G. (1987). Effects on learning of "subclinical" seizure discharges. In *Education and Epilepsy 1987*, ed. A. P. Aldenkamp, W. C. J. Alpherts, H. Meinardi & G. Stores, pp. 14–21. Lisse: Swets & Zeitlinger.

Stores, G. (1990). Electroencephalographic parameters in assessing the cognitive function of children with epilepsy. *Epilepsia* **31** (suppl 4): 45–9.

Stores, G. & Hart, J. (1976). Reading skills of children with generalized or focal epilepsy attending ordinary school. *Dev. Med. Child Neurol.* **18**: 705–16.

Tarter, R. E. (1971). Intellectual and adaptive functioning in epilepsy: a review of fifty years of research. *Dis. Nerv. Syst.* **33**: 763–70.

Tizard, B. & Margerison, J. H. (1963a). The relationship between generalized paroxysmal EEG discharges and various test situations in two epileptic patients. *J. Neurol. Neurosurg. Psychiatry* **26**: 303–13.

Tizard, B. & Margerison, J. H. (1963b). Psychological functioning during wave-spike discharges. *Br. J. Soc. Clin. Psychol.* **3**: 6–15.

Turkdogan, D., Zaimoglul, S., Yilmaz, Z. & Ozek, M. M. (1999). Cognitive and behavioral characteristics in children with central spikes. 23rd International Epilepsy Congress. *Epilepsia* **40** (suppl 2): 230.

18

Attention and alertness

Learning is dependent on three closely interrelated brain foundations: attention, memory system, and executive functioning. If one of these fundamentals fails, learning often falters. Up to 60% of children seen in an epilepsy clinic may have attention deficits (Williams *et al.*, 1992).

Attention

Alertness may be impaired in epilepsy (Stores, 1987), unrelated to the seizure type or EEG abnormality (Bruhn-Parsons & Parsons, 1977; Aldenkamp *et al.*, 1993). Approaches to tasks are similar but the search time is prolonged. More specific deficits may modify this, according to the seizure type, frequency, type of EEG abnormality, and onset age (Aldenkamp *et al.*, 1990). Impaired attention may contribute to decreased academic performance regardless of the seizure type, gender, and duration of the epilepsy (Williams *et al.*, 2000).

What is attention?

The most important question is what is meant by an attention problem? Attention, concentration, alertness, arousal, and other related terms signify different abilities. Attention refers to a general state of arousal, selection, concentration, vigilance, search time, and the triad of alertness, selectivity, and processing (Stores *et al.*, 1978).

Attention can refer to both divided attention and focused attention. A divided attention deficit means that the individual cannot handle multiple inputs. A focused attention deficit means that the child incorporates irrelevant stimuli into the thought process even when the object of attention is known.

Attention can also refer to both immediate attention and sustained attention. Immediate attention is the act of being attracted to a stimulus. Sustained attention involves the ability to maintain that attention over time. The child needs to be both sensitive to the stimulus and biased towards responding to it. Concentration is to focus and sustain attention on a specific stimulus. This is needed to gather the stimulus information for analysis, comparing similar memories, towards organizing the most appropriate motor response (Sergeant, 1996). Focused attention implies the capacity to concentrate attention on a specific target, screening out distracting stimuli. Distractibility refers to a child's attention being interrupted by a novel stimulus.

Consciousness is not vigilance. Consciousness is the immediate awareness of what is going on, allowing the individual to respond voluntarily. Vigilance is the sensitivity to novel stimuli. Selectivity signifies a child's ability to organize attention toward a specific stimulus. Switching attention implies a controlled change of attention when appropriate.

Development of attention skills

In the first four months of life, a child is most apt to attend to items in the immediate environment that have greater contrast, that have fewer edges, and that move. Thereafter, novelty becomes important, for young children tend to lose interest in repeated stimuli. By four years of age, the child's ability to voluntarily orient attention to specific items emerges. Children learn to search the environment actively rather than to be passively attracted by novelty or importance of the stimuli. Search patterns are similar. This is well established by five to six years of age (Sergeant, 1996). In middle childhood, the ability to organize a motor output response emerges as attention blends with executive functions (Halperin, 1996).

At five to ten years of age, vigilance responses change. Developmental differences in sustained attention develop at six to seven years. Focused attention skills are fully developed by around seven years of age, but the skills to sustain attention continue to develop through adolescence (Halperin, 1996). The processing rate changes especially between the ages of eight and 12 years. Between the ages of 12 and 22 years, there are virtually no differences for any type of processing (Sergeant, 1996).

Anatomy of attention

Attention depends on various functions supported by different brain regions that have become specialized and coordinated for the purposes of focusing, sustaining concentration, stabilizing, shifting, encoding, and executing. Specialization is not absolute, for when one area is damaged other structures may be able to substitute (Mirsky, 1996).

Focused attention relates to the superior temporal and inferior parietal cortices as well as the corpus striatum. Appropriate responses depend heavily on the integrity of the inferior parietal and striatal regions. Sustained attention relates to the rostral midbrain structures, including the reticular formation and thalamic nuclei. Stabilization of attentiveness appears dependent on thalamic and brainstem structures. Encoding relates more to the superior temporal cortex. The ability to shift attention relates to the prefrontal cortex and anterior cingulate gyrus. Encoding of such stimuli depends on the hippocampus and amygdala.

Disorders associated with attention problems

Disorders of attention may be inherited, acquired, or induced environmentally. Inherited problems include the primary ADHD spectrum, idiopathic seizure disorders, psychotic prodromes, and inborn metabolic disorders. Acquired damage includes perinatal insults, developmental disabilities, head injuries, acquired epilepsies, and infections. Environmental insults include poverty, exposures to alcohol or toxins, malnutrition, deprivation, and a chaotic home situation. Shy children tend to be weak in detecting and sustaining areas of attention, whereas aggressive children have problems in focusing and inhibiting responses, but both are rated as having poor concentration (Mirsky, 1996).

Attention disorders are often manifestations of difficulties in processing incoming stimuli. Either the stimulus is beyond the capability of the child's ability to respond appropriately or the child lacks the skills to handle normal stimuli. These situations can be subcategorized into a neurosensory intake problem due to a visual or auditory handicap, a subcortical processing problem in alertness and organized attentiveness, or a cortical processing impairment, as with a language or learning problem, the latter of which may be focal, as in a learning disability, or generalized, as with an abnormal intelligence. The problem may be an overwhelming environment that is too much for the child's coping skills. There is not a single ADHD but rather similar symptoms of diverse etiology (Svoboda, 1979). For example, selective attention deficits are seen more often with specific learning disabilities, whereas sustained attention deficits are more classically seen with primary ADHD, some of the latter group also showing more evidence for response organization deficits (Halperin, 1996).

Attention deficits of epilepsy

Alertness is often reduced in students, especially boys, with epilepsy (Benson, 1979; Bennett-Levy & Stores, 1984). Up to 42% of students with epilepsy have attention problems (Holdsworth & Whitmore, 1974; Hutt et al., 1977; Stores et al., 1978; Baird et al., 1980; Stores, 1981). Teacher ratings of attention do not correlate well with other measures of attentiveness and appear more apt to select the poor achievers among children with epilepsy (Stores, 1973; Stores et al., 1978; Reynolds, 1981). Children with frequent seizures are not necessarily inattentive (Holdsworth & Whitmore, 1974).

Although any of the causes of ADD can occur with epilepsy, some specific types are seen more commonly that relate to the seizure type (generalized versus partial seizures), anticonvulsant reactions, the anxieties of epilepsy, and seizure-control "awakenings." In addition, attention deficits may be due to seizure activity occurring without any clinical manifestations.

Drug reactions

Any anticonvulsant may cause or relieve attention problems, including those with excessive activity. Such reactions are more apt to occur with stronger dosages, with polypharmacy, or if the child is sensitive to the drug.

Seizure types

Attentiveness may vary with the EEG type of epilepsy (Stores *et al.*, 1978). Children with generalized seizure discharges are more apt to suffer from restlessness and inattentiveness, whereas children with focal seizure disorders are more at risk for specific learning disabilities (Ounsted & Hutt, 1964) and distractibility. Subclinical seizure disturbances may disrupt attention (Stores, 1973). Fluctuations of performance vary greatly, from retained to partially retained or completely abolished awareness during spike-wave discharges; comparable changes can be detected during subtle EEG changes, such as a simple slowing of the background activity (Erba & Cavazzuti, 1980). The capacity of the brain to handle more complex information is reduced temporarily during both generalized and probably focal epileptic discharges (Wilkus & Dodrill, 1976).

Generalized burst interruptions

Most types of epilepsy seem to affect the student's attentiveness adversely, except perhaps for true absence seizures associated with three per second spike-wave discharges. Subclinical spike-wave discharges may be accompanied by performance decrements, increased reaction time, or failure to respond. Children with generalized epilepsies and generalized EEG abnormalities perform poorly (Hovey & Kooi, 1955; Fedio & Mirsky, 1969; Mirsky *et al.*, 1960; Milstein & Stevens, 1961; Prechtl *et al.*, 1961; Tizard & Mungerson, 1963; Camfield *et al.*, 1977; Binnie, 1980) on sustained attention, on alertness (Reitan, 1974) and concentration tasks (Mirsky & Van Buren, 1965; Fedio & Mirsky, 1969), and on tests of sustained vigilance (Fairweather & Hutt, 1971). The impairment is specifically in attention capacities (Tarter, 1972). A rebound increase in paroxysmal activity after inhibition is probably due to diminished attention and the related inactivity of the non-specific mechanisms that regulate the level of cortical tone (Ricci *et al.*, 1972).

Disruption of attention is related to the symmetry, regularity, diffuse and bilateral synchrony, organization, and duration of the spike-wave burst, the proportion of spikes or polyspikes in a burst, and high-voltage maximal in the frontal-central areas (Tizard & Mungerson, 1963; Davidoff & Johnson, 1964; Mirsky & Van Buren, 1965; Hutt *et al.*, 1977; O'Donohoe, 1979). The occurrence of spike-wave bursts is not necessarily accompanied by inattention. When inattention does occur, the onset may precede the appearance of the EEG spike-wave activity, or it may appear after the onset of the bursts but not persist throughout it. Attention deficits may also be seen in the absence of EEG discharges, possibly due to a persistent disturbance or subcortical mechanisms. There appear to be independent subcortical mechanisms for attention, cortical activation, and myoclonus (Stores, 1973).

Tests requiring more complete attentiveness (reception, discrimination, motor responses) are more impaired during bursts than those that require only a part of this sequence, with motor tasks affected the least. A retrograde amnestic affect is noted (Mirsky & Van Buren, 1965).

Early-onset subcortical epilepsy involving the mesodiencephalic reticular system may produce a chronic state of impaired alertness. Generalized seizure patients perform more poorly on sustained attention behavior tasks even in the absence of spike-wave discharges. The effect of spike-wave discharges on detection of an auditory signal is not an all-or-none effect but depends on how many signals the child is attending to at the time (Ounsted & Hutt, 1964).

Children with unexplained learning difficulties may demonstrate generalized spike-wave paroxysms or generalized gross abnormalities on their EEGs without behavior changes, raising the question of whether these subclinical bursts may be associated with impairments of attention (Hutt & Fairweather, 1971; Arieff, 1974; Stores & Hart, 1976; Hutt *et al.*, 1977). Subclinical epileptiform discharges may occur without EEG evidence of its occurrence and yet may produce amnesic episodes and thus have adverse effects on learning. Spike-wave paroxysms in children slow down reaction times in a way that is likely to put them at disadvantage in timed or paced tests (Stores, 1971). The relationship between spike and wave activity and attention is a complex one. A burst is not necessarily accompanied by inattention, and vice versa. If correlated, the inattentiveness may not occur simultaneously. Inattentiveness may proceed or follow the onset of the bursts but it may not persist throughout (Ounsted & Hutt, 1964). Similarly, non-responses and paroxysmal EEGs occur together, significantly, in patients who do not have seizures, raising the question of whether such bursts are associated with episodic loss of higher functions without clinical evidence of epilepsy (Hovey & Kooi, 1955).

Cognitive and perceptual motor effects

Slowing of background rhythms is associated with poor performance on perceptuomotor tests, and is often associated with lower than normal intelligence. The child with bursts of subcortical seizure discharges arising from slow background rhythms is permanently inattentive to some degree but is also subject to episodic exacerbations. Problems in performance depend on the nature and amount of information, the rate required to process, and the age and intelligence of the child (Fairweather & Hutt, 1969; Dodrill & Wilkus, 1976; Stores *et al.*, 1978).

Responsiveness

Paroxysms generalized from the start impair responsiveness more than discharges that are generalized incompletely (Porter *et al.*, 1973). Children listening passively to an observer show longer retrograde amnesia than those actively involved in a task (Fenwick, 1981). The degree of spike-wave generalization appears to be related inversely to responsiveness. Responsiveness to visual stimuli (including visually evoked stimuli) becomes impaired 200–500 milliseconds before the onset of the three per second spike-wave discharges. Retrograde memory deficits for visual and verbal materials presented during or immediately before the spike-wave discharges have been shown (Brown *et al.*, 1974). Reaction times to auditory stimuli are normal up to within one second before a paroxysm, but only 43% are normal with the onset of the paroxysm. Responsiveness is recovered quickly after a paroxysm (Brown *et al.*, 1974; O'Donohoe, 1979).

Burst duration effect

Generalized spike-wave bursts impair awareness and responsiveness to varying degrees, depending on the duration of the discharge (Dikmen, 1980), and the rate and complexity of the material being learned (Stores & Hart, 1976). The greatest impairment may come in the early mid portion of the discharge, or intermittently throughout, or concomitant with the entire burst (Reynolds, 1981). At the spike-wave burst onset, 56% of the responses are abnormal. With short bursts, more than 50% responses to stimuli given at the burst onset are abnormal. Abnormal reaction times increase during the paroxysms, suggesting a gradual decrease of responsiveness (Porter *et al.*, 1973).

Short bursts of less than 1.5 seconds only slow performance, especially in more complex tasks, with accuracy reduced to 24% during the burst. Beyond one to 1.5 seconds, the burst disrupts performance, with prominent response omissions and slowed performance (Dikmen, 1980; Fenwick, 1981). This appears to be a reduction in the capacity to process information rather than a loss of contact (Tizard & Margerison, 1963; Reitan, 1974).

Slightly longer subclinical discharges of around two seconds or more decrease the person's capacity to process information, with slowed reaction times and reduced reactivity (Porter *et al.*, 1973), especially with more complex tasks. Even with these shorter tasks, the retrograde amnesia may persist for four to 15 seconds (Laidlaw & Reichans, 1976b). Paroxysms lasting for more than three seconds nearly always produce observable impairments of performance (Goode *et al.*, 1970; Reitan, 1974), with errors emerging one to two seconds into the spike-wave activity. Patients may resume normal performance one to two seconds before the spike-wave activity ceases (Dikmen, 1980).

Reaction time

Paroxysmal slowed reaction time results in reduced transmission of information (Fairweather & Hutt, 1971). Paroxysmal slowing of cortical activity does not appear to slow motor pursuit tests (Stores *et al.*, 1978). This effect is related to the duration of the paroxysm (Reynolds, 1981). Slowed reaction times place such children at a disadvantage on timed or paced tasks (Stores, 1971).

Decision-making

Choice reaction time latency and errors are greater with seizure bursts but faster and more accurate just before a burst (Jus & Jus, 1962; Ishiharo & Yoshii, 1967; Davidoff & Johnson, 1964; Mirsky & Van Buren, 1965; Geller & Geller, 1970; Hutt, 1972; Binnie, 1980).

Affects on responses

Spike and wave activity during a test tends to influence performance for a period of time beyond the duration of the epileptiform activity itself (Fossen & Gotlibsen, 1980). The accuracy of correct decisions in viewing visual stimuli drops to 24% during spike-wave discharges, although no detectable behavioral changes are seen for 25% of the time (Reitan, 1974).

Continuous task problems

Attention disturbances impede continuous task performance, with longer and more variable results seen in those with epilepsy (Wagenar, 1975; Mirsky *et al.*, 1960; Brittain, 1980). Maintenance of attention is partially dependent on the integrity of central midline subcortical structures more than on parts of the neopallium (Lansdell & Mirsky, 1964). Problems such as disturbance of vigilance and sustained attention may reflect differences related to the size rather than the location of the lesion, or to subcortical and "centrencephalic" functions rather than to cortical dysfunction (Dennerll, 1964). The impairment appears more on the sensory input than motor response (Stores *et al.*, 1978).

Stress influences

If a child is pushed to work at double speed, the initial frequency of spike-wave activity is lower but the subsequent increase occurs sooner (Ounsted & Hutt, 1964).

Specific seizure types

More children with generalized tonic–clonic epilepsy than absence attacks fail at school. In those who underachieve, attention problems are increased (Hutt *et al.*, 1977; Baird *et al.*, 1980). The EEG may show brief periods of unexplained confusion at times of generalized paroxysmal fast activity in individuals who may have a history of tonic seizures (Somerfill & Bruni, 1983).

Patients with absence seizures may be impaired in tasks of sustained attention (Mirsky et al., 1960; Lansdell & Mirsky, 1964; Mirsky & Van Buren, 1965) not only with attacks but also between attacks, suggesting a persistent disturbance in central subcortical functions (Mirsky & Van Buren, 1965; Stores, 1971). In brief attacks, visual stimuli reactions are delayed, while in longer attacks the stimuli are not perceived. However, both light and especially sound stimuli may terminate moderately severe absence attacks (Schwab, 1941). Reaction times are slowed (Hovey & Kooi, 1955). TCIs are more apt to be seen with classical three per second spike-wave discharges than with atypical forms. Alterations of awareness and attentiveness may precede the EEG paroxysm in some patients (Shalev & Amir, 1983). With uncontrolled absence seizures, girls have more attention problems than boys (Mirsky & Van Buren, 1965).

Some children with generalized epilepsy with myoclonic jerks are not impaired on tests of attentiveness. Children with minor motor seizures may be inattentive and overly active, but this is part of their overall developmental delays and depressed IQ (Stores, 1971).

Partial seizure

When a part of the brain is occupied by an electrical discharge, it cannot perform its normal function (Ounsted et al., 1966; Fedio & Mirsky, 1969; O'Donohoe, 1979). Frequently occurring subclinical localized cortical spikes may impair some aspects of attention (Ounsted et al., 1966; Fedio & Mirsky, 1969; Stores et al., 1978; O'Donohoe, 1979). Patients with partial seizures show the reverse of that seen with children with absence seizures, for they are impaired on tasks of shift and focus/execute attentions factors (Mirsky et al., 1960; Lansdell & Mirsky, 1964). With prolonged bursts of spiking, routine tasks are relatively unaffected but more complex tasks may be impaired (Rennick et al., 1969; Reitan, 1974). TCIs may or may not occur with focal discharges, especially longer discharges (Mirsky, 1960; Prechtl et al., 1961; Davidoff & Johnson, 1964; Hutt, 1972; Hutt & Fairweather, 1973; Brown et al., 1974; Binnie, 1980; Shalev & Amir, 1983; Quadfasel & Pruysel, 1985), sometimes preceded by brief cognitive enhancement and followed by a retrograde amnesia (Schwab, 1941; Tizard & Margerison, 1963; Davidoff & Johnson, 1964; Mirsky & Van Buren, 1965; Goode et al., 1970; Binnie, 1980).

Orientation reaction

The orientation reaction is defined as the total action of paying attention to important stimuli in preparation to deal with the situation. Characteristics of stimuli that elicit the orientation reaction include novelty, intensity, complexity, uncertainty, and surprise (O'Donohoe, 1979). Chronically discharging epileptic focis in some areas may disturb the orientation reaction by either increasing excitation of cortical-reticular connections and thus maintaining heightened arousal states, or by interfering with the normal reactivity to novel stimuli, causing inattentiveness. For example, in some children, focal epileptic seizure discharge frequencies decrease while the child is doing arithmetic (Ricci *et al.*, 1972; Stores, 1980b).

An unfamiliar stimulus activates the cortical sensory areas, such as the anterior-temporal or paroccipital areas, inhibiting excitatory collaterals via the reticular formation, thus orienting the child to the stimulus. Epileptic discharges may increase the corticoreticular excitation, thus maintaining a sustained arousal state with poor habituation to repeated stimuli, or by interfering with normal reactivity to new stimuli may cause inattentiveness even in unfamiliar situations (Stores *et al.*, 1978).

Neglect is an attention defect induced by disruption of the cortical-reticular loop, thus inhibiting arousal. Neglect is most often seen after right parietal lesions. The left hemisphere tends to mediate attention to contralateral stimuli, whereas the right hemisphere attends to both ipsilateral and contralateral stimuli. Thus, a left hemisphere lesion can still be covered by the right hemisphere, but not vice versa (Heilman & Van Den Abell, 1979).

Frontal seizures

Children with frontal lobe epileptiform abnormalities are more likely than other children with epilepsy to present with attention problems. The symptoms are of a primarily inattentive attention deficit rather than a combination of attention deficits associated with hyperactivity (Sherman *et al.*, 2000).

Complex partial seizures

Temporal lobe patients are impaired not on tasks of sustained attention (Fedio & Mirsky, 1969) but on attention aspects related to shifting and focusing in order to execute responses (Mirsky *et al.*, 1960; Lansdell & Mirsky, 1964; Mirsky, 1969). Differences are seen in activity and attention in children with unilateral temporal lobe seizure disorders, the type of environmental distraction (auditory or visual) correlating to the lateralization of the seizure focus (Stores, 1978). The child may overreact to environmental stimuli. Children with left temporal seizures tend to be inattentive and overly active in noisy settings; children with right-sided seizures tend to be visually distractable. Paradoxically, a subset of left temporal lobe children appear to be calmed in a noisy environment. If tolerated, the hyperreactivity of the temporal lobe child to environmental stimuli may be calmed by a barbiturate but not by a hydantoin, even though seizure control is obtained with the latter (Svoboda, 1979).

Modifying factors

A normal state of responsiveness is a prerequisite for attention. With epilepsy activity, a decrease in responsiveness to environmental stimuli may interfere with attention. Children who have a history of prior school or behavior difficulties, and those whose parents react maladaptively to the diagnosis of epilepsy, tend to display persistent attention deficits (Oostrom *et al.*, 2002).

Symptomatic versus idiopathic epilepsy

Children with greater brain damage have a shorter on-task performance endurance than less damaged children. Mentally subnormal children may have particular difficulty in focusing attention on one aspect of a situation, their attention being diffused over several aspects at any one time. Such children are more distractable and less able to adapt to distractions. Performance in vigilance tasks for long periods deteriorates more rapidly (Stores, 1973).

Gender

Boys have more problems than girls in sustaining attention, with variable reduced attention and acting out of classroom behaviors. They tend to be higher in motor activity but not in distractibility. Boys have trouble in tasks requiring vigilance, because they have trouble maintaining their attention (Stores, 1978; Stores *et al.*, 1978; Weingraumb, 1981). However, with uncontrolled absence seizures, girls have more attention problems (Mirsky & Van Buren, 1965).

Age onset

Children of early onset age appear to be more at risk for attention deficits.

Seizure frequency

Inattentiveness does not appear to relate to the seizure frequency, and vice versa (Hutt & Fairweather, 1973; Baird *et al.*, 1980).

Activities

The occurrence of seizures is sometimes related to particular activities or experiences (Lennox *et al.*, 1936; O'Donohoe, 1979). Tasks that require some degree of concentration or arousal (Lennox & Lennox, 1960; Stores, 1980b) and circumstances that are neither boring nor stressful may lessen seizure discharge frequency. If a task becomes stressful, the seizure discharge frequency increases and performance decreases (Ounsted and Hutt, 1964; O'Donohoe, 1979). Attention and active thinking tend to suppress generalized bursts, whereas cortical discharges of focal epilepsy may not be suppressed. This phenomenon may wear off. Suppression is generated near the beginning of each subtest (Quadfasel & Pruysel, 1955; Kooi and Hovey, 1957).

Telemetric EEGs have been used to study children in various school activities and at various academic tasks (Guey *et al.*, 1969). There is a general tendency for the EEG to desynchronize during mental work with the eyes open, but in certain tasks, such as mental arithmetic or automatic visuomotor tasks, the EEG may synchronize, suggesting a selective stimulus inhibition. Both concentration and monotony may facilitate absence seizures. Although the mechanisms differ, the EEG synchronization effect is similar (Schlack, 1980). Absence seizures occur more frequently during periods of inactivity and during school exercises. The frequency of paroxysms may increase considerably when a child is in a situation reminiscent of the classroom, which may be consistent with the general prevalence of scholastic problems (Guey *et al.*, 1969). Children vary widely in their sensitivity to discharges. Those showing greater sensitivity and a failing performance may require more aggressive anticonvulsant therapy (Dubinsky *et al.*, 1983).

Concentration

Concentration may activate epilepsy. Three factors are involved: complex decision-making, sequential decision-making, and stress (Forster, 1977). Mild deficits in cognition may be apparent when the individual has to think through a task. Transient episodes of disturbed higher integration and analytical thinking with retention of a sense of participating may be noted in testing, so that non-answer responses are occasionally given, which indicate partial loss of attention. Some of the non-answer responses might be considered "intellectual automatism" because such responses are more habitual or automatic in the situation presented than those required by the specific test goals involved. Examples include naming of the object presented or making some simple observation or association regarding it. However, transient cognitive impairments may be the cause (Hovey & Kooi, 1955). Psychologic testing utilizing EEG monitoring may help to differentiate between the entities.

Diagnosis

An epileptic child's potential capabilities may be underestimated unless the child is stimulated optimally during a period of assessment. Results obtained by a novel, arousing, formal testing procedure may not reflect a child's functional deficits in the everyday, real-life learning situation (Stores *et al.*, 1978). It can be concluded that attentional factors may be particularly vulnerable to seizure activity (Aldenkamp *et al.*, 1990).

Measures of attentiveness often include a teacher's rating of the child's attentiveness and motor activity level in the classroom, but these more often reflect the teacher's opinions rather than the child's condition; however, this does tend to select children who are underachieving (Stores, 1978). Various tests and subtests have been claimed to identify ADHD (or conditions similar to ADHD), but the observations and interpretations of the evaluator are usually of more value than the test scores. The testing conditions may suppress or incite TCIs and thus not give a true picture. Most observers do not define what they mean by an "attention problem."

Concentration may initially decrease generalized seizure discharges but increase focal discharges. As the novelty wanes, bursts appear with increasing frequency. Comprehension and retention of questions may continue even when seizure bursts occur. More difficulties occur in individuals with generalized epilepsy than with focal epilepsy in continuous performance tests, suggesting the importance of sub-cortical structures in the maintenance of attention (Dikmen, 1980). Attention is involved in that an error in calculation thought to be due to inattention is associated with an increase in paroxysmal activity (Ricci et al., 1972).

An association of generalized EEG discharges, such as seen with absence attacks, may lead to delayed answers or a transient failure to respond during simultaneous EEG intellectual testing (Hovey & Kooi, 1955; Kooi and Hovey, 1957; Binnie, 1980). Many testers would not consider these brief transitory failures during IQ tests as seizures, yet they are handicapping (Quadfasel & Pruysel, 1985; Davidoff & Johnson, 1964; Mirsky & Van Buren, 1965; Binnie, 1980).

With partial seizures and focal discharges, brief epileptiform discharges may cause deviant or depressed responses in testing. Disturbances in higher integrative mental processes are associated significantly with paroxysmal cerebral activity. These disturbances are usually manifested during psychological testing by no-answer responses and, to a less extent, by "don't know" responses and requests for repetition of the question, usually in the absence of overt seizures. Non-responses indicate transient losses of the goal idea by verbal expression of confusion or irrelevant remarks. Sometimes, non-responses or, more frequently, "don't know" responses occur in the absence of EEG bursts. Adequate answers sometimes occur along with bursts (Hovey & Kooi, 1955; Quadfasel & Pruysel, 1985; Alajouanine, 1956).

As compared with the routine clinical EEG, abnormalities decrease during task involvement, as in testing, and increase during a passive or relaxed state. Stress also brings out discharges. A child's performance variability in the classroom and in testing may reflect TCIs (Tarter, 1972).

Therapy

Epileptic children with short attention spans benefit from shorter periods of instructions. Multisensory approaches in conjunction with rote learning approaches are usually effective (Poche, 1978). The general view is that the etiology of disordered attention in children is as varied and complex as the manifestations of attention disorders themselves (Mirsky, 1996).

In children with frequent epileptiform discharges without clinical seizures, occasionally antiepileptic medication has only a limited effect on cognitive functioning, probably due to intrinsic inattention (Henricksen, 1990). Sometimes, a child with unrecognized epilepsy may tend to sit in school, learning nothing and doing nothing. When the underlying epilepsy is considered and treated, the child "awakens" and begins to investigate all they have missed out on for the past years. The teacher then notes the change and brands the child as hyperactive and inattentive, often relating this to the newly started drugs.

Situational management

Physical and mental activity seems to be an antagonist to seizures. Seizures are more apt to occur when the patient is off guard, sleeping, resting, or idling (Livingston & Berman, 1973). Therefore, maintaining optimum alertness may optimize learning.

Focusing activity

Discharges appear least when the child is concentrating and most when the child is bored (Laidlaw & Reichans, 1976a; Stores, 1976) or anxious, as with a disagreeable or stressful situation (Ounsted & Hutt, 1964; Stores, 1980b). When a task causes increased seizure activity, it is important to determine whether this is a low-motivation task or an excessively demanding task. Even a rest period after an accomplishment may trigger discharges (Guey *et al.*, 1969). More bursts occur during non-work periods than during work periods (Fairweather & Hutt, 1971). Thus, the child needs to be assigned tasks that will be non-stressful challenges. Paroxysms may occur if the child dislikes a certain task or senses an impending failure situation. The frequency of paroxysms increases considerably in situations reminiscent of the classroom context, consistent with the almost general prevalence of a variety of scholastic difficulties (Guey *et al.*, 1969). Clinical seizures, including absences, may be more frequent during specific school subject areas, which may merit evaluation of the subject area for possible performance difficulties. The relationship may also be reminiscent of a former classroom setting with emotional connotations (Stores *et al.*, 1978).

Reducing distractions

Distracting stimuli may improve the child's performance in light of spike-wave discharges (Fenwick, 1981). Spike-wave paroxysms may be both evoked and inhibited by the application of appropriate stimuli. Repeated application of specific stimuli during spike-wave paroxysms can, in certain children, more or less permanently modify the future occurrence of such paroxysms (Ounsted & Hutt, 1964). A noisy classroom may improve the performance of some children with epilepsy, paradoxically improving perceptual accuracy, perhaps by stimulating arousal (Stores *et al.*,

1978). This is seen especially in children with absence seizures, resulting in improved vigilance and less distractibility. Other generalized seizure types do not show this benefit. Thus, evaluations in a novel formal testing situation may not reflect adequately the child's everyday real-world learning situation (Weingraumb, 1981).

Children with complex partial seizures may become more distractable in an overly stimulating environment. Children with left temporal seizures may be over-stimulated by a noisy background, while children with right temporal seizures may be distracted by an excess of visual stimuli in the environment. Therefore, it is important to determine what effect, if any, the environment has on the child's performance and to respond accordingly.

Alertness and somnolence

Sleepy children are not alert. Their attention strays easily. Increased incidences of sleep problems and poor sleep exist in patients with epilepsy, often resulting in day-time lethargy as well as adjustment and behavior problems (Zaiwalla, 1989; Binnie, et al., 1990). Some children with epilepsy may have a subtle disorder of arousal mechanisms in sleep, possibly associated with impaired daytime performance (Stores, 1990). Sleep is disturbed in epilepsy by nocturnal seizures or by anomalous sleep patterns due to the epilepsy or to antiepileptic medications (Chemukar et al., 1976). The main sleep disturbance is an increase in sleep state changes, an increase in the number of awakenings, and an increase in the amount of time spent awake. A decrease in REM sleep is seen rarely (Rosen et al., 1982).

Children who have problems with sleep show a clear relationship to problems of performance on tasks involving attention, memory, motor, and cognitive skills, as well as excessive sleepiness. Tests of auditory attention may be depressed, with prominent response failures seen. Daytime alertness is reduced (Carskadon et al., 1987a; Carskadon et al., 1987b). Such children may be inattentive, off-task, lethargic, and irritable, and may seem forgetful.

Seizure-related effects

Nocturnal seizures may have detrimental effects on language functions and memory (Renier, 1987) and on alertness, possibly through the effects of disturbed sleep patterns (Declerck et al., 1989; Aldenkamp et al., 1990). Roughly one-third show seizures related to sleep, including the benign focal epilepsies of childhood. About one-third have seizures upon awakening from sleep. In adults, nearly half experience epilepsies in sleep, but in children the incidence of this is 30%. Roughly 20% experience random seizures. The stages of falling asleep are most apt to bring out CPE or benign partial seizures (Shouse, 1987). Children with CPE are most apt to have such problems associated with sleep disturbances of epilepsy (Rosen et al.,

1982). Epileptic syndromes, such as Lennox–Gastaut syndrome, may be more active in sleep, sometimes presenting as status in slow-wave sleep (Stores, 1990). Seizures with an acquired aphasia with epilepsy including ESES may be accentuated in sleep, with around 85% of patients showing continuous slow spike-wave discharges mainly during non-REM sleep (Shouse, 1987).

Sleep abnormalities are seen more often with generalized epilepsies, especially in patients with frequent, refractory seizures. Patients with generalized epilepsies retire late, have difficulty falling asleep, show frequent shifts between sleep stages, and wake unrefreshed (Chemukar et al., 1976; Binnie et al., 1990). Often, these seizures are associated with a delay to sleep onset, an increased number of awakenings, longer duration of awakenings, decreased or at least fragmented REM sleep, increased shifts between sleep stages, and a generalized reduced sleep efficiency. Such abnormalities are not seen as often with benign partial epilepsies or with bitemporal spikes. Many of the severe epileptic syndromes of childhood, including infantile spasms, present with a variety of sleep problems, even including no discernible sleep cycle (Shouse, 1987).

Seizures occur most often during non-REM sleep (Minecan et al., 2000). Effective antiepileptics tend to reduce REM sleep. If seizures are disturbing sleep patterns, then the anticonvulsant may improve sleep quality. The drugs themselves may alter normal sleep patterns. Drugs that augment the early non-REM sleep stages may reduce related seizures and improve sleep (Shouse, 1987).

Sleep disturbances in epileptic children

Sleep abnormalities are a consistent feature of epilepsy. The abnormalities can range from mild to serious, according to the severity of the seizure disorder and the association of neurologic abnormalities. Sleep instability is the most appropriate general characterization of the sleep disorders of epilepsy, with frequent stage shifts, increased awakenings, and poor sleep efficiency (Shouse, 1987). Thus, epilepsy may disturb the quality of sleep in children. Sleep fragmentation, i.e. repeated brief interruptions in the continuity of sleep with micro-arousals, may be associated with impaired performance and other behavior changes during the day (Bonnet, 1985; Levine et al., 1987; Stores, 1990).

Coexisting sleep disorders are common in epilepsy patients. Complaints of daytime drowsiness may be secondary to sleep disorders rather than to the anticonvulsants in some patients. A good history-taking may elicit a sleep-disordered breathing problem (55%) or depression (10%) due to excessive sleepiness. Some patients have a circadian rhythm sleep disorder or a delayed sleep phase syndrome, often with generalized seizures related to awakening, as with juvenile myoclonic epilepsy.

The epilepsy may fragment the sleep, resulting in repeated brief interruptions in the continuity of the sleep by small arousals, leading to impaired daytime performance and behavior (Bonnet, 1985; Levine *et al.*, 1987; Stores, 1990). Parents report more sleep disturbances in children with epilepsy than in normal children. Other problems include night terrors (in deeper sleep stages), which may be confused with complex partial seizures, especially since 47% of patients may experience epileptiform activities over the temporal lobe. Seizures may coexist with night terrors in some patients, as may headbanging, sleepwalking, and enuresis, without any direct relationship. To verify or disprove such a relationship, an EEG monitored sleep polysomnography may be needed (Shouse, 1987).

Approach

If no daytime events account for school problems in a child with epilepsy, the sleep state needs to be reviewed. A more careful review by the physician about the length, quality, and normality of sleep may reveal the answer and thus provide a route to help. Referral to a center for an overnight sleep study with full EEG monitoring may be justified (Stores, 1990).

REFERENCES

Alajouanine, T. (1956). Verbal realization in aphasia. *Brain* **79**: 1028.

Aldenkamp, A. P., Alpherts, W. C. J., Blennow, G., *et al.* (1993). Withdrawal of anti-epileptic medication in children: effects on cognitive function: the multicenter: Holmfrid study. *Neurology* **43**: 41–50.

Aldenkamp, A. P., Alpherts, W. C. J., Dekker, M. J. A., *et al.* (1990). Neuropsychological aspects of learning disabilities in epilepsy. *Epilepsia* **31** (suppl 4): 9–20.

Arieff, A. (1974). Neurology: epilepsy and learning disorders. *Illinois Med. J.* **146**: 467–70.

Baird, H. W., John, E. R., Ahn, H., *et al.* (1980). Neurometric evaluation of epileptic children who do well and poorly in school. *Electroencephalogr. Clin. Neurophysiol.* **48**: 683–93.

Bennett-Levy, J. & Stores, G. (1984). The nature of cognitive dysfunction in school-children with epilepsy. *Acta Neurol. Scand.* **69** (suppl): 79–82.

Benson, D. E. (1979). Associated neurobehavioral problems. In *Clinical Neurology and Neurosurgical Monographs: Fluent Aphasia, Alexia and Agraphia*, p. 163. New York: Churchill Livingstone.

Binnie, C. D. (1980). Deterioration of transitory cognitive impairments during epileptiform EEG discharges: problems in clinical practice. In *Epilepsy and Behavior '79*, ed. B. R. Kulig, H. Meinardi & G. Stores, pp. 91–7. Lisse: Swets & Zeitlslinger.

Binnie, C. D., Channon, S. & Marston, D. (1990). Learning disabilities in epilepsy: neurophysiological aspects. *Epilespia* **31** (suppl 4): 2–8.

Bonnet, M. H. (1985). Effects of sleep disruption on sleep, performance, and mood. *Sleep* **8**: 11–19, 85.

Brittain, H. (1980). Epilepsy and intellectual functions. In *Epilepsy and Behaivor '79*, ed. B. R. Kulig, H. Meinardi & G. Stores, pp. 2–13. Lisse: Swets & Zeitlinger.

Brown, T. R., Penry, R. S., Porter, R. S., *et al.* (1974). Responsiveness before, during and after spike-wave paroxysms. *Neurology* **24**: 659–65.

Bruhn-Parsons, A. T. & Parsons, O. A. (1977). Reaction time variability in epileptic and gbrain damaged patients. *Cortex* **13**: 373–84.

Camfield, C. S., Chaplin, S., Doyle, A. B., *et al.* (1977). Side effects of phenobarbital in toddlers: behavior and cognitive aspects. *Pediatrics* **95**: 361–5.

Carskadon, M. A., Kewenan, S. & Dement, W. C. (1987a). Nighttime sleep and daytime sleep tendency in preadolescents. In *Sleep and Its Disorders I Children*, ed. C. Guilleminault, pp. 43–52. New York: Raven Press.

Carskadon, M. A., Kewenan, S. & Dement, W. C. (1987b). Nighttime sleep and daytime sleep tendency in adolescents. In *Sleep and Its Disorders I Children*, ed. C. Guilleminault, pp. 53–66. New York: Raven Press.

Chemukar, J., Desai, A. D. & Pabini, R. (1976). The sleeping pattern and incidence of seizure discharges during whole night sleep in grand mal epileptics. *Neurol. India* **24**: 141–7.

Davidoff, R. A. & Johnson, L. C. (1964). Proxysmal EEG activity and cognitive motor perfomrance. *Electroencephalogr. Clin. Neurophysiol.* **16**: 343–54.

Declerck, A. C., Linden, I., van Oei, L. T., *et al.* (1989). Are learning problems in children with epilepsy due to a disturbed sleep. 18th International Epilepsy Congress New Delhi. *Epilepsia* **30**: 155.

Dennerll, R. D. (1964). Prediction of unilateral brain dysfunction using Wechsler test scores. *J. Consult. Psychol.* **28**: 278–84.

Dikmen, S. (1980). Neuropsychological aspects of epilepsy. In *A Multidisciplinary Handbook of Epilepsy*, ed. B. P. Hermann, pp. 236–73. Springfield, IL: Charles C. Thomas.

Dodrill, C. B. & Wilkus, R. J. (1976). Neuropsychological correlates of the electroencephalogram in epileptics. II: the waking posterior rhythms and its interactions with epileptiform activity. *Epilepsia* **17**: 101–9.

Dubinsky, B. L., Wilkening, G. N. & Minarcik, J. R. (1983). Neuropsychologic testing with concurrent electroencephalographic and simultaneous videomonitoring. *Clin. Neuropsychol.* **5**: 41.

Erba, G. & Cavazzuti, V. (1980). Rapid stimulation in continuous performance tasks under EEG monitoring. In *Advances in Epileptology the Xth Epilepsy International Symposium*, ed. J. A. Wada & J. K. Penry, p. 527. New York: Raven Press.

Fairweather, H. & Hutt, S. J. (1969). Interrelationships of EEG activity and information processing on paced and unpaced tasks in epileptic children. *Electroencephalogr. Clin. Neurophysiol.* **27**: 701–10.

Fairweather, H. & Hutt, S. J. (1971). Some effects of performance variables upon generalized spike-wave activity. *Brain* **904**: 321–6.

Fedio, P. & Mirsky, A. F. (1969). Selective intellectual deficits in children with temporal lobe or centrencephalic epilepsy. *J. Neuropsychol.* **7**: 287–300.

Fenwick, P. (1981). EEG studies. In *Epilepsy and Psychiatry*, ed. E. H. Reynolds & M. R. Trimble, pp. 242–53. New York: Churchill Livingstone.

Forster, F. M. (1977). Epilepsy evoked by higher cognitive functions: decision making epilepsy. In *Reflex Epilepsy, Behavioral therapy and Conditioned Reflexes*, pp. 124–34. Springfield, IL: Charles C. Thomas.

Fossen, A. & Gotlibsen, O. B. (1980). The measure of residual effects of CNS acting drugs on behavior. In *Epilepsy and Behaivor '79*, ed. B. R. Kulig, H. Meinardi & G. Stores, pp. 62–6. Lisse: Swets & Zeitlinger.

Geller, M. R. & Geller, A. (1970). Brief amnestic effects of spike-wave discharges. *Neurology* 290: 380–81.

Goode, D. J., Penry, J. K. & Dreifuss, F. E. (1970). Effects of paroxysmal spike-wave on continuous visual-motor performance. *Epilepsia* 22: 24–25.

Guey, J., Burreatt, M., Dravet, C. & Roger, J. (1969). A study of the rhythms of petit mal absences in children in relation to prevailing situations. *Epilepsia* 10: 441–51.

Halperin, J. M. (1996). Conceptualizing, describing, and measuring components of attention: a summary. In *Attention, Memory and Executive Functions,* ed. G. Lyon Reid & N. A. Krasnegor, pp. 119–36. Baltimore, MD: Paul H. Brookes.

Halstead, H. (1957). Abilities and behavior of epileptic children. *J. Ment. Sci.* 103: 28–47.

Heilman, K. M. & Van Den Abell, T. (1979). Right hemispheric dominance for attention. *Neurology* 29: 586.

Henricksen, O. (1990). Education and epilepsy: assessment and remediation. *Epilepsia* 31: 21–5.

Holdsworth, L. & Whitmore, K. (1974). A study of children with epilepsy attending ordinary schools: their seizure patterns progresses and behavior in school. *Dev. Med. Child Neurol.* 16: 746–58.

Hovey, H. B. & Kooi, K. A. (1955). Transient disturbances of thought processes and epilepsy. *Arch. Neurol.* 74: 287–91.

Hutt, S. J. (1972). Experimental analysis of brain activity and behavior in children with "minor" seizures. *Epilepsia* 13: 520–34.

Hutt, S. J. & Fairweather, H. (1971). Spike-wave paroxysms and information processing. *Proc. R. Soc. Med.* 64: 918–19.

Hutt, S. J. & Fairweather, H. (1973). Paced and unpaced serial response performance during two types of EEG activity. *J. Neurosurg. Sci.* 19: 85–96.

Hutt, S. J., Newton, J. & Fairweather, H. (1977). Choice reaction time and EEG time in children with epilepsy. *Neuropsychologica* 15: 257–67.

Ishiharo, T. & Yoshii, N. (1967). The interaction between paroxysmal EETG actaivities and continuous addition work of Uchida–Kraepalin psychodiagnostic test. *Med. J. Osaka Univ.* 18: 75–86.

Jus, A. & Jus, K. L. (1962). Retrograde amnesia in petit mal. *Arch. Gen. Psychiatry* 6: 163–7.

Kooi, K. A. & Hovey, H. B. (1957). Alterations in mental functions and paroxysmal cerebral activity. *Arch. Neurol. Psychiatry.* 78: 264–71.

Laidlaw, J. & Reichans, A. (1976a). Fits in childhood: education. In *A Textbook of Epilepsy*, ed. J. Laidlaw & A. Reichens, pp. 101–2. London: Churchill Livingstone.

Laidlaw, J. & Reichans, A. (1976b). Psychiatry: esp. epilespy and intellectual function. In *A Textbook of Epilepsy*, ed. J. Laidlaw & A. Reichens, pp. 145–84. London: Churchill Livingstone.

Lansdell, H. & Mirsky, A. F. (1964). Attention in focal and centrencephalic epilepsy. *Exp. Neurol.* 9: 463–9.

Lennox, W. G. & Lennox, M. E. (1960). *Epilepsy and Related Disorders.* London: Churchill Livingstone.

Lennox, W. G., Gibbs, E. A. & Gibbs, E. L. (1936). The effect on the EEG of drugs and conditions which influence seizures. *Arch. Neurol. Psychiatry* **35**: 1236–50.

Levine, B., Roiehrs T., Stepanski, E., *et al.* (1987). Fragmented sleep diminishes its recuperative value. *Sleep* **10**: 590–99.

Livingston, S. & Berman, W. (1973). Participation of epileptic patients in sports. *JAMA* **224**: 23–28.

Milstein, V. & Stevens, J. R. (1961). Verbal and conditioned avoidance learning during abnormal EEG discharge. *J. Nerv. Ment. Dis.* **132**: 50–60.

Minecan, D. N., Marzec, M., & Malow, B. A. (2000). Seizure rate variability in different stages of sleep. *Epilepsia* **41** (suppl 7): 167.

Mirsky, A. F. (1960). The relationship between paroxysmal EEG activity and performance on a vigilance task in epileptic patients. *Am. Psychol.* **156**: 486.

Mirsky, A. F. (1969). Studies of paroxysmal EEG phenomena and background EEG in relation to impaired attention. In *Attention in Neurophsyiology*, ed. C. R. Evans & T. B. Mulholland, pp. 310–22. London: Butterworth.

Mirsky, A. F. (1996). Disorders of attention, a neuropsychological perspective. In *Attention, Memory and Executive Function*, ed. G. R. Lyon & N. A. Krasnegor, pp. 71–95. Baltimore, MD: Paul H. Brookes.

Mirsky, A. F. & Van Buren, J. M. (1965). On the nature of the absence in centrencephalic epilepsy: a study of some behavioral electroencephalographic and autonomic factors. *Electroencephalogr. Clin. Neurophysiol.* **18**: 334–48.

Mirsky, A. F., Primac, D. W., Marsan, C. A., *et al.* (1960). A comparison of the psychological test performance of patients with focal and nonfocal epilepsy. *Exp. Neurol.* **2**: 75–89.

O'Donohoe, N. V. (1979). Mental handicap and epilepsy. In *Epilepsies of Childhood*, pp. 143–6. London: Butterworth.

Oostrom, K. J., Schouten, A., Kruitwagen, C. L. J., Peterson, A. C. B. & Jennekens-Schinkel, A. (2002). Attention deficits are not characteristic of schoolchildren with newly diagnosed idiopathic or cryptogenic epilepsy. *Epilepsia* **43**: 301–10.

Ounsted, C. & Hutt S. J. (1964). The effect of attentive factors on bio-electric paroxysms in epileptic children. *Proc. R. Soc. Med.* **57**: 1178.

Ounsted, C., Lindsay, J. & Norman, R. (1966). Intelligence: biological factors in temporal lobe epilepsy. In *Biological Factors in Temporal Lobe Epilepsy*, pp. 62–71. London: Heinemann.

Poche, P. (1978). Educating the child with Seizures. In *The Treatment of Epilepsy Today*, ed. G. S. Ferriss, pp. 127–41. Oradell, NJ: Medical Economics.

Porter, R. J., Penry, J. K. & Dreifuss, F. E. (1973). Responsiveness at the onset of spike-wave bursts. *Electroencephalogr. Clin. Neurophysiol.* **34**: 239–45.

Prechtl, H. F. R., Boeke, P. E. & Schut, T. (1961). The electroencephalogram and performance in epileptic patients. *Neurology* **1**: 296–302.

Quadfasel, A. F. & Pruysel, P. W. (1985). Cognitive deficits in patients with psychomotor epilepsy. *Epilepsia* **4**: 80–90.

Reitan, R. S. (1974). Psychological testing of epileptic patients. In *Handbook of Clinical Neurology*, ed. O. Magnus & A. M. Lorentz, Vol. 15, pp. 559–75. New York: American Elsevier.

Renier, W. O. (1987). Restrictive factors in the education of children with epilepsy form a medical point of view. In *Education and Epilepsy 1987*, ed. A. P. O. Aldenkamp, W. C. J. Alpherts, H. Meinardi & G. Stores, pp. 3–14. Lisse: Swets & Zeitlinger.

Rennick, P. M., Perez-Borja, C. & Rodin, E. A. (1969). Transient mental deficits associated with recurrent prolonged epileptic clouded state. *Epilepsia* **10**: 397–405.

Reynolds, E. H. (1981). The management of seizures associated with psychological disorders. In *Epilepsy and Psychiatry*, ed. E. H. Reynolds & M. R. Trimble, pp. 322–36. New York: Churchill Livingstone.

Ricci, G., Berti, G. & Cherubini, E. (1972). Changes in interictal focal activity and spike wave paroxysms during motor and mental activity. *Epilepsy* **13**: 785–94.

Rosen, I., Blennow, G., Risberg, A. M., *et al.* (1982). Quantitative evaluation of nocturnal sleep in epileptic children. In *Sleep and Epilepsy*, ed. B. M. Sterman, M. N. Shouse & P. Passouant, pp. 97–408. New York: Academic Press.

Schlack, H. G. (1980). Changes of abnormal EEG patterns during mental tasks. *Epilepsia* **21**: 205.

Schwab, R. S. (1941). The influence of visual and auditory stimuli on the electroencephalographic tracing of petit mal. *Am. J. Psychiatry* **97**: 301–12.

Sergeant, J. (1996). A theory of attention: an information processing perspective. In *Attention, Memory, and Executive Function*, ed. G. Lyon Reid & N. A. Krasnegor, pp. 57–70. Baltimore, MD: Paul H. Brookes.

Shalev, R. S. & Amir, N. (1983). Complex partial status epilepticus. *Arch. Neurol.* **40**: 90–92.

Sherman, E. M. S., Armitage, L. L., Connolly, M. B., *et al.* (2000). Behaviors symptomatic of ADHD in pediatric epilepsy: relationship to frontal lobe epileptiform abnormalities and other neurologic predictors. *Epilepsia* **41** (suppl 7): 191.

Shouse, M. N. (1987). Sleep, sleep disorders and epilepsy in children. In *Sleep and Its Disorders in Children*, ed. C. Guilleminault, pp. 291–309. New York: Raven Press.

Somerfill, E. R. & Bruni, J. (1983). Tonic status epilepticus presenting as confusional state. *Ann. Neurol.* **13**: 549–51.

Stores, G. (1971). Cognitive function in children with epilepsy. *Dev. Med. Child Neurol.* **13**: 390–93.

Stores, G. (1973). Studies of attention and seizure disorders. *Dev. Med. Child Neurol.* **15**: 376–82.

Stores, G. (1976). The investigation and managements of school children with epilepsy. *Publ. Health, Lond.* **90**: 171–7.

Stores, G. (1978). School children with epilepsy at risk for learning and behavior problems. *Dev. Med. Child Neurol.* **20**: 502–8.

Stores, G. (1980a). Educational achievement. In *Epilepsy and Behaivor '79*, ed. B. R. Kulig, H. Meinardi & G. Stores, pp. 162–8. Lisse: Swets & Zeitlinger.

Stores, G. (1980b). EEG studies in the behavioral assessment of people with epilepsy. In *Epilepsy and Behaivor '79*, ed. B. R. Kulig, H. Meinardi & G. Stores, pp. 82–90. Lisse: Swets & Zeitlinger.

Stores, G. (1981). Problems of learning and behavior in children with epilepsy. In *Epilepsy and Psychiatry*, ed. E. H. Reynolds & M. R. Trimble, pp. 33–48. New York: Churchill Livingstone.

Stores, G. (1987). Effects on learning of "subclinical" seizure discharges. In *Education and Epilepsy 1987*, ed. A. P. Aldenkamp, W. C. J. Alpherts, H. Meinardi & G. Stores, pp. 14–21. Lisse: Swets & Zeitlinger.

Stores, G. (1990). Electroencephalographic parameters in assessing the cognitive function of children with epilepsy. *Epilepsia* **31** (suppl 40): 45–9.

Stores, G. & Hart, J. (1976). Reading skills of children with generalized or focal epilepsy attending ordinary school. *Dev. Med. Child Neurol.* **18**: 705–16.

Stores, G., Hart, J. & Piran, N. (1978). Inattentiveness in school children with epilepsy. *Epilepsia* **19**: 169–75.

Svoboda, W. B. (1979). Epilepsy and learning problems. In *Learning About Epilepsy*, pp. 186–200. Baltimore, MD: University Park Press.

Svoboda, W. B. (1979). Emotional and behavioral consequences of epilepsy. In *Learning About Epilepsy*, pp. 157–84. Baltimore, MD: University Park Press.

Tarter, R. E. (1972). Intellectual and adaptive functioning in epilepsy. *Dis. Nerv. Syst.* **33**: 763–70.

Tizard, B. & Margerison, J. H. (1963). The relationship between generalized paroxysmal EEG discharges and various test situations in two epileptic patients. *J. Neurol. Neurosurg, Psychiatry* **26**: 308–13.

Tizard, B. & Mungerson, J. M. (1963). Psychological functions during wave-spike discharges. *Br. J. Soc. Clin. Psychol.* **3**: 6–15.

Wagenar, W. A. (1975). Performance of epileptic patients in continuous reaction-time situations. *Am. J. Ment. Defic.* **79**: 726–31.

Weingraumb, P. (1981). The brain: his and hers. *Discover* **April** 15–20.

Wilkus, R. J. & Dodrill, C. B. (1976). Neuropsychological correlates of the electroencephalogram in epileptics. I: topographic distribution and average rate of epileptiform activity. *Epilepsia* **17**: 89–100.

Williams, J. P., Phillips, T., Griebe, M. L., *et al.* (2000). Factors associated with academic achievement in children with controlled epilepsy. *Epilepsia* **41** (suppl 7): 246.

Williams, J., Sharp, G. B. & Griebel, M. I. (1992). Neuropsychological functioning in clinically referred children with epilepsy. *Epilepsia* **33** (suppl 3): 17.

Zaiwalla, Z. (1989). Sleep abnormalities in children with epilepsy. *Electroenicephalogr. Clin. Neurophysiol.* **782**: 29.

19

Memory

"Memory" is a term for a very wide range of phenomena that involves the storage and retrieval of information (Eccles, 1966). Difficulties in memory and concentration may impede intelligence, leading to ineffective functioning (Dreifuss, 1983).

Types of memory

Memory differs, depending on the type of stimuli and the nature of processing. Most commonly referred to are auditory and visual memory, and, to a lesser extent, emotional memory. Other senses are also linked with memory. The different forms are mediated by different yet interrelated neuroanatomic systems. Some memories may be linked in time or place of their occurrence, but others are not. Memory may be stored as interpretations or as more basic habits (O'Keefe & Nadel, 1978; Baker & Joynt, 1986).

Memories are commonly divided into immediate, recent (short-term), and remote (long-term) types (Boller, 1996).

Memory processing

Memory is a complex process consisting of sequential stages involving orientation, attention, mental tracking, learning, retention, and retrieval of both recent and remote events. Memory efficiency varies greatly between individuals (Rapin, 1985). Remembering depends on the context and frequency of the learning experience, as well as curiosity and interest in what is occurring (Kinsbourne & Caplan, 1979). Memory begins with sensory input, which triggers an anticipatory evaluation, leading to the development of a short-term memory.

Perception

Perception is the detecting and distinguishing of differences in a sensation, which requires that the person remembers the stimulus long enough to perceive important details in order to organize and interpret the information into an appropriate response (Rumbaugh & Washburn, 1966; Rapin, 1985). This depends on both attention and immediate memory. The information is processed into auditory codes (phonemes) or visual image codes (icons) (Wagner, 1996; Torgesen, 1996). These are based on low-level sensory properties processed in to higher, more abstract categories. Unless this is processed further, it is lost within 100–200 milliseconds. (visual) to two seconds (auditory). Lateralization of the basic processes begins to emerge, with the dominant hemisphere excelling in verbal processing and the non-dominant hemisphere relating to more complex visual information (Goode *et al.*, 1970).

Perceptual difficulties are common in school children and often linked with attention difficulties, especially in children with early-onset epilepsy. Such children may confuse similar numbers, letters, and words, with reversals, omissions, and sloppiness being common. Perceptual problems may relate to the epilepsy types as well as to the effects of antiepileptic drugs.

Memory storage and recall

Information to be remembered depends on attention, acquisition, consolidation, storage, and retrieval processes, which are interrelated skills. The hippocampus plays a critical role in this. The process begins with activation of low-threshold neurons specific for such memories. The systems are especially sensitive to frequent and recent experiences. The information is categorized, which creates multiple channels for access and retrieval (O'Keefe & Nadel, 1978). Executive memory works with both auditory and visual memory systems, with all three coordinated toward the development of long-term memories and habits (Torgesen, 1996).

Immediate (very short-term, episodic) memory

Immediate memory lasts for seconds to minutes, until it begins to fade rapidly (Eccles, 1966). Traces may remain for up to an hour. Immediate memory outlasts the sensory input by about 150 milliseconds, allowing extensive automatic analysis and categorization to gain understanding. Visual memory begins to fade at about one second and auditory memory in four seconds. The storage span depends on sustained electrical activation of specific neural networks (Rapin, 1985). The immediate memory traces last for up to ten seconds as bioelectrical patterns of firing bursts, which vary as per perceived differences in the stimuli (O'Keefe & Nadel, 1978; Brazier, 1979). Only during this time is retrieval possible. This temporal prolongation allows for recognition and further perceptual processing. The temporal lobe, especially the hippocampus, is involved (Torgesen, 1996).

Short-term (recent, working) memory

Short-term memory lasts minutes, declines over hours, and fades over days. Without reinforcement, non-verbal short-term memory fades within 15–30 second; verbal memories fade even faster, depending on the nature of the information. Beyond this time, performance is increasingly mediated by long-term memory systems that process the information into long-term storage (O'Keefe & Nadel, 1978). The information begins to decay unless it undergoes additional processing through rehearsal. The information may re-emerge after hours to a few days, suggesting an ongoing conversion process. The longer the information remains in short-term memory, the more likely it is to be shifted into long-term memory (Wagner, 1996).

Memory exists in two forms, ionic memory consisting of charged radicals such as electrolytes, and macromolecular memory existing as large protein structures. Short-term memory is ionic memory, found in all nerve cells as a consequence of their activities. It is temporary and usually involves a single pathway as a memory loop, continuously storing memories that are being processed (Brazier, 1979). This allows protein synthesis towards ultimate storage through rehearsal (Wagner, 1996). This begins within minutes but is ongoing over hours. Anterior mesial-temporal structures, including the hippocampal-limbic circuitry, consolidate these bits of information (Widman *et al.*, 1999). The ultimate consolidation and retention phase may take up to several months (Rapin, 1985). Short-term memory impairment does not necessarily distort long-term memory (Wagner, 1996).

The short-term memory system has a limited capacity and short duration, preserving items in the correct order. Rehearsal counteracts the decay tendency but does not enhance the capacity to remember (O'Keefe & Nadel, 1978). This memory process may be augmented by emotional intensity, by repeats of moderate intensity, or by rote repetitive input (Hart, 1975). The process may be disrupted by background noise, especially similar to noise that is being remembered, which may relate to the difficulties some children with complex partial seizures have in a noisy classroom (Torgesen, 1996).

Short-term memory is important in listening and reading comprehension (Wagner, 1996). Children with reading disability may be affected by the size of the material and its familiarity. They may have problems when they are expected to perform simultaneously and sequentially identify, compare, and blend information needed in phonetic identification (Torgesen, 1996). Interaction with long-term memory appears to be more important for reading comprehension. Auditory short-term memory disabilities are especially prominent in children with dominant or bitemporal lobe seizure disorders.

Intermittent (medium-term) memory

This is a transitional state related to conscious, vigorous, short-term memory, as in cramming for a meeting or a test. This relates to the situation and may not be retained well beyond the situation. This may be a transitional state of translation into long-term memory, in which activation of any portion of the memory activates retrieval of the remainder. Associative recall helps, such as "smelly ... feet." Meaning is generated, thus greatly facilitating recall (O'Keefe & Nadel, 1978).

Long-term (permanent, remote) memory

Long-term memory contains information in the memory stores for a long time, perhaps a lifetime (Eccles, 1966). It appears to be of unlimited capacity and to be diffuse, existing as bits of information scattered diffusely throughout the brain (Hart, 1975; Baker & Joynt, 1986); if half the brain is removed or the corpus callosum is severed, memory is not impaired (Rapin, 1985). Long-term memory comprises macromolecular permanent cellular structures (Hart, 1975), built into the fine structure of the brain by modifying educated cells (Eccles, 1966) that appear to influence or delineate specific pathways (Rapin, 1985). Perhaps this leads to some type of cellular specialization (Brazier, 1979). Glial cells appear perhaps to steer nerve extensions as well as assist in the memory-protein-building process (Hart, 1975). Thus, memory assumes a permanent, non-erasable form.

A portion of long-term memory may assume a heightened state of activation at a particular moment to be used as short-term memory. Short-term memory, rather than being a dedicated storage area, appears to be a large number of neural circuits activated temporarily for both processing and storage. As the process continues, new portions of long-term memory become active and previously activated portions decay, to return to their former resting state of inactivation (Wagner, 1996).

The memory bits are widespread throughout the brain, although they tend to cluster around the primary sensory cortices, i.e. auditory memory around the auditory cortex and visual memories around the visual cortex. The limbic system binds together these dispersed memories as a single experience. The hippocampus may be involved in long-term storage of local information, giving it a central role in memory recognition (O'Keefe & Nadel, 1978). There are integration connections between the limbic system (especially the anterior cingulate) and the prefrontal dorsal areas of the neocortex that facilitate coding of memory processes (Brazier, 1979). In complex partial epilepsy of limbic orgin in children, both short-term and long-term memories may be distorted developmentally, leading to impaired memory processing.

Recall

Recall is a complex active process of retrieval of needed information. Recall problems may be due to faulty storage (leading to retrieval omissions or distortions) or to inadequate retrieval. Retrieval may be faulty due to interference from information stored at other times, or from the intrusion of memories from other sources (Hart, 1975). Recall is influenced by motive and relies on recall strategies (Luria, 1973; Hart, 1975). Cues may help to facilitate recall (O'Keefe & Nadel, 1978).

Constant remolding of memory occurs, as newer memories replace older ones. Memories may be subject to contamination by leaking from related bits of information. People tend to fill in gaps in recall but may confuse sources, thus embedding various bits of information together. Time and place appear the most likely to fade and to be contaminated. The normal aging processes of the brain that leads to faulty or failed remembering may degrade memory. Forgetting may also be an active process, just as remembering is. Forgetting may be the result of inhibitory influences by irrelevant or interfering activities on the traces rather than a gradual decay (Luria, 1973).

The anatomy of memory

The memory system utilizes circuits within the limbic-diencephalic regions of the brain, together with closely related neocortical regions, particularly those of the anterior temporal-insular and prefrontal areas (Baker & Joynt, 1986). The limbic system, especially the hippocampus, appears related especially to short-term memory but it does play some role in long-term memory storage. Long-term memory involves the entire cortex for storage without lateralization specificity. If one hemisphere is damaged, then remote, perceptuomotor, cognitive, and short-term memories are relatively preserved but deficits are seen in visual, auditory, and tactile memory processes.

Temporal lobe and hippocampus

Memory functions are linked to the mesial portion of the temporal lobes, especially the hippocampus and connected structures. Short-term memory uses the hippocampal-limbic system to store, maintain, and retrieve new material specific memories. This is time-limited (Rapin, 1985; Baker & Joynt, 1986; Giovagnoli *et al.*, 1995). The temporal-limbic system is linked closely to all sensory and motor areas and also draws in emotionally charged memories. The anterior temporal lobe relates to antegrade memory and the consolidation of memory being established for immediate recall. The posterior temporal lobe pertains to retrograde memory and impairs retrieval of recently stored information, although other information may pass through. Recent and remote information may be served by common retrieval systems (Fenwick, 1981).

The dominant temporal lobe relates to deficits of acquisition, recall, and recognition of verbal materials (Baker & Joynt, 1986). Auditory short-term memory relates to disturbances in the area of the supramarginal angular gyrus (Warrington *et al.*, 1971). If the hippocampus is involved, the verbal memory deficit is more severe. Confrontation naming may be impaired, although less so with recent registrations. Delayed recall of stories and paired words may be impaired. This may disturb reading and word fluency. This appears to relate to more anterior and lateral disturbances.

The non-dominant temporal lobe is involved in the construction of spatial relationships and spatial memories. It either consolidates short-term memory or retrieves information once remembered (Trimble & Thompson, 1981). Lesions may produce deficits such as perceptual-spatial memories for geometric figures, topographic details, and facies, and also for melodies (Baker & Joynt, 1986).

Bilateral lesions of the hippocampus produce severe short-term memory deficits but retain long-term memories. There are general deficits affecting all forms of behaviors, such as intentions, recent actions, and so on. Problems ranging from a slight forgetfulness to severe disturbances of consciousness with total confusion for time and place may result. This may be an impairment of the handling of memory traces. The result is either a loss or a mixing of two stimuli. Luria (1973) provides an example of this mixing of stimuli. The patient is given two sentences: "The apple is growing in the garden beyond the high fence" and "The hunter killed a wolf at the edge of the forest." The patient may remember the sentences as only one sentence, such as "The hunter killed a wolf at the edge of the garden" or "Apple trees grew at the edge of the forest," thus focusing two thoughts into one.

Frontal lobe

The frontal lobe modifies memory processes and appears to organize remembering. Deep regions of the frontal lobe, along with deep regions of the temporal lobes, maintain the selectivity of memory, acting somewhat as a dynamic pacemaker, linked to other parts of the system to maintain mental processing (Brazier, 1979). The prefrontal zone of the brain appears to be involved in the active intention to memorize. Individuals with prefrontal impairments learn through stereotyped repetition, but the learning curve plateaus. This is a passive learning. Such individuals can repeat but cannot utilize aids to memory (Luria, 1973).

Memory problems arise when an event cannot be categorized for recall, which appears to be a frontal lobe function (Baker & Joynt, 1986). With frontal lobe damage, patients are not only inattentive; they also "forget to remember." Thinking is thus concrete (Trimble, 1988). Frontal lobes are immature in children. Up to age seven or eight years, normal children respond much like adults with frontal lobe damage. Patients with damage to specific zones of the frontal lobe are prone to confabulation. The confabulator picks out bits or pieces of an actual memory but confuses its true context and draws on other bits of experience to construct a story that makes sense out of it.

Parietal lobe

The parietal lobes, which are mature by six to seven years of age, are involved in short-term memory, especially spatial memory (O'Keefe & Nadel, 1978; Kurokawa *et al.*, 1980). Patients with non-dominant temporal epileptic discharges may exhibit perceptual memory problems through extension of the epileptiform field to involve the parietal lobe.

General neocortex

Long-term memory storage may occur randomly throughout the cortex. Focal lesions do not necessarily destroy a specific memory, as there appear to be other copies of the same memory in other sites (LeDoux *et al.*, 1978).

Development

One or more of the structures of the medial temporal lobes and perhaps more specifically the hippocampal formation may not be developed fully at birth, yet the medial temporal lobe structures develop early in infancy. The developing recognition ability indicates that the medial temporal lobe makes a critical contribution to visual recognition memory even at an early age (Bachevalier *et al.*, 1996). Young children remember well, particularly at short intervals. Memory improves with age (Merritt *et al.*, 1994). Even within the first few months of life the individual begins to learn predictive relationships. Predictive relationships are learned more readily than arbitrary relationships and can be learned by observations, not necessarily requiring overt motor responses. Reinforcement schedules inherently define the reliability of the perceived/predictive relationship. They can either facilitate or interfere with learning. Schedules strongly influence motivation (Rumbaugh & Washburn, 1966). At three to six months of age, infants learn by novel stimuli that a movement evokes a response (Boller, 1996). Children at three to four years tend to rely on more specific yes–no questions. Older children, by six to seven years, are able to provide spontaneously more information in response to open-ended questions (Merritt *et al.*, 1994).

Memory insults and deficits

Memory deficits, generalized or specific, may exist in storage or in retrieval. Storage may be faulty. Information may be stored but not in the correct context. Deficits in retention of old memories may also be a selective failure in context-dependent memory (O'Keefe & Nadel, 1978), in loss of memory, in confabulation in intrusion errors, and in déjà vu experiences (Baker & Joynt, 1986). Damage to one hemisphere affects short-term memory primarily. Long-term memory is affected only if a severe dementia results in bilateral loss of many brain cells (O'Keefe & Nadel, 1978). The hippocampus appears to be important in storage processing (Trimble & Thompson, 1981).

Faulty memory processing may be the result of neurotransmitter balances, caused by drugs, hormones, seizures, emotional states, or brain damage. CNS amines influence the consolidation and retrieval processes, especially in the dorsal hippocampus and upper brainstem. Norepinephrine (noradrenaline) relates to memory consolidation, as do many hormones. Dopamine is involved in memory retrieval (Brazier, 1979).

Drugs that affect the cholinergic linkage may alter the transition from short-term to long-term memory (Brazier, 1979). Anticonvulsants have the potential to interfere with memory, especially at high therapeutic dosages or in polytherapy, although the effects are usually modest and due primarily to the affect on attention. Memory tasks that do not have high attentional demands, such as memory for word lists and figure memory, are frequently insensitive to antiepileptic drug effects, whereas memory tasks with a high attentional load, such as verbal paragraph memory, are more sensitive. Children and elderly patients may be particularly sensitive to drug effects.

Physiologic states

Sleep benefits the retention of information learned during wakefulness, especially paradoxical sleep. Memory traces acquired shortly before sleep are not insulated from interference during sleep. Information processing is triggered after registration and continues during sleep in periods when necessary brain activation occurs (Brazier, 1979). Learning during waking hours results in a pattern of cells activated in the hippocampus. In sleep, these cells fire synchronously, suggesting that memory consolidation is occurring. People who have their sleep interrupted when they enter into the REM state are impaired in memory tests. Seizures and seizure medications that alter or impair restful sleep may thus impair memory processes.

Memory is reduced in affect disorders, particularly depression (Trimble, 1988). Distress occurring during an activity being remembered may interfere more with subsequent retrieval than with early encoding in the memory system (Merritt et al., 1994). Severe stresses, such as post-traumatic stress syndrome, can alter brain chemical transmitters by causing neurotransmitter imbalances.

Seizures and subclinical discharges

In epilepsy, memory disturbances, particularly for more recent events, may be seen. There is strong evidence for lateral specificity, i.e. the left hemisphere for verbal material (especially names) and the right hemisphere for non-verbal material (Trimble & Thompson, 1981). The right hippocampus appears to be vital for defects in exploration and spatial mapping (O'Keefe & Nadel, 1978).

Memory deficits of epilepsy

Epilepsy in children may impair the development of memory skills and alter lateralizations. In children with epilepsy, problems in immediate memory and delayed recall are not obvious (Davies-Eysenck, 1952). Response times are slowed. Major memory dysfunctions tend to emerge in adolescence, suggesting a particular vulnerability at this age (Macleod et al., 1978). Memory deficits are often blamed on a lack of attention and concentration (Folsom, 1953; Von Isser, 1977).

Impaired memory is associated with partial (cortical) rather than generalized seizures (Fedio & Mirsky, 1969; Glowinski, 1973; Trimble & Thompson, 1981), which is the reverse of attention functions. Memory impairments are common, even in patients with controlled seizures. All stages of the memory system can be affected (Folsom, 1953).

Generalized epilepsies

Children with generalized epilepsies have attention problems that cause them to miss out on facts (Von Isser, 1977) rather than obvious memory deficits (Stores, 1971). Children with generalized seizure disorders may show more problems with visual sequential memory than auditory memory deficits. They may also have visual perceptual difficulties, which may be linked with attention difficulties.

Generalized tonic–clonic seizures

Children with GTC seizures often have a low average memory (Quadfasel & Pruyser, 1955), although those with early onset may show weaknesses in memory and complex problem-solving (O'Leary et al., 1981). Problems with digit span, digit symbols (rote memory), and information (remote memory tasks) have been reported (Lewinski, 1947).

Absence seizures

With absence attacks, memory may be impaired primarily during rather than between attacks. The degree of memory loss for events occurring during a seizure varies from a complex amnesia to total retention of memory (Freeman et al., 1973). Memory recall may be impaired for a stimulus that precedes the discharge by up to four seconds or may be sustained for the first few seconds of the attack (Barlow, 1978). Memory may be lost especially with longer discharges and briefly afterwards (Freeman et al., 1973). Disturbances of high integrative mental processes (Kooi & Hovey, 1957) and antegrade and retrograde amnesia (Jus & Jus, 1962), impairment of sensory function and subsequently motor function (Mirsky et al., 1960), and impairment of short-term memory (Hutt & Gilbert, 1980) have all been reported with spike-wave discharges, including subclinical paroxysms. Rarely, the impairment may be perceptual, mnemonic, or motor (Gloor, 1986).

Febrile convulsions

Memory is intact in children with a history of febrile memory except for occasional weaknesses in those with seizures before age one year. Children with a neurodevelopmental delay before their first febrile convulsion are more at risk for executive function and memory problems (Chang *et al.*, 2001).

Partial epilepsies

Cortical focal seizures are most often associated with memory deficits and are less apt to present with attention problems, regardless of the seizure type, seizure frequency, or drug use (Loiseau *et al.*, 1980; Loiseau *et al.*, 1983). Patients with simple partial epilepsy or to a lesser extent with an anterior EEG focus have some memory impairments, mainly for learning, with less impairment for digit span (Macleod *et al.*, 1978). Areas much larger than the hippocampal-limbic circuitry are involved in memory dysfunctions, especially those situated frontally (Aldenkamp *et al.*, 1990). Individuals with complex partial seizures are especially at risk for memory problems (Von Isser, 1977).

Frontal lobe

Severe memory problems and attention difficulties may be caused by unilateral impairment of specific structures outside of the hippocampus (Mellanby *et al.*, 1984), such as the prefrontal cortex (Kertesz, 1983). Differences are found in verbal processes and in visual and verbal memory areas (Swartz *et al.*, 1993). Lesional epilepsy shows the greatest deficits (Lux *et al.*, 2000). Children with a frontal epileptogenic focus do not show severe neuropsychologic deficits but may have a variety of frontal dysfunctions. Intellectual functioning is relatively normal and little laterality effect is noted, except that children with left frontal foci may have a significantly impaired long-term memory (Riga *et al.*, 1998).

Temporal lobe

Children with complex partial seizures, especially those due to lesions, are especially prone to impaired memory functions, due to several problems in the verbal memory system (Mirsky *et al.*, 1960; Glowinski, 1973; Ladavas *et al.*, 1979; Hutt & Gilbert, 1980; Mayeux *et al.*, 1980; Stores, 1981; Loiseau *et al.*, 1983; Binnie *et al.*, 1990). Insults may be a small, localized deficit or a larger, more posterior, often bilateral lesion, which may be associated with a fluent aphasia (Sherwin & Efron, 1980). Verbal functions and related memory are more often depressed, especially with dominant involvement (Quadfasel & Pruyser, 1955; McIntyre *et al.*, 1976).

Short-term and recent memory are most affected, presenting as problems in the consolidation and registration phases. Even subclinical discharges may produce this interference. This is seen in integrating and memorizing verbal materials. This is unrelated to the IQ, the laterality of the discharge, the onset age, and the medications in use (Brown & Reynolds, 1981).

Hippocampal memory problems may be temporary, anterograde and prolonged, or permanent. Both temporary and permanent amnesia may follow a single seizure or a flurry of seizures. Episodic amnesia is briefly disruptive and associated with interictal spikes. The hippocampus is involved in the consolidation of memory, transferring short-term memory to long-term memory. This appears to be associated with the hilar CA3 area. Recognition memory problems correlate with hilar/dentate cell losses unilaterally. This appears to be material-specific. Thus, specific correlations seem to exist between hippocampal subfield and specific memory functions (Kortenkamp, 1996).

Mesial versus neocortical memory

Patients with more diffuse temporal seizure onset are different to those with amygdala hippocampal onset. Damage to mesial-temporal structures is less in such patients. Slightly more than half (55%) of those with amygdala–hippocampal foci have lateralized memory impairment, whereas only 20% of those with neocortical onset have lateralized memory deficits (French et al., 1992).

Surgical resection of a temporal lobe seizure focus for relief of intractable seizures may lead to improvement of intelligence and memory in some patients (Powell et al., 1975). Memory losses seen with medial-temporal lobe excision involve both antegrade and some retrograde amnesia, leaving early memories and technical skills intact (Milner & Scoville, 1957). A unilateral resection does not produce significant deficits unless there is bilateral damage. A direct relationship exists between memory deficits and the extent of damage. Patients with classic mesial-temporal sclerosis experience less memory decline postoperatively than do patients with normal or less damaged hippocampal findings. Identification of structural measures alone does not indicate an adequate means of assessing functional status (Westerveld et al., 1999; Westerveld, 2002).

Children with unilateral temporal lobe epilepsy exhibit selective verbal and visual memory deficits. The visual memory defect is apparently more important preoperatively in children than in adults with right temporal lobe epilepsy (Jambaque et al., 1992). Children with idiopathic epilepsy with complex partial seizures have improved performance in visual memory and visual motor integration over time, but children with generalized convulsive seizures do not; this is not drug-related (Bailet & Turk, 1992). There may be little, if any decrease in memory skills for children with well-controlled epilepsy when repetition is provided. Improved memory performance with recognition cues suggests that a multiple-choice format may be beneficial in learning tasks for children with epilepsy. There is a greater loss of recall over time. Recognition cues improve memory performance (Sharp *et al.*, 2000).

Dominant (left) temporal lobe epilepsy

Deficits in verbal memory are associated with left temporal lobe seizures (Fedio & Mirsky, 1969; Delaney *et al.*, 1980). These include defects of retention and learning of verbal materials (Stores, 1971). Dominant TLE patients may exhibit long-term verbal memory problems (Kurokawa *et al.*, 1980).

Dominant temporal lobe patients are significantly more impaired in learning verbal short-term knowledge, especially in the encoding and consolidation phase, and in serial information processing. They remember less verbal information and forget more rapidly. Naming problems are more prevalent with left posterior EEG abnormalities (Waxman & Geschwind, 1975; Stores, 1978; Ladavas *et al.*, 1979; Brittain, 1980; Kertesz, 1983; Mellanby *et al.*, 1984; Mungas *et al.*, 1985; Renier, 1987; Binnie, 1988; Aldenkamp *et al.*, 1990). The basic impairment may be an anomia that may contribute to the impairment of verbal learning and memory. Both circumlocution and circumstantiality may compensate for the anomia (Mayeux *et al.*, 1980). Deficits in recall of verbal material in associative learning and short prose passages are seen, as are difficulties in recalling verbal materials delivered under dichotic listening conditions (Fedio & Mirsky, 1969). Patients with left TLE show relatively few problems with visual item storage or long-term retrieval (Giovagnoli *et al.*, 1995).

A small number of people with TLE display rapid forgetting rates due to a deficit in encoding rather than the problems of consolidation usually associated with temporal lobectomy. Usually, left TLE is associated with semantic rather than encoding problems. In this group of patients, there appears to be no laterality of the encoding strategies. This suggests that deficient semantic encoding, regardless of the seizure laterality, may underlie poor word list retention in TLE (Troster *et al.*, 1991).

Patients with left hippocampal sclerosis do more poorly than those with right hippocampal sclerosis on immediate and delayed prose recall (Baxendale *et al.*, 1998). These trends are seen especially with mesial damage, which affects in particular delayed memory skills (Zimmerman *et al.*, 1951). The extent of left hippocampal neuron loss correlates significantly with impairment in learning unrelated word pairs. Intellectual and other memory scores do not correlate to hippocampal neuron loss. Hippocampal mossy fiber sprouting may contribute independently to this learning deficit (Rausch *et al.*, 1992). The deficits appear to be related to prolonged duration of the epileptic problem more than to gender or etiology (Kurokawa *et al.*, 1980).

Children with dominant TLE demonstrate significantly lower performance in verbal memory (including the retention and learning of verbal materials), mild impairment of visual-spatial memory, and lower test scores related to denomination and concept formation (Meyer & Jones, 1957; Fedio & Mirsky, 1969; Stores, 1978). Verbal reasoning and learning functions may be impaired (Reitan, 1974). Such children need to try more times to learn. A general verbal inefficiency is noted (Fedio & Mirsky, 1969; Brown & Reynolds, 1981). This is especially apparent in more complex verbal processes and in delayed recall (Delaney et al., 1980). The mild impairment in visual-spatial memory in the dominant group may be related to difficulties in using verbal mediation strategies as a means of facilitating learning and recall of non-verbal material (Battaglia, 1998). If a lesional etiology for the seizures is found, the impairments appear to be more prominent. After successful therapy, the impairment may disappear, suggesting that normal lobe functioning has been restored (Meyer & Falconer, 1960).

Non-dominant (right) temporal lobe epilepsy

People with right CPE show a deficit of learning characterized by impairment in storing visual material and consistently retrieving it from long-term memory. The problem appears to be more of storage than of retrieval (Giovagnoli et al., 1995). There is relative preservation of verbal memory and expressive speech skills (Rausch et al., 1978; Lux et al., 2000).

Right CPE is associated with visual perceptual-motor difficulties (Barlow, 1978), including the ability to discriminate and understand temporal and spatial patterns and relationships, in the appropriate sequential arrangement. This includes visual-spatial problem-solving even amid a confusing background (Milner & Scoville, 1957; Reitan, 1974; Milner, 1975). Individuals with right CPE have more problems with unfamiliar stimuli (Kimura, 1962). Recognition recall and facial recognition may also be impaired (Milner, 1968). This suggests some involvement of the right parietal lobe. Visual imagery is involved little (Read, 1981). Individuals with right CPE also may have trouble in recognizing snatches of melodies (Milner, 1968). Colors may also be appreciated differently (Lansdell, 1968).

Significant impairments of non-verbal visual memory exist in right CPE patients (Fedio & Mirsky, 1969; Stores, 1971; Doyle et al., 1974; Delaney et al., 1980; Brown & Reynolds, 1981). This includes memory for visual patterns, spatial memory, and memory for geometric designs (Zimmerman et al., 1951; Fedio & Mirsky, 1969; Milner, 1975; Delaney et al., 1980). Some patients may get around this by verbalizing the task (Milner, 1975). Reproducing designs by memory, copying figures, and working with matrices may be disturbed (Fedio & Mirsky, 1969). Reduction of the right hippocampal volume correlates with problems of delayed recall of figures (Baxendale et al., 1998).

Right CPE impairs performance in children, resulting in depressed non-verbal skills (Brown & Reynolds, 1981) manifest as subtle deficits in cognitive and perceptual problems in visual analysis. Defects in visual-spatial organization may be seen, along with impaired memory for non-verbal materials and non-verbal attention (Stores, 1971; Stores, 1976; Battaglia, 1998). These children show a significant loss in the reproducing of test designs from memory after a brief delay. Visual sequential memory may be depressed in right and in left CPE children. Right temporal lobe individuals tend to be faster in task completion, but they are more impulsive, with more errors than left CPE patients. This becomes more apparent in older children and may represent specific deficits in visual-spatial organization (McIntyre et al., 1976; Stores et al., 1978).

Bilateral temporal lobe

Patients with bilateral hippocampal damage have a loss of the ability to retain new information in long-term memory. The transition from short-term to long-term memory is impaired. This can be seen as early as eight to ten years of age. These children can hold information in short-term memory, but if distracted they cannot remember what they were doing. Such patients show continuous antegrade amnesia for the events of daily life. Some retrograde amnesia for the period immediately preceding the critical brain insult may be noted. This is not a complete loss, and certain forms of learning may be spared (Milner, 1968).

Children with hypoxic-ischemic insults in the perinatal period may be found to have severe bilateral hippocampal damage manifest by marked impairments in recall and episodic memory for everyday events but they may display relatively preserved recognition and semantic memory, i.e. memory for factual information. They may attend mainstream schools and acquire average levels in intelligence, language, and literacy skills. However, the memory impairments show up in everyday tasks, such as remembering routes, appointments, and messages, leading to problems of independence in later life. Such children also show as great an impairment of recall and episodic memory as do patients with onset of damage in later life, suggesting that they do not profit from the plasticity of early childhood (Vargha-Kahdem, 2001). Children with bitemporal epilepsy and learning disabilities tend to perform poorly in visual reception, yet often they do not display significant visual sequential memory problems (Trimble, 1980). A striking deficit in auditory sequential memory is noted.

Patient perceptions

Patients often complain of poor memory for remote events, but the complaints correlate weakly with the psychologic finding and they are able to carry out daily activities (Piazzini et al., 1998). Those with dominant temporal lobe problems complain least and have the most problems, whereas the reverse is seen with non-dominant CPE (Hendriks *et al.*, 1998). Both may manifest remote memory impairments (Bergin *et al.*, 1993). Clinical examinations often miss the problems found in memory areas on more specific testing. Often, the problem is a selective anomia from the inferior left temporal lobe (Mayeux *et al.*, 1980; Denman & Wannamaker, 1983). Remediative therapy may help the patient's functioning, resulting in more self-confidence and an increased ability to handle daily memory problems, although it may not alter the neuropsychologic test performance (Hedriks *et al.*, 1991; Westerveld *et al.*, 1999).

Epileptic amnestic syndrome

Adults may present with acute episodes of memory deficits, later found to be associated with CPE manifest by short impairments of contact and oral automatisms, not recalled by the patient. The individuals may be able to carry out ordinary and some complex activities. Interictal EEG shows hippocampal-mesial-temporal sharp activities. Selective impairment in some long-term verbal memory tasks may be found. This has not yet been reported in children (Gallasi *et al.*, 1988).

Transient cognitive deficits

Some patients experience persistent short-term memory difficulties without any history of seizures but are found to have epileptiform discharges on the EEG, although they have never experienced any episodic mental status change. Treatment with low-dosage antiepileptic monotherapy may be beneficial (Hasegawa, 2000). Discharges are sometimes divided into activity accompanied by clinical symptomatology and subclinical activity, i.e. TCIs. Cognitive impairment occurs even with subclinical discharges (Stores, 1987; Binnie *et al.*, 1987; Binnie, 1988). The acquisition phase of memory appears to be especially vulnerable if these discharges occur (Binnie *et al.*, 1987), apparently because it prevents the consolidation of acquired information.

Modifying factors

Etiology

Patients with significant lesions in the temporal lobes show material specific memory deficits dependent on the side of the pathologic findings (Durwen, 1992).

Onset age

In early-onset CPE, the right hemisphere is more likely to restitute originally left-hemisphere temporal-limbic functions than left-hemisphere neocortical functions.

The degree of restitution on either level tends to suppress originally right-hemisphere functions (Helmstaedter *et al.*, 1992).

Frequency

More frequent discharges in individuals with left-sided lesions are associated with greater verbal impairment; more discharges in subjects with right-sided lesions are associated with non-verbal impairments (Powell *et al.*, 1975; Binnie *et al.*, 1990). This may induce difficulties in elementary reading processes by obstructing the development of stable word recollection. Seizure frequency may influence learning, as may intractable epilepsies with foci in the temporal lobe.

Duration

Patients with epilepsy of long duration have worse memory scores. A greater number of seizures leads to a worsening of verbal memory. Patients with seizures in the non-dominant temporal lobe have loss of verbal memory functions in the contralateral side. The loss is progressive over time and increases with an increasing number of seizures (Sawrie *et al.*, 2000).

Antiepilepsy drugs

Reduction of anticonvulsant doses leads to significant improvement in memory performance in people with left temporal seizures, implying the influence of antiepileptic drugs on the epileptic focus (Durwen, 1992).

REFERENCES

Aldenkamp, A. P., Alpherts, W. C. J., Dekker, M. J. A., *et al.* (1990). Neuropsychological aspects of learning disabilities in epilepsy. *Epilepsia* 31 (suppl 4): 9–20.

Bachevalier, J., Malkova, L. & Beauregard, M. (1996). Multiple memory systems: a neuropsychological and developmental perspective. In *Attention, Memory and Executive Function*, ed. G. Reid Lyon & N. A. Krasnegor, pp. 185–98. Baltimore, MD: Paul H. Brookes.

Bailet, L. L. & Turk, W. R. (1992). Differential growth rates of visual memory and visual motor integration in childhood onset epilepsy. *Epilepsia* 33 (suppl 3): 8.

Baker, A. B. & Joynt, R. J. (1986). *Clinical Neurology*, Vol. 1. Philadelphia: Harper & Row.

Barlow, C. F. (1978). Risk factors of infancy and childhood: interrelationship of seizure disorders and mental retardation. In *Mental Retardation and Related Disorders*, pp. 68–75. Philadelphia: FA Davis.

Battaglia, F. M. (1998). Neuropsychological aspects of TLE in children. 3rd European Congress of Epileptology. *Epilepsia* 39 (suppl 2): 70.

Baxendale, S. A., van Paesschen, W., Thompson, P. J., *et al.* (1998). The relationship between quantitative MRI and neuropsychological functioning in temporal lobe epilepsy. *Epilepsia* 39: 158–66.

Bergin, P. S., Basendale, S. A., Thompson, P. J., *et al.* (1993). Remote memory in epilepsy. *Epilepsia* **34** (suppl 6): 70.

Binnie, C. D. (1988). Seizures, EEG discharges and cognition. In *Epilepsy, Behavior and Cognitive Function*, ed. M. R. Trimble & E. H. Reynolds, pp. 45–51. Chichester, UK: John Wiley & Sons.

Binnie, C. D., Channon, S. & Marston, D. (1990). Learning disabilities in epilepsy: neurophysiological aspects. *Epilepsia* **31** (suppl 40): 2–8.

Binnie, C. D., Kasteleijn-Nolst Trenite, D. G. A., Smit, A. M., *et al.* (1987). Interactions of epileptiform EEG discharges and cognition. *Epilepsy Res.* **1**: 239–45.

Boller, K. (1996). Conceptualizing, describing and measuring components of memory: a summary. In *Attention, Memory and Executive Function*, ed. G. Reid Lyon & N. A. Krasnegor, pp. 221–32. Baltimore, MD: Paul H. Brookes.

Brazier, M. A. B. (1979). *Brain Mechanisms in Memory and Learning.* New York: Raven Press.

Brittain, H. (1980). Epilepsy and intellectual functions. In *Epilepsy and Behavior*, ed. B. M. Kulig, H. Meinardi & G. Stores, pp. 2–13. Lisse: Swets & Zeitlinger.

Brown, S. W. & Reynolds, E. H. (1981). Cognitive impairments in epileptic patients. In *Epilepsy and Psychiatry*, ed. E. H. Reynolds & M. R. Trimble, pp. 47–163. New York: Churchill Livingstone.

Chang, Y. C., Guo, N. W., Wang, S. T., *et al.* (2001). Working memory of school-aged children with a history of febrile convulsions: a population study. *Neurology* **57**: 37–42.

Davies-Eysenck, M. (1952). Cognitive factors in epilepsy. *J. Neurol. Neurosurg. Psychiatry* **15**: 39–44.

Delaney, R. C., Rosen, A. J., Mattson, R. H., *et al.* (1980). Memory function in focal epesy: a comparison of non-surigcal unilateral temporal lobe and frontal lobe samples. *Cortex* **16**: 103–17.

Denman, S. B.& Wannamaker, B. B. (1983). Neuropsychological memory scale in temporal lobe epileptic patients. *Epilepsia* **24**: 258.

Doyle, J. C., Ornstein, R. & Galin, D. (1974). Lateralized specialization of cognitive mode III: EEG frequency analysis. *Psychophysiology* **11**: 567–78.

Dreifuss, F. E. (1983). *Pediatric Epileptology.* Boston, MA: John Wright PSG.

Durwen, H. F. (1992). Memory deficits in temporal lobe epilepsy as interactive phenomenon between epileptic focus and antiepileptic drugs. *Epilepsia* **33** (suppl 3): 138.

Eccles, J. C. (1966).*Brain and Conscious Experience.* New York: Springer-Verlag.

Fedio, P. & Mirsky, A.F. (1969). Selective intellectual deficits in children with temporal lobe or centrencephalic epilepsy. *Neuropsychologia* **7**: 287–300.

Fenwick, P. (1981). EEG studies. In *Epilepsy and Psychiatry*, ed. E. H. Reynolds & M.R. Trimble, pp. 242–53. New York: Churchill Livingstone.

Folsom, A. (1953). Psychological testing in epilepsy. I: cognitive function. *Epilepsia* **2**: 15–22.

Freeman, F. R., Douglas, E. F. O. & Penry, J. K. (1973). Environmental interaction and memory during petit mal (absence) seizures. *Pediatrics* **51**: 911–18.

French, J., Syakin, A. J., Conner, J. M., *et al.* (1992). Comparison of intracarotid amobarbital memory scores in patients with mesial versus neocortical onset temporal lobe epilepsy. *Epilepsia* **33** (suppl 3): 87.

Gallasi, R., Morreale, A., Lorusso, S., *et al.* (1988). Epilepsy presenting as memory disturbances. *Epilepsia* **29**: 624–9.

Giovagnoli, A. R., Casazza, M. & Gavanzini, G. (1995). Visual learning on a selective reminding procedure and delayed recall in patients with temporal lobe epilepsy. *Epilepsia* **36**: 704–11.

Gloor, P. (1986). Consciousness as a neurological concept in epileptology: a criical view. *Epilepsia* **27** (suppl 2): 14–26.

Glowinski, M. (1973). Cognitive deficits in temporal lobe epilepsy: an investigation of memory functioning. *J. Nerv. Ment. Dis.* **157**: 129–37.

Goode, D. J., Penry, J. K. & Dreifuss, F. E. (1970). Effects of paroxysmal spike-wave on continuous visual-motor performance. *Epilespia* **11**: 241–54.

Hart, L. A. (1975). *How the Brain Works.* New York: Basic Books.

Hasegawa, H. (2000). Persistent short term memory deficit syndrome with EEG abnormality responding to AED monotherapy. *Epilepsia* **41** (suppl 7): 239.

Helmstaedter, C., Kurthen, M., Linke, D., *et al.* (1992). Hierarchical restitution of limbic and neocortical functions in right hemispheric language dominant patients with early-onset left temporal lobe epilepsy. *Epilepsia* **33** (suppl 3): 121.

Hendriks, M. P. H., Jacobs, S., Aldenkamp, A. P., *et al.* (1998). Memory complaints and the relation with memory functions in patients with partial seizures originating form the temporal or frontal lobes. 3rd European Congress of Epileptology. *Epilepsia* **39** (suppl 2): 120.

Hutt, S. J. & Gilbert, S. (1980). Effects of evoked spike-wave discharges upon shot-term memory in patients with epilepsy. *Cortex* **16**: 443–7.

Jambaque, I., Dellatolas, G., Dulac, O., *et al.* (1992). Selective memory deficits in children with partial epilepsy. *Epilepsia* **33** (suppl 3): 8.

Jus, A. & Jus, K. L. (1962). Retrograde amnesia in petit mal. *Arch. Gen. Psychiatry* **6**: 163–7.

Kertesz, A. (1983). *Localization in Neuropsychology.* New York: Academic Press.

Kimura, D. (1962). Right temporal-lobe damage. *Arch. Neurol.* **8**: 264–71.

Kinsbourne, M. & Caplan, P. J. (1979). *Children's Learning and Attention Problems.* Boston, MA: Little Brown & Company.

Kooi, K. A. & Hovey, H. B. (1957). Alterations in mental functions and paroxysmal cerebral activity. *Arch. Neurol. Psychiatry* **1978**: 264–71.

Kortenkamp, S. R. (1996). Neuropsychologic correlates of subfield-specific hippocampal pathology. Presented at the American Epilepsy Society Conference, San Francisco, CA, 1996.

Kurokawa, T., Goya, N., Fukuyama, Y., *et al.* (1980). West syndrome and Lennox Gastaut syndrome: survey of natural history. *Pediatrics* **65**: 81–8.

Ladavas, E., Umilta, C. & Provinciali, L. (1979). Hemisphere-dependent cognitive performances in epileptic patients. *Epilepsia* **20**: 493–502.

Lansdell, M. (1968). Effect of extent of temporal lobe ablations on two lateralized deficits. *Physiol. Behav.* **3**: 271–3.

LeDoux, J. E., Barclay, L. & Premack, A. (1978). The brain and cognitive sciences. *Ann. Neurol.* **4**: 391–8.

Lewinski, R. J. (1947). The psychometric pattern. III: epilepsy. *Am. J. Orthopsych.* **17**: 714–21.

Loiseau, P., Strube, E., Broustet, D., *et al.* (1980). Evaluation of memory function in a population of epileptic patients and matched controls. *Acta Neurol. Scand.* **62** (suppl): 59–61.

Loiseau, P., Strube, E., Broustet, D., *et al.* (1983). Learning impairment in epileptic patients. *Epilepsia* **24**: 183–92.

Luria, A. R., transl. B. Haigh (1973). *The Working Brain, An Introduction to Neuropsychology.* New York: Basic Books.

Lux, S., Helmstaedter, C., Kurhten, M., Hartje, W. & Elger, C. E. (2000). Localizing value of ictal neuropsychological deficits in focal epilepsy. *Epilepsia* **41** (suppl 7): 153.

Macleod, C. M., Dekaban, A. S. & Hunt, E. (1978). Memory impairment in epileptic patients: selective effects of phenobarbital concentrations. *Science* **202**: 1102–4.

Mayer, V. & Jones, H. G. (1957). Patterns of cognitive test performance as functions of the lateral localization of cerebral abnormalities in the temporal lobe. *J. Ment. Sci.* **103**: 758–72.

Mayeux, R., Brandt, J., Rosen, J., *et al.* (1980). Interictal memory and language impairment in temporal lobe epilepsy. *Neurology* **30**: 120–25.

McIntyre, M., Pritchard, P. B., III & Lombroso, C. T. (1976). Left and right temporal epileptics: a controlled inspection of some psychological differences. *Epilepsia* **17**: 377–86.

Mellanby, J., Hawkins, C. & Wilkes, I. (1984). The relationship between seizures and amnesia in experimental epilepsy. *Acta Neurol. Scand.* **99**: 119–24.

Merritt, K. A., Ornstein, P. A. & Spicker, B. (1994). Children's memory for a salient medical procedure: implications for testimony. *Pediatrics* **94**: 17–23.

Meyer, V. & Falconer, M. A. S. (1960). Defects of learning ability with massive lesions of the temporal lobe. *J. Ment. Sci.* **106**: 472–7.

Milner, B. (1968). Visual recognition and recall after right temporal-lobe excision in man. *Neuropsychologica* **6**: 191–9.

Milner, B. (1975). Psychological aspects of focal epilepsy and its neurological management. In *Neurosurgical Management of the Epileptics: Advances in Neurology,* ed. D. P. Purpura, J. R. Penry & R. D. Walter, Vol. 8, pp. 299–321. New York: Raven Press.

Milner, B. & Scoville, W. B. (1957). Loss of recent memory after bilateral hippocampal lesions. *J. Neurol. Neurosurg. Psychiatry* **20**: 11–21.

Mirsky, A. F., Primac, D. W., Ajmone-Marsan, C., *et al.* (1960). A comparison of the psychological test performance of patients with focal and non-focal epilepsy. *Exp. Neurol.* **2**: 75–89.

Mungas, D., Ehlers, D., Walton, N. & McCutchen, C. B. (1985). Verbal learning differences in epileptic patients with left and right temporal lobe foci. *Epilepsia* **26**: 340–45.

O'Keefe, J. & Nadel, L. (1978). *The Hippocampus as a Cognitive Map.* Oxford: Oxford University Press.

O'Leary, D. S., Seidenberg, M., Berent, S., *et al.* (1981). Effects of age of onset of tonic-clonic seizures on neuropsychological performance in children. *Epilepsia* **22**: 197–204.

Piazzini, A., Canevini, M. P., Sgro, V., *et al.* (1998). Perception of memory difficulties in patients with epilepsy. 3rd European Congress of Epileptology. *Epilepsia* **39** (suppl 2): 119.

Powell, G. E., Polkey, C. E. & McMillan, T. (1975). The new Maudsley series of temporal lobectomy. I: short term cognitive effects. *Br. J. Clin. Psychol.* **24**: 109–24.

Quadfasel, A. F. & Pruyser, P. W. (1955). Cognitive deficits in patients with psychomotor epilepsy. *Epilepsia* **4**: 80–90.

Rapin, I. (1985). Brain dysfunction in children. In *Brenneman's Practice of Pediatrics,* ed. V. C. Kelley, Vol. 9, pp. 1–95. Philadelphia: Harper & Row.

Rausch, R., Babb, T. L., Ary, C. M., *et al.* (1992). Hippocampal neuron loss and mossy fiber sprouting contribute to verbal memory deficits in temporal lobe epileptic patients. *Epilepsia* **33** (suppl 3): 136.

Rausch, R., Lieb, J. P. & Crandall, P. A. (1978). Neuropsychological correlates of depth spiek activation in epielptic patients. *Arch. Neurol.* **35**: 699–705.

Read, D. E. (1981). Solving deductive-reasoning problems after unilateral temporal lobectomy. *Brain Lang.* **12**: 116–27.

Reitan, R. S. (1974). Psychological testing of epileptic patients. In *Handbook of Clinical Neurology*, ed. O. Magnus & A. M. Lorentz, Vol. 15, pp. 559–75. New York: American Elsevier.

Renier, W. O. (1987). Restrivtive factiors in the education of children with epilepsy from a medical point of view. In *Education and Epilepsy 1987*, ed. A. O. Aldenkamp, W. C. J. Alpherts, H. Meinardi & G. Stores, pp. 3–14. Lisse: Swets & Zeitlinger.

Riga, D., Saletti, V., Collino, L., *et al.* (1998). Neuropsychology of frontal epileptic activity. 3rd European Congress of Epileptology. *Epilepsia* **39** (suppl 2): 120.

Rumbaugh, D. M. & Washburn, D. A. (1966). Attention and memory in relation to learning: a comparative adaptation perspective. In *Attention, Memory and Executive Function*, ed. G. Reid Lyon & N. A. Krasnegor, pp. 199–220. Baltimore, MD: Paul H. Brookes.

Sawrie, S. M., Martin, R. C., Knowlton, R. C., *et al.* (2000). Verbal memory and temporal lobe metabolism: a quantitative FDG-PET study. *Epilepsia* **41** (suppl 7): 62.

Sharp, G. B., Williams, S. P., Griebel, M. I., *et al.* (2000). Verbal learning and memory in children with controlled seizures. *Epilepsia* **41** (suppl 7): 152.

Sherwin, I. & Efron, R. (1980). Temporal ordering deficits following anterior temporal lobectomy. *Brain Lang.* **11**: 195–203.

Stores, G. (1971). Cognitive function in children with epilepsy. *Dev. Med. Child Neurol.* **13**: 390–93.

Stores, G. (1976). The investigation and management of school children with epilepsy. *Publ. Health, Lond.* **90**: 171–7.

Stores, G. (1978). School children with epilepsy at risk for learning and behavior problems. *Dev. Med. Child Neurol.* **20**: 502–8.

Stores, G. (1981). Problems of learning and behavior in children with epilepsy. In *Epilepsy and Psychiatry*, ed. E. H. Reynolds & M. R. Trimble, pp. 33–48. New York: Churchill Livingstone.

Stores, G. (1987). Effects on learning of "subclinical" seizure discharges. In *Education and Epilepsy 1987*, ed. A. P. Aldenkamp, W. C. J. Alpherts, H. Meinardi & G. Stores, pp. 14–21. Lisse: Swets & Zeitlinger.

Stores, G., Hart, J. & Piran, N. (1978). Inattentiveness in school children with epilepsy. *Epilepsia* **19**: 169–75.

Swartz, B. E., Hlagren, E., Daims, R., Mulford, P. & Syndulko, K. (1993). Neurocognitive function in frontal lobe epilepsy. *Epilepsia* **34** (suppl 6): 33.

Torgesen, J. K. (1996). A model of memory from an information processing perspective: the special case of phonological memory. In *Attention, Memory and Executive Function*, ed. G. Reid Lyon & N. A. Krasnegor, pp. 157–84. Baltimore, MD: Paul H. Brookes.

Trimble, M. R. (1980). Anti-epileptic drugs and behavior – discussion notes. In *Epilepsy and Behavior '79*, ed. B. M. Kulig, H. Meinardi & G. Stores, pp. 76–9. Lisse: Swets & Zeitlinger.

Trimble, M. R. (1988). *Biological Psychiatry.* New York: John Wiley & Sons.

Trimble, M. R. & Thompson, P. J. (1981). Memory, anticonvulsant drugs and seizures. *Acta Neurol. Scand.* **64** (suppl): 31–41.

Troster, A. I., Barr, W. B., Warmflash, V., *et al.* (1991). The role of encoding in rapid forgetting associated with unilateral temporal lobe epilepsy. *Epilepsia* **32** (suppl 3): 73.

Vargha-Kahdem, F. (2001). Generalized versus selective cognitive impairments resulting from brain damage sustained in childhood. In *Epilepsia and Learning Disabilities*, ed. G. F. Ayala, M. Elia, C. M. Cornaggia & M. M. Trimble. *Epilepsia* **42**: 37–40.

Von Isser, A. (1977). Psycholinguistic abilities in children with epilepsy. *Exceptional Children* **February**: 270–72.

Wagner, R. K. (1996). From simple structure to complex function: major trends in the development of theories, models, and measurements of memory. In *Attention, Memory and Executive Function*, ed. G. Reid Lyon & N. A. Krasnegor, pp. 139–56. Baltimore, MD: Paul H. Brookes.

Warrington, E. K., Logue, V. & Pratt, R. T. C. (1971). The anatomical localization of selective impairment of auditory verbal short-term memory. *Neuropsychologica* **9**: 377–87.

Waxman, S. G. & Geschwind, N. (1975). The interictal behavior syndrome of temporal lobe epilepsy. *Arch. Gen. Psychiatry* **32**: 1580–86.

Westerveld, M. (2002). Inferring function from structure: relationship of magnetic resonance imaging-directed hippocampal abnormality and memory function in epilepsy. *Epilepsy Currents* **2**: 3–6.

Westerveld, M., Spencer, S. S., Stoddard, K. R., *et al.* (1999). Perceived memory impairments and objective test findings in epilepsy. *Epilepsia* **40** (suppl 7): 46.

Widman, G., Helmstaedter, C., Lehnertz, K., *et al.* (1999). Anterior mesial temporal lobe: a "working memory" structure? *Epilepsia* **40** (suppl 7): 50.

Zimmerman, F. T., Burgemeister, B. B. & Putnam, T. J. (1951). Intellectual and emotional makeup of the epileptic. *Arch. Neurol. Psychiatry* **65**: 545–56.

20

Executive functioning

Executive functioning underlies the development of learning and behavior, yet it is not well understood, especially in children (Eslinger, 1996). Problems such as early-onset epilepsy can inhibit and distort both learning and behavior by impairing brain development, especially frontal lobe function, as well as adversely altering behavioral approaches in raising the child.

Definition

Executive functioning is the ability to decide and act, or to inhibit an action, by developing and applying an appropriate problem-solving approach in order to achieve a future goal (Pennington *et al.*, 1996; Barkley, 1996). This relies on the understanding and use of various styles of thinking, such as planning and self-regulation (Borkowski & Burke, 1996).

When a child is faced by some event in the environment, the first impulse is to respond, often on an emotional basis, which may not prove rewarding. The child needs to be able to pause and consider the options based on remembered previous similar experiences. What is the goal of the response? Is it desirable? The consequences of a response need to be contemplated. The child may need to inhibit a response or defer it to a more appropriate time, when a sequenced plan of action can be developed to gain the desired goal. When the time comes, the child needs to be able to inhibit inferences that detract from the goal decided upon as the act is completed. The feedback from the environment may encourage future similar approaches or may cause the child to devise an alternate approach in the future. This all encompasses the process of executive functioning (Barkley, 1996).

Anatomy

Executive functioning is a prefrontal process including the dorsolateral regions of the frontal lobe as well as intimate ties to the basilar ganglia, the limbic system, the thalamus, and the posterior cortex. Delayed responding is mediated by the prefrontal cortical and related limbic structures, particularly the caudate in infants, and later the orbital frontal cortex itself (Barkley, 1996). The orbital and mesial-frontal areas are related to social, emotional, and motivational attributes of personality (Denckla, 1996; Pennington *et al.*, 1996).

Organization and reorganization

Brain development and especially neuronal plasticity cycles in waves through synaptic overproduction followed by pruning. Sensitive periods occur continually, being driven by diffuse waves of anatomically circulating growth factors. Each stage begins with a rapid synaptic growth within functionally differentiated neural systems, resulting in a genetically driven overproduction of synaptic connections. This is followed by environmentally driven maintenance and pruning of synaptic excessive connections (Thatcher, 1997).

The prefrontal cortex initially develops about a year behind primary sensory cortices but catches up by about four years of age. Prefrontal synaptic development persists from the fetal period to late childhood. The initial wave of development accelerates after birth, peaking at about one year of age. This is paralleled by dendritic growth and myelination. At this time, the infant is developmentally involved in tasks that do not depend on the prefrontal cortex. The second wave of synaptic development is one of exuberant synaptic connections, during which the synaptic density is 40% above the adult level. This period is from one to at least seven years of age. There is increased functional plasticity. The prefrontal lobe functions are shaped by interactions with the environment, thus refining executive functions. The excesses in synapses are eliminated during late childhood into adolescence (Huttenlocher & Dabholkar, 1997).

Executive function maturation

The basics of executive function are established in the first two to three years of early childhood (Borkowski & Burke, 1996). The child learns to analyze tasks to be performed and then to select a strategy of performance, revising the approach as needed before application. As the task is performed, the child monitors the results. Basic parenting underlies the development of this self-governed behavior.

Development of self-governed behavior basics

Initially, the child depends on the parent to guide, reinforce, and provide flexibility of choices. Thus, socioeconomic factors, parenting skills, and positive feedback are important influences (Hayes *et al.*, 1996).

Parents provide pleasure/displeasure cues before language emergence, but this merges into yes/no responses to the child's efforts. The child begins to gain rewards or admonishments for actions, which plant the concept of the association of actions with rewards and consequences, especially if the rule-givers are consistent and reinforcing. Rules are to be followed because they work, not because they are necessarily understood. Growing up in a chaotic and unpredictable environment makes this difficult.

A child learns by being told and by experiencing, drawing on established language abilities and emerging perceptive skills. This is more than just repeated experiencing or automatic behaviors; it is developing the ability to make a choice between various acceptable behaviors or developing new responses especially in new situations. An overly controlling environment may limit choosing, thus impeding the development of executive functioning.

The child learns that actions achieve goals and result in rewards or consequences. Actions are affected by rules. Actions may be motivated by enticements or altered by warnings. The child learns to pause to consider the rewards and consequences before acting. Thus, the child learns to prioritize in choosing.

Executive functioning and intelligence are affected by the feedback from parents and teachers. Thus, the child learns to develop a repertoire of strategies to be used in multiple contexts, and to note the appropriateness of strategies for certain situations. Thus, higher-order executive processes emerge, from which develops self-regulation as the basis for adaptive learning and thinking. The child learns to value strategies and achievements through self-directed actions.

The future

By school age, the child begins to develop visions into the future, imagining things that might be and things that are unwanted. These become the basis for achieving important short-term and long-term goals, setting the system of planning, developing goals and incentives towards achievement (Borkowski & Burke, 1996).

Frontal-prefrontal problems

The frontal lobes and particularly the prefrontal regions are especially related to executive functioning and to related functions, including attention and planning (Pennington, 1997).

Frontal functions

Executive function is influenced by information processing and desires. Inhibition, attention, and memory are important components (Eslinger, 1996).

Executive function

Executive function means the child needs to be able to pause (stop), look, listen, think, and plan before acting in response to a stimulus. If the child skips any or all of these intermediate stages, or if the child gets the response flow out of order, for example acts then thinks, the results may be a failure or an unwanted reaction.

Attention

Attention, memory, and execution mature with age in accuracy, in the rate of performance, in complexity, and in automaticity (Morris, 1996). Attention and executive functioning share neuropsychologic systems of analysis and are linked anatomically. The prefrontal cortex houses the executive system and links up neuroanatomically with these other brain regions, including the limbic system, and regulates them in the service of self-regulated, goal-directed, and future-oriented behavior (Barkley, 1996). This area is also involved closely in inhibition and flexibility regarding any actions that may detract from attention (Borkowski & Burke, 1996).

Memory

Executive function has three components, a working memory, an anticipation state, and an interference control that inhibits the disruption of goal-directed behavior by behaviors incompatible with it (Barkley, 1996). Working memory allows the mind to hold on to the information attended to while inhibiting any immediate response until executive action can produce the most appropriate response.

Inhibition

A subfunction of executive function includes anticipation and action preparedness, inhibition and response delay, and freedom from interferences of preceding responses such as initiation, sustaining, inhibiting or stopping, and shifting (Denckla, 1996). This can be learned (Hayes *et al.*, 1996). Delaying responses allows for further analysis, comparison with prior memories, and consideration of alternative consequences, allowing the prefrontal lobe to orchestrate the executive process. Children with ADHD and children with frontal lobe damage show delayed acquisition of executive function controls (Barkley, 1996).

Dysfunctions

Problems with these functions manifest as a variety of groups of clinical disorders. Often, language is involved in such related problems, both anatomically and functionally (Leonard, 1997).

Emotions and behavior

The frontal lobe is involved in regulating emotion. Infants with difficulties in handling stress and who are easily disturbed display a unique frontal activation pattern (Benes, 1997). The frontal lobe appears to be active in the handling of distress and the expression of negative emotions. As infants mature, there is an increased maturation of the fontal region and the ability to regulate distress increases. Such children may learn the best strategies to deal with a sensory overload and to regulate negative emotionality (Harman & Fox, 1997). Various mental disorders of childhood and adolescence tend to appear during certain stages of postnatal development. Such psychiatric disorders may be the result of developmental changes during the early and later postnatal period.

Both glutamate and gamma-aminobutyric acid (GABA) systems show extensive postnatal maturation up to and in some cases including, adulthood. The dopamine system undergoes important postnatal maturation. There may be alterations in specific interactions between two neurotransmitters within the key cortical-limbic regions, such as the prefrontal area or anterior cingulate areas, that may be involved.

Socialization

The prefrontal cortex mediates a critical role in developing and establishing capacities for social self-regulation, social awareness of others, and social self-awareness. The prefrontal cortex is important for primitive social tendencies and social development. Protracted postnatal development of the prefrontal cortex operations are responsible for higher-level or executive abilities. Interhemispheric interactions between the prefrontal cortices occur during development. Relative preservation of elementary cognitive abilities after early prefrontal cortical damage is noted (Eslinger, 1996).

Prefrontal insults

Impairments of executive function tasks are found in many neuropsychiatric and developmental disorders, a number of which are associated with or complicated by epilepsy. Executive function disorders may be inherent to and a part of the disorder, or they may be artificial or non-specific. Prefrontal cortex disturbances affect executive function. Timing of insults as related to maturation is important. Insults in other parts of the brain that connect to the frontal lobe may produce changes in both the prefrontal cortex and the non-frontal sites. The changes may be diffuse (Pennington, 1997). Myelination may be affected. Prefrontal myelination extends throughout adolescence.

Prefrontal maturation undergoes a series of changes relating to cognitive development involving programmed cell death, cell density, synaptogenesis, and synaptic density. These ongoing processes are involved in differentiating functions and then in synchronizing and integrating such functions. In young children, unlike in adults, prefrontal damage impairs intellectual development by 10 to 25 points by affecting executive functioning. This affects working memory, attention control, and organization abilities (Eslinger, 1996).

Cognitive prerequisites to psychosocial skills are important, including flexibility, empathy, and impulse control. Symbiotic linking, the conservation of new alternatives, and the anticipation of the consequences of each choice lead to a moral maturity. Planning, time-lining, decision-making, and reality-orientation lead to vocational maturation (Eslinger, 1996).

The development of executive function can be influenced actively by problems such as inborn errors of metabolism, neuronal migration deficits (as with neurofibromatosis), environmental deprivation, and other neurodevelopmental impairments (Eslinger, 1996). Many of these entities are frequently associated with epilepsy.

Brain injuries

Head injuries in childhood may result in seizures and in a variety of frontal lobe deficits common to adults. Planning skills may be deficient. Children with frontal head injuries often have difficulties in problem-solving skills, cognitive flexibility, verbal discourses, and response inhibition. Executive functions depend on the integrity of the dorsolateral frontal cortex for problem-solving, and cogntive flexibilty may be imparied with dorsolateral insults. Superior medial lesions have been associated with akinesia, speaking problems, and reduced emotions. Orbitofrontal cortex and underlying white matter tend to relate to deficits resulting in impulsivity, behavioral disinhibition, and faulty social judgments. A left frontal injury may affect both verbal and non-verbal conceptual measures, whereas a right-sided lesion may have more severe defiicts in tasks involving non-verbal or spatial components. The right frontal lobe seems to contribute to the organization of verbal information in children (Scheibel & Levin, 1997).

In congenital bilateral prefrontal damage, social feelings are shallow and limited as related to the immediate circumstances. Early left-sided damage may produce marked difficulties in social development and adaptation, often with uninhibited strong emotions, including rage reactions. Social thoughts may be simplistic (Eslinger, 1996).

Diffuse cortical sclerosis involving only one hemisphere has been associated with post-convulsive anoxic changes. It occurs in individuals who have experienced a birth injury. Shrinkage of the gyri and sulci with underlying neuronal loss and gliosis occurs in the upper cortical areas. The condition is also seen with damage in the CA sectors of the hippocampal formation. Often, neurological defects and seizure disorders are present after the initial injury at birth and may reflect a widespread occurrence of changes (Benes, 1997).

Younger children may generally be able to recover better. There may be a tendency for some to exhibit a more severe impairment when injured at an earlier age, including greater difficulties in global intellectual functioning, written language, and recognition memory. Discourse impairments are especially severe with left-sided lesions after five years of age. Some frontal mediate cognitive processes develop late in childhood. Those actively developing skills at the time of the injury are more at risk than static or matured skills. Sometimes, as injury of early childhood may emerge in mid adolescence (Scheibel & Levin, 1997).

Epilepsy

Children with frontal epileptogenic foci often do not show any severe neuropsychologic deficits. The intellectual functioning is relatively normal (Riga *et al.*, 1998) but problems of attention, organization, and planning (Zimmerman *et al.*, 1951) are more apparent. This tends to be worsened by polypharmacy and by increased seizure frequency (Sherman *et al.*, 2000). Memory problems may be severe with prefrontal lesions (Kerfesz, 1983). Frontal seizures may be overlooked or misdiagnosed.

Developmental executive function problems

Attention and perception problems are often seen with retardation. A failure to inhibit competing stimuli may affect all aspects of learning (Pennington, 1997).

Intelligence

Intelligence is influenced by but is not the same as executive functioning ability (Denckla, 1996). Gifted children especially excel in executive functioning, for they display an abundance of the process. Children who are retarded have little executive functioning. Executive functioning substructures may serve to differentiate generalized giftedness from restricted giftedness (Borkowski & Burke, 1996). Underachieving children may have a deficient executive functioning ability (Denckla, 1996).

Perceptual motor problems

In some visual motor acts, executive function exists between perception and motor acts. Motor planning and execution are linked to executive function. Usually, verbally mediated rules dominate working memories, although some children may utilize visual schemes (Denckla, 1996). Faulty executive function may impede this interation.

Attention deficits

Frontal dysfunction may be intrinsic, such as problems within the prefrontal cortex area, or extrinsic, such as problems outside of but affecting the prefrontal cortex function (Pennington, 1997). Some children with executive dysfunction present as having an attention deficit disorder, with or without hyperactivity (Denckla,

1996). Children with ADHD seem to remain delayed in the attainment of emerging executive functions. Both attention and executive function can be divided into four similar components: initiate, sustain, inhibit, and shift (Barkley, 1996).

A young preschool child with attention problems shows the uninhibited, hyperactive, and impulsive behavior pattern as the predominant feature of the disorders, but shows no more difficulties with sustained attention than do typical preschool children who have not yet developed such functions. Later, the child with such deficits shows deficits earlier in the more complex executive functions than do emerging typical children, such as poor sustained attention, poor cross-temporal organization of behavior, forgetfulness, slowed mental computation, limited self-control, limited hindsight and foresight, and eventually limited verbal fluency, problem-solving, and creativity. Adolescents with prefrontal injury or with ADHD manifest a far more complex clinical picture of deficient executive functions than preschoolers with the same disorder (Barkley, 1996).

Diagnosis

The approach appears to be to identify the important problem to be solved, to define the subgoals involved in solving the problem, to explore possible approaches to the problem from a set of potential strategies, to anticipate potential outcomes before acting on any of them, and to look back and learn from the entire problem-solving experience. This incorporates approaches of self-regulation and planning (Borkowski & Burke, 1996). Many overlapping tests are not pure and cover multiple aspects. Some children may perform poorly on a reported task of attention not because their attention system is deficient but because one or more of their perception, memory, or executive systems are deficient (Morris, 1996).

Therapy

Executive function changes a control process or sequence of central processing as a reasonable response to an objective change in an information-processing task (Borkowski & Burke, 1996). These underlying components include task analysis, strategy control of selection and revision, and strategy monitoring (Eslinger, 1996). This usually involves a knowledgeable behavioral therapist working with the school and the family in modifying or retraining the child's approaches.

In simple words, the child needs to be taught to stop, look, listen, and plan before acting. This can be done in creating situations and guiding the child through the development of responses. With each trial, alternatives of action and reasons for each need to be discussed before the action is taken. After the action is performed, the effectiveness of the action and possible other actions should be reviewed with the child. This approach can be begun by limiting the choices of responses until the child can handle more, ultimately building towards not offering choices but allowing the child to develop the response. Such approaches should be widened in the types and circumstances in which the strategies are utilized.

REFERENCES

Barkley, R. A. (1996). Linkages between attention and executive functions. In *Attention, Memory and Executive Function*, ed. G. R. Lyon & N. A. Krasnegor, pp. 307–25. Baltimore, MD: Paul H. Brookes.

Benes, F. M. (1997). Cortico-limbic circuitry and the development of psychopathology during childhood and adolescence. In *Development of the Prefrontal Cortex*, ed. N. A. Krasnegor, G. R. Lyon & P. S. Rakic-Goldman, pp. 211–40. Baltimore, MD: Paul H. Brooks.

Borkowski, J. G. & Burke, J. E. (1996). Theories, models, and measurements of executive Functioning. In *Attention, Memory and Executive Function*, ed. G. R. Lyon & N. A. Krasnegor, pp. 235–61. Baltimore, MD: Paul H. Brookes.

Denckla, M. B. (1996). A theory and model of executive function: a neuropsychological perspective. In *Attention, Memory and Executive Function*, ed. G. R. Lyon & N. A. Krasnegor, pp. 263–78. Baltimore, MD: Paul H. Brookes Publ.

Eslinger, P. J. (1996). Conceptualizing, describing, and measuring components of executive function, a summary. In *Attention, Memory and Executive Function*, ed. G. R. Lyon & N. A. Krasnegor, pp. 67–395. Baltimore, MD: Paul H. Brookes Publ.

Harman, C. & Fox, N. A. (1997). Frontal and attentional mechanisms regulating distress, experience and expression during infancy. In *Development of the Prefrontal Cortex*, ed. N. A. Krasnegor, G. R. Lyon & P. S. Rakic-Goldman, pp. 91–210. Baltimore, MD: Paul H. Brooks.

Hayes, S. C., Gifford, E. V. & Ruckstuhl, L. E., Jr (1996). Relational frame theory and executive function. In *Attention, Memory and Executive Function*, ed. G. R. Lyon & N. A. Krasnegor, pp. 279–305. Baltimore, MD: Paul H. Brookes.

Huttenlocher, P. R. & Dabholkar, A. S. (1997). Developmental anatomy of prefrontal cortex. In *Development of the Prefrontal Cortex*, ed. N. A. Krasnegor, G. R. Lyon & P. S. Rakic-Goldman, pp. 69–84. Baltimore, MD: Paul H. Brooks.

Kerfesz, A. (1983). *Localization in Neuropsychology.* New York: Academic Press.

Leonard, C. M. (1997). Language and the prefrontal cortex. In *Development of the Prefrontal Cortex*, ed. N. A. Krasnegor, G. R. Lyon & P. S. Rakic-Goldman, pp. 141–67. Baltimore, MD: Paul H. Brooks.

Morris, R. D. (1996). Relationships and distinctions among the concepts of attention, memory and executive function, a developmental perspective. In *Attention, Memory and Executive Function*, ed. G. R. Lyon & N. A. Krasnegor, pp. 1–16. Baltimore, MD: Paul H. Brookes.

Pennington, B. F. (1997). Dimensions of executive functions in normals and abnormal development. In *Development of the Prefrontal Cortex*, ed. N. A. Krasnegor, G. R. Lyon & P. S. Rakic-Goldman, pp. 265–82. Baltimore, MD: Paul H. Brooks.

Pennington, B. F., Bennetto, L., McAleer, O., et. al. (1996). Executive functions and working memory. In *Attention, Memory and Executive Function*, ed. G. R. Lyon & N. A. Krasnegor, pp. 327–48. Baltimore, MD: Paul H. Brookes.

Riga, D., Saletti, V., Collino, L., et. al. (1998). Neuropsychology of frontal epileptic activity. 3rd European Congress of Epileptology. *Epilepsia* **39** (suppl 20): 120.

Scheibel, R. S. & Levin, H. S. (1997). Frontal lobe dysfunction following closed head injury in children: findings from neuropsychological brain imaging. In *Development of the Prefrontal Cortex*, ed. N. A. Krasnegor, G. R. Lyon & P. S. Rakic-Goldman, pp. 241–64. Baltimore, MD: Paul H. Brooks.

Sherman, E. M. S., Armitage, L. L., Connolly, M. B., *et al.* (2000). Behaviors symptomatic of ADHD in pediatric epilepsy: relationship to frontal lobe epileptiform abnormalities and other neurologic predictors. *Epilepsia* **41** (suppl 7): 191.

Thatcher, R. W. (1997). Human frontal lobe development: a theory of cyclical cortical reorganization. In *Development of the Prefrontal Cortex*, ed. N. A. Krasnegor, G. R. Lyon & P. S. Rakic-Goldman, pp. 85–116. Baltimore, MD: Paul H. Brooks.

Zimmerman, F. T., Burgemeister, B. B. & Putnam, T. J. (1951). Intellectual and emotional makeup of the epileptic. *Arch. Neurol. Psychiatry* **65**: 545–56.

21

Academics

Learning difficulties occur in up to 50% of children with epilepsy (Rutter *et al.*, 1970; Stores, 1978; Stores, 1987; Thompson, 1987; Aldenkamp *et al.*, 1990). This leads to the children falling behind in school subjects, dropping school grades, and eventually an increased number of students leaving school early, unprepared for earning a living.

Learning problems

Academic problems arise from specific cognitive deficiencies rather than any generalized cognitive dysfunction. Such problems include reduced attention span (Fairweather & Hutt, 1969; Rugland, 1990a), impaired memory (Stores, 1973; Stores, 1981; Stores & Hart, 1976), poor abstract reasoning (Knight & Tymchuck, 1968), perceptual difficulties, and slowed inefficient processing (Fairweather & Hutt, 1969; Waxman & Geschwind, 1975; Brittain, 1980; Kupke & Lewis, 1985; Dodrill, 1987; Aldenkamp, 1987; Beaumont, 1987; Oxley & Stores, 1987; Aldenkamp *et al.*, 1990). These are manifest as difficulties in reading, writing, arithmetic, and other academic activities. Such problems tend to persist, especially if not remediated. Family variables such as parental income, educational levels, and psychosocial stressors do not account for the problems (Bailet & Turk, 2000).

Subgroups

There may be subgroups of children with learning disabilities identified in epileptic children, each of which display deficient reading skills and require a different form of treatment (Strang & Rourke, 1985; Aldenkamp *et al.*, 1990).

Some children with a temporal lobe dysfunction display a memory deficiency type with problems in short-term memory and memory span, leading to disorders in the stabilization and consolidation of the word image (Strang & Rourke, 1985; Aldenkamp *et al.*, 1990).

Some children have an attention deficit type of problem with underachievement, seen especially with a high frequency of tonic–clonic seizures. Such children are distractable. On the Wechsler Intelligence Scale for Children, revised (WISC-r), problems in coding, digit span, and arithmetic are seen. It can be concluded that attentional factors may be particularly vulnerable to seizure activity (Aldenkamp *et al.*, 1990).

Another group displays a slowness of information processing, especially in complex tasks. These children underachieve, especially in arithmetic. This often relates to detrimental effects of polytherapy and long-term treatment, as with phenytoin. Other factors include the seizure type, seizure frequency, type of EEG abnormality, and onset age (Aldenkamp, 1987; Aldenkamp *et al.*, 1990).

Some children display a problem-solving type of disorder. There is a disturbance of higher-order cognitive processing, such as concept formation and logical thinking, decision-making, and verbal reasoning. This is common. It may be related directly to epileptic factors (Strang & Rourke, 1985; Aldenkamp *et al.*, 1990).

Some children may show a decreased capacity for systematic mental operation, leading to specific underachievement in arithmetic. This has also been seen in the general population of learning-disabled children with an arithmetic disability (Strang & Rourke, 1985; Aldenkamp *et al.*, 1990).

Auditory-verbal processing

Children with epilepsy may perform less well in verbal tasks (Trimble, 1990). Auditory perception and language-processing disabilities as well as difficulties in attention and concentration are noted (Fairweather & Hutt, 1969; Rugland, 1990a). Memory problems, especially auditory, are perhaps the most significant problems reported (Stores & Hart, 1976; Stores, 1973; Stores, 1981; Bailet & Turk, 2000). If considered for surgery, the absence of early brain injury is predictive of a decrease in verbal learning after anterior temporal lobotomy, although there is a contralateral improvement in right temporal lobe patients (Saykin *et al.*, 1993).

Visual motor processing

Perceptual problems are more common yet are often overlooked in children with epilepsy, especially children with non-dominant complex parietal seizures, suggesting an involvement spread to the parietal area. An early-onset non-dominant temporal-parietal seizure focus is a significant risk for the development of perceptual motor problems and visual memory difficulties. An early-onset dominant left temporal lobe focus may result in less impairing language problems than anticipated but may be associated with perceptual motor and visual memory deficits. In early life, the left-sided insult may be overcome in part by transferring developing language functions to the non-dominant side, but at the sacrifice of some perceptual skill development (Waxman and Geschwind, 1975; Brittain, 1980; Kupke & Lewis, 1985; Aldenkamp, 1987; Beuamont, 1987; Dodrill, 1987; Oxley & Stores, 1987; Aldenkamp *et al.*, 1990).

Academic performance

Children with epilepsy show lower academic achievement scores relative to their IQ, with particular difficulties in reading (including comprehension and word recognition) and even more in spelling and arithmetic (Seidenberg *et al.*, 1986; Trimble, 1990). These children perform worse than their siblings in most aspects and are more apt to repeat grades (Bailet & Turk, 2000). Boys with epilepsy tend to do badly in spelling, arithmetic, and reading comprehension (Weintraub, 1981); whereas girls with epilepsy do better than epileptic boys in most areas, except math.

Reading

Many children with epilepsy underachieve significantly in reading relative to their basic intelligence (Rutter *et al.*, 1970; Laidlaw & Reichens, 1976; Wechsler, 1973; Stores, 1976; Trimble, 1990). This cannot be accounted for by absences from school (Laidlaw & Reichens, 1976).

Teachers report that children with epilepsy have no more reading problems than their siblings, but in formal testing the child with epilepsy is about 11 months behind their siblings (Long & Moore, 1979; Weintraub, 1981) and about 12–23 months behind classmates in reading (Rutter *et al.*, 1970; Weintraub, 1981). Children with uncomplicated epilepsies tend to be of average intelligence but about one year behind in reading due to specific reading impairments (Stores & Hart, 1976; Long & Moore, 1979; Stores, 1987). About 18% are delayed in reading by at least two years, irrespective of their level of intelligence (Green & Hartlage, 1970; Rutter *et al.*, 1970; Rutter & Yule, 1975; Stores, 1976; Stores & Hart, 1976; Long & Moore, 1979; Baird *et al.*, 1980; Stores, 1981; Weintraub, 1981; Stores, 1987). Even in a residential school placement, 91% of children with epilepsy were found to be at least 28 months behind in reading and 64% were retarded readers, i.e. more than 28 months behind and significantly below predicted levels (Weintraub, 1981). The incidence of dyslexia in adults who have grown up with epilepsy is about four times that in the normal population, especially in left-handed women (Schacter *et al.*, 1991).

The outlook for children whose reading is more than two standard deviations from predictions is poor (Rutter, 1974). Impairment of verbal ability of these children sometimes leads to reading problems that interfere with the total educational process (Poche, 1978). The underachieving child is more likely to suffer from disabilities in schools where educational failure results in segregation and replacement. Factors to be considered include the attainment of class peers, the degree of mainstreaming, and the extent to which teaching is individualized rather than group-based (Rutter, 1974).

Causes

Children with epilepsy perform less well in verbal tests and show a higher than expected frequency of reading retardation (Trimble, 1990). Early studies noted differences in automatic reading in the speed and accuracy as well as in reading comprehension and recall of ideas, possibly reflecting a failure of concentration and recent memory (Fox, 1931–3). There may exist independent types of learning problems in reading-disabled children (Strang & Rourke, 1985). These types are divided between auditory and visual channels of learning as well as the visual-auditory integration form. There are a variety of subtypes for each channel, including perception (or discrimination) memory and visual sequential memory, as well as comprehension types. Reading problems may be caused by defects in several levels of information processing, such as visual scanning and recognition, the ability to transform information from one modality to another, phonetic attack skills, linguistic reasoning, and comprehension (Boder, 1973; Fisk & Rourke, 1979; Rourke, 1985; Ceci, 1986; Aldenkamp *et al.*, 1990). Major subgroups of reading difficulties include a disturbed phonetic type and a disturbed visual processing type. Both show deficient reading, but each type requires a different form of treatment (Strang & Rourke, 1985). It has been theorized that such problems may relate to anomalous brain structures in dyslexic patients, including dysplasias (Schacter *et al.*, 1991).

The reading skills of epileptic boys, regardless of their type of epilepsy, are often inferior to those of epileptic girls, a gender difference not seen in non-epileptic children (Stores & Hart, 1976). Reading problems do not tend to be seen in girls with epilepsy (Berger, 1971). Early-age seizure onset is also associated with poorer reading comprehension (Seidenberg *et al.*, 1986).

Seizure types

The accuracy and comprehension reading skills of children with an idiopathic generalized epilepsy and seizure subclinical discharges appear no worse than those of children without epilepsy (Berger, 1971; Stores & Hart, 1976). Children who have both generalized tonic–clonic and absence seizures are more apt to have reading problems (Seidenberg *et al.*, 1986). Children with progressive myoclonic epilepsy may present with dyslexia without any aphasic findings at the onset, although prior speech delays may be noted (Piras *et al.*, 1991).

Focal spike abnormalities are more apt to be related to impairments of reading, especially if the left temporal lobe is involved. Children are significantly depressed in reading accuracy (Berger, 1971; Stores & Hart, 1976) but not necessarily in reading comprehension, although for comprehension left-hemispheric spike foci are more impairing than right-sided discharges. No verbal performance discrepancies on the WISC or relating to the degree of behavioral disturbances are found to explain these differences (Stores & Hart, 1976). Reading factors relative to depressed performance include male gender, left temporal lobe discharge, and reliance on phenytoin for more than two years (Stores, 1976; Stores *et al.*, 1978).

Laterality

The laterality of epileptic foci correlates with cognitive functioning. Children, especially boys, with clearly left-sided epileptic foci show a lower performance on reading and arithmetic tests than children with right-sided foci (Stores & Hart, 1976; Stores *et al.*, 1978; Weintraub, 1981; Camfield *et al.*, 1984; Kasteleijn-Nolst Trenite *et al.*, 1990; Rugland, 1990a). Children with left-hemispheric lesions of onset before age ten, despite normal language development, may lag behind, with impairments of syntax and semantics (Van der Vlugth & Bakker, 1980). More problems with anxiety, attention, and excessive activity are seen in this group (Trimble, 1983).

Children with right temporal spike discharges especially with right-hemispheric lesions, may also have reading problems (Trimble, 1983). Problems in reading and writing acquisition and in integrating graphemes and phonemes may be noted (Van der Vlugth & Bakker, 1980).

Subclinical discharges

Children with localized or clearly lateralized left-sided epileptiform discharges without obvious clinical signs show poorer reading performance than children with localized or clearly lateralized right-sided discharges. Subclinical discharges significantly impair reading performance during the discharge, resulting in repetitions, corrections, hesitations, omissions, and additions (Kasteleijn-Nolst Trenite *et al.*, 1988).

Epileptiform discharges increase during performance of academic tasks. Nearly all children show an increase in epileptiform discharge rate during reading and sometimes also arithmetic. During reading, a greater increase in the discharge rate over the right hemisphere than over the left is noted. The discharges remain subclinical. Epileptiform discharges occur less frequently and with a shorter total duration over the left hemisphere than the right, suggesting that cognitive tasks suppress epileptiform discharges when they activate a region of the brain within the epileptogenic zone. Discharges from other epileptogenic zones not activated directly by the tasks are increased (Wilkins, 1986; Kasteleijn-Nolst Trenite *et al.*, 1988; Kasteleijn-Nolst Trenite *et al.*, 1990).

Medication effect

Antiepileptic medication may lead to improvement within six to 12 months in children with focal seizures. Children on medication do better on reading scores, memory tasks, and visual-motor skills. Used properly, antiepileptic therapy shows no deleterious effects (Mandlebaum *et al.*, 1993). Children on phenytoin for more than two years have more reading problems (Berger, 1971) in both accuracy and comprehension compared with children on other medications (Stores & Hart, 1976).

Reading epilepsy

In some people, the very act of reading may induce a seizure, presenting as jaw or body jerking (sometimes with vocalization), violent movements, or simply dropping the book when reading. The reader may lose their place when reading. If the patient continues to read, a major seizure may occur. The unfamiliarity and/or emotional content of the reading may be important. Reading may provoke absence-like attacks and also bursts of diffuse polyspike and wave discharges of short duration (Critchley *et al.*, 1959–60; Forster & Daily, 1973). Spike-wave discharges may occur both with reading and with talking, unrelated to any specific word or phonemic element. In some patients, focal discharges in the temporal lobe, or occasionally the frontal or parietal-occipital lobe, may be seen. Reading music or braille may also induce seizures (Brooks & Jirauch, 1971; Forster & Daily, 1973).

Reading epilepsy is classified as sensory precipitated reflex epilepsy, potentially provoking seizures by a variety of complex mechanisms. This may involve repetitive proprioceptive impulses to eye or oral articulation movements, attention/concentration, pattern sensitivity, emotional factors, surprise or startling, or a communication complication, depending on the individual. Reading epilepsy may be inherited, perhaps as an autosomal dominant disorder with genetically determined threshold sensitivity, although the presence of a family history is found in only a few cases (Brooks & Jirauch, 1971; Ramani, 1983). Once the dysrhythmia begins, it occurs with increasing frequency if reading is continued (Critchley *et al.*, 1959–60; Forster *et al.*, 1969; Forster, 1977a).

Reading epilepsy can be divided into two categories, primary and secondary, i.e. those patients only with reading epilepsy when reading and those who also have seizures at other times (Bickford *et al.*, 1956; Fairweather & Hutt, 1971; Forster, 1977a).

Primary reading epilepsy

Some individuals have epileptic attacks only when reading (Forster *et al.*, 1969; Ramani, 1983), without any cause ever being found. Reading-induced epilepsy, often of childhood onset, is an idiopathic generalized seizure preceded by myoclonus of the jaw (Forster *et al.*, 1969; Brooks & Jirauch, 1971; Hall & Marshall, 1980). The precipitant appears to be higher cognitive processes associated with language functioning (Ramani, 1983), although the exact mechanism remains undetermined (Vanderzant *et al.*, 1982). Familiarity with the material being read lessens the tendency (Forster, 1977a).

Two distinct subtypes have been noted: seizures with a short latency onset after five to ten minutes of reading, and seizures after prolonged reading of 30–40 minutes (Browne *et al.*, 1975). The warning aura may be an inability to get over a word, or a feeling like one may swallow one's tongue, or a complaint of spots before the eyes or of blurred vision, all without any jaw jerking. The aura may present with visual difficulties such as letters or words appearing out of place (Critchley *et al.*, 1959–60).

Primary reading epilepsy is the objective or subjective feeling of brief movement (often jerking) or spasms of the jaw, throat, or a limb experienced only while reading. There may be vocalization or an initial pause. If the reading is continued, the jaw jerking increases in frequency and severity until consciousness is lost, with the onset of the generalized major motor seizure. Cessation of reading abolishes this phenomenon (Critchley *et al.*, 1959–60; Forster *et al.*, 1969; Brooks & Jirauch, 1971; Forster, 1977a; Login & Kolakovich, 1978).

The resting EEG is normal, but it becomes active during reading (Forster *et al.*, 1969; Brooks & Jirauch, 1971); with the jaw jerking (Login & Kolakovich, 1978), a bilaterally synchronous three to six per second spike or polyspike-wave discharge emerges, increasing in frequency if reading is continued. The EEG abnormalities may be focal in some patients and generalized in others (Forster *et al.*, 1969; Brooks & Jirauch, 1971; Ramani, 1983). Focal discharges may be parietal-occipital areas in some patients (Critchley *et al.*, 1959–60) and frontal in others, with a tendency to be lateralized to the dominant hemisphere. In some people, the triggering stimulus may be simple and stereotypic, such as by a specific word, with the evoked EEG abnormality being focal cortical (Forster, 1977; Ramani, 1983).

Secondary reading epilepsy

Secondary reading epilepsy, seen in both children and adults (Critchley *et al.*, 1959–60), is part of a much more generalized epilepsy disorder in which seizures occur during or are precipitated by reading (Forster *et al.*, 1969). The stimulus is more complex, such as seizures induced by language rather than by a specific word (Ramani, 1983).

Reading meaningful but unfamiliar material usually precipitates the seizures at any point within 40 minutes. Substitution of an unfamiliar word into familiar and memorized material may even precipitate a seizure, as may reading a foreign language, braille, or numbers (Math calculation, however, does not precipitate seizures.) Seizures come when reading aloud and also with silent reading, without movements of the oral-glossal muscles. Occasionally, the act of reading does not trigger seizures but listening to playback of what was read does. Concentration-induced seizures may also occur with reading epilepsy. This can also be seen with card games but not with childhood games (Forster, 1977b).

The EEG discharge is more diffuse, generalized in nature, and presumably of subcortical origin. There may be simple and complex forms, primarily generalized in simple reflex forms and focal cortical in the more complex reflex forms. Not all reading epilepsies are of the complex type. Patients with a simple visual or proprioceptive input present with seizures of a simple type with a bilaterally synchronized spike or spike-wave discharge, maximum anterior, which may build up to a major seizure (Ramani, 1983). Patterns may also precipitate absence-like attacks (Critchley *et al.*, 1959–60). In others, complex language processing is responsible. The focal EEG abnormality often involves specifically the frontal-temporal regions of the dominant hemisphere (Ramani, 1983).

Individuals with birth injuries may have reading-evoked seizures, often with preceding subjective sensations. Before each attack, the words might appear to be out of place and the letters interchanged, just prior to the right-sided to generalized motor seizure. The EEG may show reading-provoked isolated sharp waves in the left occipital area from childhood onward. A unilateral lesion, especially of the right hemisphere, may be invoked in secondary reading epilepsies (Critchley *et al.*, 1959–60).

Medication is the only therapy, although reading epilepsy tends to be rather refractory to anticonvulsants. Valproate and clonazepam may be effective, especially with generalized forms of reading epilepsy (Forster, 1977a; Login & Kolakovich, 1978; Hall & Marshall, 1980; Login, 1981; Vanderzant *et al.*, 1982).

Spelling

Children, particularly boys, with epilepsy may have even more difficulties in spelling and math than with reading (Bagley, 1971; Green & Hartlage, 1970; Green & Hartlage, 1971; Weintraub, 1981; Jelnnekens-Schinkel *et al.*, 1987). Children with mixed absence-generalized tonic–clonic seizures are particularly disadvantaged (Seidenberg *et al.*, 1986). Children with a past history of febrile convulsions, whether treated or not, may have more spelling disorders (Camfield *et al.*, 1979).

Arithmetic

Delays in arithmetic skills comprise the most common and most impaired area of academic functioning (Green & Hartlage, 1970; Green & Hartlage, 1971). Early seizure onset, increased lifetime seizure total, and the presence of generalized seizures relate to poorer arithmetic achievement as well as spelling difficulties (Seidenberg *et al.*, 1986). Children with epilepsy have particular difficulties in acquiring arithmetic skills, often performing about one to two years behind their peers, even in uncomplicated cases of epilepsy (Bagley, 1970; Green & Hartlage, 1970; Green & Hartlage, 1971; Poche, 1978). A variety of learning disabilities may affect arithmetic, including problems of perceptual discrimination, spatial ordering, attention, and memory skills. Math problems become especially apparent in Piaget's concrete operations stage of development of the seven- to 11-year-old, in which the grasp of numerical and spatial reasoning as well as the cause and effect concept becomes most important (Haskell, 2000). Math struggles become most prominent in the adolescent years (Aldenkamp, 1983; Aldenkamp, 1987; Bagley, 1970; Bagley, 1971; Green & Hartlage, 1970; Green & Hartlage, 1971; Ross & West, 1978; Seidenberg *et al.*, 1986; Weintraub, 1981).

Gender

Both girls and boys have problems with arithmetic (Seidenberg *et al.*, 1986). Gender differences have been noted in math aptitude and achievement, especially by adolescence. Girls excel in computation, while boys excel in tasks requiring mathematical reasoning ability (Fox, 1931–3). The gender differences increase through high school years (Benbow & Stanley, 1980; Benbow & Stanley, 1981), when math courses involve more perceptual-spatial aspects, with geometry, trigonometry, etc. (Collins, 1951). Problems in concentration and recent memory are often blamed for depressions in written math as compared with oral math (Fox, 1931–3).

Seizure types

Children with generalized seizures, especially those with both absence and generalized tonic–clonic seizures, perform more poorly than children with partial seizures. People with multiple seizure types are at increased risk for various aspects of psychological functioning (Seidenberg *et al.*, 1986). Arithmetic is not thought to be influenced by the lateralization of discharges (Kasteleijn-Nolste Trenite *et al.*, 1988; Kasteleijn-Nolste Trenite *et al.*, 1990), yet children with left-sided epileptic foci have lower performance on arithmetic tests than children with right-sided foci, including lower scores on mental arithmetic (Stores & Hart, 1976; Camfield *et al.*, 1984). Even if learned, math skills are often applied poorly in practical situations. Subclinical epileptiform discharges increase during performance of academic tasks, especially with reading but also frequently with arithmetic (Wilkins, 1986; Kateleijn-Nolst Trenite *et al.*, 1988).

Math processing

Reading involves primarily one language, the alphabet, whereas math involves three languages, the alphabetical language, the numerical language, and the operational language of plus, minus, divide, and multiply. Arithmetic is a more complex task, involving multiple cognitive operations, both verbal and spatial, requiring activity of both hemispheres. Arithmetic operations require the functioning of a large number of higher mental processes that reside largely in the left hemisphere. The right hemisphere is capable of only simple addition. The right hemisphere is capable of more complex math operations and perhaps also with a greater degree of accuracy. Language is a higher mental process involved in arithmetic operations. The identification or expression of numbers rather than calculation is the math operation related to language. Cortical lesions disturbing language often disturb number identification, although calculations may remain intact. Lesions associated with memory also interfere with math operations, most prominently those involving division and subtraction and calculations that involve remembering math tables, although the ability to perform at least simple addition may be preserved (Kateleijn-Nolst Trenite et al., 1990). Calculation deficits are especially pronounced even when the ability to count or identify numbers is preserved (Ojemann, 1974). Memory deficits may impair the learning and recall of multiplication tables.

A decreased capacity for systematic mental operations may contribute to the specific underachievement in arithmetic, similar to that found in non-epileptic learning-disabled children with an arithmetic disability (Aldenkamp et al., 1990; Strang & Rourke, 1985). Children with epilepsy tend to be slightly behind in numerical reasoning (Halstead, 1957; Heijbel & Behman, 1975). Slowed information processing may be noted, especially in complex task configurations, with underachievement in arithmetic. This appears to be related to detrimental effects of polytherapy and long-term treatment with phenytoin (Aldenkamp, 1983; Aldenkamp, 1987). The lack of concentration in children with epilepsy accounts for the poor results seen in written math as compared with oral math (Fox, 1931–3).

Math-induced seizures

Many children with epilepsy show an increase in the epileptiform discharge rate during reading or arithmetic (Kateleijn-Nolst Trenite et al., 1988). Seizures may be induced by any type of cognitive activity involving math, including reading numbers (Forster, 1977a), mental arithmetic, and related intelligence test subtests (Fenwick, 1981). Seizures that appear during arithmetic may be due to concentration, hand movements, or the mental activity involved in the computation task (Forster & Daily, 1973; Forster, 1977b).

Generalized convulsions

Patients with generalized convulsions precipitated by arithmetic (Wilkins et al., 1982) and by concentration (Aarts et al., 1984) demonstrate EEG discharges only during specific intellectually demanding activities. The incidence of epileptiform EEG activity is increased by cognitive tasks activating the specific cognitive region and decreased by cognitive activity that involves other brain regions (Wilkins, 1986). Some individuals who have a history of struggles in math experience generalized tonic–clonic seizures associated with generalized spike-wave activity and also often have absence seizures. Easy arithmetic tasks, including simple math calculations, produce the three per second spike-wave bursts. Harder problems produce a loss of consciousness. Still harder problems produce a generalized seizure. Some patients may give any answer quickly to successfully avoid the discharges (Ingvar & Nyman, 1962).

Mental arithmetic may induce subclinical generalized epileptiform activity. Tasks involving multiplication, division, and the manipulation of spatial information are especially apt to bring out such epileptiform activity. Few if any discharges occur with addition and subtraction. Tasks involving the retention of numerical information in short-term memory, such as the immediate repetition of a series of eight digits, do not activate the discharges. There may be a history of generalized shaking without loss of consciousness beginning around age 12 years (Wilkins *et al.*, 1982).

Focal convulsions

Mathematical calculations and even the act of focusing attention on an arithmetic problem may lead to a seizure of focal onset, such as with a right frontal spiking. The seizure symptoms may be a minor motor type or they may present as generalized tonic–clonic activity. There may be a history of below-average intelligence, with difficulties in math calculations and perhaps other areas, such as verbal abstractions. Activation occurs principally with mental or written calculation but rarely when listening to the presentation of math problems, when picturing numbers in problem form, when working simple math problems, or with immediate digit recall. Attacks may be seen occasionally in activities dealing with numbers, such as in dialing a telephone or when knitting and counting the stitches. No activation may be seen with reading, writing, reciting, revisualization, or recalling numbers or other symbols. Major antiepileptics may have only a moderate effect (Ingvar & Nyman, 1962; Wiebers *et al.*, 1979).

Drawing and writing

Handwriting problems, which slow performance and lower the functioning level, may be seen in the classroom, especially in written efforts (Forster, 1977a; Jelnnekens-Schinkel *et al.*, 1987). Hypergraphia (excessive writing) may be seen with temporal lobe foci (Waxman & Geschwind, 1975; Aldenkamp *et al.*, 1990).

Children with epilepsy may struggle with drawing, which may be the result of several types of disorders. Children with right-hemispheric problems may have difficulties in incorporating spatial information into their drawing, leading to disproportion and faulty articulation of parts of the drawing. Those with left-hemispheric problems seem to have difficulties in planning the drawing, leading to simplified versions (Warrington *et al.*, 1966).

Writing-induced seizures

Seizures may also occur when writing, even when the child is blindfolded. Taking shorthand does not produce seizures, but transcribing shorthand to typing may do so. Playing the piano may also trigger seizures. The seizures appear as abnormal movements, clonic jerking, or tonic freezing of the writing hand (Forster & Daily, 1973; Forster, 1977a).

Other problems

Speed of information processing, memory, vigilance alertness, sustained and focused attention, and motor fluency are important cognitive domains that are especially vulnerable to epileptic factors. Other areas of deficit are in language and problem-solving, and there may be perceptual and motor difficulties (Waxman and Geschwind, 1975; Kupke & Lewis, 1985; Brittain, 1980; Aldenkamp, 1987; Beaumont, 1987; Dodrill, 1987; Oxley & Stores, 1987; Aldenkamp *et al.*, 1990).

Modifying factors

Modifying factors include underlying brain abnormalities, pre-existing learning disabilities, specific attention and memory deficits, and psychological adjustment factors (Bailet & Turk, 2000). Risk predictors include a history of status and the child's neuropsychological profile and behavior more than seizure and medical variables (Warner *et al.*, 1991).

Idiopathic versus symptomatic seizures

Children with symptomatic epilepsies are more prone to having learning disabilities than those with idiopathic epilepsies, especially if the seizures are of preschool onset. The brain scans may be abnormal, or coexistent medical conditions may be present (Bailet & Turk, 2000). Some children with focal epilepsy and generalized epilepsy are found to have heterotopias especially in the left hemisphere in the area of the planum temporale (Galaburda & Kemper, 1979).

Gender

Boys with epilepsy do badly in spelling, arithmetic, and reading comprehension, and girls with epilepsy generally do better than boys with epilepsy, except in arithmetic. Children with both absence and generalized tonic–clonic seizures seem particularly disadvantaged (Seidenberg *et al.*, 1986).

Age of onset

Children whose seizures develop before five years of age perform significantly worse in verbal and performance IQ areas. The performance of children with secondarily generalized seizures is worse than those with simple and complex partial seizures (Collins, 1951; Keith *et al.*, 1955; O'Leary *et al.*, 1983; Rodin *et al.*, 1986; Rugland, 1990a).

Frequency

The effect of seizure frequency on academic abilites in children with learning is debated (Bailet & Turk, 2000). Cognitive activity is believed to reduce the frequency of spontaneous epileptiform EEG discharges (Guey *et al.*, 1967; Vidart & Geier, 1977). The frequency is lowest in performance at the child's own level than in tasks of greater or lesser difficulty (Hutt *et al.*, 1977). The discharge rate may be lower at rest than during performance of difficult scholastic tasks (Kateleijn-Nolst Trenite *et al.*, 1988).

Duration

There is an inverse correlation between the duration of seizures and the child's intelligence (Farwell *et al.*, 1985; Rugland, 1990a).

REFERENCES

Aarts, J. H. P., Binnie, C. D., Smit, A. M., *et al.* (1984). Selective cognitive impairment during focal and generalized epileptiform EEG activity. *Brain Dev.* **107**: 293–308.

Aldenkamp, A. P. (1983). Epilepsy and learning behavior. In *Advances in epileptology: The XIVth International Epilepsy Symposium*, ed. M. Parsonage, R. H. E. Grant, A. G. Craig & A. A. Ward, Jr, pp. 221–9. New York: Raven Press.

Aldenkamp, A. P. (1987). Learning disabilities in epilepsy. In *Education and Epilepsy* 1987, ed. A. P. Aldenkamp, W. C. J. Alpherts, H. Meinardi & G. Stores, pp. 21–38. Lisse: Swets & Zeitlinger.

Aldenkamp, A. P., Alpherts, W. C. J., Dekker, M. J. A., *et al.* (1990). Neuropsychological aspects of learning disabilities in epilepsy. *Epilepsia* **31** (suppl 4): 9–20.

Bagley, C. R. (1970). The educational performance of children with epilepsy. *Br. J. Educ. Psychol.* **140**: 82–3.

Bagley, C. (1971). *The Social Psychology of the child with Epilepsy*. London: Kegan Paul.

Bailet, L. L. & Turk, W. R. (2000). The impact of childhood epilepsy on neurocognitive and behavioral performance: a prospective longitudinal study. *Epilepsia* **41**: 426–31.

Baird, H. W., John, E. R. Ahn, H., *et al.* (1980). Neurometric evaluation of epileptic children who do well and poorly in school. *Electroencephalog. Clin. Neurophysiol.* **48**: 583–93.

Beaumanoir, A., Ballism T., Varfis, G., *et al.* (1964). Benign epilepsy of childhood with Rolandic spikes. *Epilepsia* **15**: 301–15.

Beaumont, M. E. (1987). *Epilepsy and Learning: Understanding the Learning Difficulties Experienced by Children with Epilepsy*. Melbourne: National Epilepsy Association of Australia.

Benbow, D. P. & Stanley, J. C. (1980). Sex differences in mathematical ability: fact or artifact? *Science* **210**: 1262–3.

Benbow, C. P. & Stanley, J. C. (1981). Mathematical ability: is sex a factor? (a response). *Science* **212**: 114–21.

Berger, H. (1971). An unusual manifestation of Tegretol (carbamazepine) toxicity. *Ann. Intern. Med.* **74**: 449–50.

Bickford, R. G., Whelan, J. L., Klass, D. W. & Corbin, K. B., *et al.* (1956). Reading epilepsy. *Trans. Am. Neurol. Assoc.* **31**: 100.

Boder, E. (1973). Developmental dyslexia: a diagnostic approach based on three atypical reading–spelling patterns. *Dev. Med. Child Neurol.* **15**: 664–87.

Brittain, H. (1980). Epilepsy and intellectual functions. In *Epilepsy and Behaivor*, ed. B. M. Kulig, H. Meiinardi & G. Stores, pp. 2–13. Lisse: Swets & Zeitlinger.

Browne, T. R., Dreifuss, R. E., Dyken, P. R., *et al.* (1975). Ethosuximide in the treatment of absence (petit mal) seizures. *Neurology* **25**: 515–24.

Brooks, J. E. & Jirauch, P. M. (1971). Primary reading epilepsy: a misnomer. *Arch. Neurol.* **25**: 97–104.

Camfield, C. S., Chaplin, S., Doyle, A. V., *et al.* (1979). Side effects of phenobarbital in toddlers: behavior and cognitive aspects. *J. Pediatr.* **93**: 361–5.

Camfield, P. E., Gates, R., Ronen, G., *et al.* (1984). Comparison of cognitive ability, personality profile and school success in epileptic children with pure right versus left temporal lobe EEG foci. *Ann. Neurol.* **15**: 1122–6.

Ceci, S. J. (1986). *Handbook of Cognitive and Neurophysiological Aspects of Learning Disabilities.* London: Lawrence Erlbaum.

Collins, A. L. (1951). Epileptic intelligence. *J. Consult. Psychol.* **165**: 393–9.

Critchley, M., Cobb, W. & Sears, T. A. (1959–60). On reading epilepsy. *Epilepsia* **1**: 403–17.

Dodrill, C. B. (1987). Aspects of antiepileptic treatment in children. *Epilepsia* **29** (suppl 3): 10–14.

Fairweather, H. & Hutt, S. J. (1969). Interrelationship of EEG activity and information processing on paced and self–paced tasks in epileptic children. *Electroencephalogr. Clin. Neurophysiol.* **27**: 701–10.

Fairweather, H. & Hutt, S. J. (1971). Some effects of performance variables upon generalized spike-wave activity. *Brain* **904**: 321–6.

Farwell, J. R., Dodrill, B. B. & Batzel, L. W. (1985). Neuropsychological abilities of children with epilepsy. *Epilepsia* **26**: 395–400.

Fenwick, P. (1981). Precipitation and inhibition of seizures. In *Epilepsy and Psychiatry*, ed. E. H. Reynolds & M. R. Trimble, pp. 306–21. New York: Churchill Livingstone.

Fisk, J. & Rourke, B. P. (1979). Identification of subtypes of learning disabilities at three age levels: a neuropsychological, multivarient approach. *J. Clin. Neuropsycholl.* **4**: 289–309.

Forster, F. M. (1977a). Reflex epilepsy, behavior therapy and conditioned reflexes. In *Reflex Epilepsy, Behavior Therapy and Conditioned Reflexes*, pp. 94–123. Springfield, IL: Charles C. Thomas.

Forster, F. M. (1977b). Epilepsy evoked by higher cognitive functions: decision making epilepsy. In *Reflex Epilepsy, Behavior Therapy and Conditioned Reflexes*, pp. 124–34. Springfield, IL: Charles C. Thomas.

Forster, F. M. & Daily, R. F. (1973). Reading epilepsy in identical twins. *Trans. Ann. Neurol. Assoc.* **98**: 186–8.

Forster, F. M., Paulsen, W. A. & Baughman, F. A., Jr. (1969). Clinical therapeutic conditioning in reading epilepsy. *Neurology* **19**: 717–23.

Fox, J. T. (1931–3). The response of epileptic children to mental and educational tests. *Br. Med. Psych.* **4**: 235–48.

Galaburda, A. M. & Kemper, T. L. (1979). Cytoarchitectonic abnormalities in developmental dyslexia: a case study. *Ann. Neurol.* **6**: 94–100.

Green, J. B. & Hartlage, L. C. (1970). Comparitive performance of epileptic and non-epileptic children and adolescents on academic, communicative and social skills. Presented at the 3rd European Symposium on Epilepsy.

Green, J. B. & Hartlage, L. C. (1971). Comparative performance of epileptic and non-epileptic children and adolescents. *Dis. Nerv. Syst.* **32**: 418–21.

Guey, J., Charles, C., Coquery, C., *et al.* (1967). Study of psychological defects of ethosuximide (Zarontin) on 25 children suffering from petit mal epilepsy. *Epilepsia* **8**: 2129–41.

Hall, J. H. & Marshall, P. C. (1980). Clonazepam therapy in reading epilepsy. *Neurology* **30**: 550–51.

Halstead, H. (1957). Abilities and behavior of epileptic children. *J. Ment. Sci.* **103**: 28–47.

Haskell, S. H. (2000). The determinants of arithmetic skills in young children: some observations. *Eur. Child Adolesc. Psychiatry* **9**: 77–86.

Heijbel, J. & Behman, M. (1975). Benign epilepsy of children with centrotemporal EEG foci: intelligence, behavior and school adjustment. *Epilepsia* **16**: 679–87.

Hutt, S. J., Newton, S. & Fairweather, H. (1977). Choice reaction time and EEG activity in children with epilepsy. *Neuropsychologia* **15**: 257–67.

Ingvar, D. H. & Nyman, C. E. (1962). Epilespia arithmetices, a trigger mechanism in a case of epilepsy. *Neurology* **12**: 282–7.

Jelnnekens-Schinkel, A., Linsschooten-Duikersloot, E. M. E. M., Bourma, P. A. D., Peters, A. C. B. & Stijnen, T. H. (1987). Spelling errors made by children with mild epilepsy: writing-to-dictation. *Epilepsia* **28**: 555–63.

Kasteleijn-Nolst Trenite, D. G. N., Bakker, D. J., Binnie, C. D., *et al.* (1988). Psychological effects of epileptiform EEG discharges. I: scholastic skills. *Epilepsy Res.* **2**: 111–16.

Kasteleijn-Nolst Trenite, D. G. N., Siebelink, B. M., Beerends, S. G. C., *et al.* (1990). Lateralized effects of subclinical epileptiform EEG discharges on scholastic performance in children. *Epilepsia* **31**: 740–46.

Keith, H., Evert, J. C., Green, M. W., *et al.* (1955). Mental status of children with convulsive disorders. *Neurology* **5**: 419–25.

Knight, R. M. & Tymchuk, A. J. (1968). An evaluation of the Halstead-Reitan Category Text for children. *Cortex* **4**: 403–13.

Kupke, T. & Lewis, R. (1985). WAIS and neuropsychological tests, common and unique variance with in an epileptic population. *J. Clin. Exp. Neuropsychol.* **7**: 353–66.

Laidlaw, J. & Richens, A. (1976). Fits in childhood: education. In *A Textbook of Epilepsy*, pp. 101–2. New York: Churchill Livingstone.

Login, I. S. (1981). Clonazepam therapy in reading epilepsy. *Neurology* **31**: 115.

Login, I. S. & Kolakovich, T. M. (1978). Successful treatment of primary reading epilepsy with clonazepam. *Ann. Neurol.* **4**: 155–6.

Long, G. G. & Moore, J. R. (1979). Parental expectations for their epileptic children. *J. Child Psychol. Psychiatry* **20**: 299–312.

Mandelbaum, D. E., Burack, G. D. & Daswani, A. A. (1993). Effects of seizure type and medication on psychological functioning in epileptic children. *Epilepsia* **34** (suppl 6): 72.

Ojemann, G. A. (1974). Mental arithmetic during human thalamic stimulation. *Neuropsychologia* **12**: 1–10.

O'Leary, D. S., Lovell, M. R., Sackellares, J. C., *et al.* (1983). Effects of age of onset on partial and generalized seizures on neurophysiological performance in children. *J. Nerv. Ment. Dis.* **171**: 624–9.

Oxley, J. & Stores, G. (1987). *Epilepsy and Education.* London: Medical Tribune Group.

Piras, M. R., Sechi, G. P., Mutani, R., *et al.* (1991). Developmental surface dyslexia in progressive myoclonic epilepsy. 19th International Epilepsy Congress. *Epilepsia* **32** (suppl 1): 25.

Poche, P. (1978). Educating the child with seizures. In *The Treatment of Epilepsy Today*, ed. G. S. Ferriss, pp. 127–41. Oradell, NJ: Medical Economic Co. Book Division.

Ramani, V. (1983). Primary reading epilepsy. *Arch. Neurol.* **40**: 49–51.

Rodin, E. A., Schmaltz, S. & Twitty, G. (1986). Intellectual functions of patients with childhood-onset epilepsy. *Dev. Med. Child Neurol.* **28**: 250–53.

Rourke, B. P. (1985). *Neuropsychology of Learning Disabilities: Essentials of Subtype Analysis.* New York: Guildford Press.

Rugland, A. L. (1990a). Neuropsychological assessment of cognitive functioning in children with epilepsy. *Epilepsia* **31** (suppl 4): 41–4.

Rugland, A. (1990b). Subclinical epileptogenic activity. In *Pediatric Epilepsy*, ed. M. Sillarpaa, S. I. Johnanessen, G. Blennow & M. Dam, pp. 217–23. London: Wrightson Biomedical.

Rutter, M. (1974). Emotional disorder and educational underachievement. *Arch. Dis. Child.* **48**: 249–56.

Rutter, M. & Yule, W. (1975). The concept of specific reading retardation. *J. Child. Psychol. Psychiatry* **16**: 181–97.

Rutter, M., Graham, P. & Yule, W. (1970). A neuropsychiatric study in childhood. In *Clinics in Developmental Medicine* 35/36, pp. 237–55. London: Spastics Society and Heinemann.

Saykin, A. J., Maerlender, A. C., Moran, M., *et al.* (1993). Level and patterns of changes in verbal learning after anterotemporal lobectomy: effects of early risk factors. *Epilepsia* **34** (suppl 6): 91.

Schacter, S. C., Galaburda, A. M. & Ransil, B. J. (1991). Epilepsy: associations with developmental dyslexia, gender, and handedness. *Epilepsia* **32** (suppl 3): 74–5.

Seidenberg, M., Beck, N., Geisser, M., *et al.* (1986). Academic achievement of children with epilepsy. *Epilepsia* **27**: 753–9.

Stores, G. (1973). Studies of attention and seizure disorders. *Dev. Med. Child Neurol.* **15**: 376–82.

Stores, G. (1976). The investigation and management of school children with epilepsy. *Publ. Health, Lond.* **90**: 171–7.

Stores, G. (1978). School children with epilepsy at risk for learning and behavior problems. *Dev. Med. Child Neurol.* **20**: 502–8.

Stores, G. (1981). Problems of learning and behavior in children with epilepsy. In *Epilepsy and Psychiatry*, ed. E. H. Reynolds & M. R. Trimble, pp. 33–48. New York: Churchill Livingstone.

Stores, G. (1987). Effects on learning of "subclinical" seizure discharges. In *Education and Epilepsy 1987*, ed. A. P. Aldenkamp, W. C. J. Alpherts, H. Meinardi & G. Stores, pp. 14–21. Lisse: Swets & Zeitlinger.

Stores, G. & Hart, J. (1976). Reading skills of children with generalized and focal epilepsy attending ordinary school. *Dev. Med. Child Neurol.* **18**: 705–16.

Stores, G., Hart, J. & Piran, N. (1978). Inattentiveness in school children with epilepsy. *Epilepsia* **19**: 169–75.

Strang, J. & Rourke, B. P. (1985). Adaptive behavior of children who exhibit specific arithmetic disabilities and associated neuropsychological abilities and deficits. In *Neuropsychology of Learning Disabilities. Essentials of Subtype Analysis*, ed. B. P. Rourke, pp. 302–31. New York: Guildford Press.

Thompson, P. J. (1987). Educational attainment in children and young people with epilepsy. In *Epilepsy and Education*, ed. J. Oxley & G. Stores, pp. 15–24. London: Medical Tribute Group.

Trimble, M. R. (1983). Anticonvulsant drugs and psychosocial development: phenobarbitone, sodium valproate and benzodiazepines. In *Antiepileptic Drug Therapy in Pediatrics*, ed. P. M. Morselli, C. E. Pippinger & J. Penry, pp. 201–71. New York: Raven Press.

Trimble, M. R. (1990). Antiepileptic drugs, cognitive function and behavior in children: evidence from recent studies. *Epilepsia* **31** (suppl 4): 30–35.

Van der Vlugth, H. & Bakker, D. (1980). Lateralization of brain function in persons with epilepsy. In *Epilepsy and Behavior '79*, ed. B. M. Kulig, H. Meinardi & G. Stores, pp. 30–35. Lisse: Swets & Zeitlinger.

Vanderzant, C., Fiitz, R., Holmes, G., *et al.* (1982). Treatment of primary reading epilepsy with valproic acid. *Arch. Neurol.* **39**: 452–3.

Vidart, L. & Geier, S. (1977). Enrigistrements tele'encephalographiques chex des sujets epileptiques pendant le travail. *Rev. Neurol.* **117**: 475–80.

Warner, M. H., Dodrill, C., Batzel, L. W., *et al.* (1991). Early predictors of academic and psychosocial functioning in adolescents with a history of seizures. *Epilepsia* **32** (suppl 3): 75.

Warrington, E. K., James, M. & Kinsbourne, M. (1966). Drawing disability in relation to laterality of cerebral lesion. *Brain* **89**: 53–82.

Waxman, S. G. & Geschwind, N. (1975). The interictal behavior syndrome of temporal lobe epilepsy. *Arch. Gen. Psychiatry* **32**: 1580–86.

Wechsler, A. F. (1973). The effect of organic brain disease on recall of emotionally charged versus neutral narrative texts. *Neurology* **23**: 130–35.

Weintraub, P. (1981). The brain: his and hers. *Discover* **April**: 15–20.

Wiebers, D. O., Westmoreland, B. F. & Klass, D. W. (1979). EEG activation and mathematical calculation. *Neurology* **29**: 1499–1503.

Wilkins, A. J. (1986). On the manner in which sensory and cognitive processes contribute to epileptogenisis and are disrupted by it. *Acta Neurol. Scand.* **74** (suppl 109): 91–5.

Wilkins, A. J., Zifkin, B., Andermann, F., *et al.* (1982). Seizures induced by thinking. *Ann. Neurol.* **11**: 608–12.

22

Antiepileptic medication effects

In 1948, William Lennox observed: "Many physicians, attempting to extinguish seizures, only succeed in drowning the intellectual process of the patient." The goal of therapy is to stop the seizures without stopping the patient's functioning. With antiepileptic medications, the question concerns not the best drug for the seizure type but rather the best drug for the child.

Anticonvulsants

The goal of modern drug treatment for epilepsy should be the cessation of seizures but also the prevention of cognitive and behavior dysfunctions (Billard, 1999). All anticonvulsant drugs impair cognitive functions to some degree, although some do so more than others. The longer a drug is in use, the longer becomes the list of side effects associated with it. No single drug causes problems in every patient. No drug can be assumed to never cause any cognitive impairment (Bourgeois, 2002). Adverse effects on learning and behavior usually appear by one month after beginning an antiepileptic medication (Henricksen, 1990). The effects of antiepileptic drugs on brain development and cognitive functioning need to be considered when choosing which antiepileptic to use (Alpherts & Aldenkamp, 1990; Blennow et al., 1990; Rugland, 1990; Trimble, 1990).

Adverse effects

Antiepileptic medications at excessive dosages impair both behavior and cognition, even if used alone (Matthews & Harley, 1975; Stores & Piran, 1978; Bourgeois et al., 1983; Reila, 1998). Although drug levels can be checked, the standard therapeutic ranges signify only a level needed and tolerated in many patients; there are exceptions. Some patients need and tolerate more drug, but others need and tolerate less. Levels need to be compared with the child's functioning (Stores, 1976). Even at accepted therapeutic levels, some individuals may be overly sensitive to the adverse effects of a medication. This may be overcome in some patients by lowering dosage, but in others it may be overcome only by stopping the medication.

Use of multiple anticonvulsants simultaneously (polypharmacy) tends to accentuate cognitive and behavior problems (Reynolds & Shorvon, 1981; Trimble & Thompson, 1984a). Performance is suppressed, but this may not be apparent until the drugs are withdrawn, with improvements in more than 50% (Shorvon & Reynolds, 1979; Thompson & Huppert, 1980; Reynolds & Shorvon, 1981; Thompson & Trimble, 1982a; Thompson & Trimble, 1982b; Trimble & Thompson, 1983; Giordani *et al.*, 1985; Blennow *et al.*, 1990; Trimble, 1990). Children on polypharmacy may have more problems (Thompson & Trimble, 1983; Butlin *et al.*, 1984; Cull, 1988; Rugland, 1990; Trimble, 1988; Trimble, 1990) with attention, perception, memory, and retrieval, as well as difficulty in problem-solving, with consequently slowed performance (Schain, 1983; Trimble & Cull, 1990). This can be overcome by reducing the drug load (Aldenkamp *et al.*, 1993). The golden rule of anticonvulsant therapy remains to use as few drugs and in as small a dose as possible (Addy, 1987). If polytherapy proves necessary, increased awareness of how the drugs work may serve to avoid duplicated brain effects, approaching seizure control by selecting medications that work in differing ways so as to avoid increasing adverse tendencies.

Drug effects on cognition

All anticonvulsants have been associated with adverse effects on cognition in some but not all children (Aldenkamp, 2001; Stores, 1990). Drug effects differ between children more than between adults (Trimble & Thompson, 1981; Thompson & Trimble, 1982a; Thompson & Trimble, 1982b; Dodson, 1988; Aldenkamp *et al.*, 1990; Trimble, 1990; Trimble & Reynolds, 1976). About 1% experience cognitive side effects after drug initiation, but if recognized these effects are usually reversible (Aldenkamp, 2001).

Age effects

The elderly, the neurodevelopmentally evolving child, and the fetus may be more at risk for the cognitive side effects of antiepileptic medications (Meador, 2002). In elderly patients, metabolism may be more sluggish, whereas in preschool children, metabolism is more rapid, requiring higher dosages and more frequent dosing. In children under four years of age, and in girls with menses, some drugs such as phenytoin may be metabolized erratically (Aldenkamp *et al.*, 1993).

Intrauterine exposure

In utero exposure to antiepileptic drugs at dosages required to produce somatic malformation and at clinically relevant blood levels can impair neurodevelopment (Loring & Meador, 2001). Motor and mental development postnatally may be slowed (Thomas *et al.*, 2001). Barbiturates, phenytoin, clonazepam, and valproate are neurotoxic to the developing brain, resulting in reduced neuron numbers and reduced enzyme systems, including GABA. Phenobarbital reduces dendritic branching at high level. Partial recovery may be seen following removal from exposure. The children of mothers on polypharmacy show a proportional increase in neurologic dysfunctions and lowered intelligence (Koch *et al.*, 1999; Reinisch *et al.*, 1995; Vinten *et al.*, 2001).

Problems

The principal psychologic disturbances include depression or deterioration of learning and intelligence, which may emerge with introduction of the drug or may be a gradual, chronic, insidious effect.

Intelligence

All established antiepileptic drugs may have adverse, often subtle, cognitive effects on intelligence, although with differing frequencies (Trimble & Reynolds, 1976; Trimble & Thompson, 1981; Trimble & Thompson, 1983; Aldenkamp, 2001; Cornaggia & Gobbi, 2001).

Deterioration

With chronic drug usage, even at therapeutic levels, a subtle, slow deterioration of intelligence, emotions, or behaviors may occur. The problem can usually but not always be overcome by switching to another anticonvulsant drug (Svoboda, 1979).

Learning disabilities

Children appear to be at special risks for cognitive side effects of antiepileptic drugs. The most common problem areas include attention, perception memory, and performance speed (Macleod *et al.*, 1978; Meador, 2001; Meador, 2002). These side effects are more apt to occur at high drug levels, but they may be seen with therapeutic blood ranges (Hartlage *et al.*, 1980; Trimble & Thompson, 1983). The effects may be drug-precipitated problems or drug-induced aggravation of underlying problems (Cornaggia & Gobbi, 2001). Underlying learning disabilities may be improved by altering the choice or dosage of the anticonvulsant medication (Hosking *et al.*, 1993). With some children, the drug may speed up performance but at the sacrifice of accuracy (Blennow *et al.*, 1990).

Attention problems

Almost any drug that affects the nervous system is capable of inducing some type of attention and vigilance problem in children (Besag, 2001; Meador, 2002).

Teachers' impressions

Teachers perceive at least one-third of children with epilepsy as having poor concentration and mental processing and to be less alert than their normal peers (Bennett-Levy & Stores, 1984). However, teachers receive little information on the medications being used, especially in those children whose seizures are controlled and whose medications are tolerated well (Gadow, 1982).

Treatment versus no treatment

The risks and benefits of treatment should be weighed against the risks and benefits of uncontrolled seizures. Only 30–40% of children presenting with their first seizure will have recurrences (Shinnar, 1991). Benign seizure types such as simple febrile seizures, benign focal seizures, and photosensitive seizures may not require treatment, for the medications may be more impairing than the seizures (Pellock, 1990). Potentially recurring seizures or subclinical EEG activity associated with adverse related functions may be treated. Treatment should be continued only if the benefit of reduced epileptiform activity can be demonstrated and if adverse cognitive effects of the drug can be avoided (Henricksen, 1990). The child must be monitored closely for any adverse effects; if such effects arise, the child should be reassessed with the therapy optimized. Most children (70–75%) who remain seizure-free for two to four years can come off medication (Shinnar *et al.*, 1985), although those with neurologic abnormalities may be less apt to become medication free (Pellock, 1990).

Older anticonvulsants

The older, established antiepileptic drugs, based largely on the barbiturate model, have both neural and systemic problems. Systemic concerns included rashes and liver, kidney, and blood reactions. Neural reactions, often subtle, include sedation, attention problems, perceptual difficulties, memory difficulties, and cognition impairments. The drug effects often emerge within a few months and almost always before six months of taking the drug (Dodrill, 1998; Meador *et al.*, 1995). Some higher cognitive effects may emerge only with chronic treatment and may persist even after the drug is stopped (Gallassi *et al.*, 1988).

Barbiturates
Phenobarbital

Phenobarbital is inexpensive, is relatively safe, and can be given as a once-daily dosage. Like any drug, the use of it requires close monitoring for any side effects (Jeavons, 1977).

Phenobarbital is a sedative and may depress intelligence and performance (Stores, 1975). In younger children on phenobarbital, development is delayed (Trimble, 1983; Farwell *et al.*, 1990). At higher doses, the drug may produce memory and comprehension problems, slow performance, and interfere with attention and concentration (Stores, 1975; Camfield *et al.*, 1977; Hartlage *et al.*, 1980; Trimble, 1980; Trimble & Corbett, 1980; Stores, 1981; Reynolds, 1981; McCuiston *et al.*, 1983; Rodin *et al.*, 1986). Younger children, neurologically impaired children, and elderly patients are especially sensitive to these effects. Intellectual changes begin to emerge by six months in younger children, with early reduction of performance and full-scale IQ (Wapner *et al.*, 1962; Vining *et al.*, 1987; Dodson, 1988; Meador *et al.*, 1995). By 12 months, changes are subtle (Trimble & Cull, 1990), although a reduced comprehension may emerge, persistent a year later (Farwell *et al.*, 1990). When discontinued, some recovery in fine motor skills, short-term memory, and attention may be noted (Giordani *et al.*, 1983). Intellectual depression, academic performance, and P300 cognitive evoked potential delays may persist into the early grade-school years (Trimble & Corbett, 1980; Trimble, 1983; Vining *et al.*, 1983; Dodson, 1988; Vining, 1990; Chen *et al.*, 2001; Bourgeois, 2002).

Intellectual decline may occur in younger children, especially at high dosages (Stores, 1981; Bourgeois *et al.*, 1983; Rodin *et al.*, 1986; Aldenkamp *et al.*, 1990). If the dose is corrected, intelligence recovers (Matthews & Harley, 1975; Trimble, 1983; Trimble & Corbett, 1980). Barbiturates may cause a folate deficiency and declining intelligence, which can be corrected by folate replacement therapy (Wolf, 1979).

Male children born to mothers on phenobarbital show a lower verbal and total intelligence. Higher fetal exposures are associated with a reduced neuron density and complexity, possibly related to a reduction of calcium in the growing brain tissue, interfering with trophic changes in molecules and thus blocking transmitter activity as with spontaneous activities.

Attention, especially vigilance, concentration, and sustained attention skills can be affected, especially at high dosages, although some tolerance may develop in days to weeks (Trimble & Corbett, 1980). Some children continue to have sustained attention problems (Kimura, 1961; Stores, 1971; Potolicchio *et al.*, 1985). Some children are distractible, with difficulties filtering out extraneous stimuli, probably representing a cortical mechanism disturbance (Mirsky & Kornetsky, 1964; Stores, 1971; Stores, 1973; Dreifuss, 1983). Younger children may become overly excitable and overly active, although paradoxically some children may calm down (Kimura, 1961; Laidlaw & Richens, 1976). Visual perceptual-motor discrimination, perceptual memory, and fine motor tasks and speed may be impaired at higher dosages, which can be reversed by reduction of the dosage (Matthews & Harley, 1975). The problem may be apparent in arithmetic, picture completion, and block design IQ subtests (Hutt *et al.*, 1968; Reynolds, 1981; Theodore & Porter, 1983; Thompson & Huppert, 1980; Hartlage *et al.*, 1980; Aldenkamp, 2001).

Both auditory and visual short-term memory, but not long-term memory, may be depressed, especially at higher serum concentrations but also with therapeutic levels. Scanning and response times are slowed (Camfield *et al.*, 1977; Turner, 1977;

Macleod *et al.*, 1978; Camfield *et al.*, 1979; Dikmen, 1980; Theodore & Porter, 1983; Aldenkamp, 2001). This may occur acutely or chronically (Wolf *et al.*, 1981). Changing medication or reducing polypharmacy may overcome this (Giordani *et al.*, 1983).

Learning disabilities, with a depressed performance and full scale, have been noted with the barbiturates and primidone, especially at higher dosages. This appears to be related to the adverse effects on perceptual discrimination and memory functions (Hutt *et al.*, 1968; Reynolds & Travers, 1974; Camfield *et al.*, 1977; Thompson & Huppert, 1980; Trimble, 1980; Reynolds, 1981; Theodore & Porter, 1983; Vining *et al.*, 1983; Mitchell & Chavez, 1987; Vining *et al.*, 1987, Trimble, 1990; Bourgeois, 2002). At low dosages, visual scanning in a noisy setting and category decision-making may be impaired (Thompson & Huppert, 1980). At higher levels, verbal learning at all stages of auditory processing, especially discrimination and memory, is impaired, although not as much as visual motor processing (Somerfield-Ziskind & Ziskind, 1940; Matthews & Harley, 1975). Reading scores are significantly lower, but spelling and arithmetic tests are not, although arithmetic subtests of IQ testing may be impaired (Jus & Jus, 1962; Dodrill, 1998).

Primidone

Primidone is mostly metabolized to phenobarbital so the drugs produce similar behavior and cognitive side effects (Hartlage *et al.*, 1980; Trimble & Corbett, 1980; Dreifuss, 1983). Prenatal exposure to primidone is associated with a lowering of the resultant IQ in the child, inversely related to the primidone level (Koch *et al.*, 1999). The drug can depress or deteriorate intelligence (Trimble, 1983; Trimble & Corbett, 1980; Corbett *et al.*, 1985; Trimble, 1990; Trimble & Cull, 1990). Attention, concentration, and coordination problems (Macleod *et al.*, 1978; Stores, 1975; Trimble, 1980; Gadow, 1982) are noted, as are perceptual motor problems (Theodore & Porter, 1983; Rodin *et al.*, 1986) and short-term memory problems (Macleod *et al.*, 1978). These occur especially with higher levels of the drug (Thompson & Huppert, 1980). Discontinuing primidone may produce dramatic improvements in mental and motor performance in children (Theodore & Porter, 1983).

Phenytoin

The problems associated with the barbiturates were thought to be avoidable by switching to phenytoin, despite the latter drug's cosmetic side effects of hirsutism, gingival hypertrophy, and coarser facial features (Thompson & Trimble, 1982a; Thompson & Trimble, 1982b; Theodore & Porter, 1983; Ozdirim *et al.*, 1978; Thompson, 1983).

Intellectual depression or decline may be seen with phenytoin therapeutic levels, especially at higher serum levels (Barlow, 1978; Thompson & Trimble, 1981;

Thompson & Trimble, 1982a; Thompson & Trimble, 1982b; Reynolds, 1983; Thompson, 1983; Aldenkamp, 2001). The changes may be subtle (Thompson et al., 1981). Developmental delays may be seen in younger children (Matthews & Harley, 1975; Vallarta et al., 1976; Dodrill, 1976; Dodrill, 1980; Lindsay et al., 1980; Trimble, 1980). Problem areas include concentration, perception, perceptual memory, and motor speed (Nolte et al., 1980; Trimble, 1980; Trimble & Corbett, 1980; Trimble, 1980; Thompson & Huppert, 1980; Reynolds, 1981; Corbett et al., 1985; Rodin et al., 1986). Children on phenytoin seem to be most vulnerable to learning adverse effects. Stopping the drug usually leads to a slow recovery (Theodore & Porter, 1983; Gallassi et al., 1988; Blennow et al., 1990).

Intellectual deterioration may be seen with chronic therapy, especially at high serum levels (Corbett et al., 1985; Rodin et al., 1986). There may be no other signs of intoxication (Rosen, 1968; Reynolds, 1983). If this persists, only 50% may recover fully (Nolte et al., 1980). A progressive but partially reversible phenytoin encephalopathy can occur without other clinical signs of toxicity (Glaserm, 1972), especially in mentally retarded children, at normal therapeutic ranges (Vallarta et al., 1974; Trimble, 1990). This relates to depressed serum and red blood cell folate levels; it responds to replacement therapy (Trimble & Corbett, 1980; Trimble & Cull, 1990; Trimble, 1990).

Children born to mothers on phenytoin, especially as part of polypharmacy, may have a slightly depressed intelligence (Koch et al., 1999). Phenytoin reduces neurons and beta-alanine, especially those involved in GABA, in the fetus. Acetylcholine may be reduced. A fetal hydantoin syndrome has been described, with congenital defects and characteristic facies.

Attention and concentration impairments, including problems in sustained attention, are seen with phenytoin at therapeutic serum levels (Laidlaw & Richens, 1976; Stores, 1978; Gadow, 1982; Trimble, 1983; Riva et al., 1991; Duncan et al., 1990; Aldenkamp et al., 2001). Performance improves when the drug is discontinued (Duncan et al., 1990). Visual perceptual deterioration, especially discrimination, may be worse (Dodrill, 1975). There is an inverse relationship between the speed of response and the number of errors (Blennow et al., 1990).

Impairments have been reported in visual and verbal short-term memories in children, especially with higher drug levels (Stores & Hart, 1976; Vining et al., 1979; Hartlage et al., 1980; Thompson et al., 1981; Thompson & Trimble, 1982a; Thompson & Trimble, 1982b; Dreifuss, 1983). The speed of recall is slowed, which affects decision-making (Reynolds, 1981; Thompson et al., 1981; Trimble, 1982; Thompson, 1983; Trimble, 1983; Andrewes et al., 1986). Information processing and reaction times are slowed. Visual evoked responses show this effect to emerge gradually over time (Green et al., 1982; Aldenkamp et al., 1990; Blennow et al., 1990). Motor-related tasks are more affected than higher mental functions (Macleod et al., 1978).

Children on phenytoin may experience major learning difficulties, especially at high serum levels of the drug (Trimble, 1990; Trimble & Cull, 1990). Reading delays are seen, especially in boys with focal seizures, who may be two years behind their peers (Stores, 1975; Stores, 1976; Stores, 1978; Stores, 1979; Stores & Hart, 1976; Thompson & Trimble, 1982a; Thompson & Trimble, 1982b; Thompson, 1983; Trimble, 1983; Wilson *et al.*, 1983; Corbett *et al.*, 1985). This may relate to the visual perceptual and memory deficits (Trimble, 1982). Changing to another medication may lead to improvements in schoolwork (Reynolds & Travers, 1974; Reynolds, 1981; Thompson, 1983, Rosen, 1986).

Carbamazepine

Children switched to carbamazepine may learn better (Trimble & Thompson, 1985; Vining, 1990; Aldenkamp, 2001). Benefits began to appear by three months and emerge fully by six months (Thompson & Trimble, 1982a; Thompson & Trimble, 1982b). Negative effects emerge more gradually and persist long after the drug is discontinued (Gallassi *et al.*, 1988).

Carbamazepine causes little if any cognitive impairment (Martin *et al.*, 1965; Rett, 1976; Trimble, 1990). Memory scanning and new information learning may be slowed at high dosages. Intellectual deterioration is rarely seen (O'Dougherty *et al.*, 1987). Children with complex partial epilepsy show more improvement than those with generalized seizures (Aman *et al.*, 1990). Cognitive complaints are more apt to appear when the EEG background appears slowed (Salinsky *et al.*, 2000).

Attention and attentiveness improve in children on carbamazepine (Jeavons, 1977; Schain *et al.*, 1977; Zavyazkina, 1998), with improved in-seat activity, attention span, motor steadiness, and task-specific response times (Bourgeois, 2002). At higher serum levels, problems in attention and mental speed as well as difficulties in problem-solving, concentration, and sustained attention appear (Dodrill, 1976; O'Dougherty *et al.*, 1987; Gallassi *et al.*, 1988; Blennow *et al.*, 1990). Problems cease when the drug is discontinued (Gallassi *et al.*, 1988; Blennow *et al.*, 1990; Aldenkamp, 2001).

Perceptual recognition, organization, visual-motor skills, and eye–hand coordination may improve (Martin *et al.*, 1965; Puente, 1975; Trimble & Thompson, 1983; Aman *et al.*, 1990; Trimble, 1990), although declines have been seen in drawing figures, visual search and scanning, and visual recall (Bourgeois, 2002). Improvements occur more in children with partial seizures than in those with generalized seizures, the latter children being messier in performance (Trimble, 1990; Thompson & Trimble, 1982a; Thompson & Trimble, 1982b). Auditory and visual response times improve at low and peak levels. Response times are longer with higher blood levels (O'Dougherty *et al.*, 1987; Trimble, 1990). The P300 evoked potentials show a prolonged stimulation-evaluation time (Goldberg & Burdick, 2001). With complex partial seizures, performance may be more rapid but at the expense of accuracy, especially in more complex tasks (O'Dougherty *et al.*, 1987; Mitchell *et al.*, 1988; Aman *et al.*, 1990; Zavyazkina, 1998; Blennow *et al.*, 1990; Trimble, 1990). More errors of commissions than omissions occur (Trimble, 1990). Motor speed and visual-motor coordination, more than mental speed, are increased (Trimble & Thompson, 1983; Trimble, 1987; Reinvang *et al.*, 1991). Slowing may occur at higher blood levels (Trimble & Corbett, 1980), unrelated to the derived epoxide levels (Camfield *et al.*, 1986).

Mild impairments in memory may be seen, although memory processing may be more rapid (Aldenkamp, 2001; Dodrill, 1976; Forsythe *et al.*, 1991). At lower blood levels, memory scanning is faster but the error rate is increased. At higher blood levels, the error rate falls as the scanning time is slowed (O'Dougherty *et al.*, 1987; Aman *et al.*, 1990; Blennow *et al.*, 1990). Immediate and short-term visual and verbal memory as well as decision-making may be impeded (Reynolds, 1981; Panel, 1998; Goldberg & Burdick, 2001). Memory problems correlate with the duration of carbamazepine treatment (Reinvang *et al.*, 1991; Trimble, 1987). In children on carbamazepine, the memory impairments show up in the first six months but are more definite after one year of treatment (Forsythe *et al.*, 1991). The long-release form of carbamazepine, providing a more stable pattern of cognitive functioning, appears to benefit long-term memory (Aldenkamp *et al.*, 1987; Zavyazkina, 1998). Carbamazepine may benefit or may produce subtle learning deficits (Goldberg & Burdick, 2001). Children on carbamazepine perform higher in reading (Bailet & Turk, 1991; Bailet & Turk, 2000). There is a 22% improvement in school marks for arithmetic, especially in those children of average or above-average intelligence (Trimble & Cull, 1990).

Valproate

Valproate is a non-sedative, broad-spectrum drug that was once felt to be relatively free of side effects involving school performance (Dreifuss, 1983). The drug was initially thought to improve mental efficiency, alertness-attentiveness (in 68%), and school performance (in 36%), perhaps by replacing drugs with more side effects (Sonnen *et al.*, 1975; Thompson & Trimble, 1982a; Thompson & Trimble, 1983; Trimble, 1983; Lairy & Goas, 1985; Trimble, 1990; Bourgeois, 2002). However, it does have subtle effects when given with other anticonvulsants, by augmenting their side effects.

Valproate may produce cognitive impairments at high dosage (Thompson & Trimble, 1982c; Thompson & Trimble, 1983; Trimble, 1990; Gendron *et al.*, 1991; Aldenkamp, 2001; Bourgeois, 2002). These occur early in therapy and are reversible by reducing the dosage (Rutter & Yule, 1975; Browne, 1980). Occasionally, an encephalopathy with stupor is seen (Trimble & Cull, 1980) when given in combination or as monotherapy (Sackellares *et al.*, 1979; Pakalnis *et al.*, 1989). The serum levels are within the range of usual tolerance and the liver functions remain normal (Trimble, 1990), except for an elevated ammonia level in some patients, especially if the child is also on phenobarbital (Reynolds, 1981; Trimble, 1983). Valproate exposure in utero may be associated with increased cognitive impairment rate, more behavior problems, and more special educational needs in the child (Vinten *et al.*, 2001).

Once thought to benefit alertness (Fenelon *et al.*, 1972; Stores, 1975; Coulter *et al.*, 1980; Potolicchio *et al.*, 1985; Trimble & Cull, 1990), valproate has now been found to cause subtle attention problems (Goldberg & Burdick, 2001), impairing concentration (Aman *et al.*, 1987; Gallassi *et al.*, 1990) and sustained attention (Hara & Fukuyama, 1989), especially at higher levels with more severe types of epilepsy. This may be of delayed appearance. These effects are reversible (Gallassi *et al.*, 1990).

Like other anticonvulsants, valproate may produce mild to moderate impairments in visual-motor processes, including slower performance and mental speed (Coenen *et al.*, 1991; Aldenkamp, 2001). The reaction time may be improved, especially in shorter tasks (Jeavens & Clark, 1974; Harding & Pullen, 1977; Harding *et al.*, 1980), but may be slowed at higher dosage, with impairments in motor speed of decision-making, visual scanning, and picture memory, especially with polypharmacy (Aman *et al.*, 1987; Trimble, 1990; Thompson *et al.*, 1981; Thompson & Trimble, 1982c; Aman *et al.*, 1987; Trimble, 1990; Thompson & Trimble, 1983). Visual-spatial processing is spared (Goldberg & Burdick, 2001). Children on valproate perform faster but at the expense of accuracy (Blennow *et al.*, 1990).

Adverse effects on memory, including coding, digit matching, and semantic memory, have been noted only at high doses (Thompson & Trimble, 1983; Trimble, 1983; Goldberg & Burdick, 2001). These effects are reversible (Aman *et al.*, 1987; Gallassi *et al.*, 1990). Minimal effects on learning are reported (Sommerbeck *et al.*, 1977). Children on valproate may have modest reading problems and near-significant mathematics problems (Bailet & Turk, 1991).

Diones

This is an older group of drugs used primarily for absence seizures. Due to major reactions in children on diones, these drugs have been phased out, the last to be discontinued being trimethadione. No major learning problems were emphasized.

Succinimides

Ethosuximide is used primarily for absence seizures and is now the principle drug of this group still in use. Initially, rather than any intellectual impairment or deterioration, improvements in verbal skills were reported (Stores, 1975; Browne *et al.*,

1975; Ladavas *et al.*, 1979). In some patients, adverse effects, including lowered intellectual efficiency, have been noted (Laidlaw & Richens, 1976; Theodore & Porter, 1983; Stores, 1975; Nolte *et al.*, 1980; Trimble & Corbett, 1980; Trimble, 1980). Occasionally, intellectual decline and depressed comprehension have been seen in older children and adolescents (Guey *et al.*, 1967; Browne *et al.*, 1974; Stores, 1975). Occasional slowness, perseverations, depressed short-term memory, and perceptual-spatial difficulties have been seen (Browne *et al.*, 1974; Hartlage *et al.*, 1980; Blennow *et al.*, 1990). Alertness may be depressed. Auditory and visual reaction times may be prolonged. The faster the response, the greater the number of errors seen. Ethosuximide is generally felt to be free of adverse effects on school performance (Dreifuss, 1983), with authors some reporting improvements (Dreifuss, 1983; Stores, 1971) but others reporting deterioration (Trimble, 1990; Trimble & Cull, 1990; Trimble & Reynolds, 1976).

Benzodiazepines

Benzodiazepines may produce unwanted behaviors and drowsiness in 13–91% of children, especially if the medication is increased rapidly. These drugs need to be discontinued very slowly to prevent seizure aggravation.

Clonazepam impairs both intellect and behavior (Trimble & Cull, 1990). Attention, concentration, and cognitive functioning may deteriorate (Sato *et al.*, 1977; Dreifuss, 1983). Psychomotor speed, the accuracy of movements, and reaction time may also decline (Trimble, 1983).

Nitrazepam has been of benefit to children with myoclonic seizures, especially infantile myoclonic spasms. When the seizures are controlled, behavior improves. In children who were not previously retarded, academic accuracy may improve dramatically (Mayeux *et al.*, 1980).

Clobazam is likely to impair cognitive performance and to provoke behavioral disturbances (Trimble & Cull, 1990), although it is less sedative than other benzodiazepines, with fewer memory and psychomotor effects. With Lennox-Gastaut syndrome, clobazam may produce some benefits in psychomotor arousal, increased attentiveness, purposeful activity, and participation in schoolwork. The drug seems to have little effect on cognitive skills (Trimble, 1983), although an occasional child may seem more alert, with fewer cognitive difficulties and reduced seizure frequency (Farrell *et al.*, 1984). Slowing of mental processing speed becomes significant only when the task demands are increased (Trimble & Thompson, 1983).

Other drugs

Bromides were once used for seizures, being one of the earliest drug approaches to epilepsy. The problems that resulted were of deterioration of mentation, due to intoxication. Psychoses and neuroses appeared to be aggravated. Sedation was common (Waxman & Geschwind, 1975). This experience contributed to the concept of an association of epilepsy, mental deterioration, and psychiatric disorders.

Clorazepate is sedative even at low dosages, and thus is often initiated slowly (Bourgeois *et al.*, 1983).

Chlorothiazide occasionally may be sedative, especially in children (Mirsky, 1960).

New antiepileptic drugs

The newer drugs primarily target neurotransmitter actions (Meador, 2002). These drugs show more CNS side effects than systemic effects. Although released mainly for partial seizures, many of these drugs have proven to have a broader range of action. However, the need to start with low dosages and increase the dosage gradually to avoid the initial sensitivity symptoms, of sedation, memory impairments, and language problems is important. If this rule is followed, early sensitivity side effects are often transient and minimized. The effects on the various aspects of learning are still being studied, especially in children.

Felbamate may produce an alerting effect at home and in learning at school, but an occasional child becomes agitated and hyperactive. Some have problems sleeping at night, leading to daytime sleepiness, which interferes with learning.

Flunarizine, in early studies, shows some sedative and memory problems.

Gabapentin is a safe drug used in the treatment of partial seizures with minimal cognitive effects noted (Dodrill, 1998; Leach *et al.*, 1997; Meador *et al.*, 1999; Turrentine *et al.*, 1999; Aldenkamp, 2001; Loring & Meador, 2001; Meador, 2002). At high dosages, drowsiness may be seen. Chronic treatment may induce slowing of the EEG background and cognitive complaints (Salinsky *et al.*, 2000; Aldenkamp, 2001).

Lamotrigine is an antiepileptic drug with a wide spectrum of efficacy used in the treatment of partial seizures and both primary and secondary generalized seizures. Lamotrigine has minimal cognitive side effects and may show an improvement in performance as a psychotropic effect (Banks & Beran, 1991; Meador *et al.*, 2000; Aldenkamp, 2001; Meador, Loring *et al.*, 2001; Goldberg & Burdick, 2001; Loring & Meador, 2001; Bourgeois, 2002; Meador, 2002). Occasional reports of concentration disturbances (Aldenkamp, 1997; Aldenkamp, 2001) and memory problems (Dodrill, 1998) have been noted. Lamotrigine may protect against hippocampal CA3 layer cell loss and reduce surrounding damage (Goldberg & Burdick, 2001). Some children on lamotrigine demonstrate an improvement in learning and behavior independent of seizure control (Hosking *et al.*, 1993).

Levetiracetam usually shows no changes in cognition (Dodrill, 1998; Goldberg & Burdick, 2001; Loring & Meador, 2001). Sleepiness (21%) and possibly modest cognitive/memory problems (6%) and coordination problems may be seen

(Aldenkamp, 2001). Sleepiness is the most common problem with this drug in children (Mandelbaum *et al.*, 2001; Wilner, 2002).

Losigamone has reportedly been linked with occasional confusion, sleepiness, and insomnia.

Oxcarbamazepine is touted as having no cognitive effects. It may help to focus attention and speed (Aldenkamp, 2001). Oxcarbamazepine shows no deleterious effects in adults (Aikia *et al.*, 1992). Reaction times may be slowed (Loring & Meador, 2001). Memory appears to be unaffected. Psychomotor performance and concentration seem to be improved. In the first week of treatment, patients feel more clear-minded and quick-thinking (Curran *et al.*, 1991).

Progabide produces significant memory impairment in handling new information (Gutierrez *et al.*, 1984).

Rufinamide may improve cognitive function at lower doses but possibly impair short-term memory at higher doses (Aldenkamp, 2001).

Sulthiame may impair more complex cognitive functioning requiring sustained attention and concentration, resulting in poorer performance in areas requiring motor responses (Stores, 1975; Blank & Anderson, 1983; Dikmen, 1980).

Stiripentol may produce a significant improvement in attention tasks (Levy *et al.*, 1984).

Tiagabine is effective for partial seizures and has shown minimal cognitive and behavior side effects (Dodrill, 1998; Loring & Meador, 2001; Bourgeois, 2002; Meador, 2002). Improvements in verbal fluency, faster psychomotor speed, and quicker responses have been noted (Dodrill *et al.*, 1997; Aikia *et al.*, 1999; Aldenkamp, 2001; Bourgeois, 2002). Problems with sleepiness, somnolence, and insomnia have been reported. At high dosages, tiagabine may produce a prolonged non-convulsive status state of altered awareness, with EEG demonstration of bifrontal sharp and slow-wave discharges. This may represent an excessive activity at GABA-B receptors in the thalamic-cortical circuits (Concepcion *et al.*, 2000).

Topiramate blocks the spread of partial and generalized seizures. This is a potent drug with multiple avenues of action, potentially producing both benefits and adverse reactions. A variety of cognitive problems may be seen if the drug is started and increased too rapidly, or if it is given at higher doses, or if the patient had difficulties before introduction of the drug (Dodrill, 1998). Some patients (75%) experience an initial sensitivity to the drug for the first few months, with usually mild to moderate transient cognitive problems related to frontal lobe dysfunctions (Baeta *et al.*, 2000). These include problems of attention, concentration, vigilance, memory, and word naming (Aldenkamp, 2001).

Some individuals experience a decline in intelligence, especially verbal intelligence (Thompson *et al.*, 1999), with a significant deterioration of verbal processing affecting both verbal learning and verbal fluency (Ahmed *et al.*, 1998; Farnham *et al.*, 1999; Thompson *et al.*, 1999). Working memory and visual-motor processing may also be affected (Reynolds, 1985; Baeta *et al.*, 2000). This may be part of the initiation sensitivity (Martin *et al.*, 1999; Aldenkamp *et al.*, 2000; Meador, 2001; Bourgeois, 2002), but it may not relate to any rapid titration or dosage (Ahmed *et al.*, 1998; Farnham *et al.*, 1999; Thompson *et al.*, 1999). The changes are reversible when topiramate is stopped. Generally, introducing topiramate slowly can reduce the chances of cognitive impairments (Martin *et al.*, 1999; Aldenkamp *et al.*, 2000; Meador, 2001; Bourgeois *et al.*, 2002). Patients on topiramate must be monitored closely (Dodrill, 1998). Younger children often tolerate the drug better, with fewer cognitive side effects seen (Panel, 1998).

Topiramate can induce non-convulsive status, presenting with confusion and decreased consciousness. The EEG shows diffuse spikes polyspike, and slow-spike wave complexes. A dramatic improvement over a few days occurs after stopping the drug (Raza & Fiol, 2000).

Topiramate may produce deficits in attention and concentration difficulties (6–14%) for at least the first month (Aldenkamp *et al.*, 2000; Bourgeois, 2002; Goldberg & Burdick, 2001; Martin *et al.*, 1999; Meador, 2001). Psychomotor slowing (Goldberg & Burdick, 2001) and incoordination may be seen (40%), which does not appear to be dose-related (Ahmed *et al.*, 1998). Topiramate is effective for cognitively impaired individuals, with improvement in adverse behaviors in 24%, but 20% of patients may experience cognitive or motor slowing, and 8% may have adverse behavior responses (Doherty & Gates, 1999).

Impairment of verbal memory, affecting both digit span and word-finding (Meador, 2002), is a dose-titration-related reaction (Burton & Harden, 1996; Cornaggia & Gobbi, 2001) that may persist for at least the first month or two (Aldenkamp *et al.*, 2000; Martin *et al.*, 1999; Meador, 2001). The word-finding difficulties are seen especially under stress, and more often if the patient is on polypharmacy (13%) (Reynolds, 1985). When the drug is discontinued, improvements are seen in digit span, language comprehension, both verbal and figure fluency, and in math and naming skills (Sviklas *et al.*, 1999). Topiramate can be effective as an add-on drug in learning-disabled children with difficult-to-control seizures. About 14% of learning-disabled children may not tolerate the drug, which is the same as in those without learning disabilities (Kelly *et al.*, 2002).

Vigabatrin (gamma vinyl gaba) shows minimal to no cognitive effects in most patients (Aldenkamp, 2001; Dodrill *et al.*, 1993; Dodrill, 1998; Gilham *et al.*, 1993; Meador, 2002; Trimble *et al.*, 1991). Confusional states may be seen (Reila, 1998). Reported side effects of vigabatrin have generally been mild and transient, not requiring alteration of the drug regimen. Initiation problems of drowsiness (29%), insomnia, and fatigue are often transient (Dodrill, 1998). No significant intellectual problems and some improvements have been reported (Caner *et al.*, 1991). Addition of vigabatrin to other anticonvulsants results in a decreased response time in tests of central cognitive processing ability pertaining to arithmetic (McQuire *et al.*, 1991). In children, attention, including sustained concentration and mental processing (Kalviainen *et al.*, 1991), has been seen to improve (McQuire *et al.*, 1991). In mentally retarded children, a hyperkinetic syndrome may be seen (Aldenkamp, 2001; Jampaque *et al.*, 1991). Memory problems have been seen, especially in patients with complex partial epilepsy. These problems are principally an anomia that was not noted previously (McQuire *et al.*, 1991).

Although greeted initially with great expectations, after a lengthy trial due to concerns of cerebral vacuolar formation seen in animal studies, vigabatrin was limited and withdrawn in the USA when findings of visual field losses were noted.

Zonisamide is a newer antiepileptic drug released for complex partial seizures. It may impair specific cognitive functions, including the acquisition and consolidation of new information and verbal learning. This may be a dose-related effect, with tolerance observed over time (Goldberg & Burdick, 2001; Berent *et al.*, 1987). Cognitive problems (19.5%) include confusion (15.5%), slowed thinking (13.6%), sluggishness (7%), drowsiness (14–24%), sleep disturbances or insomnia (6–10%), and tremor. Both adults and children on the drug may have problems with attention and concentration (3%). Visual perceptual learning is impaired (Goldberg & Burdick, 2001). Lethargy and hyperactivity may be seen. Memory difficulties are infrequent (1.9%). Learning is impaired in 2.5–5% (Mandelbaum *et al.*, 2001). The initial sedation and learning impairment may be tolerated within the first half-year (Loring & Meador, 2001).

REFERENCES

Addy, D. P. (1987). Cognitive function in children with epilepsy. *Dev. Med. Child Neurol.* **29**: 394–404.

Ahmed, M., Besag, F., Fowler, M., *et al.* (1998). Efficacy and safety of topiramate in patients with severe epilepsy and learning disabilities. 3rd European Congress of Epileptology. *Epilepsia* **39** (suppl 2): 3.

Aikia, M., Kalviainen, R. & Riekinen, P. P. J., Sr (1999). The cognitive effects of initial tiagabine monotherapy. *Epilepsia* **40** (suppl 7): 51.

Aikia, M., Kalvianen, R., Sivenius, J., *et al.* (1992). Cognitive effects of oxycarbamazepine and phenytoin monotherapy in newly diagnosed epilepsy: one year follow-up. *Epilepsy Res.* **1**: 199–203.

Aldenkamp, A. P. (1997). Effect of seizures and epileptiform discharges on cognitive function. *Epilepsia* **38** (suppl 1): 52–5.

Aldenkamp, A. P. (2001). Effects of antiepileptic drugs on cognition. In *Epilepsia and Learning Disabilities*, ed. G. F. Ayala, M. Elia, C. M. Cornaggia & M. M. Trimble. *Epilepsia* **42**: 46–9.

Aldenkamp, A. P., Alpherts, W. C. J., Blennow, G., *et al.* (1993). Withdrawal of antiepileptic medication in children-effects on cognitive function: the Multicenter Holmfrid study. *Neurology* **43**: 41–50.

Aldenkamp A. P., Alpherts, W. C. J., Dekker, M. J. A. *et al.* (1990). Neuropsychological aspects of learning disabilities in epilepsy. *Epilepsia* **31** (suppl 4): 9–20.

Aldenkamp, A. P., Alpherts, W. C. J., Moerland, M. C. P., *et al.* (1987). Controlled release carbamazepine: cognitive side-effects in patients with epilepsy. *Epilepsia* **28**: 507–14.

Aldenkamp, A. P., Baker, G., Mulder, O. G., *et al.* (2000). A multicenter, randomized clinical study to evaluate the effect on cognitive function of topiramate compared with valproate as add-on therapy to carbamazepine in patients with partial-onset seizures. *Epilepsia* **41**: 1167–78.

Alpherts, W. C. J. & Aldenkamp, P. A. (1990). Computerized neuropsychological assessment of cognitive functioning in children with epilepsy. *Epilepsia* **31** (suppl 4): 35–40.

Aman, M. G., Werry, J. S., Paxton, J. W. & Turbott, S. H. (1987). Effects of sodium valproate on psychomotor performance in children as a function of drug concentration, fluctuations in concentration and diagnosis. *Epilepsia* **28**: 115–24.

Aman, M. G., Werry, J. S., Paxton, J. W., *et al.* (1990). Effects of carbamazepine on psychomotor performance in children as a function of dose, concentration, seizure type and time of mediation. *Epilepsia* **31**: 51–60.

Andrewes, D. G., Bullen, J. G., Tomlinson, L., *et al.* (1986). A comparative study of the cognitive effects of phenytoin and carbamazepine in new referrals with epilepsy. *Epilepsia* **27**: 128–34.

Baeta, E. M., Santana, I. M., Castro, G., *et al.* (2000). Topiramate therapy in patients with intractable epilepsy: cognitive effects. *Epilepsia* **41** (suppl 7): 234.

Bailet, L. L. & Turk, W. R. (1991). The influence of antiepileptic therapy on academic achievement in childhood-onset epilepsy. *Epilepsia* **32** (suppl 3): 73.

Bailet, L. L. & Turk, W. R. (2000). The impact of childhood epilepsy on neurocognitive and behavior performance: a prospective longitudinal study. *Epilepsia* **41**: 426–31.

Banks, G. K. & Beran, R. G. (1991). Neuropsychological assessment in Lamotrigine treated epileptic patients. *Clin. Exp. Neurol.* **28**: 230–37.

Barlow, C. F. (1978). Risk factors of infancy and childhood: interrelationship of seizure disorders and mental retardation. In *Mental Retardation and Related Disorders*, pp. 68–75. Philadelphia: F. A. Davis.

Bennett-Levy, J. & Stores, G. (1984). The nature of cognitive dysfunction in schoolchildren with epilepsy. *Acta Neurol. Scand.* **69** (suppl 99): 79–82.

Berent, S., Sackellares, J. C., Giordani, B., *et al.* (1987). Zonisamide (CI-912) and cognition: results from preliminary study. *Epilepsia* **28**: 61–7.

Besag, F. C. (2001). Treatment of state-dependent learning disabilities. In *Epilepsia and Learning Disabilities*, ed. G. F. Ayala, M. Elia, C. M. Cornaggia & M. M. Trimble. *Epilepsia* **42**: 46–9.

Billard, C. (1999). Anti-epileptic drugs and cognitive function. In *Childhood Epilepsies and Brain Development*, ed. A. Nehlig, J. Motte, S. L. Moshe & P. Plouin, pp. 279–88. London: John Libbey & Co.

Blank, J. R. & Anderson, R. J. (1983). The effects of anticonvulsant drugs on rehabilitation and employment of epileptics. *J. Rehabil.* **49**: 61–3.

Blennow, G., Heijbel, J., Sandstedt, P., *et al.* (1990). Discontinuation of antiepileptic drugs in children who have outgrown epilepsy: effects on cognitive function. *Epilepsia* **31** (suppl 4): 50–53.

Bourgeois, B. F. D. (2002). Differential cognitive effects of antiepileptic drugs. *J. Child Neurol.* **17**: 2828–33.

Bourgeois, B. F. D., Presky, A. I., Palkes, H. S., *et al.* (1983). Intelligence in epilepsy: a prospective study in children. *Ann. Neurol.* **14**: 438–44.

Browne, T. R. (1980). Drug therapy: valproic acid. *N. Engl. J. Med.* **302**: 661–4.

Browne, T. R., Dreifuss, F. E., Dyken, P. R., *et al.* (1975). Ethosuximide (Zarontin) in the treatment of absence (petit mal) seizures. *Neurology* **25**: 515–24.

Browne, T. R., Penry, S. K., Porter, R. & Dreifuss, F. (1974). Responsiveness before, during and after spike-wave paroxysms. *Neurology* **24**: 59–66.

Burton, L. A. & Harden, C. (1996). Effect of topiramate on attention. *Epilepsy Res.* **27**: 29–32.

Butlin, A. I., Danta, G. & Cook, M. L. (1984). Anticonvulsant effects on the memory performance of epileptics. *Clin. Exp. Neurol.* **20**: 27–35.

Camfield, P. R., Camfield, C. S., Gates, R., *et al.* (1986). Changes in serum carbamazepine or carbamazepine-10-11-epoxide levels do not alter reaction time in children with stable epilepsy. *Ann. Neurol.* **20**: 428.

Camfield, C. S., Chaplin, S., Doyle, A. B., *et al.* (1977). Side effects of phenobarbital in toddlers: behavior and cognitive aspects. *Pediatrics* **95**: 361–5.

Camfield, C. S., Chaplin, S. & Doyle, A. B. (1979). Side effect of phenobarbital in toddlers: behavior and cognitive aspects. *J. Pediatr.* **95**: 361–5.

Caner, A. R., Comargo, C. H. P., Cukiert, A., *et al.* (1991). Cognitive effects of vigabatrin. 19th International Epilepsy Congress. *Epilepsia* **32** (suppl 1): 102–3.

Chen, Y., Chi Chow, J. & Lee, I. (2001). Comparison of the cognitive effect of antiepileptic drugs in seizure-free children with epilepsy before and after drug withdrawal. *Epilepsy Res.* **44**: 65–70.

Coenen, A. M. I., Groothasen, J., van Luijtellar, E. L. J. M., *et al.* (1991). Effects of discontinuation of carbamazepine and valproate on cognitive functioning in children. 19th International Epilepsy Congress. *Epilepsia* **32** (suppl 1): 56–7.

Concepcion, S., Werz, M. A., Avery, J., *et al.* (2000). Tiagabine induced spike-wave stupor in patients with partial epilepsy. *Epilepsia* **41** (suppl 7): 104.

Corbett, J. A., Trimble, M. R. & Nichol, T. C. (1985). Behavioral and cognitive impairments in children with epilepsy: the long-term effects of anticonvulsant therapy. *J. Am. Acad. Child Psychiatry* **24**: 17–23.

Cornaggia, C. M. & Gobbi, G. (2001). Learning disability in epilepsy: definitions and classification. In *Epilepsia and Learning Disabilities*, ed. G. F. Ayala, M. Elia, C. M. Cornaggia & M. M. Trimble. *Epilepsia* **42**: 2–5.

Coulter, D. L. III, Wu, H. & Allen, R. J. (1980). Valproic acid therapy in childhood epilepsy. *JAMA* **44**: 788.

Cull, C. A. (1988). Cognitive function and behavior in children. In *Epilepsy, Behavior and Cognitive Function*, ed. M. R. Trimble & E. H. Reynolds, pp. 97–111. Chichester, UK: John Wiley & Sons.

Curran, H. V., Java, R. & Luder, M. H. (1991). Cognitive and psychomotor effects of oxcarbamazepine. 19th International Epilepsy Congress, Rio De Janeiro, Brazil. *Epilepsia* **32** (suppl 1): 56.

Dikmen, S. (1980). Neuropsychological aspects of epilepsy. In *A Multidisciplinary Handbook of Epilepsy*, ed. B. P. Hermann, pp. 236–73. Springfield, IL: Charles C. Thomas.

Dodrill, C. B. (1975). Diphenylhydantoin serum levels, toxicity and neuropsychological performance in patients with epilepsy. *Epilepsia* **16**: 593–600.

Dodrill, C. B. (1976). Psychology. In *Textbook of Epilepsy*, ed. J. Laidlaw & A. Reichens, Vol. II, pp. 282–91, New York: Churchill Livingstone.

Dodrill, C. B. (1980). Neuropsychological evaluation in epilepsy. In *Epilepsy: A Window to Brain Mechanisms*, ed. J. S. Lockard & A. A. Ward, Jr, pp. 231–41. New York: Raven Press.

Dodrill, C. B. (1998). The effects of seizures and various AEDs on cognition. Presented at the American Epilepsy Society Conference, San Diego, CA, 1998.

Dodson, W. E. (1988). Aspects of antiepileptic treatment in children. *Epilepsia* **29** (suppl 3): 10–14.

Doherty, K. T. & Gates, J. R. (1999). Use of topiramate in the cognitively impaired. *Epilepsia* **40** (suppl 7): 62.

Dreifuss, F. E. (1983). *Pediatric Epileptology*. Boston, MA: John Wright PSG Inc.

Duncan, J. S., Shorvon, S. D. & Trimble, M. R. (1990). Effects of removal of phenytoin, carbamazepine and valproate on cognitive function. *Epilepsia* **31**: 584–91.

Farnham, S. J., Reisse, G. L., Gustafson, M., *et al.* (1999). Effect of topiramate on cognitive test performance. *Epilepsia* **40** (suppl 7): 52.

Farrell, K., Jan, J. E., Julian, J. V., *et al.* (1984). Clobazam in children with intractable seizures. *Epilepsia* **25**: 657.

Farwell, J. R., Lee, Y. J., Hirtz, D. G., *et al.* (1990). Phenobarbital for febrile seizures – effects on intelligence and on seizure recurrence. *N. Engl. J. Med.* **322**: 364–9.

Fenelon, B., Holland, J. T. & Johnson, C. (1972). Spatial organization of the EEG in children with reading disabilities: a study using nitrazepam. *Cortex* **8**: 444–64.

Forsythe, I. Butler, R., Berg, I. & McGuire, R. (1991). Cognitive impairment in new cases of epilepsy randomly assigned to carbamazepine, phenytoin and sodium valproate. *Dev. Med. Child Neurol.* **33**: 524–34.

Gadow, K. D. (1982). School involvement in the treatment of seizure disorders. *Epilepsia* **23**: 215–24.

Gallassi, R., Morreale, A., Lorusso, S., *et al.* (1988). Carbamazepine and phenytoin, comparison of cognitive effects in epileptic patients during monotherapy and withdrawal. *Arch. Neurol.* **45**: 892–4.

Gallassi, R., Morreale, A., Lorusso, S., *et al.* (1990). Cognitive effects of valproate. *Epilepsy Res.* **5**: 160–64.

Gendron, C. N., Garnett, W. R., Culbert, J., *et al.* (1991). The association between valproate serum concentrations and cognitive function. *Epilepsia* **32** (suppl 3): 49.

Gillham, R. A., Blacklaw, J., McKel, P. J., *et al.* (1993). Effect of vigabatrin on sedation and cognitive function in patients with refractory epilepsy. *J. Neurol. Neurosurg. Psychiatry* **56**: 1271–5.

Giordani, B., Berent, S., Sackellares, J. C., *et al.* (1985). Intelligence test performance of patients with partial and generalized seizures. *Epilepsia* **26**: 37–42.

Giordani, B., Sackallares, J. C., Miller, S., *et al.* (1983). Improvements in neuropsychological performance in patients with refractory seizures after intensive diagnostic and therapeutic intervention. *Neurology* **33**: 489–93.

Glaser, G. H. (1972). Diphenylhydantoin toxicity. In *Antiepileptic Drugs*, ed. D. M. Woodbury, J. K. Penry & R. P. Schmidt, pp. 219–26 . New York: Raven Press.

Goldberg, J. F. & Burdick, K. E. (2001). Cognitive side effects of anticonvulsants. *J. Clin. Psychiatry* **62** (suppl 14): 10–15.

Green, J. B., Walcoff, M. & Lucke, J. F. (1982). Phenytoin prolongs far-field somatosensory and auditory evoked potential interpeak latencies. *Neurology* **32**: 58–88.

Guey, J., Charles, C., Coquery, C., *et al.* (1967). Study of psychological defects of ethosuximide (Zarontin) on 25 children suffering from petit mal epilepsy. *Epilepsia* **8**: 129–41.

Gutierrez, A., Dreifuss, F. E., Santilli, N., *et al.* (1984). Psychiatric symptoms associated with progabide. *Epilepsia* **25**: 657.

Hara, H. & Fukuyama, Y. (1989). Sustained attention during the interictal period of mentally normal children with epilepsy or febrile convulsions and the influence of anticonvulsants and seizures on attention. *Jpn. J. Psychiatry Neurol.* **43**: 411–16.

Harding, G. F. A. & Pullen, J. J. (1977). The effect of sodium valproate in the EEG , the photosensitive range, the CNV and reaction time. *Electroencephalogr. Clin. Neurophysiol.* **43**: 465.

Harding, G. F. A., Pullen, J. J. & Drasdo, N. (1980). The effect of sodium valproate and other anticonvulsants on performance in children and adolescents. In *The Place of Sodium Valproate in the Treatment of Epilepsy*, ed. M. J. Parsonage & A. D. S. Caldwell, pp. 61–71. London: Royal Society of Medicine and Academic Press.

Hartlage, L. C., Stovall, K. & Kocack, B. (1980). Behavioral correlates of anticonvulsant blood levels. *Epilepsia* **21**: 185.

Henricksen, O. (1990). Education and epilepsy: assessment and remediation. *Epilepsia* **31** (suppl 4): 21–5.

Hosking, G., Spencer, S. & Yuen, A. W. C. (1993). Lamotrigine in children with severe developmental abnormalities in a pediatric population with refractory seizures. *Epilepsia* **34** (suppl 6): 42.

Hutt, S. J., Jackson, P. M., Belsham, A. & Higgers, G. (1968). Perceptual motor behavior in relation to blood phenobarbital level: a preliminary report. *Dev. Med. Child Neurol.* **10**: 626–32.

Jampaque, I., Dellatolas, G., Dulac, O., *et al.* (1991). Verbal and visual memory impaired in children with epilepsy. *Neuropsychologia* **31**: 1321–7.

Jeavens, P. M. (1977). Choice of drug therapy in epilepsy. *Practitioner* **219**: 542–56.

Jeavens, P. M. & Clark, J. E. (1974). Sodium valproate in the treatment of epilepsy. *Br. Med. J.* **2**: 584–6.

Jus, A. & Jus, K. (1962). Retrograde amnesia in petit mal. *Arch. Gen. Psychiatry* **6**: 163–7.

Kalviainen, R., Aikia, M., Partanen, J., *et al.* (1991). Randomized controlled pilot study of vigabatrin versus carbamazepine monotherapy in newly diagnosed patients with epilepsy: an interim report. *J. Child Neurol.* **6**: 60–69.

Kelly, K., Stephen, L. J., Sills, G. J., *et al.* (2002). Topiramate in patients with learning disability and refractory epilepsy. *Epilepsia* **43**: 399–402.

Kimura, D. (1961). Cerebral dominance and the perception of verbal stimuli. *Can. J. Psychol.* **15**: 166–71.

Koch, S., Titze, K., Zimmermann, R. B., *et al.* (1999). Long-term neuropsychological consequences of maternal epilepsy and anticonvulsant treatment during pregnancy for school-age children and adolescents. *Epilepsia* **40**: 1237–43.

Ladadavas, E., Umilta, C. & Provinciali, L. (1979). Hemisphere dependent cognitive performances in epileptic patients. *Epilepsia* **20**: 493–502.

Laidlaw, J. & Richens, A. (1976). Fits in childhood: education. In *A textbook of Epilepsy*, ed. J. Laidlaw & A. Richens, pp. 101–2, London: Churchill Livingstone.

Lairy, G. C. & Goas, A. L. (1985). Epilepsy in child psychiatry: effects of treatment by dipropylacetic acid. *Electroencephalogr. Clin. Neurophysiol.* **43**: 557–8.

Leach, J. P., Girvan, J., Paul, A., *et al.* (1997). Gabapentin and cognition: a double blind, dose ranging, placebo-controlled study in refractory epilepsy. *J. Neurol. Neurosurg. Psychiatry* **62**: 372–6.

Levy, R. H., Loiseau, P., Guyot, M., *et al.* (1984). Stirpental kinetics in epileptic patients: non-linearity and interactions. *Epilepsia* **25**: 675.

Lindsay, J., Ounsted, C. & Richards, P. (1980). Long-term outcome I children with temporal lobe seizures IV Genetic factors, febrile convulsions and remission of seizures. *Dev. Med. Child Neurol.* **22**: 429–39.

Loring, D. W. & Meador, K. J. (2001). Cognitive and behavior effects of epilepsy treatment. *Epilepsia* **42** (suppl 8): 24–32.

MacLeod, C. M., Dekaban, A. S. & Hunt, E. (1978). Memory impairment in epileptic patients: selective effects of phenobarbital concentration. *Science* **202**: 1102–4.

Mandelbaum, D. E., Kugler, S. L., Wenger, E. C., *et al.* (2001). Clinical experience with levetiracetam and Zonisamide in children with uncontrolled epilepsy. *Epilepsia* **42** (supp 7): 183.

Martin, N. F., Movarrekhi, M. & Gisiger, M. G. (1965). Etude de quelques effets du Tegretol sur une population d'enfants epilepticques. *Schweiz Med. Wochenschr.* **95**: 982–9.

Matthews, C. G. & Harley, J. P. (1975). Cognitive and motor-sensory performances in toxic and non-toxic epileptic subjects. *Neurology* **25**: 184–8.

Mayeux, R., Brandt, J., Rosen, J., *et al.* (1980). Interictal memory and language impairment in temporal lobe epilepsy. *Neurology* **30**: 120–25.

McCuiston, M., Hartlage, L. C. & Noonan, M. (1983). Stability of correlations between serum phenobarbital levels and neuropsychological test performance. *Clin. Neuropsychol.* **5**: 46.

McQuire, A. M., Duncan, J. S. & Trimble, M. S. (1991). Effects of vigabatrin on cognitive function and mood when used as add-on therapy in patients with intractable epilepsy. *Epilepsia* **33**: 128–34.

Meador, K. J. (2001). The effects of antiepileptic drugs on memory. *Epilepsia* **42** (suppl 7): 219.

Meador, K. J. (2002). Cognitive outcomes and predictive factors in epilepsy. *Neurology* **58** (suppl 5): 21–8.

Meador, K. J., Kamin, M., Hulihan, J., *et al.* (2001). Cognitive functions in adults with epilepsy: effect of topiramate and valproate added to carbamazepine. *Epilepsia* **42** (suppl 2): 75.

Meador, K. J., Loring, D. W., Moore, E. E., *et al.* (1995). Comparative cognitive effects of pheno-barbital, phenytoin, and valproate in healthy adults. *Neurology* **45**: 1494–9.

Meador, K. J., Loring, D. W., Ray, P. G., *et al.* (1999). Differential cognitive effects of carbamazepine and gabapentin. *Epilepsia* **40**: 1279–85.

Meador, K. J., Loring, D. W., Ray, P. G., *et al.* (2000). Effects of carbamazepine and lamotrigine on interrelation of neuropsychological measures. *Epilepsia* **41** (suppl 7): 235.

Meador, K. J., Loring, D. W., Ray, P. G., *et al.* (2001). Differential cognitive and behavioral effects of carbamazepine and lamotrigine. *Neurology* **56**: 1177–82.

Mirsky, A. F. (1960). The relationship between paroxysmal EEG activity and performance on a vigilance task in epileptic patients. *Am. Psychol.* **15**: 486.

Mirsky, A. F. & Kornetsky, C. (1964). On the dissimilar effects of drugs on the digit symbol substation and continuous performance tests. *Psychopharmacologia* **5**: 161–77.

Mitchell, W. G. & Chavez, J. M. (1987). Carbamazepine versus phenobarbital for partial onset seizures in children. *Epilepsia* **28**: 56–60.

Mitchell, W. G., Chavez, J. M., Zhon, Y., *et al.* (1988). Carbamazepine influences reaction time and impulsivity in children with epilepsy. *Epilepsia* **29**: 681.

Nolte, R., Wetzel, B., Brugmann, G., *et al.* (1980). Effects of phenytoin and primidone mono-therapy on mental performance in children. In *Antiepileptic Therapy: Advances in Drug Monitoring*, ed. S. I. Johannesen, P. L. Morselli, C. E. Pippenger, *et al.*, pp. 81–6. New York: Raven Press.

O'Dougherty, M., Wright, F. S., Cox, S., *et al.* (1987). Carbamazepine plasma concentration relationship to cognitive impairment. *Arch. Neurol.* **44**: 853–6, 863–7.

Ozdirim, E., Renda, Y. & Epur, S. (1978). Effects of phenytoin and phenobarbital upon the behavior of epileptic children. In *Advances in Epileptology 1977: Psychology, Pharmacotherapy and New Diagnostic Approaches*, ed. H. Meinardi & A. Rowan, pp. 120–23. Amsterdam: Swets & Zeitlinger.

Pakalnis, A., Drake, M. E. & Denio, I. (1989). Valproate associated encephalopathy. *J. Epilepsy* **2**: 41–4.

Panel (1998). Questions and answers. Presented at the American Epilepsy Society Conference, San Diego, CA, 1998.

Pellock, J. M. (1990). Risk vs. benefits of antiepileptic drug therapy. *Int. Pediatr.* **5**: 177–81.

Potolicchio, S. J., Jr, Gut, A. M. & Beaumanoir, A. (1985). Alertness in epileptics: pharmacological and psychometric study. *Electroencephalogr. Clin. Neurophysiol.* **43**: 541.

Puente, R. M. (1975). The use of carbamazepine in the treatment of behavioral disorders in children. In *Epileptic Seizures – Behavior – Pain*, ed. W. Berkmayer, pp. 243–52. Baltimore, MD: University Park Press.

Raza, A. M. M. & Fiol, M. (2000). Topirimate can cause non-convulsive status epilepticus. *Epilepsia* **41** (suppl 7): 220.

Reila, A. R. (1998). Special population: cognitive concerns in neorates, the mentally handicapped, and school-aged children. Presented at the American Epilepsy Society Conference, San Diego, CA, 1998.

Reinisch, J. M., Sanders, S. A., Mortensen, E. L., *et al.* (1995). In utero exposure to phenobarbital and intelligence deficits in adult men. *JAMA* **274**: 1518–25.

Reinvang, I., Bjartvei, S., Johannessen, S. I., *et al.* (1991). Cognitive function and time-of-day variation in serum carbamazepine concentrations in epileptic patients treated with monotherapy. *Epilepsia* **32**: 116–21.

Rett, A. (1976). The so-called psychoatropic effect of Tegretol in the treatment of convulsions of cerebral oigin in children. In *Epileptic Seizures – Behaivor – Pain*, ed. W. Birkmayer, pp. 194–204. Bern: Hans Huber.

Reynolds, E. H. (1981). Biological factors in psychological disorders associated with epilepsy. In *Epilepsy and Psychiatry*, ed. E. H. Reynolds & M. R. Trimble, pp. 264–90. New York: Churchill Livingstone.

Reynolds, E. H. (1983). Mental effects of antiepileptic medication: a review. *Epilepsia* **14** (suppl 2): 85–95.

Reynolds, E. H. (1985). Antiepileptic drugs and psychopathology. In *The Psychopharmacology of Epilepsy*, ed. M. R. Trimble, pp. 49–65. Chichester, UK: John Wiley & Sons.

Reynolds, E. H. & Shorvon, S. D. (1981). Monotherapy or polytherapy for epilepsy? *Epilepsia* **22**: 1–10.

Reynolds, E. H. & Travers, R. D. (1974). Serum anticonvulsant concentrations in epileptic patients with mental symptoms. *Br. J. Psychiatry* **124**: 440–45.

Riva, D., Milani, N., Pantaleoni, C., *et al.* (1991). The influence of antiepileptic drugs on cognitive functions in children. 19th International Epilepsy Congress. *Epilepsia* **32** (suppl 1): 57.

Rodin, E. A., Choon So Run, Kitano, H., *et al.* (1976). A comparison of the effectiveness of primidone versus carbamazepine in epileptic out patients. *J. Nerv. Ment. Dis.* **163**: 41–6.

Rodin, E. A., Schmaltz, S. & Twirty, G. (1986). Intellectual functions of patients with childhood-onset epilepsy. *Dev. Med. Child Neurol.* **28**: 25–33.

Rosen, J. A. (1968). Dilantin dementia. *Trans. Am. Neurol. Assoc.* **93**: 273.

Rugland, A. L. (1990). Neuropsychological assessment of cognitive functioning in children with epilepsy. *Epilepsia* **31** (suppl 4): 41–4.

Rutter, M. & Yule, W. (1975). The concept of specific reading retardation. *J. Child Psychol. Psychiatry* **16**: 181–97.

Sackellares, J. C., Soo, I. I. & Dreifuss, F. E. (1979). Stupor followed by administration of valproic acid in patients receiving other anti-epileptic drugs. *Epilepsia* **20**: 697–703.

Salinsky, M. C., Binder, L. M., Oken, B. S., *et al.* (2000). Effects of chronic gabapentin and carbamazepine treatment on EEG, alertness and cognition in healthy volunteers. *Epilepsia* **41** (suppl 7): 151.

Sato, S., Penry, J., Dreifuss, F. E., *et al.* (1977). Clonazepam in the treatment of absence seizures: a double-blind clinical trial. *Neurology* **27**: 371.

Schain, R. J. (1983). Carbamazepine and cognitive functioning. In *Antiepileptic Drug Therapy*, ed. P. L. Morselli, C. E. Pippenger & J. K. Penry, pp. 189–91. New York: Raven Press.

Schain, R. J., Ward, J. W. & Guthrie, D. (1977). Carbamazepine as an anticonvulsant in children. *Neurology* **27**: 476–80.

Shinnar, S. (1991). Treatment decisions in childhood epilepsy. In *Epilepsy in Childhood and Its Treatment*, ed. W. E. Dodson & J. M. Pellock, pp. 215–22. New York: Demos.

Shinnar, S., Vining, P. G., Mellits, E. D., *et al.* (1985). Discontinuing antiepileptic medication in children with epilepsy after two years without seizures. *N. Engl. J. Med.* **313**: 976–80.

Shorvon, S. D. & Reynolds, E. H. (1979). Reduction of polypharmacy for epilepsy *Br. Med. J.* **2**: 1023–5.

Somerfield-Ziskind, E. & Ziskind, E. (1940). Effect of phenobarbital on the mentality of epileptic patients. *Arch. Neurol. Psychiatry* **43**: 70–79.

Sommerbeck, K. W., Theilgaard, A., Rusmussen, K. E., *et al.* (1977). Valproate sodium: evaluation of so-called psychotropic effects: a controlled study. *Epilepsia* **18**: 159–67.

Sonnen, A. E. H., Zelvelder, W. H. & Bruens, J. H. (1975). A double blind study of the influence of dipropylacetate on behavior. *Acta. Neurol. Scand. Suppl.* **60**: 43–7.

Stores, G. (1971). Cognitive function in children with epilepsy. *Dev. Med. Child Neurol.* **13**: 390–92.

Stores, G. (1973). Studies of attention and seizure disorders. *Dev. Med. Child Neurol.* **15**: 376–82.

Stores, G. (1975). Behavioral effects of antiepileptic drugs. *Dev. Med. Child Neurol.* **17**: 647–58.

Stores, G. (1976). The investigation and management of school children with epilepsy. *Publ. Health, Lond.* **90**: 171–7.

Stores, G. (1978). School children with epilepsy at risk for learning and behavior problems. *Dev. Med. Child Neurol.* **20**: 502–8.

Stores, G. (1981). Problems of learning and behavior in children with epilepsy. In *Epilepsy and Psychiatry*, ed. E. H. Reynolds & M. R. Trimble, pp. 33–48. New York: Churchill Livingstone.

Stores, G. (1990). Electroencephalographic parameters in assessing the cognitive function of children with epilepsy. *Epilepsia* **31** (suppl 4): 45–9.

Stores, G. & Hart, J. (1976). Reading skills of children with generalized or focal epilepsy attending ordinary school. *Dev. Med. Child Neurol.* **18**: 705–16.

Stores, G. & Piran, N. (1978). Dependency of different types in school children with epilepsy. *Psychol. Med.* **8**: 441.

Svoboda W. B. (1979). Anticonvulsant side effects: idiosyncratic reactions. In *Learning About Epilepsy*, p. 129. Baltimore, MD: University Park Press.

Theodore, W. H. & Porter, R. J. (1983). Removal of sedative–hypnotic antiepileptic drugs from the regimens of patients with intractable epilepsy. *Ann. Neurol.* **13**: 320–24.

Thompson, P. J. (1983). Phenytoin and psychosocial development. In *Antiepileptic Drug Therapy in Pediatrics*, ed. P. Morselli, C. E. Pippinger & J. K. Penry, pp. 193–200. New York: Raven Press.

Thompson, P. J. & Huppert, F. (1980). Problems in the development of measures to test cognitive performance in adult epileptic patients. In *Epilepsy and Behaivor '79*, ed. B. M. Kulig, H. Meinardi & G. Stores, pp. 37–42. Lisse: Swets & Zeitlinger.

Thompson, P. J. & Trimble, M. R. (1981). Sodium valproate and cognitive functioning in normal volunteers. *Br. J. Clin. Pharmacol.* **12**: 819–24.

Thompson, P. J. & Trimble, M. R. (1982a). Anticonvulsant drugs and cognitive functions. *Epilepsia* **23**: 531–44.

Thompson, P. J. & Trimble, M. R. (1982b). Comparative effects of anticonvulsants on cognitive functioning. *Br. J. Clin. Pract.* **18** (suppl): 154–6.

Thompson, P. J. & Trimble, M. R. (1982c). Sodium valproate and cognitive functioning in normal volunteers. *Br. J. Clin. Pharmacol.* **12**: 819–24.

Thompson, P. J. & Trimble, M. R. (1983). Anticonvulsant serum levels: relationship to impairments of cognitive functioning. *J. Neurol. Neurosurg. Psychiatry* **46**: 227–33.

Thompson, P. J., Cross, G., Baxendale, S. A., *et al.* (1999). Changes in intellect and verbal processing in association with topiramate treatment. *Epilepsia* **40** (suppl 7): 50.

Thompson, P. J., Huppert, F. & Trimble, M. R. (1981). Phenytoin and cognitive functions: effect on normal volunteers and implications of epilepsy. *Br. J. Clin. Psychol.* **20**: 155–62.

Trimble, M. (1980). Antiepileptic drugs and behaivor – discussion notes. In *Epilepsy and Behaivor '79*, ed. B. M. Kulig, E. Meinardi & G. Stores, pp. 76–9. Lisse: Swets & Zeitlinger.

Trimble, M. R. (1982). Anticonvulsant drugs and hysterical seizures. In *Pseudoseizures*, ed. T. L. Riley & A. Roy, pp. 148–58. Baltimore, MD: Williams & Wilkins.

Trimble, M. R. (1983). Anticonvulsant drugs and psychosocial development: phenobarbitone, sodium valproate and benzodiazepines. In *Antiepilepsy Drug Therapy in Pediatrics*, ed. P. L. Morselli, C. E. Pippenger & J. K. Penry, pp. 201–12. New York: Raven Press.

Trimble, M. R. (1987). Anticonvulsant drugs and cognitive function: a review of the literature. *Epilepsia* **28**: 37–45.

Trimble, M. R. (1988). Anticonvulsant drugs: mood and cognitive functions. In *Epilepsy, Behaivor and Cognitive Function*, ed. M. R. Trimble & E. H. Reynolds, pp. 135–45. Chichester, UK: John Wiley & Sons.

Trimble, M. R. (1990). Antiepileptic drugs, cognitive function and behavior in children: evidence from recent studies. *Epilepsia* **31** (suppl 4): 30–4.

Trimble, M. R. & Corbett, J. A. (1980a). Behavioral and cognitive disturbances in epileptic children. *Irish Med. J.* **73** (suppl): 21–8.

Trimble, M. R. & Corbett, J. A. (1980b). Anticonvulsant drugs and cognitive function. In *Advances in Epileptology: The Xth Epilepsy International Symposium*, ed. J. A. Wada & J. K. Penry, pp. 113–20. New York: Raven Press.

Trimble, M. R. & Cull, C. (1990). Children of school age: the influence of antiepileptic drugs on behavior and intellect. *Epilepsia* **29** (suppl 3): 13–19.

Trimble M. R. Reynolds, E. H. (1976). Anticonvulsant drugs and mental symptoms. *Psychol. Med.* **6**: 169–78.

Trimble, M. R. & Thompson, P. J. (1981). Memory, anticonvulsant drugs and seizures. *Acta Neurol. Scand.* **64** (suppl 89): 31–41.

Trimble, M. R. & Thompson, P. J. (1983). Anticonvulsant drugs, cognitive function and behavior. *Epilespia* **24** (suppl 1): 55–63.

Trimble, M. R. & Thompson, P. J. (1984a). Anticonvulsant drugs and cognitive function. *Epilepsia* **25**: 642.

Trimble, M. R. & Thompson, P. J. (1984b). Sodium valproate and cognitive function. *Epilepsia* **25** (suppl 1): 60–4.

Trimble, M. R. & Thompson, P. J. (1985). Anticonvulsant drugs and cognitive function. *Ann. Neurol.* **18**: 412.

Turner, M. (1977). Appearance, disappearance and migration of EEG foci in child hood. *Electroencephalogr. Clin. Neurophysiol.* **43**: 578.

Turrentine, L. K. A., Martin, R. C., Gilliam, F. G., *et al.* (1999). Differential cognitive effects of carbamazepine and gabapentin in healthy senior adults. *Epilepsia* **40** (suppl 7): 83.

Vallarta, J. M., Bell, D. B. & Reichert, A. (1976). Progressive encephalopathy due to chronic hydantoin intoxication. *Am. J. Dis. Child* **128**: 27–34.

Vining, E. P. G. (1990). Cognitive and behavioral side effects of antiepileptic drugs. *Int. Pediatr.* **5**: 182.

Vining, E. P. G., Botsford, E. & Freeman, J. M. (1979). Valproate sodium in refractory seizures. *Am. J. Dis. Child* **133**: 274–6.

Vining, E. P. G., Mellits, E. D., Cataldo, M. F., *et al.* (1983). Effects of phenobarbital and sodium valproate on neuropsychological functions and behavior. *Ann. Neurol.* **14**: 360.

Vining, E. P. G., Mellits, E. D., Dorsen, M. M., *et al.* (1987). Psychologic and behavioral effects of antiepileptic drugs in children: a double blind comparison between phenobarbital and valproic acid. *Pediatrics* **80**: 165–74.

Vinten, J., Gorry, J. & Baker, G. A. (2001). The long-term neuropsychological development of children exposed to antiepileptic drugs in utero. The Liverpool and Manchester Neurodevelopmental Study Group. *Epilepsia* **42** (suppl 7): 293–4.

Wapner, I., Thurston, D. L. & Hollowach, J. (1962). Phenobarbital: its effects on learning in epileptic children. *JAMA* **182**: 937.

Waxman, S. G. & Geschwind, N. (1975). The interictal behavior syndrome of temporal lobe epilepsy. *Arch. Gen. Psychiatry* **32**: 1580–86.

Wilner, A. (2002). Antiepileptic reduces seizures in children and adults. *CNS News* **4**: 16.

Wilson, A., Petty, R., Perry, A., *et al.* (1983). Paroxysmal language disturbance in an epileptic treated with clobazam. *Neurology* **33**: 652–4.

Wolf, S. M. (1979). Controversies in the treatment of febrile convulsions. *Neurology* **29**: 287–90.

Zavyazkina, N. (1998). Carbamazepine effect on cognitive functions of patients with epilepsy. 3rd European Congress of Epileptology. *Epilepsia* **39** (suppl 2): 120.

23

Effects of other therapies

When tolerated medications do not control the seizures, other approaches such as surgical, dietary, and psychologic treatments must be considered. Such approaches may prevent further loss of intellectual functioning, but they do not overcome epilepsy-related problems that are already present.

Surgery

Surgery is an option if the seizure is localized, arising from a non-vital brain region. The risk of any significant cognitive decline is generally reduced because the tissue to be resected is dysfunctional (Loring & Meador, 2001). The basic surgical approaches are to isolate or remove the seizure focus or to prevent the spread. A damaged brain area that produces seizures is less likely to retain desired functions than epileptic foci that are otherwise intact. Cognition may be preserved or partially recovered by early intervention. A higher rate of cognitive impairments is found in children with intractable epilepsy, independent of the epilepsy duration. Epilepsy surgery can be of benefit by significantly decreasing the seizures in 50–90% of children as well as reducing use of anticonvulsants. Few differences exist in cognitive performance between children with intractable seizures who are surgical candidates and those who are not (Smith *et al.*, 2002).

The risks of the surgery should be balanced against the risks of continued seizures on cognition, quality of life, injury, and death. With a modern evaluation, the risk of developing a severe memory loss is less because preoperative imaging of contralateral hippocampal atrophy and sclerosis would contraindicate surgery. The risks of these less severe deficits can be predicted (Meador, 2002).

Considerations

Early surgical intervention for epilepsy may minimize or prevent the developmental lags, intellectual decline, and psychosocial consequences seen in adults with chronic epilepsy. If temporal lobe epilepsy is allowed to continue through adolescence, cognition and self-image are fully established, and further improvements are not apt to occur (Westerveld *et al.*, 1993; Matsuzaka *et al.*, 2001).

There are different time windows for the reconstitution and compensation of mesial and cortical aspects of memory. Whereas memory recovery appears to be restricted by decreasing plasticity and physiological aging, mesial functions seem to be reconstituted by contralateral mesial structures over a much longer period (Helmstaedter & Elger, 1998).

The laterality of the surgery has no effect on the outcome. Epilepsy surgery does not result in changes in cognitive performance beyond those seen over time in children with intractable seizures. There are minimal cognitive risks to surgery, yet the surgery probably should not be expected to produce cognitive performance benefits, at least in the first years (Smith *et al.*, 2000).

Temporal and cortical approaches

Factors that help to predict the seizure outcome include the initial symptoms of the seizure, the normality of the EEG between seizures, the site of the seizure focus, the side of the brain where language is located, the amount of brain tissue removed, the EEG patterns during the surgery, and the identification of the seizure boundary. Operating on a temporal lobe, especially the deeper portions, without checking out the temporal lobe function on the other side can lead to a possible loss of all acute memory functions. It is important to localize memory functions to determine how safe the surgery will be and how far to operate (Rausch, 1981).

With a temporal lobectomy, there is a risk of material-specific verbal memory decline with left temporal lobe resection and a decline in visuospatial memory losses with right-sided resection. There is also a risk for global memory deficits after unilateral resection, especially if significant damage exists in the contralateral temporal lobe (Loring & Meador, 2001). The laterality and site of the seizure focus are less apt to correlate with the type of memory deficit in children being considered for seizure surgery than in children with medically controlled seizures, suggesting that the severity of the seizure disorder may play a role in the expression of the memory deficit (Smith *et al.*, 2002). Less pronounced hemispheric differences are found in school-age children after a temporal lobectomy than in adults. Children may a have a lower risk of memory deterioration, which may be due to their larger potential for cerebral plasticity. This decreases with maturation (Lendt *et al.*, 1999).

The intracarotid amobarbital tests (WADA test) can predict verbal but not visuospatial memory changes that occur after anterior temporal lobotomies. Injection ipsilateral to the seizure focus demonstrates a relationship to verbal memory findings and the postoperative verbal memory changes, when relying primarily on the contralateral hemisphere (Chiaravalloti & Glosser, 2001). In children, the use of verbally oriented memory stimuli such as printed words, arithmetic problems, and repetition of a nursery rhyme diminishes the capacity of the WADA test to predict lateralized seizure onset in children with seizures originating in the left hemisphere.

Using real objects as memory stimuli during the WADA procedure may be superior to using memory stimuli presented on cards for predicting the side of seizure onset (Lee *et al.*, 2001). Other approaches, including functional imaging studies, are proving successful alternatives in localization and lateralization the Wada test. Injection of a variety of isotopic substances during activation of various brain functions localized to the functional sites can be detected by rapid MRI or PET scanning techniques.

Learning disorders must be considered both preoperatively and postoperatively in rehabilitation. Preoperatively, one must consider the effect that the surgical approach to the epileptic focus may have on learning processes. Ablation of an epileptogenic area often produces a positive effect because it eliminates the negative consequences of the epileptic discharges. However, if the epileptogenic focus has not completely lost its own primary function, the same ablation may lead to an augmented functional deficit (Cornaggia & Gobbi, 2001).

Frontal lobe surgery

Whether with a frontal lobe seizure focus or as the postoperative results of frontal lobe seizure surgery, difficulties in continuous tasks that depend on feedback from a prior response to make the next choice, such as mazes and sorting tasks, may be noted. Speech and speech fluency may be reduced with left frontal lobotomies (Dikmen, 1980).

Diminished problem-solving skills and an impairment in verbal intelligence may be seen in patients undergoing extensive frontal lobectomy for cryptogenic epilepsy. When a tumor is excised, there may be improvement in verbal functioning (Hempel *et al.*, 2001). Both frontal and temporal resections may lead to memory changes of a comparable degree but due to different mechanisms, possibly representing different levels of information processing (Chelune *et al.*, 1993; Durwen, 1991).

Temporal lobe surgery

The average age of a patient undergoing temporal lobectomy is about 20 years, although it seldom takes that long to determine whether a patient is refractory to medical therapy (Meador, 2002). There is no great difference between a temporal neocortical lesionectomy and an en bloc temporal lobectomy including mesial-basal structures, suggesting that the lesionectomy also produces widespread disruption of neuronal pathways. The chief difference is that in lesionectomy patients, the performance IQ is improved (Hempel *et al.*, 2001).

Risks and predictors

The hippocampus, a frequent source of epilepsy, is the part of the temporal lobe that is involved in acute memory. Chronic epilepsy may lead to cell death in the hippocampus, from which the brain attempts to recover by reorganizing the remaining cells and their connections. Key functions may be shifted. This tends to lead to further memory loss, changes in emotions, an increased tendency toward further seizures, and also a greater likelihood that the normal brain functions (such as language and memory) may be shifted from their normal location.

Typically, the type of memory deficits seen postoperatively relate to the side that was operated on. More bothersome verbal memory problems occur after surgery on the language-dominant side, while problems with non-verbal memories may follow surgery on the non-dominant side. Risks are greater with later age of onset of epilepsy and the absence of atrophy or gliosis in the hippocampus or other mesial-temporal lobe structures on the side of the resection (Meador, 2002; Sass *et al.*, 1994; Seidenberg *et al.*, 1996; Trenerry *et al.*, 1993).

Patients with higher intellectual functions and intact verbal memory skills preoperatively, especially with less hippocampal atrophy, show the greatest losses of verbal memory postoperatively (Chelune *et al.*, 1991; Loring & Meador, 2001). Tumor patients may show stable or improved verbal IQ, verbal fluency, and problem-solving postoperatively, but occasionally they may experience a mild decline in confrontation naming. With cryptogenic epilepsy, a decline in verbal fluency is frequently seen, including a slight decline in problem-solving as well as in verbal IQ and confrontation naming. Improved self-awareness and social judgment are seen in children (Hempel *et al.*, 2001).

Risks are higher in patients with high preoperative verbal memory, without hippocampal atrophy and without preoperative dysfunction of the target temporal lobe, by WADA or by PET. The lack of hippocampal atrophy suggests that there remains significant functional capacity despite the epileptogenic process. Mesial-temporal lobe sclerosis on the side contralateral to the target surgical site limits the chances of any functional shift. Dissociation of functional measures such as WADA, PET, MRI, or fMRI in the wrong direction is another concern (Loring & Meador, 2001; Meador, 2002). Mesial-temporal lobe sclerosis on the side contralateral to the planned surgery is another risk factor, since this limits the chances of a function shift. The risk is increased if functional assessments suggest greater preoperative functional adequacy of the left temporal lobe and lower functionality reserve in the right temporal lobe.

Patients who are not seizure-free after a left temporal lobectomy are more likely to show greater verbal memory impairments than those without postoperative seizures, although verbal memory impairment may be present in seizure-free patients (Loring & Meador, 2001).

Surgical approaches

The surgeon may remove the entire temporal lobe or only the epileptogenic portion of it or limit the resection to the amygdala and hippocampus.

Total lobectomy

Removal of the entire temporal lobe on one side does not affect old memory but affects memories acquired in the previous few days to weeks. Unless shifted to the right side, removal of the left dominant temporal lobe results in verbal memory problems in learning new items, as related to the hippocampus. Unrelated word pairs are a problem. Delayed recall is impaired severely. Logical recall is reduced in some patients. There may be difficulties in word-finding, especially of names. Such patients may be trained to use visual imagery to substitute for auditory memory (Grote *et al.*, 1991).

Partial lobectomy

Removing only a small amount of brain tissue that involves the hippocampus can lead to deficits of associative learning, i.e. learning of facts related to other facts. Removal of a larger section including a portion of temporal neocortex may also affect more complex language. Even if only the surface is removed, there is the risk of not remembering the names of items and people (Blakemore & Falconer, 1967).

Hippocampectomy

A left-selective amygdalohippocampectomy can lead to a significant decline in memory function postoperatively. Older adults, especially males, with a later onset of seizures and with a better preoperative performance are at greater risk to show memory losses. A right-selective amygdalohippocampectomy shows a lesser degree of impairment, if any, in non-verbal memory (Gleissner *et al.*, 2002).

Cognitive effects

Postoperatively, the general intelligence is relatively unimpaired (Meyer & Yates, 1955) and may even be improved in some patients (Powell *et al.*, 1975), due to the elimination of disruptive effects of the seizures and a reduction in the antiepileptic medication (Loring & Meador, 2001). With surgery on the dominant temporal lobe, there may be a transient depression of verbal IQ or of performance intelligence in the non-dominant temporal lobe, but recovery to the preoperative status is usually seen within a year (Blakemore & Falconer, 1967; Delaney *et al.*, 1980; Dikmen, 1980). Poor seizure relief and an absence of pathology leads more often to a lower presurgical intelligence and further depression post-lobectomy, especially if both factors are present (Chiaravalloti & Glosser, 2001; Shurtleff *et al.*, 2001).

Resection on the dominant left temporal lobe results in a lower verbal and full-scale intelligence and depressed delayed memory scores, with higher-performance intelligence (Chelune *et al.*, 1993). Subtle non-verbal impairments may result from resection of the non-dominant right temporal lobe (Blakemore & Falconer, 1967), although in some patients both verbal and performance intelligence improve (Klove & Matthews, 1967).

Memory effects

Both right temporal lobe and left temporal lobe patients are at risk for memory decline postoperatively. A significant decline in verbal memory may be seen, taking the form of poor recall of short stories, difficulties with word-listing learning tasks, and difficulties in learning and recalling unrelated word pairs (Chiaravalloti & Glosser, 2001). A postoperative decline in memory is mostly the result of the removal of functioning brain that plays a role in memory before surgery (Helmstaedter & Elger, 1998).

Not all patients have equally severe memory changes after surgery (Loring & Meador, 2001). Those with injury earlier in life have a greater sparing of language than memory functions, possibly related to a reorganization of brain functioning after damage to critical temporal lobe structures early in life. A larger resection may produce no more cognitive decrements than a smaller resection when the hippocampal tissue that is removed is dysfunctional. Patients with extensive atrophy of the contralateral hippocampus have more severe cognitive deficits after surgery, presumably due to the inability of contralateral brain structures to compensate for resected tissue (Chiaravalloti & Glosser, 2001).

Postoperative recovery of verbal learning and memory is related to plasticity and neuronal compensation, which is independent of pathology and the seizure outcome. The older the patient at the time of surgery, the less is their ability to compensate. Learning and data acquisition are unchanged or even improved in patients younger than 15 years who are operated on in the period in which contralateral or ipsilateral restitution of impaired left hemisphere functions can be assumed. Impaired verbal short-term or working memory can be compensated for somewhat by other left hemispheric functions (Helmstaedter & Elger, 1998).

Immediate memory is impaired selectively after bilateral hippocampal pathology, even if this pathology is sustained perinatally. The rescuing of speech and basic communication abilities is often achieved at the cost of non-verbal cognitive functions being crowded out. Early unilateral brain damage leading to hemispherectomy places a heavy cost on intellectual ability, thus setting limits on the ultimate development of all aspects of cognitive function (Vargha-Kahdem, 2001).

Following a temporal lobectomy with maximal attempts to spare hippocampal tissue, immediate memory performance decreases by 15% and delayed memory remains the same. With a more radial approach, immediate memory decreases by 30% and delayed memory decreases by 44%. Selective hippocampal sparing leads to less verbal memory deficit following a dominant lobectomy (Grote *et al.*, 1991). Patients who become seizure-free after surgery tend to experience fewer specific memory deficits (Chiaravalloti & Glosser, 2001).

Follow-up one year later shows improvement of some memory functions and continued impairment of others, reflecting the degree of seizure control and the state of the remaining temporal lobe. Uncontrolled seizures interfere with memory functions in the remaining contralateral temporal lobe. Other variables include the age of the patient at operation and the side of the resection (Novelly *et al.*, 1984). Memory problems may continue to improve for one to two years. A rise in function may be seen by the fifth postoperative year. Up to 12 years later, a remarkable degree of late recovery is noted. Verbal memory scales remain inferior to non-dominant temporal lobe memory. The overall recover is related inversely to the age of the patient at surgery and the incidence of postoperative seizures (Milner, 1968).

Left temporal resection

Auditory memory problems related to a dominant left temporal lobectomy include the registration and retention of verbal impressions. Short-term memory recall and associated paired learning skills may be a problem for up to several years postoperatively (Blakemore & Falconer, 1967). Written word fluency may be intact (Milner, 1975; Novelly *et al.*, 1984). Individuals may have problems in following the gist of more complicated verbal materials, such as in a novel or at a lecture, possibly due to problems with categorizing materials involved in the retention of materials in short-term memory. Difficulties in recalling names from given categories are seen. Problems with initial organization and categorization are seen (Novally *et al.*, 1984). Verbal encoding strategies display significantly more false recognition errors postoperatively (Rausch, 1981). Immediate and delayed visual memory, including visual imagery, remain intact and may even be improved (Read, 1981; Novelly *et al.*, 1984). Memory problems may be primarily for words rather than numbers, thus math abilities are not unaffected (Serafetindes, 1969). Memory defects appear to be mostly for words heard or read, although word fluency may not change (Novelly *et al.*, 1984). This may be present but not appreciated preoperatively (Milner, 1968).

Right temporal resection

In non-dominant right temporal lobectomy candidates, preoperatively patients have problems with copying or recall. Postoperatively, they may have problems with recall but their copying normalizes. Slight visuospatial memory defects with a slight verbal memory improvement may be seen, including disturbed learning for new unfamiliar faces, musical compositions, and designs and patterns (Chiaravalloti & Glosser, 2001).

Bilateral temporal ablation

Medial temporal lobe resections bilaterally result in a persistent impairment of recent memory whenever the removal is carried far enough posterior to damage portions of the anterior hippocampus and hippocampal gyrus. The degree of memory loss appears to depend on the extent of the hippocampal removal. Removal of only the uncus and amygdala bilaterally does not appear to cause memory impairments

(Milner & Scoville, 1957). When a global and persistent amnesic syndrome follows a unilateral temporal lobectomy, it may be assumed that surgery removed the remaining functioning tissue of a bilateral hippocampal lesion. Bilateral loss of the hippocampus and the hippocampal gyrus causes severe, lasting short-term memory loss. Verbal relearning after temporal lobectomy can be accelerated by slower presentation of material and by the use of prelearned associations (Stores, 1971).

Perception

There are less significant differences in the level of performance between right and left temporal lobectomy patients in visual-spatial organization and memory functions. Postoperative improvement is seen in both groups (Stanulis & Fogel, 1984).

With a right temporal lobectomy, problems in visual recognition may occur, suggesting that some patients are not encoding the visually presented material normally. A supposed failure of visual encoding may cause a patient to focus more on the auditory channels (Rausch, 1981). If the excision extends far back along the inferior surface of the temporal lobe, spatial abilities may be disturbed more. Injury to the parietal lobe results in severe impairments of visual-spatial orientation. The recall and recognition of visual and auditory patterns that cannot be coded easily with words as well as the learning of style mazes (whether visual or proprioceptive guided) are problematic. Deficits in complex visual pattern-solving and mild perceptual deficits may occur. These effects are subtle and often can be demonstrated only when normal perceptual cues are reduced (Milner, 1975).

Children

In children with intractable epilepsies, developmental quotients progressively decrease with age, often due to continued frequent seizures. Surgical intervention may halt the decline in developmental intellectual quotient and allow the recovery of this postoperatively (Matsuzaka *et al.*, 2001).

Less pronounced hemispheric differences are seen in school-age children with temporal lobe epilepsy as compared with adults. Children may a have a lower risk of memory deterioration after temporal lobectomy due to their larger potential for cerebral plasticity (Lendt *et al.*, 1999). Some children may improve in IQ and memory tests (Powell *et al.*, 1975; Binnie *et al.*, 1990).

Preadolescent children who undergo a temporal lobectomy for intractable seizures may experience a short-term memory problem that is a function of the pathology (Snyder *et al.*, 2001). Postoperative losses also occur in recognition memory. Children, particularly those with a left temporal focus, may show significantly reduced language performance (Gotman, 2001). Children and adolescents, like adults, may experience decrements in verbal learning abilities, although some may gain skills. List learning but not story memory is affected. The higher the presurgical functioning, the more likely the child is to experience losses (Shurtleff *et al.*, 2001). Memory may not change in follow-up after surgery, whereas language performance and attention improve significantly three months and one year, respectively, after surgery. Poor seizure control appears to be the decisive factor for children with losses in memory (Lendt *et al.*, 1999).

Follow-up

Postoperative rehabilitation must take into account the developmental level of the individual, which may require weeks to months of intensive specialist input (Cornaggia & Gobbi, 2001). In planning, it is best to anticipate potential deficits and to be prepared to remediate these than to be surprised.

Neocortical excision

Excisions in the other parts of the brain, i.e. the parietal or occipital lobes and the posterior-frontal lobe, are associated more with deficits in sensory, special sensory, or motor functions, respectively. Some visual perceptual problems may be associated with non-dominant parietal resections. In children especially, subsequent problems with learning skills are often less impairing than after frontal or temporal resection (Kitchen *et al.*, 1993).

Multiple pial resection

Multiple subpial resections tend to minimize the surgical effects on cortical function in eloquent language or primary motor or sensory regions, while decreasing the spread of seizure activity in the horizontal plain (Loring & Meador, 2001).

Hemispherectomy

A hemispherectomy is usually performed for intractable seizures related to a significantly damaged or underdeveloped brain hemisphere or with a progressive problem such as Rasmussen's encephalitis. In an effort to control seizures that threaten the remaining functions of the involved hemisphere, the removal of the hemisphere may allow recovery of cognitive functions beyond those anticipated in the child. The uncontrollable seizures usually will have resulted in the shift of such functions to the opposite hemisphere. Such an approach is desirable as early as possible before brain maturation, otherwise the potential for such plasticity is lost. However, too often in a child, consideration of such an extreme is often postponed in fear of potential loss of skills. Once the seizures have been controlled, partial recovery of functions is not unusual. Even a hemiplegia may be lessened postoperatively. However, this requires an active rehabilitative program and family support. With selected patients, after a thorough evaluation, earlier surgery may allow a better functional chance.

Corpus callosotomy

The corpus callosum joins the two cerebral hemispheres, allowing the interchange of information to facilitate learning and to coordinate responses. Surgery is often considered to lessen seizure frequency and spread, limiting the focus to one hemisphere rather than allowing secondary generalization, i.e. to stop the spread of the seizures and thus to prevent a localized focus from producing big seizures. Patients tolerate a two-stage approach better than a complete one-stage callosotomy. In the two-stage approach, the anterior portion is severed first, and about a half-year later the remaining posterior portion and hippocampal connections are severed. Subtle speech and motor neurologic deficits may follow the first operation (Loring & Meador, 2001) and some incoordination between the two body sides may follow the second (Cukiert *et al.*, 2001). Some problems appear to be due to the disconnection of the two hemispheres and some due to traction on the hemisphere during the surgery.

In children, acute syndromes are infrequent, but if present recovery is rapid. Transient language and communication problems are the most common. Attention problems are often improved but occasionally may be worsened. Memory problems may emerge in some patients, possibly as the result of disconnection of previously damaged lobes in which part of the language-related functions are transferred to the other side. The memory problems may persist and worsen, especially if present preoperatively.

Coordination of motor acts between the two body sides may be impaired, such that body recognition and awareness between the two sides are no longer coordinated (Cukiert *et al.*, 2001). This may improve in time, especially in children who seem able to adjust without much difficulty (Loring & Meador, 2001). Some children have problems in imitating movements and gestures for the first few months, but they appear to compensate eventually.

Reading problems without writing problems (dyslexia without agraphia) may be seen in a poorly dominant hemisphere with occipital damage and a splenium section. Rarely, a person may have problems reading things to one side but not on the other, which may persist. Left-hand and left-hemispheric dominance may contribute to a dysgraphia, but right-hand and right-hemispheric dominance may also go to a dysgraphia.

Vagus nerve stimulation

Vagal nerve stimulation (VNS) has shown no adverse cognitive effects and may have positive behavior benefits. However, it has much less probability of yielding a seizure-free state than surgery (Meador, 2002). Its mode of seizure control is not understood. No validated changes in attention, motor functioning, short-term memory, learning and memory, or executive functions have been confirmed.

Attention may improve in some patients, and arousal may be increased during VNS treatment. Possible induced impairments include recognition impairments or reduction of figure-memory performance, the latter possibly being related to increased effects of the left VNS on brain concentration. Possible stimulation-related enhanced word-recognition memory during a retention interval has been mentioned (Hoppe *et al.*, 1999). Initially, no differences are noted in objective memory testing, but a mild improvement in the total number of words recalled may be seen (Ravdin *et al.*, 2000).

Diet

In developmentally delayed children, significant gains in all areas except gross motor skills are noted about one month after initiating a ketogenic diet. Advances in receptive communications and fine motor skills are noted by four to six months. Sustained improvement in receptive language may be responsible for reports of improved alertness (Noldy-MacLedan *et al.*, 2001).

REFERENCES

Binnie, C. D., Channon, S. & Marston, D. (1990). Learning disabilities in epilepsy: neurophysiological aspects. *Epilepsia* **31** (suppl 4): 2–8.

Blakemore, C. B. & Falconer, M. I. A. (1967). Long-term effects of anterior temporal lobectomy on certain cognitive functions. *J. Neurol. Neurosurg. Psychiatry* **30**: 364–7.

Chelune, G. J., Van Ness, P. C., Naugle, R. I., *et al.* (1993). Comparison of memory deficits after frontal and temporal lobe epilepsy surgery. *Epilepsia* **34** (suppl 6): 101.

Chiaravalloti, N. D. & Glosser, G. (2001). Material-specific memory changes after anterior temporal lobectomy as predicted by the intracarotid amobarbital test. *Epilepsia* **42**: 902–11.

Cornaggia, C. M. & Gobbi, G. (2001). Learning disability in epilepsy: definitions and classification. In *Epilepsia and Learning Disabilities*, ed. G. F. Ayala, M. Elia, C. M. Cornaggia & M. M. Trimble. *Epilepsia* **42**: 2–5.

Cukiert, M., Canar-Cukiert, A. R., *et al.*, (2001). Neuropsychological effects of anterior callosal sections. *Epilepsia* **42** (suppl 7): 249.

Delaney, R. C., Rosen, A. J., Mattson, R. H., *et al.* (1980). Memory function in focal epilepsy: a comparison of non-surgical unilateral temporal lobe and frontal lobe samples. *Cortex* **16**: 103–17.

Dikmen, S. (1980). Neuropsychological aspects of epilepsy. In *Multidisciplinary Handbook of Epilepsy*, ed. B. P. Herman, pp. 236–73. Springfield, IL: Charles C. Thomas.

Durwen, H. F. (1991). Comparison of verbal memory performance in therapy-resistant left temporal lobe epilepsy patients before and after left temporal lobe resection. 19th International Epilepsy Conference. *Epilepsia* **32** (suppl 10): 39.

Gleissner, U., Helmstaedter, C., Schramm, J., *et al.* (2002). Memory outcome after selective amygdalohippocampectomy: a study in 140 patients with temporal lobe epilepsy. *Epilepsia* **43**: 87–95.

Gotman, M. (2001). Learning and memory before and after resection from temporal lobes. *Epilepsia* **42** (suppl 7): 219.

Grote, C. L., Morrell, F. & Whisler, W. W. (1991). Verbal memory following dominant hippocampal resection: a comparison of two approaches. *Epilepsia* **32** (suppl 3): 87.

Helmstaedter, C. & Elger, C. E. (1998). Functional plasticity after left anterior temporal lobectomy: reconstruction and compensation of verbal memory functions. *Epilepsia* **39**: 399–406.

Hempel, A., Risse, G. L., Frost, M. D., *et al.* (2001). Neuropsychological outcomes of dominant frontal topectomy in children and adolescents. *Epilepsia* **42** (suppl 7): 160.

Hoppe, C., Helmstaaedter, C. & Elger, C. E. (1999). Cognitive effects of acute and chronic vagus nerve stimulus – a reply to Clark *et al. Epilepsia* **40** (suppl 7): 84.

Kitchen, N. D., Thompson, P. J., Fish, D. R., *et al.* (1993). Neuropsychological sequelae after temporal neocortical lesionectomy: comparison with temporal lobectomy. *Epilepsia* **34** (suppl 6): 71.

Klove, H. & Matthews, C. G. (1967). Differential psychological performance in major motor, psychomotor and mixed seizure classification of known and unknown etiology. *Epilepsia* **8**: 117–28.

Lee, G. P., Park, Y. D., Hempel, A., *et al.* (2001). Effect of WADA method in predicting lateralized impairment in pediatric epilepsy surgery candidates. *Epilepsia* **42** (suppl 7): 160–61.

Lendt, M., Helmstaedtet, C. & Elger, C. E. (1999). Pre- and postoperative neuropsychological profiles in children and adolescents with temporal lobe epilepsy. *Epilepsia* **40**: 1543–50.

Loring, D. W. & Meador, K. J. (2001). Cognitive and behavior effects of epilepsy treatment. *Epilepsia* **42** (suppl 8): 24–32.

Matsuzaka, T., Baba, H., Matsuo, A., *et al.* (2001). Developmental assessment based surgical intervention for intractable epilepsies in infants and young children. Proceedings of the 33rd Congress of the Japan Epilepsy Society. *Epilepsia* **42** (suppl 6): 9–12.

Meador, K. J. (2002). Cognitive outcomes and predictive factors in epilepsy. *Neurology* **58**: (suppl 5): 21–8.

Meyer, V. & Yates, V. J. (1955). Intellectual changes following temporal lobectomy for psychomotor epilepsy. *J. Neurol. Neurosurg. Psychiatry* **18**: 44–52.

Milner, B. (1968). Disorders of memory after brain lesions in man. Preface: material specific and generalized memory loss. *Neuropsychologica* **6**: 175–7.

Milner, B. (1975). Psychological aspects of focal epilepsy and its neurosurgical management. In *Neurosurgical Management of the Epilepsies*, ed. D. P. Purpura, J. K. Penry & R. D. Walter, Vol. 8, pp. 299–321. New York: Raven Press.

Milner, B. & Scoville, W. B. (1957). Loss of recent memory after bilateral hippocampal lesions. *J. Neurol. Neurosurg. Psychiatry* **20**: 11–21.

Noldy-MacLedan, N. E., Hansen, J. & Curtis, R. (2001). Neurodevelopmental advances in children on the ketogenic diet: a pilot study. *Epilepsia* **42** (suppl 7): 161.

Novelly, R. A., Augustine, E. A., Mattson, R. H., *et al.* (1984). Selective memory improvement and impairment in temporal lobectomy for epilepsy. *Ann. Neurol.* **15**: 64–7.

Powell, G. E., Polkey, C. E. & McMillan, T. (1975). The new Maudsley series of temporal lobectomy. I: short-term cognitive effects. *Br. J. Clin. Psychol.* **24**: 109–24.

Rausch, R. (1981). Lateralization of temporal lobe dysfunction and verbal encoding *Brain Lang.* **12**: 92–100.

Ravdin, L. S. D., Harden, C. L., Correa, D. D., *et al.* (2000). Memory and mood following vagus nerve stimulation for intractable epilepsy. *Epilepsia* **41** (suppl 7): 136.

Read, D. E. (1981). Solving deductive reasoning problems after unilateral temporal lobectomy. *Brain Lang.* **12**: 116–27.

Sass, K. J., Westerveld, M., Buchanan, C. P., *et al.* (1994). Degree of hippocampal neuron loss determines severity of verbal memory decrease after left anteromesiotemporal lobectomy. *Epilepsia* **35**: 1179–86.

Seidenberg, M., Hermann, B. P., Dohan, F. C., Jr, *et al.* (1996). Hippocampal sclerosis and verbal encoding ability following anterior temporal lobectomy. *Neuropsychology* **34**: 699–708.

Serafetindes, E. A. (1969). Memory for words and memory for numbers. *J. Learn. Disabil.* **2**: 142–3.

Shurtleff, H. A., Bournival, B. D., Ellenbogen, R. G., *et al.* (2001). Verbal learning changes in children/adolescents after temporal lobectomy (TLE). *Epilepsia* **42** (suppl 7): 199.

Smith, M. L., Elliott, I. M. & Lach, L. (2002). Cognitive skills in children with intractable epilepsy: comparison of surgical and nonsurgical candidates. *Epilepsia* **46**: 621–7.

Smith, M. L., Lach, L. M. & Elliot, I. M. (2000). Reasoning, remembering, and academics in children with epilepsy: does surgery make a difference? *Epilepsia* **41** (suppl 7): 81.

Snyder, T. J., Sinclair, D. B., McKean, J. D., *et al.* (2001). Memory morbidity post temporal lobectomy in preadolescent children. *Epilepsia* **42** (suppl 7): 163.

Stanulis, R. G. & Fogel, G. (1984). Changes in visual spatial organization and memory ion epilepsy patients following temporal lobectomy. *Epilepsia* **25**: 665.

Stores, G. (1971). Cognitive function in children with epilepsy. *Dev. Med. Child Neurol.* **13**: 390–92.

Trenerry, M. R., Jack, C. R., Jr, Ivnik, R. J., *et al.* (1993). MRI hippocampal volumes and memory function before and after temporal lobectomy. *Neurology* **43**: 1800–805.

Vargha-Kahdem, F. (2001). Generalized versus selective cognitive impairments resulting from brain damage sustained in childhood. In *Epilepsia and Learning Disabilities*, ed. G. F. Ayala, M. Elia, C. M. Cornaggia & M. M. Trimble. *Epilepsia* **42**: 37–40.

Westerveld, M., Zawacki, T., Spencer, S. S., *et al.* (1993). Epilepsy surgery in children and adolescents. *Epilepsia* **34** (suppl 6): 36.

24

Diagnosis

Children with epilepsy are at risk for learning problems. Cognitive impairment is the link between epilepsy and the inability to learn in school (Aldenkamp *et al.*, 1990). Epilepsy may cause dysfunction of a given specific performance that coincides with the cortical area involved, without causing mental retardation. When cognitive performance has not definitely been acquired, a dysfunction in a specific cognitive performance may cause an imbalance of the complex system of cognitive development. True mental retardation may improve if the specific cognitive dysfunction is treated adequately early (Cornaggia & Gobbi, 2001).

A proper assessment of the complex situation is difficult, requiring the collaboration of physician, psychologist, teacher, and family. The child should at least be screened, even if not evaluated formally, using appropriate observations and tests as part of the initial evaluation and in follow-up, especially if the history and/or school reports indicate possible problems. Children with difficult seizure problems and learning difficulties may need to be referred to a specialized epilepsy center to insure the best possible assessment. Although most children with epilepsy benefit from medication, excessive medication may cause learning difficulties even in a well-functioning child with benign absence seizures (Henricksen, 1990). For some patients with medication-resistant seizures, earlier surgery may be beneficial and may prevent the learning and social handicaps that may otherwise emerge.

Early signs of learning disabilities

In children with inherited learning disabilities and with very early-onset seizures that lead to later learning disabilities, there may be early signs suggestive of later learning disabilities (Svoboda, 1979). These learning problem risks may show up as poor sucking and feeding in the neonate, as crawling and coordination problems in infancy, or as speech problems in the toddler. The preschool child may be slow to learn numbers, letters, nursery rhymes, names, or addresses. The child might not like to color, to cut, or to read. The child may be slowed and confused at tying, buttoning, or dressing. Such children may be delayed in telling the time, clumsy in sports, or superficial in cleaning their room.

In first grade, the child is most apt to have reading problems. Frustrations may cause behaviors that lead to mislabeling a child as having an attention deficit. By third grade, spelling and math problems may become major issues.

Often, in grading papers, the teacher sums up the correct or incorrect answers, but does not take time to note the reason for the incorrect answers. Mistakes may mask the signs of learning disabilities. If misspellings are really substitutions of similar but incorrect letters, such as a "b" for "d" or "p," "brid" for "bird," or "no" for "on," the child may have a spatial problem. If the mistake is the substitution of similar letters except for a small detail, such as "v" and "y" or "m" and "n" or "h," the child may have a problem in detail discrimination. Both of these are visual perception problems, which are more common than realized in children with epilepsy. If the child has the right letters but out of order, such as "sotp" for "stop," there may be a sequencing problem. This can also be seen by mistakes in writing, when the child gets all the words right but writes them out of order.

Children who can say the right answers but struggle in writing them most probably have a problem. Similarly, the child who can write an answer but cannot say it may have a problem. Language problems may be manifest in children who confuse what they hear or who have problems in explaining their ideas.

Math problems also yield clues. Reversals and detail confusions may be seen in recognizing numbers and operational signs. If problems arise by adding six plus five to get 14, because the child confused six with nine, the child may have spatial difficulties. Overlooking details, such as not differentiating eight from three or five, or seeing 432 as 42, suggests problems in perceptual discrimination. Sequencing problems can be seen when the child sees 4021 as 4201 or 4210. The child may confuse plus, multiplication, and division signs and thus perform the incorrect operation. Spatial confusions may manifest in confusions of columns in working problems, especially in carrying and borrowing, when a child may stray into an adjacent column. Some children do not seem to remember math tables. Mistakes do not just happen repeatedly; they are usually the product of a faulty technique, which needs to be discovered.

If problems continue to go unrecognized, by adolescence the child's frustrations often trigger acting out behaviors. The child may give up and do nothing, attempt to run away figuratively, seek to avoid efforts, become angry and aggressive, develop anxiety-based physical complains, or become discouraged, even to the point of attempting suicide. Delinquency is not an uncommon consequence of untreated learning disabilities.

Considerations

Whenever a student is underachieving, especially in specific situations or in certain subjects, the possibility of a learning disability should be considered. Such academic struggles should not be excused as the result of a behavior problem, of the medication in use, or of the fact that the seizure problem exists (Aldenkamp *et al.*, 1990).

Underachievement may be classified according to the scholastic skill involved. If the child underachieves in only certain subjects, there may be an underlying learning disability or associated prior emotional trauma as a cause (Rutter, 1977). Emotional factors to be explored include the attitudes of the parents and teachers, task-associated behavior and emotional problems, and problems with attention, which may be secondary to the frustration and struggles to learn (Wirt *et al.*, 1977).

Emotional and behavior disorders may be a symptomatic expression of a cognitive impairment in individuals with epilepsy. Behavior and mood disorders may be the cause of a reduced learning ability. Complex partial epilepsies have been linked to interictal affective and personality disturbances, self-destructive behaviors (Kanemoto *et al.*, 1999), and, after decades in a few patients, psychotic states (Cornaggia & Gobbi, 2001). Similarly, mental health personnel need to look closely for possible underlying causes for childhood behavior problems in the evaluation, lest they end up treating only the symptoms and not the cause.

The doctor's office

In caring for children with epilepsy, the doctor's prime duty is to look for the cause and alleviate it if possible. If seizures continue, the epilepsy must be classified so that treatment with the best antiepileptic drug for the child can be initiated, always at the lowest possible dose and accompanied by close monitoring for side effects. If a second or third drug is required, one needs to watch even more closely to insure that the side effects do not add to the burden of the epilepsy (Henricksen, 1990).

At each and every visit, as well as whenever problems arise, the physician should seek not just to determine seizure control and medication intake but also to inquire about school performance and behavior. Any hint of problems should be pursued (Svoboda, 1979).

The approach to learning disabilities in epilepsy concentrates first on analyzing the differential effects of the epileptic factors on cognitive function. The impact of seizure activity, localization of the epileptogenic foci, and the antiepileptic treatment on cognitive functioning need to be evaluated. If available, computerized neuropsychologic testing may be most useful in addressing issues of learning disabilities in children with epilepsy, including test–retest variation, deterioration, and the supposed specificity of learning disabilities (Aldenkamp *et al.*, 1990).

Classroom observations

The teacher and psychologist need to collaborate in detecting specific learning disabilities as early as possible and in providing special education services as soon as needed. Adverse behaviors in certain academic areas or classes may suggest underlying frustrations or stresses that need to be evaluated. The teacher and the psychologist can often begin to make the diagnosis by analyzing the mistakes to determine what kind of errors are being made. Perhaps it is best to save the faulty papers, rather than the excellent ones, to analyze for mistake trends. A child with epilepsy can have any form of learning disability (Strang, 1987). The assessment is the basis for appropriate remedial education.

Observation made during the classroom performance may be used in evaluation of learning disabilities. Important issues that may be detected include significant error types in classroom efforts, test–retest variation, deterioration, and the specificity of learning disabilities (Aldenkamp *et al.*, 1990). The teacher's ratings of inattentiveness in the classroom often do not correlate with cognitive tests for measuring attention (Stores, 1987).

If the parent is not getting answers because the school authorities find nothing, the parent needs to persist in asking why the child with seizures struggles in reading even though they have been assured that the IQ is adequate and there are no apparent problems. When the answer to this is found, the response should begin the child on a road to learning.

Formal evaluation

Most studies of cognition in children with epilepsy rely on intelligence testing, such as the Wechlser Intelligence Score for Children (WISC). Such tests give an indication of the child's level of functioning, yet they may not be sensitive to all neurologic impairments or reflect the way the child performs in school. Subtle disturbances of memory, perception, and attention may not be detected (Holmes, 1987). A test battery should be chosen to address the at-risk areas as well as suspected weak areas. Any evaluation should be made under optimum conditions, although simulating the conditions in which the academic problems and related behaviors emerge may be more productive. The evaluator(s) should be aware of the relationships between the seizure types, the medications, the problems, and the behaviors.

Basic evaluation

Selection of the child for screening and/or testing, with the family's approval, should be made because of a seizure that occurred in school or during a school activity or when the parents voluntarily identify the child as having some form of epilepsy. The basics of educational testing should include a basic comprehensive intelligence test, academic tests, and, especially in children with epilepsy, tests of perception and memory, all performed with close observation of the child's alertness and performance styles. The evaluator should be alert to any possible mini-seizures during the evaluation, noting any alterations in test performance. Such testing should be performed after the antiepileptic medications have been optimized and should be performed with full awareness of when the child's last seizure occurred.

IQ testing

The Wechsler intelligence test group, i.e. the Wechsler Adult Intelligence Scales (WAIS), the Wechsler Intelligence Scales for Children, revised (WISC-r), and the Wechsler Preschool and Primary Scale of Intelligence (WIPPSI), are tests of intelligence, not of brain function. Some of the subtests that are indicated as performance subtests are not purely non-verbal in nature (Zimmerman *et al.*, 1951). Attention factors may be particularly vulnerable to seizure activity and may skew such subtests as coding (Aldenkamp *et al.*, 1990). The goal of the testing is to gain a better understanding of the child's difficulties in learning, so as to develop an individualized program to overcome those difficulties.

The basic IQ test may be supplemented by tests of language, of fine and gross motor processes (as in perceptual-motor tests), and of memory. Various psycholinguistic (learning processing) tests may be helpful. Observing how the tasks are performed may be as informative as the test scores themselves.

Academic performance

There has been a tendency towards overinterpreting what the tests really say. On tests such as the Wide Range Achievement Test (WRAT), the common thought is that this evaluates reading, arithmetic, and spelling. However, the reading is actually vocabulary identification, i.e. reading a list of words rather than reading paragraphs for comprehension. Thus, the WRAT does not test reading, although numerous studies have interpreted it as doing so. The WRAT may well be supplemented by a test of reading comprehension. If mistakes are noted, they should be analyzed to determine the reason for the mistake. The testing should be correlated with classroom observations and should include coverage of the areas of difficulties. Samples of class work efforts bearing examples of the errors noted are valuable in analysis.

Behavior screens

Various screens for entities such as childhood depression, ADHD, or more global childhood emotional disturbances may be used, but it must be realized that these only raise questions. If a problem is indicated, referral for more expert evaluation is needed. ADHD screens, for example, are more apt to identify underachievement than ADHD. More often, simple observations in the testing situations as well as in the classroom, combined with a parent interview, can be most informative.

A major center may have a set assessment battery in children, including tests such as the Reitan Neuropsychologic Battery, WISC-r, Peabody Individual Achievement Test, a child behavioral checklist, the Self Concept Scale, and a children's epilepsy battery adapted for the parents (Hawkins *et al.*, 1985). These are useful in general studies of the epilepsy population, but a child with difficulties needs a more individualized choice of tests. In the smaller medical or mental health centers, psychologist's office, or usual school setting, such a battery is not readily available. Much, however, can be obtained by using a simple battery including the WISC-r, the WRAT augmented by a test of reading comprehension, and a childhood behavioral checklist. Further testing obtained through speech and language services, pediatric occupational therapists, and physical therapists may address perceptual motor processing.

Special tests

Tests such as the Halstead Reitan Battery consist of simple sensory and motor tasks for the hands and are unrelated to educational levels. More complex tasks used to assess higher cognitive functions are reasonably objective but have been criticized for their insensitivity to focal and lateralized brain damage. The Luria–Nebraska Battery of neuropsychiatric tests has been criticized for its subjectivity and lack of normals for children initially. Thus, the examiner tends to choose subtests from a variety of subtests, including the WAIS or WISC-r, but the results are inconsistent and difficult to compare due to variances in procedural changes in the same battery (Rugland, 1990a).

Some children can perform adequately in the calm and quiet setting of a testing room, but when stressed by the examiner or asked to perform in a more distracting setting resembling the classroom their performance may deteriorate markedly. Adding this situation to the testing status may demonstrate the problems that the child may be experiencing. The evaluator should be aware that in some children a seizure might be precipitated. Such testing may reveal additional needs in coping with stress that the child may have.

Psycholinguistic testing

Tests of cognitive processing have occasionally been utilized in children with epilepsy, such as the Illinois Test of Psycholinguistic Abilities. In one study, no differences were found comparing children with absence epilepsy with children with other seizure types (Von Isser, 1977). A larger group of learning-disabled children subdivided into roughly 25 children in each of five groups of generalized tonic–clonic, absence, myoclonic, complex partial (left, right, and bilateral), and past febrile convulsions were evaluated using a psycholinguistic profile augmented by visual perceptual and auditory discrimination testing. Many had visual perceptual problems. Children with complex partial seizures had a significantly higher incidence of auditory memory and sequential memory problems, especially if the left temporal lobe was involved.

A trained educational psychologist may use a battery such as the WISC-r, the PIAT or WRAT plus tests of reading comprehension, the KEY Math tests plus the Frostig Tests of Visual Perception, the Wepman Tests of Auditory Perception, and the Illinois Test of Psycholinguistic Abilities as tools, analyzing the observed performance and the types of errors noted as well as the raw scores in developing an individualized educational program in coordination with the child's school teachers.

A lengthy and critical discussion of various testing approaches is covered by Dodson *et al.* (1991).

Electroencephalographic studies

In childhood epilepsy, it is important to establish the location and extent of the focus and any underlying lesion, as this may be indicate the sort of specific learning disability to expect and lead to more appropriate management (Henricksen, 1990).

Routine electroencephalography

In addition to a routine wake and sleep EEG, including fasting, hyperventilation, and photic stimulation, it is important to try to simulate the conditions during which the seizures occur. Thus, if the seizures seem to occur with the performance of certain academic efforts, such as reading, math calculation, or writing, the task should be performed during the EEG testing using unfamiliar reading passages or more difficult math problems to simulate the triggering academic processes. Sometimes, EEG abnormalities are noted only when the patient is involved in the tasks that produce the symptoms (Binnie, 2001). Long-term recordings, sometimes with video monitoring and telemetry (Binnie *et al.*, 1990) or by using outpatient cassette recordings, may be useful to demonstrate relationships (Stores & Bergel, 1989; Stores, 1990). Such testing, especially if combined with a computerized neuropsychological battery, makes it possible to demonstrate the relationships between epileptic discharges and various activities, and to evaluate whether such discharges influence performance (Stores, 1987; Binnie, 1988).

If seizures are of concern as contributing to the performance and yet the regular EEG is normal, an overnight study may be indicated to check for nocturnal activations, especially if there is a history of intellectual or language regression. If there is a history of sleep disturbances, a sleep study may be considered, especially if the underachieving child repeatedly arrives at school in a sleepy state (Stores, 1990).

Merely to diagnose an EEG abnormality without correlation to the academic problem may be more impairing, especially if the EEG study is overread. Children have been seen at epilepsy centers burdened by unnecessary drugs, with resultant behavior and cognitive difficulties, and who have, in review, been found to have had misread normal EEGs or in some cases EEG abnormalities unrelated to the events for which they were ordered. Tapering off the medications and reviewing the original situations often leads to correct diagnoses and more appropriate help.

Computerized electroencephalographic neuropsychometrics

Observations of how the child reacts and how the performance is affected by stress introduced in the testing often will not only bring out weak areas in academic performance but also will indicate needs in handling similar stresses in the classroom. Subtle pauses or inconsistent errors may suggest subclinical seizures affecting the testing. If this is the case, ideally an EEG should be run during testing. Functional testing is desirable because the amount of epileptic activity on a standard EEG, where the patient is lying down with eyes closed, does not necessarily reflect the situation at school (Henricksen, 1990). EEG recordings during psychological testing are desirable if available (Stores, 1987; Binnie, 1988), especially for children who show inconsistent performance in learning behavior. Computerized neuropsychologic assessment has been developed to simultaneously register EEG and performance via a cognitive test battery (Aldenkamp *et al.*, 1990). This is ideal for such situations but is not readily available due to costs and the lack of technical expertise.

Computer-aided neuropsychological assessment is especially useful from age eight onwards. Measures of reaction time, motor speed, information processing, and memory are most often evaluated. Performance speed increases with age. Differences in information processing emerge at about 12 years of age and beyond, unrelated to frontal lobe maturation (Alpherts & Aldenkamp, 1990).

Such approaches indicate that subclinical discharges may impair performance in 61% of patients on simple and choice reaction times, even with bursts lasting only one second (Rugland, 1990b). Individual epileptiform EEG discharges may be accompanied by a momentary disruption of adaptive cerebral function as TCIs (Aarts *et al.*, 1984). Short one- to two-second generalized discharges may occur without apparent effect on performance, whereas focal discharges of even shorter duration sometimes influence a patient's response. However, the findings suggest that all epileptiform discharges disturb functioning to some extent if the test batteries are sufficiently sensitive (Henricksen, 1990).

This valuable research tool needs to be available at least at epilepsy centers providing comprehensive care to children with epilepsy so that the school problems can be diagnosed and remediated more accurately.

Other tests

A child with focal epilepsy should have an MRI scan, especially if there is a language, learning, or behavior problem. A child with epilepsy who has a deterioration of functions without apparent cause should definitely have an MRI scan to rule out a treatable lesion and to help understand and localize cognitive problems.

The P300 cognitive evoked potential is a late event-related potential occurring after presentation of novel stimuli as an extended brain stem auditory evoked response testing of hearing. The derived waveform is influenced by ongoing initial cognitive activity. The brain generation of this potential may be inked to the hippocampal formation and amygdala. With left temporal EEG seizures, the P300 latency is longer and lower amplitudes may be derived. This is not seen in patients with generalized seizures. Delayed P300 has been associated with disturbances of cognitive processing. This may relate to temporal lobe dysfunction of the seizure type (Syrigou-Papavasiliou *et al.*, 1985). Individuals who have difficulties especially in auditory processing in the decoding phase, and individuals with difficulties appearing in noisy situations, may show such P300 abnormalities. Such testing may aid both in the confirmation and understanding of such relationships. The information may be translated into remedial approaches for those experiencing learning difficulties.

A lesion demonstrated by MRI, or, to a lesser extent, hippocampal atrophy renders a hemisphere unlikely to become dominant, but epileptogenic foci can coexist with apparently normal neuropsychologic function, whereas with non-lesional epilepsy language may remain ipsilateral (Kanazawa *et al.*, 2000).

Operative considerations

Children with medication-resistant epilepsy are at risk for further cognitive skill regressions and emergence of behavior problems due to the insults of recurring seizures (as well as subclinical discharges) and a heavy medication load. For such children, earlier surgery may preserve intelligence and emotional intactness. A complete neuropsychologic test is expensive but important when planning a surgical approach, although the results are more appropriate to brain localization than to school learning. Combined with PET and fMRI non-invasive techniques, important cognitive activities and risks can be determined. Then, more precise localization of the epileptiform discharges can be obtained by placing electrodes on, in, or beneath the brain, including further testing using both verbal and spatial stimuli to evaluate language and memory. Thus, surgical approaches for those patients who can benefit have been rendered more precise in avoiding vital learning areas while providing surgical relief.

Prognosis

A good outcome may be obtained in those children who display indications of possible learning problems and are evaluated promptly for such difficulties. If the difficulties are tested and verified properly, the result must be a reasonable remediative program. Information to the school and the parents concerning the child's abilities and limitations may be as important as seizure control. If the problems are diagnosed and treated successfully, the child can be motivated to learn, self-esteem improves, and the psychosocial problems diminish (Henricksen, 1990).

REFERENCES

Aarts, J. H. P., Binnie, C. D., Smith, A. M., *et al.* (1984). Selective cognitive impairment during focal and generalized epileptiform EEG activity. *Brain* **107**: 293–308.

Aldenkamp, A. P., Alpherts, W. C. J. & Dekker, M. J. A. (1990). Neuropsychological aspects of learning disabilities in epilepsy. *Epilespia* **31** (suppl 4): 9–20.

Alpherts, W. C. J. & Aldenkamp, A. P. (1990). Computerized neuropsychological assessment of cognitive functioning in children with epilepsy. *Epilespia* **31** (suppl 4): 35–40.

Binnie, C. D. (1988). Seizures, EEG discharges and cognition. In *Epilepsy, Behavior and Cogntive Function*, ed. M. R. Trimble & E. H. Reynolds, pp. 45–51. London: John Wiley & Sons.

Binnie, C. D. (2001). Panel Discussion I. In *Epilepsia and Learning Disabilities*, ed. G. F Ayala, M. Elia, C. M. Cornaggia & M. R. Trimble. *Epilespia* **42**: 2–5.

Binnie, C. D., Chanon, S. & Maston, D. (1990). Learning disabilities in epilepsy: neuropsychological aspects. *Epilespia* **31** (suppl 4): 2–8.

Cornaggia, C. M. & Gobbi, G. (2001). Learning disability in epilepsy: definitions and classification. In *Epilepsia and Learning Disability*, ed. G. F. Ayala, M. Elia, C. M. Cornaggia & M. R. Trimble. *Epilespia* **42**: 2–5.

Dodson, W. W., Kinsbourne, M. & Hildbrunner, B. (1991). *The Assessment of Cognitive Function in Epilepsy*. New York: Demos.

Hawkins, R. C. II, Hubler, D. W. & Geis, S. (1985). Neuropsychological assessment as a component of comprehensive treatment planning with seizure-disordered children. *Epilespia* **26**: 529.

Henricksen, O. (1990). Education and epilepsy: assessment and remediation. *Epilepsia* **31** (suppl 4): 21–5.

Holmes, G. L. (1987). Psychosocial factors in childhood epilepsy. In *Diagnosis and Management of Epilepsy in Children*, pp. 112–24. Philadelphia: W. B. Saunders.

Kanazawa, O., Yoshino, M., Sasagawa, M., *et al.* (2000). VIQ-PIQ discrepancies in partial epilepsy on the relation to lateralities of focal MRI lesions, P3 peaks and focal spikes. Proceedings of the 32nd Congress of Japan Epilepsy Society. *Epilespia* **41** (suppl 9): 64.

Kanemoto, K., Kawasaki, J. & Mori, E. (1999). Violence and epilepsy: a close correlation between violence and postictal psychoses. *Epilespia* **40**: 107–9.

Rugland, A. L. (1990a). Neuropsychological assessment of cognitive functioning in children with epilepsy. *Epilespia* **31** (suppl 4): 41–4.

Rugland, A. (1990b). Subclinical epileptogenic activity. In *Pediatric Epilepsy*, ed. M. Sillarpaa, S. I. Johnanessen, G. Blennow & M. Dam, pp. 217–23. London: Wrightson Biomedical.

Rutter, M. (1977). Brain-damage syndromes. I: childhood: concepts and findings. *J. Child Psychol. Psychiatry* **18**: 1–21.

Stores, G. (1987). Effects of learning of "subclinical" seizure discharges. In *Education and Epilepsy 1987*, ed. A. P. Aldenkamp, W. C. J. Alpherts, H. Mienardi & G. Stores, pp. 14–21. Lisse: Swets & Zeitlinger.

Stores, G. (1990). Electroencephalographic parameters in assessing the cognitive function of children with epilepsy. *Epilespia* **31** (suppl 4): 5–49.

Stores, G. & Bergel, N. (1989). Clinical utility of cassette EEG in children with seizure disorders. In *Ambulatory EEG Monitoring*, ed. J. S. Ebersole, pp. 129–39. New York: Raven Press.

Strang, J. D. (1987). Educational and related treatment considerations concerning the child with epilepsy: a developmental approach. In *Education and Epilepsy*, ed. A. P. Aldenkamp, W. C. J. Alpherts, H. Meinardi & G. Stores, pp. 118–34. Lisse: Swets & Zeitlinger.

Svoboda, W. B. (1979). Epilepsy and learning problems. In *Learning About Epilepsy*, pp. 186–200. Baltimore, MD: University Park Press.

Syrigou-Papavasiliou, A., LeWitt, P. A., Green, V., *et al.* (1985). P300 and temporal lobe epilepsy. *Epilespia* **26**: 528.

Von Isser, A. (1977). Psycholinguistic abilities in children with epilepsy. *Exceptional Children* **February**: 270–72.

Wirt, R. D., Lachar, D., Klinedinst, J. K., *et al.* (1977). *Multidimensional Description of Child Personality: AS Manual for the Personality Inventory for Children*. Los Angeles: Western Psychological Services.

Zimmerman, F. T., Burgemeister, B. B. & Putnam, T. J. (1951). Intellectual and emotional makeup of the epileptic. *Arch. Neurol. Psychiatry* **65**: 545–56.

25

Gaining help

Children with intractable epilepsy often require special educational services because of progressive educational and psychosocial handicaps combined with a devastating seizure problem (Dam, 1990). Special education services may be warranted until better control is achieved. The main goals in working with such children is to prepare them for the demands of adulthood in terms of being able to care for themselves and to be self-supporting.

Learning problems may be reversible or permanent. Drug-induced and epilepsy-induced learning problems are potentially reversible, with consequent improvement in functioning resulting in a significant improvement in the quality of life (Besag, 2001). Even with learning disabilities of a more permanent nature, such as those from seizures causing brain damage, in children the plasticity of the brain may allow partial recovery of function (Henricksen, 1990).

Successfully overcoming a learning disability requires the combination of appropriate medical care working closely with educational experts. Unfortunately, proposals for practical treatment are seldom based on a multidisciplinary approach (Aldenkamp, 1987; Aldenkamp et al., 1990; Radley, 1987; Renier, 1987; Thompson, 1987).

Federal recommendations

The Federal Commission for the Control of Epilepsy and Its Consequences (1978) identified the learning consequences of epilepsy in childhood, resulting in a series of recommendations. The report noted:

The primary responsibility for providing the best possible education for handicapped children rests with the schools. If aware of their problems, schools can take a number of specific actions to help assure that handicapped children do indeed receive the education to which they are entitled . . .

Teachers believe children with epilepsy have twice as many problems . . . such as lack of concentration, restlessness, and fidgeting . . . as their classmates. The same problems that interfere with school performance also prevent employment of people with epilepsy . . . The informed teacher will realize that the child with epilepsy may also have learning disabilities and will provide the extra help needed ... Whether in a special or regular classroom situation though, the teacher must be alert to the special problems and needs of the child with epilepsy ... aware, for instance, that absence seizures can reduce learning time so that a child will require extra help ... and must work closely with parents, counselors, school psychologists, and the child to assure the best possible learning situation ...

Children who had epilepsy only had little problems in school. It was those who had related problems, either intellectual impairment or emotional problems, who had difficulty ... Since social ostracism is one of the major problems confronting children with epilepsy, it is important to contain these children in regular classroom situations, whenever possible. For some children such placement may not be suitable; however, there have never been systematic studies to determine under what conditions special placement may be advantageous for the child with epilepsy.

The medical setting

The medical setting is often the place to initiate search for help for educational problems and to monitor the effectiveness of such help, as well as to monitor the effectiveness and tolerance of the medical management. Dreifuss (personal communication) once noted that even experts in epilepsy often overlook subtle intoxication states. This is one of the major reasons that blood levels of anticonvulsant drugs are important and must be interpreted in light of the child's functioning. Subtle changes in alertness and cognition caused by medication may be difficult to detect, especially if the child originally suffered from frequent brief seizures. A computerized test battery, if available, may be administered repeatedly as it helps to optimize the medication therapy. Drug side effects should not replace the seizure adversities. Treatment of subclinical discharges, if initiated, should be continued only if the benefit of reduced epileptiform activity can be demonstrated and if adverse cognitive effects of the drug can be avoided (Henricksen, 1990).

A proper assessment of the complex situation is difficult, requiring the collaboration of a physician, a psychologist, and a teacher. All members of the team, be it a specialized team at an epilepsy center or a community team consisting of the child's treating physician, the child's teacher, and the school psychologist, should cooperatively communicate their observations, concerns, and suggestions in a common jargon. Any testing performed locally should be reviewed by the medical center team and impressions shared with the local facilities. Children with difficult seizure problems and learning difficulties may best be referred to a comprehensive epilepsy center to insure the best possible assessment. Information to the school and the parents concerning the patient's abilities and limitations may be as important as seizure control (Henricksen, 1990).

The school setting

School systems and teachers need information about the child, including the epilepsy type and medication, to allow them to meet the child's special educational needs (Aldenkamp *et al.*, 1990). If the teacher suspects the possibly of difficulties in learning or seizure problems, the teacher, working with the parents, needs to refer the child for evaluation and then be prepared to follow up the child in helping with any problems and needs that are identified in the team approach.

Needs

Children with epilepsy should be placed in the least restrictive schooling environment so that social, emotional, and educational requirements can be met in a setting best suited to the individual's present needs and future development. Personal assessment and monitoring of programs form an equally important part of the child's educational program in an integrated school (Aldenkamp *et al.*, 1990).

Educational placement

Specialized teaching should be started early, when necessary, with the patient integrated into a normal school if possible. Good functioning in a special educational placement is preferable to marginal functioning in a regular class. Placement should always be in the most appropriate program to meet the child's needs, within the least restrictive setting. Given two programs of equal appropriateness, one should always choose the least restrictive setting (Henricksen, 1990).

Studies have shown that the most important factor in education is the teacher, not new building's or modern audiovisual equipment or even the most fancy of computerized equipment. An alert and interested teacher is often the best monitor of the child's function, provided the teacher has the support of and close communication with the physician (Svoboda, 1979).

Support services

Subgroups of children with epilepsy have special needs with regard to the type of educational supports. Improvements in attention after sensory stimulation may be seen in these children (Stores, 1978). Some children seem to be chronically underaroused, and stimulation by the introduction of extra noise through earphones has an alerting effect on performance. This may relate to the observation that a high level of arousal generally reduces epileptiform activity Extra stimulation may also benefit drug-induced slowing of information processing (Aldenkamp *et al.*, 1990). However, some children cannot tolerate environmental stimuli and may require a less distracting learning placement until they can be taught to cope with normal background stimuli.

Participants in a program for memory improvement for people with epilepsy show a significant improvement on some objective memory tests three months after discontinuing therapy. This can help with life functioning, giving more self-confidence and increased ability to cope with daily memory problems (Aldenkamp et al., 1990). Similar approaches have been effective with children through learning disability approaches. When given the chance, children do respond well to good remediative programs. The school may need to involve a speech pathologist to help with communication and memory problems, occupational and physical therapists to help with the motor tasks, and a behavior specialist to help with the behavior reactions often seen when tasks become difficult. The parents should be involved, for they need to continue with the same therapies during weekends, on vacations, and when activities at home involve similar areas. Some epilepsy centers use outreach educational epilepsy specialists to work with local schools to develop more appropriate programs for children with epilepsy.

Emotional support

Epilepsy is regarded as one example of a potential, associated, or contributory factor impairing adaptive behavior (Blennow et al., 1990; Henricksen, 1990; Trimble, 1990). Psychosocial problems are common among children with epilepsy. These problems may be caused partially by school issues and partially by the seizures. Psychosocial problems may increase seizure frequency and school difficulties. Certain children are caught up in a vicious circle, with seizures leading to learning difficulties and then to psychosocial problems and eventually more seizures. The problem is magnified if the child also has an attention deficit disorder. Adverse effects of anticonvulsants may accentuate this cycle, whether in excessive dosage or excessive number of drugs (Thompson & Trimble, 1982; Tomlinson et al., 1982; Rugland et al., 1987).

It is important to consider the environmental influences in the home and school settings. At home, the family characteristics, the parenting style, the parental expectations, the degrees to which the child's special parenting needs are met, the social-cultural environmental aspects, and the presence of a facilitative environment are all influences. Key aspects of the school setting that should be considered include the educational placement, the educational program, the teacher expectations, the teacher interactional style, and the availability and quality of special educational resources (Gourley, 1990).

Impaired cognitive functioning impedes the development of age-appropriate adaptive behavior, thus adding to the epileptic burden in children. Detailed neuropsychological assessment can detect underlying ability-related impairments that contribute to the behaviors and serve as a base for a multidisciplinary treatment program tailored to the individual needs of the child. Maladaptive behaviors need to be identified, treated directly, or, whenever possible, prevented, because such behaviors may exacerbate the effects of cognitive deficiencies. Behaviors will always be shaped by environmental influences. Multiple factors typically underlie the behaviors. These will interfere with the development and expression of adaptive behavior unless corrected (Aldenkamp *et al.*, 1990; Gourley, 1990).

Employment

Employed epileptic patients tend to have a higher intelligence, a better neuropsychologic test performance, fewer neurologic and EEG abnormalities, and a better work history than unemployed epileptics. No differences in seizure etiology, frequency, severity, or type are noted. Discrimination against epilepsy and undereducation are major inhibitors to successful employment (Rodin *et al.*, 1972). Adults with epilepsy are often set in their ways: those who want to work will work, and those who do not, usually do not get jobs. The impact of seizure control through surgery improves the quality of employment, not the quantity of those employed. In a three-year project at the West Virginia State Vocational Rehabilitation Center at Institute West Virginia, people with epilepsy and normal intelligence without any additional handicaps were worked with towards improving employability. A significant degree of academic underachievement and behavioral disabilities that were previously unrecognized were found to be creating problems sufficient to prevent employment. Initial evaluations using such tests as the Wide Range Achievement Tests tended to give misleading indications of reading skills, whereas reading tests for comprehension and application were found to show major delays interfering with day-to-day functioning of the young adults. A significant number of the people in this program were dropped because of frustration temper outbursts resulting from their chronic academic failures.

Programs that become involved with young adolescents with epilepsy as part of the educational program to assess employment potentials and needs as part of the educational planning are valuable. These prevocational programs can merge into vocational preparation training in later schooling to prepare the teenager for adulthood employment. Thus, education, vocational training, and interpersonal relationships are combined into a common program (Svoboda, 1979).

Treatment plan (individualized educational plan)

If a child is not achieving up to expectation, the school should try to discover why. This should lead to various tests of intellectual and academic function. When such tests do not indicate the reason, the school authorities may tend to blame the problem on behavior. Misbehavior in class is most often a symptom of frustration, not the cause of learning problems (Palfrey *et al.*, 1978; Svoboda, 1979).

US law

In the USA, under public law 94-142, any child with educational handicaps is entitled to the most appropriate education in the least restrictive setting, regardless of the handicap. Legislative and judicial decisions have modified this to be "a reasonable education in the least restrictive placement" by subsequent rulings, both legislative and judicial. The principles of PL 94-142 and the subsequent modifying law PL 99-457 is that every school-age individual must be served at no cost to the child. The state must have a program to identify such children. This is referred to as Child Find. The laws prescribe testing that must be non-discriminatory in evaluation and appropriate placements. The programs must be individualized to meet the specific needs of each child with an individualized educational plan. The parents have the right to protest against the state or local school district's actions if they feel that they are discriminatory, inappropriate, or unfair. The parents, legal guardians, or appointed surrogates are to be involved at each step. They must give consent to each stage of the legally defined special educational process. They must be notified in advance of key district actions and meetings and must be encouraged to participate in developing the plan (Purvis, 1991). For the child with epilepsy, the emphasis remains on the educational handicap but the categorization is often under "other medical impairments."

PL 99-457 extended the rights and protections to three- to five-year-old children with disabilities. An individual family service plan needs to be developed and reviewed on an annual basis, with a documented update every six months. Federal policies for early intervention programs for infants who are disabled or at risk are prescribed in the law. Every state must develop an Interagency Coordinating Council of appropriate state and local agencies relevant to the welfare of the disabled child (Purvis, 1991). This provides for developmental help to those infants and toddlers with devastating epileptic syndromes who are at risk for developmental disablement as part of their epilepsy.

Process

This begins with a review of the history. A parent intake interview and a neuropsychological assessment are then obtained. This is prepared as a parent feedback, with intervention strategies and other parental influences discussed. The decision is then made regarding other needed assessments. A remedial educational conference is then held, which is followed by a treatment planning conference, if the two are not combined. This ends up with a treatment plan to be enacted (Scheiber, 1977; Aldenkamp *et al.*, 1990).

Learning deficiencies can impair the development of adaptive behavior. This should be a part of the evaluation. Adaptive behavior assessment for treatment planning purposes begins with a general adaptive behavior assessment, a maladaptive assessment, special education limitations suspected and confirmed if present, cognitive and physical performance capacity assessment, treatment and training influences and their effects, and the environmental influences in the home, community, and school (Aldenkamp *et al.*, 1990; Gourley, 1990). The assessment of epilepsy regarding an individual's social inclusion should be discussed. The quality of care within the school environment should be addressed, as should the ability of the environment to supply prescribed treatment and to administer rescue medications. Specialist provision should address the room environment, support services such as psychological or behavioral supports, and possibly investigative services (Kerr & Bowley, 2001).

School systems and teachers need information about the child to allow them to meet the child's special educational needs. In both the UK and the Netherlands, mobile epilepsy teams have provided special help and educational supports (Aldenkamp *et al.*, 1990). Programs using remediation for function training have been developed especially for disorders of problem-solving and cognitive style and are in evaluation (Aldenkamp, 1987; Moerland, 1987), including instructional guides for teachers and parents published in the Netherlands and Australia. In the USA, the Epilepsy Foundation of America School Alert Kit has provided basic educational information on epilepsy to teachers and pupils (Aldenkamp *et al.*, 1990).

The number of children referred to special education for epilepsy in the UK decreased by 80% over the latter part of the twentieth century. Mental handicaps and behavior disorders are the most common reasons for referral, with seizures accounting for only 21% of referred cases (Thompson, 1987).

Parental involvement: a right and a duty

Under the US Public Law 94-142, the Right to an Education for All Handicapped Children, the parents have both a right and a duty to be involved in their child's education. The physician serves as the advocate for the young patient and should be kept abreast of the process of educating the child. The physician needs to be active in sharing information and concerns with the school and should have a copy of the current individualized educational plan in the medical files (Palfrey *et al.*, 1978; Svoboda, 1979).

Working with schools

The concept can be expensive when a restrictive educational system meets single-minded parents bearing excessive demands. More money may be spent in administration and appeals than in education. When parents and educators work together, often a reasonable program can be established at far less expense. The care plan should address all three aspects of the remediative team: the medical, the educational, and the home. A good sharing communication should be established between all. The health providers should assist in the communication of the individual's seizures and in the communication of an individual's response to treatment and the treatment history. Barriers to the acceptance of epilepsy and the assessment of the impact of epilepsy on an individual's social inclusion should be discussed (Kerr & Bowley, 2001) and, whenever possible, minimized.

The health providers should assist in continuing communication of the individual's seizures and in the communication of an individual's response to treatment and the treatment history (Kerr & Bowley, 2001). Pharmacokinetic features show greater interpatient variability in children than in adults (Aldenkamp *et al.*, 1990; Dodson, 1988). The teacher and support staff will be watching the child daily and may be able to catch subtle changes suggesting a drug reaction. Such observations should be relayed to the physician. Similarly, the physician should let the teachers know of any changes in medications and the possible effects of any new medications, realizing that the school staff may tend to overdiagnose such reactions. Objective monitoring is desirable but is often difficult to obtain in children with behavioral reactions.

The quality of care should be addressed, as should the ability of the environment to supply prescribed treatment and to administer rescue mediations. Specialist provision should address the room environment, support services such as psychological or behavioral supports, as well as possibly investigative services. The family needs to consider respite services, education, training, and overall support (Kerr & Bowley, 2001).

Results

The long-range goal is to prepare the child for adulthood in terms of self-care and earning a living. When given the most appropriate education to meet their needs, children with epilepsy do well, especially if the remedial help is begun early, before repeated frustrations and failures have taken hold.

REFERENCES

Aldenkamp, A. P. (1987). Learning disabilities in epilepsy. In *Education and Epilepsy*, ed. A. P. Aldenkamp, W. C. J. Alpherts, H. Meinardi & G. Stores, pp. 21–38. Lisse: Swets & Zeitlinger.

Aldenkamp, A. P., Alpherts, W. C. J., Dekker, M. J. A., *et al.* (1990). Neuropsychological aspects of learning disabilities in epilepsy. *Epilepsia* **31** (suppl 4): 9–20.

Besag, F. C. (2001). Treatment of state-dependent learning disabilities. In *Epilepsy and Learning Disabilities*, ed. G. F. Ayala, M. Elia, C. M. Cornaggia & M. R. Trimble. *Epilespia* **42** (suppl 10): 46–9.

Blennow, G. , Heijbel, J., Sandstedt P., *et al.* (1990). Discontinuation of antiepileptic drugs to children who have outgrown epilepsy: effects on cognitive function. *Epilepsia* **31** (suppl 4): 50–53.

Commission for the Control of Epilepsy and Its Consequences (1977–8). *Plan for Nationwide Action on Epilepsy*, Vol. I, Chapters 3, 8, and 11. Bethesda, MD: National Institutes of Neurological and Communicative Disorders and Stroke.

Dam, M. (1990). Children with epilepsy: the effects of seizures, syndromes and etiological factors on cognitive functioning *Epilespia* **31** (suppl 4): 26–9.

Dodson, W. E. (1988). Aspects of antiepileptic treatment in children. *Epilepsia* **29** (suppl 3): 10–14.

Gourley, R. (1990). Educational policies. *Epilepsia* **31** (suppl 4): 59–60.

Henricksen, O. (1990). Education and epilepsy: assessment and remediation. *Epilepsia* **31** (suppl 4): 21–5.

Kerr, M. & Bowley, C. (2001). Multidisciplinary and multi-agency contributions to care for those with learning disability who have epilepsy. In *Epilepsia and Learning Disabilities*, ed. G. F. Ayala, M. Elia, C. M. Cornaggia & M. R. Trimble *Epilepsia* **42**: 46–9.

Moerland, C. (1987). Subtypes of learning disabilities in epilepsy. In *Education and Epilepsy*, eds. A. P. Aldenkamp, W. C. J. Alperts, H. Meinardi & G. Stores, pp. 38–50. Lisse: Swets & Zeitlinger.

Palfrey, J. S., Mervis, R. C. & Butler, J. A. (1978). New directions in the evolution of handicapped law: the physician's role on Public Law 94–142. *N. Engl. J. Med.* **298**: 891.

Purvis, P. O. (1991). The public laws for education of the disabled – the pediatrician's role. *Dev. Behav. Pediatr.* **12**: 327–39.

Radley, R. (1987). The educational needs of children with epilepsy. In *Epilepsy and Eduaction 1987*, ed. J. Oxley & G. Stores, pp. 9–15, London: Medical Tribune Group.

Renier, W. O. (1987). Restrictive factors in the education of children with epilepsy from a medical point of view. In *Education and Epilepsy 1987*, ed. A. P. Aldenkamp, W. C. J. Alpherts, H. Meinardi & G. Stores, pp. 3–14. Lisse: Swets & Zeitlinger.

Rodin, E. A., Rennick, P., Dennerll, R., *et al.* (1972). Vocational and educational problems of epileptic patients. *Epilepsia* **13**: 149–60.

Rugland, A. L., Bjornaes, H., Henricksen, O., *et al.* (1987). The development of computerized tests as a routine procedure in clinical EEG practice for the evolution of cognitive changes in patients with epilepsy. 17th Epilepsy International Congress. *Epilepsia* **28** (suppl): 207.

Scheiber, B. (1977). You have rights – use them! In *Closer Look, Special issue of Fall*. Washington, DC: National Information Center for the Handicapped.

Stores, G. (1978). Schoolchildren with epilepsy at risk for learning and behavior problems. *Dev. Med. Child Neurol.* **20**: 502–8.

Svoboda, W. B. (1979). Epilepsy and learning problems. In *Learning About Epilepsy*, pp. 186–200. Baltimore, MD: University Park Press.

Thompson, P. J. (1987). Educational attainment in children and young people with epilepsy. In *Epilepsy and Education 1987*, ed. J. Oxley & G. Stores, pp. 15–24. London: Medical Tribune Group.

Thompson, P. J. & Trimble, M. R. (1982). Anticonvulsant drugs and cognitive functions. *Epilepsia* **23**: 531–44.

Tomlinson, L., Andrews, D. G., Merrifield, E., *et al.* (1982). The effects of antiepileptic drugs on cognitive and motor functions. *Br. J. Clin. Pract.* **18** (suppl): 177–83.

Trimble, M. R. (1990). Antiepileptic drugs, cognitive function and behavior in children, evidence from recent studies. *Epilepsia* **31**(suppl 4): 30–34.

26

Frustrations of learning problems

Psychosocial problems are common in children with epilepsy. These problems may lead to an increase in the seizure frequency as well as contributing to school problems. Many children with uncontrolled epilepsy have to cope not only with the seizures and subclinical discharges but also with underlying brain damage, drug effects, and the psychosocial problems, which in combination tend to cause or heighten learning difficulties (Henricksen, 1990). The child is increasingly frustrated and impeded in the development of age-appropriate adaptive behaviors.

Behavior affects learning

Learning disorders may be associated with behavior disorders such as conduct disorders, major depressive disorders, dysthymic disorders, and oppositional defiant disorders in 10–15% of cases in the non-epileptic population (Cornaggia & Gobbi, 2001). These same disorders are seen with increased frequency in children with epilepsy.

Emotional and behavior disorders may be a symptomatic expression of cognitive impairment in individuals with epilepsy. Behavior and mood disorders may cause reduced learning processing. There is a correlation between temporal lobe epilepsy and interictal affective and personality disturbances (Perini et al., 1996). Directed violence and self-destructive behavior have been described (Kanemoto et al., 1999) in postictal psychoses (Cornaggia & Gobbi, 2001).

Epileptic child underachievers tend to be depressed (Bagley, 1970; Rutter et al., 1970; Palkes et al., 1982). Depression may impede mental processing, resulting in a more globally impaired cognitive profile, thereby obscuring the localizing value of IQ testing results. Patients with more diffuse impairments may be at a greater risk for depression. The same relationships are not seen between anxiety and cognition despite the high frequency of anxiety in the patient population (Stoddard et al., 1999).

The most common learning disabilities seen in children with epilepsy are memory problems and perceptual difficulties. Various learning disabilities seem to relate to different types of behavioral traits, which themselves become handicapping.

Children with higher-order learning disabilities, particularly in problem-solving, are often noted. Some have progressively declining IQs and were hyperactive when young, with a tendency to become hypoactive as they grow older. They are often blamed as being poorly motivated (Aldenkamp *et al.*, 1990; Gourley, 1990).

In learning, the children often have problems adjusting to new tasks, in shifting from one task to another, and in following sequences of steps. They may have problems performing everyday tasks. They have difficulties in learned behaviors, especially in selecting, retrieving, and applying information. Such difficulties emerge in acquiring and storing new forms of behaviors. This leads to behavior disintegration.

Learning disabilities affect behavior

Experts in learning disabilities have noted that specific behaviors seem to relate to specific types of learning disabilities, often as a result of dealing with the struggles to learn.

Auditory-verbal processing problems
Perception

Children with auditory-perceptual handicaps often have difficulty listening, particularly in group situations. Such children seem to be easily confused and inattentive. They often give poor responses to spoken orders. They are frustrated in their efforts to talk. Some children are felt to display autistic mannerisms and may be mislabeled as such. Some children may seem to be controlling lest they have to listen to others giving orders. They may become keyed up in noisy settings.

Memory

Children with auditory memory problems often forget what they have been told and thus are frequently scolded for not carrying out orders. They may get into trouble if they forget what they were previously told to do or not do. They are easily frustrated in lecture-style classes, and their frustration often comes out in undesirable behaviors. Memory problems, especially subtle ones, are common, particularly in children with epilepsy when the site involves the dominant temporal-frontal lobes.

Reception

Children with problems in understanding what they hear may be excessively active yet may also be inhibited, sometimes acting negativistic with temper explosion. They seem to be confused and preservative. They may appear to be uninvolved and socially superficial. They may fear new or strange places. They tend to be either loners or domineering leaders who do not allow others to give directions. They tend to feel left out, sensitive, and easily hurt. At times they may be grandiose and overly dramatic, with histrionic behaviors manifest.

Association

The child with problems in associations does not seem to learn from previous experiences. They misbehave and do not seem to learn from prior scolding and punishments. They do not associate what was forbidden in prior situations with the present situation. They may have a poor sense of humor.

Expression

Children with verbal expression problems often seem quiet, friendly, shy, and withdrawn. They may become easily frustrated, with a resultant explosive temper. They respond to but often do not initiate social interactions. The parents tend to be overprotective, with reduced discipline manifest.

Visual-motor processing problems

Perception

Visual perceptual problems, i.e. confusing similar items, symbols, letters, numbers, or other such details that differ only in small details, in spatial rotation, or slightly in form, are common findings in younger children with epilepsy who are found to have difficulties in school. Some of their behavior problems may originate with the perceptual problems (Frostig, 1963; Frostig, 1973; Frostig & Maslow, 1961).

Children with visual-spatial disorders are often found to have problems in interpersonal areas and in terms of socialization (Strang & Rourke, 1985). Children who do not perceive clearly what they see on the written page also tend to not perceive well when told to clean their rooms and to not perceive body language, including emotional facial expressions. Thus, they do not heed body language cues, tending to blunder in and subsequently receiving unexpected responses. After repeated failures, they tend to withdraw from social interactions, leading to an underdeveloped social sense.

Marianne Frostig has written much to enable the understanding of some of the basics of many of the frustration behaviors that develop in children with perception problems (Frostig & Maslow, 1961; Frostig, 1963; Frostig et al., 1963; Frostig; 1964; Frostig & Horn, 1964; Frostig, 1966; Frostig, 1970; Frostig, 1973; Frostig & Maslow, 1973). Inadequate perceptive abilities may lead to the development of unclear social relationships that are often superficial, unrefined, and immature. Such children tend to be emotionally rigid in defense, which leads to an inability to perceive others adequately and to handle new situations. Such children have difficulty accepting other people's points of view. They do not share feelings. They divorce their own frustration hostility from the picture they have of others. They may project their own feelings of helplessness and frustration, believing that others, not they, are aggressive, when indeed it is the perceptually handicapped child that tends to be stubborn, unbending, hateful, and prejudiced. If their rigid defense is challenged, they may react chaotically.

Children with perceptual problems develop a poor body image inherently related to a poor body awareness sense. Such children feel clumsy, put together wrong, and that they cannot do anything right. When they try something, they may show performance problems due to the perceptual difficulties, which reinforces a poor self-concept. They are clumsy at sports, poor at table manners, unsuccessful at cleaning their room, and fail at school.

The child, because of failures and clumsiness, often develops a poor body image. The child has experienced repeated performance failures, leading to isolation born of experiences of exclusion and rejection. These contribute to a loss of self-confidence and of loss of self-esteem. Such children often seem anxious, depressed, or grieving their failures. They may act out aggressively, which only results in counter-aggression in a vicious cycle. This becomes emotionally stressful, which may present as inattentiveness, undermotivation, and restlessness. Eventually, there is a behavioral disintegration.

Some children may seem disorganized but develop a rigid defense. Such children may be self-centered, accepting only their own ideas. They project feelings of hostility, helplessness, and frustration; if they are crossed or their self-centered concepts are challenged, they may react violently.

This self-centered, rigid, aggressive behavioral may take one of three aspects. Social relationships may be unclear, superficial, unintelligence, and unrefined, leading to both social and emotional maladjustments and resulting in difficulties in relating to other people. Some children continue in a continued emotional turmoil, which appears to be chaotic. Others may adopt a superficial rigidity, their facade disintegrating into chaotic behavior when they are stressed. The protection state tends to become the rigid chaotic state. A rigid insistence on sameness may emerge, but still there is a struggle to cope. If this sameness demand is challenged, the child may disintegrate from the rigid state to one of chaotic behavior.

Behavior problems may result in attention-getting actions that are often aggressive or hostile. Some children develop a chronic anxiety state with nervous habits, withdrawal, physical complaints, or fantasizing. They may be frigid and look around fearfully. Some children retreat into a defeatism, with loss of interest and refusal to try.

Generally, children with perception problems may be misdiagnosed as having ADHD, because they present with inattentiveness and excesses of energy with an emotional lability, difficult social interactions, and behavior problems.

Expression

Children with problems in manual expressions tend to be slow and clumsy in their manual responses. They often become self-conscious and inhibited, being disinclined to take part in any physical activity that may show off their incoordination. Some may compensate by becoming the clumsy clown to distract attention from their performance failures. Such children are particularly disadvantaged if they are in a family or environment that places much value on physical abilities such as sports, dancing, or gymnastics.

Frustrations and failures

As the child experiences failure after failure while those around are commended for successes, their motivation to learn is transformed into a motivation towards avoiding tasks that are frustrating, overwhelming, or potential failures. Such children may seek the easiest way out of a task. They work to avoid criticism and failure rather than to perform correctly and productively. Some may develop more complicating behaviors such as deviant and distorted school performance, refusal to perform, tricks to avoid schoolwork, or a school phobia or truancy. Eventually, such children tend to avoid anything that requires effort, that may prove frustrating, or that may demonstrate the weaknesses and shortcomings. The child becomes convinced that he or she is stupid by the admonitions of teachers and the taunts of peers.

The frustrations of those trying to teach the child are often transferred to the child, who may react with inattention and distractibility, loss of motivation and learning enthusiasm, restlessness or hyperactivity, avoidance efforts, or secondary emotional problems. Such children may appear to be indifferent, apathetic, or disinterested, or to make no effort. Some may act the clown to distract from the tasks at hand. Other children may give up in a defeated attitude and avoid participation. They are often described as inactive, withdrawn, or shy. Some children become resentful and angry and develop a temper, with bullying or aggressive behavior. A high percentage of children arrested for delinquent behaviors are found to have learning disabilities. Still other children become depressed and discouraged, withdrawing, developing physical pains to escape the classroom to the nurse's office or the sickbed, or often being in tears. They have no confidence. Mental health personnel may actively treat the reactions but not recognize the underlying causes.

The school setting

Teachers describe many epileptic children as inattentive, distractable, restless, constantly fidgeting, or displaying poor concentration. This may be due to a behavioral problem, unrecognized seizures, a disturbed learning process, or a drug reaction.

Behavior problems are far more apt to be the consequences than the cause of learning difficulties. The frustrations of effortful failures are overwhelming (Svoboda, 1979).

Some children diagnosed as having ADHD or autism may be affected by undiagnosed manifestations of epilepsy. Undiagnosed severe epileptic conditions, such as frontal lobe epilepsies with subclinical specific EEG activity including rapid activity lasting between one and 1.5 seconds, are subsequently associated with the onset of severe behavioral disturbances (sometimes with psychotic symptoms), or schizophrenia-like or autism-like syndromes, in both children and adults (Cornaggia & Gobbi, 2001).

Academic frustrations

In epileptic children, reading and math delays are found to be associated with behavior disorders, particularly aggression (Laidlaw & Richens, 1976). Behavior disorders are most likely to be a consequence than a cause of reading problems. Almost all children who underachieve educationally have behavior problems, whereas only 25% with educational underachievement have primary behavior problems. Depressed reading achievement is more common in children with personality deficits (Long & Moore, 1979). There appears to be an association between reading struggles and maladjustment (Bagley, 1970; Rutter *et al.*, 1970; Palkes *et al.*, 1982), including antisocial disorders and conduct problems. Of children with specific reading retardation, 25% showed antisocial behaviors in the eyes of teachers. Children showing persistent aggression or conduct disorders are often found to have low attainment in all subjects (Rutter, 1974).

Does underachievement lead to a conduct disorder, or vice versa? An emotional disorder is not the primary cause of a severe reading retardation, although it may be a secondary influence. When children, especially smart children, have difficulties in reading or fail to learn to read, they are likely to be faced continually with negative responses to their failures. School becomes a negative experience, strongly associated with failure and with adverse responses to failure socially. By the time people begin to consider whether the child needs help, the child is likely to have given up. The remedial teacher is faced with a discouraged, miserable child who lacks confidence and feels that success in any area is not possible (Rutter, 1974).

Summary

The child with epilepsy often presents with an integrated collection of seizures, medication reactions, learning difficulties, and behavior difficulties. It is very difficult to treat only one or two aspects successfully. To be effective, one needs to treat in a comprehensive manner all of the problems together. This takes teamwork.

REFERENCES

Aldenkamp, A. P., Alpherts, W. C. J., Dekker, M. J. A., *et al.* (1990). Neuropsychological aspects of learning disabilities in epilepsy. *Epilepsia* **31** (suppl 4): 9–20.

Bagley, C. R. (1970). The educational performance of children with epilepsy. *Br. J. Educ. Psychol.* **140**: 82–3.

Cornaggia, C. M. & Gobbi, G. (2001). Learning disability in epilepsy: definitions and classification. In *Epilepsia and Learning Disabilities*, ed. G. F. Ayala, M. Elia, C. M. Cornaggia & M. R. Trimble. *Epilepsia* **42**: 2–5.

Frostig, M. (1963). Visual perception in the brain-injured child. *Am. J. Orthopsychiatry* **33**: 665–71.

Frostig, M. (1964). *The Frostig Program for the Development of Visual Perception.* Chicago: Follett.

Frostig, M. (1966). *Developmental Test of Visual Perception.* Palo Alto, CA: Consulting Psychologists Press.

Frostig, M. (1970). *The Developmental Program in Visual Perception.* Ohio: Teaching Guide Follet.

Frostig, M. (1973). *Learning Problems in the Classroom: Prevention and Remediation.* New York: Grune and Stratton.

Frostig, M. & Horn, H. (1964). *The Frostig Program for the Development of Visual Perception.* Chicago: Follett.

Frostig, M. & Maslow, R. (1961). Visual perception and early education. In *Learning Disabilities: Introduction to Educational and Medical Management*, ed. L. Tarnopol, pp. 217–37. Springfield, IL: Chas C. Thomas.

Frostig, M. & Maslow, P. (1973). *Learning Problems in the Classroom.* New York: Grune and Stratton.

Frostig, M., Lefever, W. & Wittlesey, J. (1963). Disturbance in visual perception. *J. Educ. Res.* **57**: 160–62.

Gourley, R. (1990). Educational policies. *Epilepsia* **31** (suppl 4): 59–60.

Henricksen, O. (1990). Education and epilepsy: assessment and remediation. *Epilepsia* **31** (suppl 4): 21–5.

Kanemoto, K., Kawasaki, J. & Mori, E. (1999). Violence and epilepsy: a close relation between violence and post-ictal psychosis. *Epilepsia* **40**: 107–9.

Laidlaw, J. & Richens, A. (1976). Fits in children: education. In *A Textbook of Epilepsy*, pp. 101–2. London & New York: Churchill Livingstone.

Long, C. G. & Moore, L. (1979). Parental expectations for their epileptic children. *J. Child Psychol. Psychiatry* **20**: 299–312.

Palkes, H. S., Prensky, A. L., Bourgeois, B. F. D., *et al.* (1982). Intelligence of epileptic children: a prospective study. *Ann. Neurol.* **12**: 206.

Perini, G. I., Tosin, C., Carraro, C., *et al.* (1996). Interictal mood and personality disorders in temporal lobe epilepsy and juvenile myoclonic epilepsy. *J. Neurol. Neurosurg. Psychiatry* **61**: 601–5.

Rutter, M. (1974). Emotional disorder and educational underachievement. *Arch. Dis. Child* **48**: 249–56.

Rutter, E. M., Graham, P. & Yule, W. A. (1970). A neuropsychiatric study in childhood. *Clin. Dev. Med.* **3**: 237–55.

Stoddard, K. R., Westerveld, M., Ayotte, S. L., Spencer, D. D. & Spencer, S. S. (1999). Negative affect and neuropsychological test performance. *Epilepsia* **40** (suppl 7): 49.

Strang, J. D. & Rourke, B. P. (1985). Adaptive behavior of children who exhibit specific arithmetic disabilities and associated neuropsychological abilities and deficits. In *Neuropsychology of Learning Disabilites: Essentials of Subtype Analysis*, ed. B. P. Rourke, pp. 302–27. New York: Guildford Press.

Svoboda, W. B. (1979). Epilepsy and learning problems. In *Learning About Epilepsy*, pp. 186–200. Baltimore, MD: University Park Press.

Part III

Behavior problems

27

Mental health needs

About 30% of patients with epilepsy have some kind of psychiatric symptom (Onuma, 2000). The Federal Commission for the Control of Epilepsy and Its Consequences (1978) found that around 52% have major emotional problems. This surpasses the incidence seen in individuals with known brain damage, such as cerebral palsy. Help from mental health specialists knowledgeable about epilepsy is not readily available.

Epilepsy in children results in an increased risk for behavioral, emotional, psychiatric, and social impairments, occurring at a higher frequency than in people with other chronic illnesses, than in people who are visually or hearing handicapped, and much higher than in healthy children (Smith *et al.*, 2002). Psychiatric disorders occur in 5–10% of the general pediatric population, 16% of those with chronic medical disorders, 29% of children with idiopathic epilepsy, and 58% of symptomatic epilepsy (Rutter *et al.*, 1970; Connolly *et al.*, 1984). This increased incidence is seen in both newly diagnosed and chronic epilepsy (Hoare, 1984). Various studies show that 21–27% of children with epilepsy have behavior disturbances. The frequency is increased if the epilepsy is complicated by other neurologic problems (Holdsworth & Whitmore, 1974; Mellor & Lowit, 1977). Teachers report a 21% incidence of deviant behaviors, such as aggressive, objectionable, truculent, spiteful, bullying, and attention-seeking behaviors (Holdsworth & Whitmore, 1974). Anxiety and depression a prominent in epileptic children with family functioning variables found to be influential (Ettinger *et al.*, 1998). The incidence of significant behavior problems in pediatric neurology epilepsy clinic is even higher, at 36–50%, although such clinics often attract the more difficult epilepsy cases (Hinton & Knights, 1969; Whitehouse, 1971).

The problems

Children are children first and epileptic second. A child goes through the normal developmental struggles of growing up. Epilepsy only accentuates or distorts these struggles. Children are born with inherited traits that are thereafter influenced by their environment, including important others. The effect of epilepsy can be divided into exogenous factors (influences) and endogenous factors (brain changes).

Exogenous factors

Society expects certain things to be present in a person with epilepsy and thus influences the developing child to fulfill these expectations. Children tend to adapt to the expectations that others have of them. Exogenous influences from the child's family, school, and peers shape the developing child's personality, social interactions, and self-concepts. These influences often mirror the stigmatizing beliefs that are seen with epilepsy. These factors shape psychosocial development in the growing child.

The personality emerges over developmental stages. Epilepsy may distort this development. A child with epilepsy may exhibit defects later on in life, one of which is difficulties in adaptation. Later psychiatric labels may have prior developmental antecedents. The epilepsy influences a behavior on which the emergent self depends. Resultant personality traits may represent the chronicity, the impediment, whether voluntary or involuntary, the frequency, and the impaired functioning of the individual .

Parental influences

The parents' evolving concerns influence their parenting styles.

Child's self-concept

The child's self-concepts are derived from attitudes of important others in their life. Negative attitudes towards the child are disruptive to self-esteem, which can be catastrophic. Some claim epilepsy as an excuse for failures or faults. If at some later time the epilepsy is controlled through medication or surgery, the child then no longer has an excuse for their failures. Some retreat into non-epileptic events and some develop other psychiatric conditions.

School

Lowered expectations and experienced frustrations and failures reflect a reduced self-concept, especially if cognitive deficits are present.

Peers

A young child may be concerned when their classmate falls unconscious in a seizure, but the next day, after parents have explained about epilepsy, the child may return with a now negative attitude towards the epileptic child. This inhibits social development.

Endogenous factors

Endogenous problems are commonly thought to originate from chemical imbalances of the brain, although in part these can also be the result of persistent exogenous influences. Although the process may originate in childhood, often the symptoms emerge in late adolescence or adulthood. Generally, although infrequent presentations are seen in childhood, the major psychiatric disturbances may emerge an average of 20 years after the onset of epilepsy in childhood.

Pediatric presentations

Common pediatric problems associated with epilepsy include attention deficits, anxiety, depression, conduct disorders, and temper. Many patients have emotional problems that may be included in mixed disorders of conduct and emotions (Onuma, 2000). Epileptic adolescents show decreased social competence and increased behavior problems compared with controls. Males show more problems than females (Batzel *et al.*, 1984).

Attention deficit disorder with or without hyperactivity

ADHD is a widely debated entity. Does it exist or is it just an extreme variant of normal? Is it a single entity or a cluster of entities? Why do the frequencies of diagnosis vary so widely, i.e. why do some US states prescribe a stimulant three times more frequently than other states? Even within a state, some counties may prescribe a stimulant up to ten times more frequently an in other counties. Some nations use primarily behavior approaches to this entity.

Anxiety

The capriciousness of convulsions and reflected worries of the parents create many anxieties in a child. Anxiety may build up to precipitate a seizure breakthrough.

Depression

Only in the past 20 years has the concept of childhood depression been accepted. The diagnosis is often overlooked because the presentation is different to that in adults. Many children diagnosed as having ADHD but who respond to an antidepressant far better than to a stimulant may be depressed. It is estimated that up to 25% of those with ADHD may be bipolar.

Conduct disorders

Conduct disorder in relation to epilepsy needs special consideration. The essential feature is the repetitive and persistent pattern of conduct in which the basic rights of others or major age-appropriate social norms and rules are violated. The conduct is more serious than the ordinary mischief and pranks, manifested either by physical violence against people or property or by non-aggressive patterns such as truancy or substance abuse. These behaviors may be confined to the family context. Poor frustration tolerance, irritability, temper outbursts, and provocative recklessness are often present. Academic achievement is frequently low. Aberrant behavior or conduct disorder is often seen in juvenile epilepsy (Onuma, 2000).

Temper outbursts

Frustrated children have tempers that can become extreme. A tendency has been to blame these as epileptic. The legal profession has adapted this as an excuse for illegal acts.

Psychiatric problems primarily of adulthood

In adults, dementia, paranoid psychoses, depression, neurosis, hysteria, and pseudo-seizures occur more often in the course of the disease than chance combination would suggest (Onuma, 2000). Some of the major disorders appear to have delayed onset. A child with a chronic epileptic condition, often complex-partial, by late adolescence to young adulthood, begins to experience the major psychiatric condition, be it a psychosis or a bipolar disorder. The delay, averaging around 20 years from seizure onset to psychiatric disorder onset, suggests seizure-induced changes in the brain affect the neurotransmitter system. Some of these episodic disturbances may be subdivided into preictal, ictal, postictal, and interictal events especially, suggesting a close relationship to seizure activity. Although seen infrequently, these problems may also appear in children.

Non-epileptic events

Non-epileptic events are often overlooked until they become firmly established. Children and adults may have these, although the causes and outlook may be somewhat different. Arriving at the correct diagnosis of a non-epileptic event opens the door to diagnose the psychiatric condition causing the presentation.

Modifying factors

Location of the brain dysfunction

The site of the disturbance of the brain may or may not distort the functions related to that portion of the brain involved, i.e. left brain lesions affect language-related skills, which may distort social interactions and may relate to learning disabilities. There is an increased incidence of thought disorders in this population. By comparison, right-hemispheric dysfunctions may cause perceptual motor learning disorders. There is an increased incidence of emotional mood problems and a different personality disorder in this group. The part of the hemisphere involved may relate to the type of dysfunction more apt to be seen. Frontal lobe disturbances may affect organization, recall, and social interactions. Frontal-temporal lobe limbic disturbances may be related to emotionality as well as hyperactivity and temper outbursts (Lindsay *et al.*, 1979). Left temporal involvement can affect language understanding, expression, and memory; right temporal-parietal involvement can affect perception and details. Bilateral brain involvement would place a person at higher risks for learning disabilities and emotional problems.

Age of onset

An insult in the brain of the developing child may distort development and thus lead to disturbed functions. An insult to the brain in the older child or adult usually causes a skill loss, but the loss of a skill itself can produce an emotional reaction that can be handicapping.

Problems in behavior are present at the time of the onset of seizures and are more prominent in boys with prior unrecognized seizures. Prior to the use of antiepileptic medication or to the emergence of psychosocial reactions to the seizures, unrecognized seizures adversely affect a child's behavior. Such problems included internalizing problems, anxiety/depression, attention difficulties, and thought difficulties (Dunn *et al.*, 1999). Earlier onset leads to a longer exposure to the exogenous factors and a longer duration for endogenous processes to build up.

Cause of the brain dysfunction

The cause may be inherited, acquired, or idiopathic. Normal brains may show abnormal functions, as with epilepsy, learning disabilities, etc. If brain damage is found, it tends to worsen the dysfunction, i.e. those with a specific problem such as epilepsy or a learning disability usually have a more severe manifestation of a dysfunction than those without brain damage. Both types can be helped, however.

Nature of the brain dysfunction

In looking at dysfunctions with a seizure disorder, the problems may relate to the seizure discharge itself, the nature of the brain insult causing the seizure, if present, the effect of the medications used to treat the seizures, and the management of the person's condition. Even patients without brain damage may have problems. It appears that the management is the most important aspect, but all factors are important in shaping the patient's functioning.

Chronicity

Some children may grow up with epilepsy yet not develop major psychiatric problems until late adolescent or, more frequently, young adulthood. Often, there is a

20-year interim history between the epilepsy onset and the emotional disturbance emergence. This is seen especially in complex partial epilepsy. What factors are there with this condition that may be treated earlier to avoid the later psychiatric disorder?

Medication effects

The drug effects must be considered on seizure control and on both learning and behaviors. Depression and psychoses may be triggered. The drugs may help or hinder behavior. For example, carbamazepine and valproic acid may have positive effects but also occasionally negative effects on behavior. These drugs are less apt to affect learning, but if the drug level is too high or too low, learning, emotions, and behavior may be disturbed. The mere changing from a proprietary brand of carbamazepine to a generic form has been associated with deterioration of seizure control, emotions, and learning in 50% due to altered absorption and inadequate variable blood levels; in these patients, use of generics is not good. Longer-acting forms of the drugs may level out variations and smooth out emotionality.

A shaping social stigma

The terms "epilepsy" and "epileptic" as used in society have carried negative connotations. This has bred prejudicial attitudes towards inclusion of individuals with epilepsy in social activity, sports, and employment. This begins in the school years or even earlier. These attitudes carry over into expectations and thus tend to be negative reinforcers. Children with epilepsy often have problems in adapting, and to be burdened with societal prejudicial views is an even heaver load to bear.

Management

Once considered together, neurology and psychiatry have now split over the past century. The European model of neurology has tended to blend psychiatry and neurology, while the American model has tended to separate them out. A patient with epilepsy and behavior problems in Europe may be cared for by either a practicing neurologist or a psychiatrist, whereas in the USA the same individual might be referred to a neurologist for seizure care and to a psychiatrist for mental health care. The field of epilepsy is now reuniting the two fields into a common ground, and each specially is using the other's drugs to treat their own group of patients.

Prevention through early recognition

Exogenous factors may be preventable through early counseling and guidance. Endogenous factors often take years to emerge but may display subtle earlier signs that can lead to earlier diagnosis and thus possible lessening of the impact.

Treat the symptoms or the cause?

Exogenous problems are best treated behaviorally. Medications treat symptoms. Behavior approaches treat causes. Medications may be used temporarily for severe presentations.

Endogenous problems may be due to altered brain chemistry and therefore may be rebalanced by medications, but studies by the National Institutes of Mental Health have suggested that "talk therapy" may also alter brain chemistries. Adverse behavioral approaches such as post-traumatic stress syndrome have been shown to produce altered neural chemistries. Beneficial behavioral approaches may similarly normalize imbalances. Medication may balance some imbalances but may create other imbalances. At this point, a combination of therapies (behavior plus medication) may be best.

Which is it?

The question often arises as to whether an episodic event is a seizure or misbehavior. This has been brought up especially in adults who have committed acts of violence (Delgado-Escueta *et al.*, 1981). Generally, any abnormal behavior that is part of a seizure discharge is characterized by being unplanned and unprepared for. Seizure events usually last less than one to two minutes. One may see simple, vague, non-directed movements. Consciousness is usually impaired. The patient may be forgetful after the event. Events that do not meet these criteria are usually not seizures and should not be treated as such without further proof. However, there are exceptions to each observation. Prolonged seizures, such as febrile convulsions, generalized tonic–clonic attacks in children, and epileptic status, may last longer. Movements may be more complex and at times directed, if they are in reaction to a hallucination for example. In a simple partial seizure, consciousness remains intact by definition.

REFERENCES

Batzel, L. Q., Dodrill, C. B. & Farwell, J. R. (1984). Social competence and behavior problems in normal and epileptic adolescents. *Epilepsia* 25: 648.

Commission for the Control of Epilepsy and Its Consequences (197–8). *Plan for Nationwide Action on Epilepsy*. Bethesda, MD: National Institutes of Neurological and Communicative Disorders and Stroke.

Connolly, J., Freeman, R., Dodrill, C. & Batzel, L. (1984). Psychiatric status in adolescents with epilepsy. *Epilepsia* 25: 646.

Delgado-Escueta, A. V., Matson, R. H., King, L., *et al.* (1981). The nature of aggression during epileptic seizures. *N. Engl. J. Med.* 305: 711–17.

Dunn, D. W., Austin, J., Hustser, G. A., Rose, D. F. & Harezlak, J. (1999). Which children with new-onset seizures are at risk for behavior problems? *Epilepsia* **40** (suppl 7): 56.

Ettinger, A. B., Wiesbrot, D. M., Nolan, E. E., *et al.* (1998). Symptoms of depression and anxiety in pediatric epilepsy patients. *Epilepsia* **39**: 595–9.

Hinton, G. G. & Knights, R. M. (1969). Neurological and psychological characteristics of 100 children with seizures. In *Proceedings of the First Congress of the International Association for the Scientific Study of Mental Deficiency*, ed. B. Richard, pp. 315–56. London: Michael Jackson.

Hoare, P. (1984). The development of psychiatric disorders among school children with epilepsy. *Dev. Med. Child Neurol.* **26**: 3–13.

Holdsworth, L. & Whitmore, K. (1974). A study of children with epilepsy attending ordinary school. II: information and attitudes held by their teachers. *Dev. Med. Child Neurol.* **16**: 759–65.

Lindsay, J., Ounsted, C. & Richards, P. (1979). Long term outcome in children with temporal lobe seizures. III: psychiatric aspects in childhood and adult life. *Dev. Med. Child Neurol.* **21**: 630–36.

Mellor, D. H. & Lowit, I. (1977). A study of intellectual function in children with epilepsy attending ordinary schools. In *Epilepsy, The Eighth International Symposium*, J. K. Penry, pp. 291–4. New York: Raven Press.

Onuma, T. (2000). Classification of psychiatric symptoms in patients with epilepsy. Proceedings of the 32nd Congress of Japan Epilepsy Society. *Epilepsia* **41** (suppl 9): 43–8.

Rutter, M., Graham, P. & Yule, W. (1970). A neuropsychiatric study in childhood. In *Clinics in Developmental Medicine*. London: Spastics Society and Heinemann.

Smith, M. L., Elliott, I. M. & Lach, L. (2002). Cognitive skills in children with intractable epilepsy: comparisons of surgical and nonsurgical candidates. *Epilepsia* **46**: 631–7.

Whitehouse, D. (1971). Psychological and neurological correlates of seizure disorders. *Johns Hopkins Med. J.* **129**: 36–42.

28

Psychologic development

There are two definitions of normal. The psychologist defines "normal" as the standard and calls everything else abnormal, i.e. imperfect. Doctors, parents, and teachers use the term "normal" to describe a child who seems likely to grow up to be a satisfactory member of society in spite of the fact that symptoms and signs of inconvenient behavior are clearly present (Winnicott, 1964). A normal child can employ any or all of the devices that nature has provided in defense against anxiety and intolerable conflict. An abnormal child shows a limitation and rigidity to employ symptoms and a positive lack of relationships between the symptoms and what can be expected in the ways of help (Winnicott, 1984).

Differences arise when there is a fundamental clash between the reality of the external world and the child's inner world of feelings. Differences also arise with the discovery that with excitement go destructive thoughts. The child must decide between the peace of mind of restraint versus the eagerness of satisfaction of desires. The child begins to create an inner world in which battles are lost and won, a world in which magic holds sway. The child's play may allow glimpses of this inner world (Winnicott, 1984).

Behavior lateralization and localization

There is no strict localization for various emotions and consequent behaviors. The frontotemporal limbic system is often spoken of as the primitive brain, subject to more emotions than cognition. The temporal lobe has been described as the bridge between neurology and psychiatry, a bridge that no one is quite sure in which direction the patient is traveling on at any one time.

There are subtle tendencies that are more lateralized than localized, and disturbances of the involved hemisphere may distort the manifestation of the emotion.

Left versus right hemispheric tendencies

Localization-related epilepsy and the laterality of the focus are related to behavior disturbances that may adversely affect learning, ranging from behavior disorders (Stores, 1987) and aggression (Ounsted et al., 1966) to frank psychoses

(Flor-Henry, 1972). Intellectual disturbances are seen more with left hemisphere damage, whereas right-hemispheric lesions, especially frontal lobe damage, are more likely to result in affective or behavioral disorders and somatic complaints. Sexual abnormalities and criminal behaviors are associated especially with the frontal lobe (Laidlaw & Richens, 1976).

Left-hemispheric lesions are associated more closely with major psychiatric disabilities, especially those involving the temporal lobe. However, there tend to be more psychologic disturbances with right frontal and left parietal lesions. Psychologic disorders of left temporal lobe lesions are significant, even in the absence of neurologic deficits (Laidlaw & Reichens, 1976). This raises the question of the relationship between dominant temporal-frontal subtle language deficits and psychiatric problems. Problems of misunderstanding and/or being misunderstood often lead to behavior problems. This may cause the individual to feel unsure of their own abilities and to feel controlled by others or by forces beyond their control. In this insecurity, a person may tend to become overly detailed in speech and writing, often augmenting efforts with note-taking. One characteristic is to become stuck in details yet to never complete work. Problems with communication with others may cause an individual to either try to control the conversational activities or to withdraw and avoid. Such individuals may also not function well in a noisy situation and tend to fidget due to problems concentrating. Having experienced numerous misinterpretations, the individual begins to feel that things tend to be their own fault, as others don't necessarily have the same problems. Thoughts may be distorted, even to the extreme. Thus, when such behaviors appear, one needs to look closely at the basic languages functioning, especially under stress.

The right hemisphere interprets the mood of spoken language and notes the details of unspoken language, i.e. body language. Disturbances to the right hemisphere may distort these basic abilities. Impulsivity and acting on first impressions are common. The patient may misinterpret the mood of others. Even more, the individual may not perceive the details of body language, such as "back off" cues, and may rush in only to be rebuffed. Because such an individual is less detail-oriented, they tend to rush through activities, making errors, which are unnoticed. When confronted, the individual may even deny such faults. Environmental distractions are prominent. The patient's actions tend to lead to rejections and gradually the self-image suffers, although one trick may be to fall back on numerous approaches to try to defend the image.

Mood disorders of depression and mania tend to be associated with left temporal foci.

Frontal lobe

The frontal lobe, an area often involved in the impact of a head trauma, is one of the least understood brain portions, especially in developing children. Since patients can function after removal of the prefrontal lobe, it has been thought of to be less necessary. Developmentally, however, the frontal lobe acts as the conductor to the orchestra of the brain, selecting the players (i.e. stimulating development in the parietal and temporal lobes especially) and then orchestrating them to work as a unit. It executes the functioning of the brain in planning and organization. Early damage may impair intellectual functioning, although the other portions of the brain remain intact. Seizures are more often misinterpreted and sometimes mistaken for non-epileptic events. Teachers have less understanding of the concepts of executive functioning than is needed to teach children with special problems.

Neurochemical changes

The development of the brain and brain functions parallels developmental changes and maturation of the neurochemical system. The neurotransmitter balance is also evolving towards maturity. With preadolescence and especially with adolescence, the hormones have a marked change on the developing brain, including both cognitive and especially emotional aspects.

Psychosocial development in children

Children are reflections of their parents and, to a lesser degree, their family, teachers, and peers. Premature self-awareness is no healthier than delayed awareness (Winnicott, 1984).

In terms of psychology, Erikson (1965) has divided the ages of man into eight stages, five of which pertain to childhood and adolescence. The development of epilepsy strongly affects the developmental processes of each stage.

Trust and mistrust

This is an age of constant tasting and testing the relationship with the outside world. Positive interactions develop trust; negative interactions result in mistrust. This is the main challenge of early infancy. Hopefully, the infant is born into a facilitating environment that should be able to adjust progressively to the individual's needs (Winnicott, 1984).

Infants involved in the sensorimotor phase of learning are working out their sense of trust versus mistrust and of attachment versus anxiety. Mother is important. Mothers cuddle children and talk about how good it feels. Fathers rough-house the child, talking about what the future will be like. Both approaches are important. A child under emotional stress may withdraw, become apathetic, or fail to thrive. A child deprived of such bonding experiences and feeling touch may also withdraw into an apathetic state.

The infant already begins to lay down styles for classroom behavior. The influential keys at this stage are of attention and response from the parent. The lack of attention may lead to withdrawal, self-stimulation, inability to focus, preoccupation with fantasy, or inability to form close relationships. A faulty response to the infant's efforts may result in an inability or unwillingness to respond to unfamiliar challenges or a fear of failure.

This relates to the initial development of executive functions, helping the child to learn to make choices. Consistent reactions strengthen executive choices. Erratic reactions result in faulty executive organization.

A child with early seizures often persists in infantilization. The parents are driven by the fear that the child will grow up to succumb to the seizures, i.e. a vulnerable child syndrome, which the child may later acquire. This may lead to a Peter Pan syndrome, in which the child avoids growing up in order to avoid adulthood. Parental attention may be more on the medical condition than on the child. Depending on the seizure control, the parents' responses and reactions toward the child and the seizures may vacillate, impairing the development of executive planning.

Autonomy versus shame and doubt

In late infancy, the child becomes aware of individuality rather than being a mere extension of the parent and family. The baby tests this by trying out its own decisions and desires. If the feedback is negative, the developing negative self-concept becomes negative; if positive, the infant becomes more confident. This stage is decisive for other developing concepts of love and hate, cooperation and willfulness, freedom of self-expression and its suppression. The toddler, especially in the "terrible twos," is highly involved in this developmental process. Imagination may take hold as the toddler goes through the stage of magical thinking and TV hero worship, only to be brought back to the reality of daily experiences.

The toddler is involved in the sense of autonomy versus the sense of shame and doubt in this preoperational cognitive stage of thinking. The toddler discovers individualization, i.e. of being a separate individual from the parents. The child does not have to use the potty just because mother says so, or eat something disliked despite the mother's wishes. Thus, the child initiates the mother into the terrible twos. Problems of separation anxiety and passive aggressive reactions may be seen. Boys tend to be more aggressive and girls more passive in play.

If the responses to a child's initiatives are disorderly and erratic, the child may develop an inability to follow through and to complete tasks. Disruptive outbursts may become controlling. A child may be intolerant to frustrations in efforts or may become defiant of authorities. Young children tend to be distractable. If the child's efforts do not meet self-expectations, the child may destroy the effort (Swap, 1974). When a parent smothers the infant with epilepsy who is trying to be one's self by overprotective restraints, the infant may react with passive dependency or defiance. Children with epilepsy may hear the message of being an epileptic child, i.e. not normal, and that children with epilepsy cannot do certain things, giving such children a handicapped self-image from early in life.

Initiative versus guilt

Given confidence, the child begins to test out drives and desires. Sociability emerges, with new activities and new interests. The child experiences societal limits, approvals, encouragement. Social institutions at home, at school, and at play offer children an economic ethos in the form of adult ideals to replace the heroes of fairy tales.

This is the age of curiosity. If the child has learned to be stifled in exploratory efforts, a fear of looking or of exploring may emerge or an extreme independence may be displayed. Some children respond with overzealous exploration beyond normal limits in risk-taking behaviors (Swap, 1974). The child with epilepsy may be overly protected and overly restrained, prohibited from interactions in the usual activities of childhood, thus losing out on the experiences that help to develop initiative and accomplishment. Often, such children cease to try, especially if warned persistently that it might be dangerous because of the seizures; a few, however, still may try the risk-taking route.

Industry versus inferiority

As the child starts school, the child learns to win recognition by producing, thus becoming anxious to produce and please. If efforts tend to be met with failures, the child develops a poor self-image and may cease trying.

By the early school years, the child enters into concrete operations style of thinking, with the struggle of initiative versus guilt being prominent. Peer groups are most important. The child models after super heroes, and fantasy is often soothing. A child with epilepsy may seek to be a superhero, invulnerable to the dangers that the epilepsy threatens to bring. Problems may show up as school refusal, aggressive behaviors, learning problems, and attention/hyperactivity problems of various types. A temper may emerge if the child is crossed.

At this age, the child is engrossed by social contacts and the mastery of achievement. Early failures and negative feedback often lead to low achievement. The child becomes overly dependent on others' approval or initiatives, becoming a follower. Socially, failures lead to low self-esteem, isolation, difficulties with sharing in competition, and inappropriate social behaviors. Aggression and teasing may be seen (Swap, 1974). Socialization skills may remain underdeveloped.

The child evolves through these early stages into a latency period, which is a period of teachability and socialization with peers, although usually it becomes same-sex socialization. In adolescence, socialization begins to be towards the opposite sex (Winnicott, 1984).

In the later school years, there is the sense of industry versus inferiority, as concrete operations of thinking merge into abstractions. Emotional reactions often present as more recognizable depression or as rebellious behavior, manifest as an oppositional disorder merging into a conduct disorder.

The child with epilepsy, especially if treated as a fragile, handicapped, child, who has to take pills and keep seeing doctors often tends to adapt to the image given. The occurrence of seizures in class can be an exclamation point to accentuate "differentness." To such negativity a child often responds by dependency and withdrawal, although some may rebel to the portrayal and to the taking of medication.

Identity versus role confusion

Puberty, with its major body, mind, and sexual changes, brings about a recapitulation of the early psychological developmental stages as part of an emerging sense of self and of being, from which comes doing (Winnicott, 1984).

With the onset of puberty, the child undergoes a repeat review of the earlier stages, with peers often replacing parents as the guide. The young adolescent tends to re-evaluate their role in the society of their peers in terms of trust and mistrust. Work efforts are towards autonomy of self as an individual, not a family member. The adolescent seeks group independence, i.e. to be unique yet a part of a peer clique. Teenagers explore new activities, with attempts to establish their own ideals, often met by the response of peer encouragement and adult disapproval. Accomplishments in school or sports become important, and failures can be a catastrophe, as can exclusion from participation because of epilepsy.

The teenager's main role is in seeking to determine a role in life. Questions such as "Who am I?," "Where am I going?," and "What am I doing here?" become important in interactions with peers. How the teenager answers these questions depends greatly on the feedback received in growing up.

The adolescent strives toward independence, yearning for freedom from the parents at a rate faster than some parents are ready to yield. The growing adolescent needs understanding, not criticism. Growth comes through experiences and the individual understanding of such experiences. The adolescent is most anxious for experiences. The parents need to see the child as a separate entity and know when to let go. The child should not be held under a burden of gratitude or obligation. Parental retention of a child in a state of dependence breeds either a state of submissive dependence or rebellion, as does an overcontrolling parent. If a parent does not accept their part in the independence effort, the child is forced to go elsewhere for such support. The child strives to become a separate individual, not the parent image. Parents may impede the independence striving by trying to fit the child into their own envision needs, to make the child become a parent, a perpetual child, a lover, or a patient (Wickes, 1966).

The child may stand up to the authoritative dominant parent or they may remain submissive. The child can retain the role of a subservient or become rebellious or even overmimic the parent. Conversely, a weak parent is a weak role model for the child to emulate or to see other role models. A child who doubts their own abilities to face the world may return to the safety of the dependency of the home or may transfer the dependency to another authority figure (Wickes, 1966). Some adolescents vacillate between excessive independence (rebellion) to excessive dependency (clinging), and remain at this point, frozen in this stage of adolescent maturation for years or even decades.

At the time the adolescent is coming to grips with a changing body, an emerging sexuality, and the challenge of new freedoms, the teenager is torn in a vacillation between the ways of the past and the intriguing challenges of the future. This vacillation is perplexing to the adolescent and even more so to the parents (Wickes, 1966).

If epilepsy enters into the picture, the child may be overwhelmed and restricted, with a self-view as disabled. Issues of independence and overdependency arise in the adolescence while the parents are grappling with fears of letting go, especially if they are still overly protective.

Problems due to developmental distortions

The effects of seizures at various ages must be understood in light of the developmental processes in which the child is challenged at the age, and the roles that parents, teachers, and peers play. The impact of an adverse experience with epilepsy may be to throw the child back to an earlier, safer age, an age at which the child was able to cope. Similarly, parents may retreat to a learned age at which they could cope better. Such developmental stagnations and regressions are often brought out if the complications of epilepsy arise along with the seizure challenges.

Dependency versus rebellion

Overindulgent, overprotective, and over-restrictive parents linked with an insecure, anxious, and discouraged child who has a low self-concept tend to keep the child immature, and dependence becomes a negative, self-perpetuating inhibition (Svoboda, 1979). The child and parent may share a common fear of the child's growing-up. If the epilepsy attacks remain uncontrolled, the child tends to become more dependent on others for help. The rejecting attitudes of society tend to discourage any attempts toward independence. Part of the adolescent crisis is the struggle between dependence and independence, with the latter being the desired goal. The epileptic child is more handicapped in this struggle. If the seizures are a chronic problem, the child may not be able to cope with this struggle, retreating back to dependency. This is especially true if the seizures have been present since early childhood. If the seizures begin during the adolescent period, the teenager is often able to make the transition to independence, although the trip may be rough and marked by rebelliousness. Some stagnate between dependence and interdependence for decades (Svoboda, 1979).

The patient's family, friends, and physician can encourage this striving toward independence by continually stressing responsibility and involvement by the seizure patient in the their own seizure management. The patient should be familiar with the details of the medications and the seizure status. The adolescent should assume primary responsibility for the medications, although the parents remain the resource for the purchase of the medications. Beginning vocational planning and guidance can encourage responsibility even in the earlier years with the parents; in the adolescent period, this orientation becomes the major thrust.

Developmental perspectives

Epilepsy can distort psychological development at the age of onset and thereafter. The type of resultant behavior is related to the age of impact of the seizure disorder.

Infancy and early childhood

Seizures occurring during infancy may affect the earliest developmental sense of identify and how the parents relate to a child. The parent fear of separation from a child can be intense and may produce problems of anxiety in childhood. Over-protectiveness emerges. Subsequently, the parents may experience severe anxiety when a toddler exhibits normal climbing and exploratory behaviors, which in turn may suppress normal curiosity, an essential element of later learning (Weisbrot & Ettinger, 2001).

Epilepsy affects the child's earliest developing sense of identity. Parents may be fearful of separating from their infant. This may lead to a separation anxiety in the child. The parents' anxieties tend to be shared with the young child (Weisbrot & Ettinger, 2001).

Early-onset epilepsies may compromise development, with delays in cognition and difficulties in language and behavior manifest. Seizures are said to occur in one-third of children with pervasive developmental disorders such as autism and Asperger's syndrome (Weisbrot & Ettinger, 2001). Seizures occur in about one-third of children with pervasive developmental disorder and may be a factor in behavior regression.

Middle childhood

Academic problems and an increased incidence of ADHD emerge with epilepsy. Up to 68% of children with epilepsy experience academic problems. More than twice as many children with epilepsy have reading delays compared with non-epileptic children.

Early onset of seizures, brain damage, epilepsy severity, and anticonvulsant toxicity are all said to contribute to intellectual deterioration, which parents fear (Weisbrot & Ettinger, 2001). In later childhood, problems of learning and ADHD may emerge in epileptic children (Rutter *et al.*, 1970). This tarnishes the self-image, as failure after failure greet the young student and the parents. The clinician should routinely assess cognitive functioning in pediatric epilepsy patients, and, when indicated, consider referral for neuropsychological testing. Subtle signs of impairment may be overlooked at a critical time for intellectual development (Weisbrot & Ettinger, 2001).

Adolescence

Adolescence is a period of development of the sense of identity and the movement toward independence from parents. Adolescents continue to vacillate between dependency and self-sufficiency. The onset of epilepsy in adolescence is highly disruptive. More intense family conflicts and acting out behaviors may occur (Weisbrot & Ettinger, 2001). The teenager rebels against being told to take the medication and being forbidden to partake in sporting and social activities because of the epilepsy.

In adolescence, complex partial epilepsy becomes more frequent. This disrupts normal adolescent yearning for greater independence from the family. Emotional changes may be induced by seizures affecting the limbic system as a seat of emotions, accentuating an already over-reactive adolescent emotionality. This may be difficult to differentiate from natural shifts in mood or true depressive episodes. Teenagers with epilepsy may have more adjustment problems, sexual identity issues, and body image distortions than their peers (Viberg *et al.*, 1987), although one study demonstrated no differences in the rate of psychopathology in adolescents with temporal lobe epilepsy compared with teens with asthma. Cosmetic side effects from medication, such as weight gain and hair loss, can add to the negative self-image. Restriction from driving, which limits independence, is a great vexation to the teenage epileptic patient (Weisbrot & Ettinger, 2001).

REFERENCES

Erickson, E. H. (1965). Eight ages of man. In *Childhood and Society*, 2nd edn, pp. 147–74. New York: W. W. Norton.

Flor-Henry, P. (1972). Ictal and interictal psychiatric manifestations in epilepsy: specific or non-specific *Epilespia* **13**: 733–83.

Laidlow, J. & Richens, A. (1976). Psychiatry. In *Textbook of Epilepsy*, pp. 151–2. New York: Churchill Livingstone.

Ounsted, C., Lindsay, J. & Norman, R. E. (1966). Biological factors in temporal lobe epilepsy *Dev. Med. Child Neurol. Suppl* 22.

Rutter, M., Graham, P. & Yule, W. A. (1970). *A Neuropsychiatric Study in Childhood*. Philadelphia: J. B. Lippincott.

Stores, G. (1987). Effect on learning of "subclinical" seizure discharges In *Education and Epilepsy*, ed. A. P. Aldenkamp, W. C. J. Alpherts, H. Meinardi & G. Stores, pp. 14–20. Lisse: Swets & Zeitlinger.

Svoboda, W. B. (1979). Emotional and behavioral consequences of epilepsy. In *Learning About Epilepsy*, pp. 167–84. Baltimore, MD: University Park Press.

Swap, S. M. (1974). Disturbing classroom behaviors: a developmental and ecological view. *Exceptional Children* **41**: 163–72.

Viberg, M., Blennow, G. & Polsky, B. (1987). Epilepsy in adolescence: implications for the development of personality. *Epilespia* **28**: 542–6.

Weisbrot, D. M. & Ettinger, A. B. (2001). Psychiatric aspects of pediatric epilepsy. In *Primary Issues in Psychiatry*, ed. A. B. Ettinger & A. M. Kanner, pp. 127–46. Philadelphia: Lippincott Williams & Wilkins.

Wickes, F. G. (1966). Adolescence. In *The Inner World of Childhood*, pp. 100–123. New York: New American Library/Appleton Century.

Winnicott, D. W. (1964). What do we mean by the normal child? In *The Child, the Family and the Outside World*, pp. 124–30. New York: Addison-Wesley.

Winnicott, D. W. (1984). The concept of a healthy individual. In *Home Is Where We Start From*, pp. 21–34. New York: WW Norton & Co.

29

Seizure types and modifying factors

In children, a relationship between neuropsychological functioning and psychopathology exists. Children with impaired cognition tend to be more aggressive and have more mental disorders but show less social competency than children who are neurologically intact (Hermann, 1982). Pathology of the limbic system rather than complex partial seizures appears to be the more significant factor in predisposing patients with seizures to psychopathology. Both the psychopathology and seizure disorders appear to arise from cerebral damage rather than from the seizures themselves (Stevens & Hermann, 1981).

Neurologic basis of ictal behavior

Two things happen in seizures: some discharges activate behaviors and some discharges interfere with behavior processes (Gloor, 1986). The type of behaviors manifest relates to the area of the brain involved in the discharge. The temporal lobe, especially the limbic portion, i.e. the hippocampus and amygdala, is most important.

Activation may manifest as hallucinations, memories and illusions, ideational concepts, affects, or sexual responses. The substrate of these appears to be the temporal lobe. The lateral cortex may be involved, but the limbic system, especially the amygdala, is most important. More complex experiences are multicortical in specific sites of origin. The intensity, however, is less localized and more widespread.

Inhibitions, i.e. negative activities, include impaired consciousness during which the patient is non-responsive and afterwards does not remember. Ictal aphasias often present as confusion, a lack of initiation of voluntary movements, inattention, ictal amnesias during which the patient may be able to carry out an ongoing action, and a confusional state with slowed mentation and psychiatric symptoms such as with petit mal seizures. This confusional state appears to involve an alternating excitation–inhibition of the thalamus, as with absence or complex partial status. These can occasionally present with problems of hostile aggressiveness and negativity, perhaps with hallucinations, disorientation, minor jerks, and apnea. Behaviors can be normal in between. The variability of experiences is notable.

Neurochemical foundations of ictal behavior

Meldrum (1983) has reviewed the neurochemical foundations of ictal behavior. Although seizures differ in manifestation, they appear to be similar on a biochemical basis. With cerebral seizures, there is increased cerebral blood flow, focal or generalized; increased metabolism, especially of glucose and oxygen; changes in the energy metabolism; very rapid ionic changes, including potassium efflux, calcium influx, and changes in sodium, magnesium, and water; secondary-messenger changes; and changes of neurotransmitters. Ionic changes favor epileptic discharges but, if extreme, block synaptic dendrites.

Ictal autonomic changes occur within seconds. The blood pressure rises. There is an increased cerebral blood flow within minutes, with increased blood pressure and increased cerebral blood flow, principally through vasodilation. In focal seizures, the main changes are focal, although there are some changes in other related areas. Thus, a focal seizure may activate areas distant from the inciting epileptiform discharge.

Energy changes lead to receptor changes, especially increasing sensitivity in the glutamate cycle. Messenger changes occur within the first few seconds of a seizure onset and peak within a minute. It may take these changes from 90 minutes to five hours to induce psychopathology. However, there is also a regionalized inhibition or delay of protein synthesis, which may affect recovery and repair.

Neurotransmitter changes occur. GABA turnover is enhanced. Glutamate and aspartate content is reduced through release. Monoamines are increased, with an increase in norepinephrine turnover. The initial changes, if any, are mild but if the patient enters into status late increases may be marked.

The effects these changes have on seizure behaviors, especially through repetition, are not well understood. Neurotransmitters are a major target of research in the study of psychopharmacology.

Ictal phases

Interictal discharges awake inhibitory interactions. The discharge site is surrounded by an inhibitory halo, which may affect other brain functions in that area. Ictal metabolic enhancements include an increase in excitation, with pathologic changes enhancing function. Ictal inhibition produces generalized or specific nuclear or pathway changes, leading to a cessation of function. Postictally, in the recovery phase, there are continued changes in the metabolites, in ionic changes, and in neurotransmitters. Unequal recovery is seen within interrelated areas. A postictal depression of neuronal function occurs. With very brief seizures, there may be an increase in potassium or changes in GABA inhibition. Metabolic effects are more prominent with prolonged seizures and may influence emotional processes.

Metabolism

Engel (1983) has contributed much to our understanding of the neurobiology of interictal behaviors. There is evidence against a single focus in chronic complex partial epilepsy. Epileptic discharges take time to develop. There are usually eventually multiple sites, which in evolution may tend to migrate locally as well as to distant areas. Ictal onset originates from more than one site. The side of the ictal onset may be diffuse rather than the site of the interictal discharge. Interictal hypometabolism may involve larger areas. Seizures and auras may continue after the removal of the epileptic lesion. Bilateral lesions may be necessary for the manifestations of some spontaneous seizures. In many patients, focal seizures with cortical focal lesions show more diffuse hypometabolism. Most patients show thalamic hypometabolism. PET scans may reveal diffuse inhibition with focal lesions, including some on the contralateral side in the hippocampus. This is a GABA-related mechanism as an active interictal inhibitory process serving to protect the brain from damage. Thus, one can envision an epileptic process as a changing, evolving process recruiting both adjacent and distant areas of the brain. Consequently, the dysfunctions of epilepsy, both cognitive and behavioral, may be changing, evolving, and expanding.

There is a correlation between specific cognitive functions and focal hypometabolism of partial seizures. Neuropsychological testing connects dysfunction with hypometabolism of the ictus. Chronic seizures may lead to unusual inter-hemispheric relationships, i.e. the left temporal and right frontal hypometabolism, or the left frontal and left occipital areas. In patients with corpus callosotomy, hypometabolism resolves. Hypometabolism is more dominant in patients with psychoses. Behavioral dysfunction, although located more diffusely, is affected similarly by such changes.

Seizure types

Behavior problems may vary according to the seizure type, the extent, lateralization, and location of the brain involved, and the number of years that the seizure problem has been present. More often, the emotional and behavioral problems are mild, with no major handicapping or at least no recognized impact on the patient's life. These problems may distort the patient's reactions and responses sufficiently to create discontent, frustration, and adjustment problems. This may be due to the interactions and effects on the centers of emotion (the limbic system) and the sensory learning areas of the brain surface. Many studies tend to accentuate deviant behaviors more than their frequency of occurrence or the degree of handicapping of the behavior. These can best be looked at as increased tendencies and not absolute associations.

Generalized seizures

Specific seizures may lead to specific behavior tendencies. Generalized seizure patients are thought to be more prone to problems with poor attention, incomplete work, omissions in learning, fidgeting, and frank hyperactivity. The type of seizures has an important relationship to behavior and personality disorders (Holmes, 1987). Some reports suggest an occasional association between certain traits and seizure types in children.

Tonic–clonic epilepsy

GTC seizures occur as often in children with behavior disorders as in those with subnormal intelligence. The seizures do not appear to predispose the children to behavior or intellectual handicaps (Holdsworth & Whitmore, 1974). Certain behaviors, such as temper tantrums and behavioral personality aberrations, may be more prominent with idiopathic GTC epilepsy. Immature actions and difficulties in maintaining effective social contacts may be noted (Zimmerman et al., 1951). Behavior problems and personality disorders are seen more often on awakening in GTC patients than in those with late-onset or sleep-associated seizures. Patients with awaking epilepsy may tend to be more superficial, suggestible, easily led, hot tempered, and infantile, while those with sleep epilepsy may be more pedantic, persistent, industrious, and hypochondriacal (Sillanpaa, 1973).

Patients with GTC seizures are not a homogeneous group. Those with brain damage are more apt to have mental changes. Behavior and personality changes may be present in forms similar to those found in more pronounced degree in complex partial epilepsy, but these are not well documented. Some patients may display increased restlessness and irritability hours or even days before an attack. Even with seizure control, a patient may still display episodes of irritability. Children may display a protracted misbehavior, which occasionally follows a series of closely spaced grand mal seizures. Postictal psychoses typically appear following a silent interval of one or more days and may be severe enough to require hospitalization. These are not uncommon in adults, but they are rare in children (Blumer, 1977).

Absence epilepsy

Individuals with absence epilepsy are generally free of any marked behavior disturbances, possibly due to the lack of involvement of temporal-limbic structures (Blumer, 1977). Childhood absence epilepsy may be associated with poor sibling relationships, reduced social outings, and emotional difficulties (Caplan et al., 1991; Caplan et al., 1992; Weisbrot & Ettinger, 1998; Weisbrot & Ettinger, 2001). Such children may be somewhat passive and, if disturbed, tend to show neurotic symptoms. These symptoms, including nightmares, nail-biting, and thumb-sucking, much like those with awakening epilepsy, occur in up to 25%. Such habits may relate to school difficulties (Sillanpaa, 1973).

Both boys and girls with absence seizures may have anxiety. With typical three per second spike-wave discharges, only the boys show anxiety. Children with absences seem not to experience the social isolation seen with other seizure types of epilepsy (Stores, 1977), yet many show poor social adaptation (Ounsted *et al.*, 1966; Louiseau *et al.*, 1983; Dam, 1990). Individuals with absence seizures have the fewest personality deviations of all patients with epilepsy. Character disorders are uncommon, regardless of whether the spells are idiopathic or symptomatic (Zimmerman *et al.*, 1951).

Myoclonic epilepsy

The patient with myoclonic seizures may be thought to appear emotionally weak, unstable, and self-centered. Such patients, like those with complex partial epilepsy, seem to be more vulnerable and less able to cope with life.

Juvenile myoclonic epilepsy

Patients of normal intelligence are described as having tendencies to show engaging but emotionally unstable, fairly immature personalities, wavering between camaraderie and mistrust, which may cause difficulties in social adaptation. Controlled psychological and sociological studies confirm this by frequently displaying neurotic character traits (Dam, 1990; Janz, 1969; Janz & Christian, 1957). Juvenile myoclonic epilepsy patients may show a tendency towards irresponsibility and impaired impulse control, neglect of duties, emotional instability, quick temper, and distractibility (Caplan *et al.*, 1991; Caplan *et al.*, 1992; Weisbrot & Ettinger, 1998; Weisbrot & Ettinger, 2001).

Progressive myoclonic epilepsy

Mental symptoms, intellectual deterioration, and psychotic features are especially emphasized soon after the first neurologic features of Lafora myoclonic epilepsy, often about the same time as the GTC seizures appear. In non-Lafora types, personality features emerge when the disorder becomes disabling. The patient may become infantile, dependent, and mood-labile, with outbursts of aggressiveness and depression. Lability of mood may emerge conspicuously as related to the physical condition, as the patient may be euphoric or prone to depression, which may present as apathy. Apathy, but not dementia, has been reported in the non-Lafora type. Psychotic symptoms are not usually seen (Koskiniemi, 1974).

Epileptic syndromes
Febrile seizures

Behavior disorders, particularly hyperactivity, may be seen in children treated for prolonged periods for febrile convulsions (Wolf *et al.*, 1981).

West's syndrome of infantile spasms

West's infantile spasms are associated with severe cognitive impairments, developmental delays, and impaired social interactions, worsened with poor seizure control (Caplan *et al.*, 1991; Caplan *et al.*, 1992; Weisbrot & Ettinger, 1998; Weisbrot & Ettinger, 2001).

Lennox–Gastaut syndrome

Lennox–Gastaut syndrome is associated with behavioral difficulties common to mental retardation, such as hyperactivity (Caplan *et al.*, 1991; Caplan *et al.*, 1992; Weisbrot & Ettinger, 1998; Weisbrot & Ettinger, 2001). Three groups of later psychiatric problems are seen: minimally disturbed patients, patients with personality disorders, and psychotic patients (Beaumanoir *et al.*, 1988). In a group of 40 children, in follow-up half the group demonstrated behavior problems, with hyperactivity aggressiveness, or frankly psychotic behavior seen (Aicardi & Gomes, 1988).

Landau–Kleffner syndrome of acquired aphasia with epilepsy

Landau–Kleffner syndrome is associated with behavior disturbances, including hyperactivity, aggression, depression, and psychoses (see Chapter 5) (Caplan *et al.*, 1991; Caplan *et al.*, 1992; Weisbrot & Ettinger, 1998; Weisbrot & Ettinger, 2001).

Epilepsy with electrical status epilepticus during slow sleep

Epilepsy with electrical status epilepticus during slow sleep is usually accompanied by a progressive functional deterioration. Secondary behavior problems include hyperactivity, aggression, and psychoses. This entity is associated with inattention hyperactivity impulsiveness, a loss of sense of danger, aggressiveness, mood changes, disinhibition, mouthing of objects, reduced play, and preservations. Subtle cognitive changes may occur first (Caplan *et al.*, 1991; Caplan *et al.*, 1992; Weisbrot & Ettinger, 1998; Weisbrot & Ettinger, 2001).

Partial epilepsies

Localization and laterality of the epileptic focus relate to behavior disturbances, including behavior disorders (Stores, 1987), aggression (Ounsted *et al.*, 1966), and frank psychoses (Flor-Henry, 1972; Binnie *et al.*, 1990). Left-hemispheric damage is associated more closely with psychiatric disabilities, especially those involving temporal lobe lesions, particularly on the left (Giordani *et al.*, 1983). Frank depressive episodes and bipolar presentations are more often localized to the left frontal-temporal lobe. Affective disorders, behavior problems, and somatic complaints are more often related to right-hemispheric damage, especially involving the frontal lobe.

Most children with unilateral CPE show no significant cognitive or emotional difficulties. When such emotional problems exist, they are often seen with a cognitive deficit. Cognitive, personality, and school difficulties are distributed equally between left and right CPE (Camfield *et al.*, 1982).

Simple partial epilepsies

There is a lower incidence of behavioral changes in patients with simple partial seizures compared with those with complex partial temporal seizures, for, as with absence seizures, there is usually no involvement of the limbic system. However, with extensive brain damage and epilepsy, the risk for psychiatric disturbances is bound to increase. Such children may display episodic rage reactions similar or identical to the onset frequently observed in complex partial seizures (Blumer, 1977). Simple partial epilepsy can produce distressing symptoms leading to behavior reactions. With simple partial epilepsy, behavior symptoms may persist in status (Engel *et al.*, 1978).

Benign central-temporal (Rolandic) epilepsy

Benign Rolandic epilepsy was initially thought to be associated with normal psychological functioning (Caplan *et al.*, 1991; Caplan *et al.*, 1992; Weisbrot & Ettinger, 1998; Weisbrot & Ettinger, 2001). This condition occurs in about 8.5% of healthy schoolchildren (Tiodze & Lomashvili, 1991), presenting as a simple partial seizure (20%), or as complex partial seizures (21%), or as secondarily generalized seizures (59%) (Giordani *et al.*, 1999). The condition does not appear to impair social ultimate adjustments of children (Loiseau *et al.*, 1983).

Further studies of these children reveal that what is thought of as benign may be only relatively benign. The children may have an average intelligence, yet 15% are in special education and 5% are using ADHD medication. Attention-related scores are depressed (Giordani *et al.*, 1999), with hyperactivity reported (5.8–13.3%). Social adaptation is dependent mainly on the behavior deviations (Tiodze & Lomashvili, 1991). Behavior ratings show elevations in psychosomatic complaints and in learning problems. Risks for selective cognitive and behavioral difficulties appear to be increased. Variability in performance indicates the need for cognitive monitoring of these children (Giordani *et al.*, 1999).

Complex partial epilepsy

Complex partial seizures with involvement of the limbic system carry a high risk for behavior and personality disorders, with a higher rate of psychiatric problems

(Holmes, 1987). Temporal lobe epilepsy is associated more often with attention deficits, hyperactivity, antisocial behavior, aggression, schizophrenia-like psychoses, formal thought disorders, communication deficits, increased aggression, sexual dysfunction, maladaptive social behaviors, and behavioral disinhibition (Caplan *et al.*, 1991; Caplan *et al.*, 1992; Weisbrot & Ettinger, 1998; Weisbrot & Ettinger, 2001). Some patients with complex partial seizures tend to be emotionally disturbed but free of clinical seizures (Blumer, 1977). Seizure patients with complex partial epilepsy seem to have more difficulties in coping. Such patients may be the most difficult to rehabilitate. Studies in children with this condition are limited.

Severe maladjustments resulting from serious behavioral and psychological disturbances along with incomplete control of CPE affect about 75% of the patients (Bray, 1962). Affective liability may be seen in over-reaction to colors and in content characteristics (Whitehouse, 1976). Complex partial epilepsy patients have the strongest inclinations toward tensions, conflicts, and ambivalence between self-controls and acting out, leading to neurotic symptoms. Wide variability is seen (Whitehouse, 1976).

CPE may be characterized by specific behavior disturbances (Fedio & Mirsky, 1969). Patients with complex partial seizures of temporal lobe origin may be at increased risk for specific personality traits, including excessive aggression, violence, psychoses, and other antisocial behaviors (Holmes, 1987). Adolescents as well as adults with chronic CPE may show personality changes, which are characteristic and reasonably consistent, such as excessive sensitivity, irritability, aggressiveness, depressed sexual behavior, preoccupation with religion, and hypergraphia (extensive detailed writing and drawing) (Barlow, 1978). Aggression is seen more often with right CPE than with left CPE. Affective disorders are seen more often with right CPE, although this is debated. Left CPE is associated with schizophrenic-like illnesses and an increased risk for educational and behavior problems (Stores, 1981).

Neuroses, neurotic or hysterical symptoms, and behavior changes in pure CPE occur more frequently. Symptoms of an organic psycho-syndrome (dementia, irritability, states of confusion, deterioration of memory, etc.) predominate in combined types (Sillanpaa, 1973). This is probably a limbic disorder, often with preictal or postictal timing, although interictal mood irritably is also common.

Psychotic states are prevalent in the two forms. Changes of slowness, preservation, and apathy are more common than irritability, impulsivity, or hyperkinesia (Sillanpaa, 1973). Episodic psychoses may appear with or follow a seizure, or they may arise between seizures. Patients with CPE may suffer psychotic episodes with forced normalization of the EEG (Engel *et al.*, 1978). Later psychoses tend to develop as the CPE seizures are controlled (Reynolds, 1981).

A wide range of patterns of psychological diagnosis in children has been noted, including psychotic, hyperactive, neurotic, and retardation (Bray, 1962). Marked depressive mood, hysterical manifestations, paranoid trends, and psychotic reactions are not common in childhood temporal lobe seizures, but they do occur occasionally. In the pediatric age group, hyperactivity and angry outbursts are more prominent. In older adolescents and young adults, these may become more prominent while outbursts of rage may lessen (Blumer, 1977).

Epileptic boys seem especially predisposed to behavior complications. Persistent left CPE is associated with emotional dependency. Boys are especially apt to develop other types of disturbed behavior (Stores, 1978). Such children are described as shy, immature, schizoid, and inadequate. Occasionally, aggressive traits and symptoms of anxiety are noted in children (Berger, 1971). Temper tantrums are common (Barlow, 1978).

Psychologic problems have been seen in as many as 85% of children with temporal lobe seizures. In follow-up, 10% develop a schizophreniform psychosis, 6% have been treated for anxiety or depression, and 14% exhibit antisocial behaviors. In one study, over half of the children with antisocial behaviors had been in court for more than one offense, usually aggression in the form of assault or major property damage. This was a higher rate than in most studies (Lindsay et al., 1979). By adulthood, about 70% of those not severely retarded were psychiatrically healthy, but 10% developed schizophrenia-like psychoses. All had left CPE (Williams & Mostofsky, 1982).

Thirty percent of children with CPE demonstrate psychotic behavior, especially associated with bilateral temporal lobe abnormalities. In one study, no children with anterior temporal spike foci were found to be disturbed enough to be considered as psychotic (Brett, 1966). All psychotic children have either a unilateral mid-temporal spike focus or spike foci rising independently in both temporal lobes. Most children with bilateral abnormalities are psychotic. The common neurologic findings are restricted to mild speech disorders, possibly relating to the expressive language functions of the temporal lobe (Bray, 1962).

Dominant complex partial epilepsy
The highest risk group are boys with left temporal lobe epilepsy, with problems such as behavior disorders (Stores, 1987), aggression (Ounsted et al., 1966), and psychoses (Flor-Henry, 1972). Boys with left temporal lobe epileptic foci, unlike girls, experience anxiety, inattention, social isolation, and overactivity (Stores, 1977).

Traits seen in this group include less impulsivity but more emotional sensitivity (McIntyre et al., 1976; Stores, 1978). Individuals with left temporal lobe epilepsy may tend to make unusual interpretations of verbal representations in their affective states. This may affect discernment of verbal affect cues, impacting on interpersonal relationships. This may lead to adverse psychopathology. There is greater potential for verbal communication disturbances, which may be related to atypical affective labeling (McIntyre *et al.*, 1976). Patients with dominant temporal lobe dysfunction tend to misunderstand others and be easily hurt, thus tending to withdraw and become secretive. They may become bogged down with details. They tend to feel that their environment controls them. They tend to minimize good qualities and maximize their faults.

In adults, a left temporal epileptic focus may result in specific sequelae in the patient's personality, leading to social introversion. Impairment or impoverishment of interpersonal relationships is characteristic. The ability to correctly discern verbal affective cues may be important in the formation and maintenance of successful interpersonal relationships. These patients fail to detect the intended meaning of an affective laden message and thus are more likely to have difficulties in interpersonal interactions. They may be considered to be psychiatrically disturbed. Left temporal lobe patients are found to be more likely to experience difficulties in some aspects of their verbal communication of affect (McIntyre *et al.*, 1976).

Patients with left temporal lobe epilepsy are characterized by increased dependency, less external composedness, higher depressive drive and mood, more nervousness, higher recall for information and experience exchange, and a higher tendency to perseverate. No differences in cognitive and psychosocial status are seen. The evaluation of personality features contributes to the lateralization and counseling of patients with temporal lobe epilepsy considered for epilepsy surgery (Feddersen *et al.*, 2000).

There is an increased psychiatric disability with temporal lobe epilepsy in children (Rutter *et al.*, 1970) especially in boys with a left-sided focus (Stores, 1977; Trimble, 1988). A poor psychopathologic outcome is seen in children with hyperactivity or a rage reaction history, for 14% develop antisocial behavior as adults, including court convictions or aggression. A disordered home environment does not seem to have a predictive value on the outcome (Ounsted & Lindsay, 1981; Trimble, 1988).

Non-dominant complex partial epilepsy
The emotional problems tend to be of externally directed emotions, with hyperactivity, impulsivity, and inattention noted (McIntyre *et al.*, 1976; Stores, 1978). There are misunderstandings of social cues and facial expressions. The child may exhibit impulsive acting out of emotional feelings, including aggression and anger. If the individual develops a major psychiatric disturbance, it is more apt to be a mania or a depression than a thought disturbance such as schizophrenia. The personality disorders associated with right temporal lobe epilepsy may demonstrate rigidity, aggression, obsessional traits, disruptive behavior, and turbulent behavior (Andermann, 1994). Boys with right temporal lobe foci are more apt to report problems of anxiety; this is not seen with girls (Stores, 1977).

Frontal lobe complex partial epilepsy

Patients with frontal lobe epilepsy may demonstrate more thought disorders (Caplan *et al.*, 1991; Caplan *et al.*, 1992; Weisbrot & Ettinger, 1998; Weisbrot & Ettinger, 2001). Frontal lobe complex partial seizures may be associated with postictal psychoses. An increase in seizure frequency may lead to succeeding psychoses of a paranoid or schizophrenic nature. Predisposing factors include an organic dissembling delusional state. The patient usually has an intractable form of epilepsy. There may be bilateral involvement, including bitemporal independent foci. Often, structural lesions or foreign tissue is found as the cause. The precipitating factors may be an increase in complex partial activation if drug reduction is performed too rapidly. Transient use of haloperidol may be beneficial.

Subclinical seizure discharges

Interictal epileptiform activity

Binnie (1995) discussed the importance of interictal and subclinical discharges and their behavior correlates. EEGs are often overinterpreted: spikes are not seizures, and the responses are not related to the abnormal EEG. It is recognized increasingly, however, that subclinical discharges, whether of hippocampal or neocortical origin, can produce transient disturbances of functioning, depending on the type of activity and discharge (see Chapter 17).

Discharge impairments

Binnie noted that the presence of subictal epileptiform activity might augment behavior with an intense, unstable, affective bias. In adults, a considerable number of affectively ill patients who have epilepsy-related mood disorders and who have not experienced manifest convulsions have been studied. Roughly 10% of patients in one clinic were found to have a final diagnosis of subictal and interictal affective illnesses, whereas only 3.8% arrived with that diagnosis. About 50% were diagnosed as bipolar, 30% as atypical or dysthymic, and 10% as having unipolar affective disorders. Bipolar affective syndromes are part of a spectrum that begins with typical bipolar illnesses, passes through rapid-cycling lithium-refractory states, and ends in labile, rapidly changing mood disorders that are either subictal or interictal in nature. Most patients are clinically recognizable in that they has had a history of epilepsy, an abnormal EEG, or an interictal symptom profile that has been described. Proper treatment of subictal affective states and rapid-cycling primary bipolar illness is critical because this syndrome is accompanied by a high suicidal rate. The antiepileptic mediations, particularly the limbic anticonvulsant carbamazepine, are effective for many of these patients, in combination with psychiatric antidepressants or lithium salts (Himmelhoch, 1984).

Medication responsiveness

In issuing medications, the prescriber must consider the potential effects of the anticonvulsant. Is the handicap of the drug more or less than the impairment of subclinical seizures? Interictal spikes may not respond to many anticonvulsants: do these respond to antiepileptic drugs or to other therapies (Binnie, 1995)? Is a benefit seen related to discharge control or to the psychotropic benefit of the antiepileptic drug?

Modifying factors

CNS variables that have been debated include the seizure type, age of onset, age of recurrence, degree of seizure control, duration of epilepsy, etiology, aura type, gender, and the neuropsychological status (Neugebauer *et al.*, 1991). Medication variables include antiepileptic drug type, polytherapy, and antiepileptic drug toxicity. Psychosocial variables include fear of seizures, perceived stigma, perceived discrimination, adjustment to epilepsy, feelings of lack of control over one's life, social support, socioeconomic status, and the childhood home environment (Weisbrot & Ettinger, 1998).

Endogenous factors, such as a migration defect, an encephalomalacia, an inborn error of metabolism, chromosomal aberrations, and genetic syndromes, may underlie psychopathology in seizures. Impairments of neuropsychologic functioning later on are seen more often with symptomatic than with idiopathic epilepsy (Klove & Matthews, 1967). Hamartomas perhaps are more related to psychoses, especially if in the hippocampus. XXY males display rage and violence, especially with an ectodermal dysplasia. The psychologic problems are probably an interrelated mixture of multiple factors, varying with each person.

Location

Location considerations include whether the epileptic focus is limbic or non-limbic as well as the laterality of the lesion. Most authors refer to limbic involvement underlying endogenous psychiatric conditions.

Gender

Girls with epilepsy have more problems than boys with epilepsy. However, there is a general tendency for boys to be more vulnerable than girls to various types of stresses in life (Rutter *et al.*, 1970).

Age of onset

Earlier age of onset of seizures appears to be associated with more severe subsequent behavior deficits (Klove & Matthews, 1967). Seizure problems beginning in early childhood are more often associated with personality and character disorders, problems in getting along with others, aggressive acting out behaviors, and hyper-activity. Seizures beginning in adolescence or early adulthood are more apt to be associated with depression and discouragement. Patients with a seizure problem of long duration seem to have more emotional and behavior problems than those with seizures of recent onset. In a survey of children with newly diagnosed seizure problems, 32.6% had behavior problems and 25.8% had clinical behavior problems, suggesting that problems are already present in some children (Austin *et al.*, 1999).

Seizure frequency and duration

Seizure frequency is a very powerful predictor of behavioral problems (Besag, 2001). In about 75% of adults, undesirable life events appear to be unrelated to the seizure frequency. Patients with a seizure problem of long duration seem to have more emotional and behavior problems than those with seizures of recent onset.

Effects of therapy

Indirect effects include altered endocrine function and sleep patterns. Sleep especially REM sleep stages, may be altered by seizures. Abrupt control-induced cessation may produce a behavior confusion state.

Other exogenous factors

Perales (1999) noted that important exogenous factors to consider include the effects of medications or surgery, the response of the family and community in terms of self-esteem, self-image, self-confidence, and the ability of the patient to participate in the family and then the community. Family variables of decreased communication and consultation with medical personnel, increased family stress, and decreased extended family social support are associated with increased behavior problems (Austin *et al.*, 1991).

Postictal period

Schacter (1996) noted that the postictal period may be one of confusion, depression, difficulty in talking, embarrassment, exhaustion, fear, frustration, headache, loneliness, memory loss, nausea, pain, perceptual alterations, sleep, thirst, and weakness. Some of these factors are direct consequences of the seizure event and some are the results of the psychosocial reactions. The postictal state is often more handicapping than the seizure itself, especially if a dysfunction is present. Exhaustion and the need for sleep often continue beyond the duration of the seizure. Patients cannot function for up to 12–24 hours. The postictal state can be terrifying, with fear and loneliness. Everything seems distant in time and space. A powerful sense of anguish, pain, and loneliness may be present. Postictal depression is infrequent and is probably multifactorial, being both biological and psychological in origin. It can be disappointment because of the recurrent loss of control. Perceptual alterations may split the mind, with one side dashing scene to scene and the other whirling and gnashing in chaotic colors, with weird shapes and movements. These symptoms may last for up to an hour. Such experiences, especially if repeated; may have significant influences on the psychiatric state. A child may be perplexed by such episodes and fearful of recurrence.

Fisher (1996) reviewed the physiology of the postictal period. Following a seizure, there is a refractory period with transmitter depletion. There is an initial refractory period followed by a hypoexcitability for a period of time. However, the cells can still fire. The sodium pump is turned on to create the hypopolarization state. The refractory period of glutamate desensitization with transmitter depletion leads to an inhibitory hierarchy being activated, resulting in hyperpolarizing pumps with increased potassium and hydrogen and blood flow changes. Neurotransmitter excesses of opiates and adenosine occur. The cerebral blood flow relates to metabolism, but this is altered after a seizure. Cerebral blood flow and metabolism dissociate during and after a seizure.

Trimble (1996) commented that in many cases, the patient is often more handicapped postictally than ictally. Postictal psychopathological events include automatisms and fugues, clouding of consciousness, delirium, and twilight states, behaviors that represent more of a chemical change than an electrical change. Postictal behavioral disinhibition is seen when the patient appears to be conscious and exhibiting partial control of what they are doing. This can be seen especially with frontal seizures.

Elger (1996) reported that mood disturbances might develop, including depression (34%), fear (10%), exhaustion (8%), aggression (6%), and nervousness (4%). Full recovery from the postictal period may take at least one to two hours.

Schacter (1996) added that a postictal psychosis is most often seen with recalcitrant epilepsy, especially with bilateral representation and a medial temporal origin. Postictal psychoses occur rarely but can be disturbing. It is not known why a postictal state is longer when a tumor is found. Patients with amygdala atrophy seem to have a prolonged postictal state as opposed to those with others. To prevent postictal psychoses, generally one seeks to avoid neuroleptics, which can worsen the situation.

REFERENCES

Aicardi, J. & Gomes, AL. (1988). The Lennox–Gastaut syndrome: clinical and electroencephalographic features. In *The Lennox Gastaut Syndrome*, ed. E. Neidermeyer & R. Degen, pp. 25–46. New York: Alan R. Liss.

Andermann, F. (1994). Psychiatric illnesses in epilepsy. Presented at the American Epilepsy Society Conference, 1994.

Austin, J. K., Dunn, D. W., Huster, G. A., et al. (1999). Correlates of behavior problems in children with new-onset seizures. *Epilepsia* **40** (suppl 7): 75.

Austin, J. Risinger, M. W. & McNelis, A. (1991). Family, seizure and gender variables associated with child behavior problems. *Epilepsia* **32** (suppl 3): 29.

Barlow, C. F. (1978). Risk factors of infancy and childhood: interrelationship of seizure disorders and mental retardation. In *Mental Retardation and Related Disorders*, pp. 768–75. Philadelphia: F. A. Davis.

Beaumanoir, A., Foletti, G., Migistris, M., et al. (1988). Status epilepticus in the Lennox–Gastaut syndrome. In *The Lennox Gastaut Syndrome*, ed. E. Neidermeye & R. Degen, pp. 283–99. New York: Alan R. Liss.

Berger, H. (1971). An unusual manifestation of Tegretol (carbamazepine) toxicity. *Ann. Intern. Med.* **4**: 449–50.

Besag, F. C. (2001). Treatment of state-dependent learning disabilities. In *Epilepsia and Learning Disabilities*, ed. G. F. Ayala, M. Elia, C. M. Cornaggia & M. M. Trimble. *Epilepsia* **42**: 46–9.

Binnie, C. D. (1995). Behavioral correlates of interictal spikes. Presented at the American Epilepsy Society Conference, 1995.

Binnie, C. D. Channon, S. & Marston, D. (1990). Learning disabilities in epilepsy: neurophysiological aspects. *Epilepsia* **31** (suppl 4): 2–8.

Blumer, D. (1977). Neuropsychiatric aspects of psychomotor and other forms of epilepsy in childhood. In *Comprehensive Management of Epilepsy in Infancy, Childhood and Adolescence*, ed. S. Livingston, pp. 486–97. Springfield, IL: Charles C. Thomas.

Bray, P. F. (1962). Temporal lobe syndromes in children. *Pediatrics* **70**: 517–38.

Brett, E. M. (1966). Minor epileptic status. *J. Neurol. Sci.* **3**: 52–75.

Camfield, P. R., Ronen, G. M., Gates, R. D., et al. (1982). Temporal lobe epiepsy in children: comparison of cognitive ability, personality profile and school success in children with pure right versus left EEG foci. *Ann. Neurol.* **12**: 205.

Caplan, R., Guthrie, D., Shields, W. D., et al. (1992). Formal thought disorder in pediatric complex partial seizure disorders. *J. Child Psychol. Psychiatry* **33**: 1399–412.

Caplan, R., Shields, W. D., Mori, L., et al. (1991). Middle childhood onset of interictal psychoses: case studies. *J. Acad. Child Adolesc. Psychiatry* **30**: 893–6.

Dam, M. (1990). Children with epilepsy: the effects of seizures, syndromes and etiological factors on cognitive functioning. *Epilepsia* **31** (suppl 4): 26–9.

Elger, C. E. (1996). Postictal cognition. Presented at the American Epilepsy Society Conference, 1996.

Engel, J., Jr (1983). Basic mechanisms of epilepsy. In *Contemporary Neurology Series: Seizures and Epilepsy*, pp. 71–111. Philadelphia: F. A. Davis.

Engel, J., Ludwick, B. I. & Fetell, M. (1978). Prolonged partial complex status epilepticus EEG and behavior observations. *Neurology* **28**: 863–9.

Feddersen, B., Runge, U., Herzer, R., et al. (2000). Concerning psychopathology in focus epilepsies with unilateral temporal focus. *Epilepsia* **41** (suppl 7): 158.

Fedio, P. & Mirsky, A. F. (1969). Selective intellectual deficits in children with temporal lobe or centrencephalic epilepsy. *J. Neuropsychol.* **7**: 287–300.

Fisher, R. S. (1996). Physiology and pharmacology of the postictal state. Presented at the American Epilepsy Society Conference, 1996.

Flor-Henry, P. (1972). Ictal and inter-ictal psychiatric manifestations in epilepsy: specific or non-specific. *Epilepsia* **13**: 733–83.

Giordani, B., Berent, S., Sackellares, J. C., *et al.* (1983). Intelligence and academic achievement in patients with partial, generalized and partial secondary generalized seizures. *Epilepsia* **24**: 258.

Giordani, B. J., Laughrin, D. M., Berent, S., *et al.* (1999). Children with benign epilepsy with centrotemporal spikes (BECTS): cognitive and behavioral features. *Epilepsia* **40** (suppl 7): 128.

Gloor, P. (1986). Consciousness as a neurological concept in epileptology: a critical view. *Epilepsia* **27** (suppl 2): 14–26.

Hermann, B. P. (1982). Neuropsychosocial functioning and psychopathology. I: children with epilepsy. *Epilepsia* **23**: 545–54.

Himmelhoch, J. M. (1984). Major mood disorders related to epileptic changes. In *Psychiatric Aspects of Epilepsy*, ed. D. Blumer, pp. 271–94. Washington, DC: American Psychiatric Press.

Holdsworth, L. & Whitmore, K. (1974). A study of children with epilepsy attending ordinary schools. I: their seizure patterns, progress, and behavior in schools. *Dev. Med. Child Neurol.* **16**: 746–58.

Holmes, G. L. (1987). *Psychosocial Factors in Childhood Epilepsy*, pp. 112–24. Philadelphia: W. B. Saunders.

Janz, D. (1969). *Die Epilepsien*. Stuttgart: Theme.

Janz, C. D. & Christian, W. (1957). Impulsiv-petit mal. *Dtsch. Z. Nervenheilkd* **176**: 348–86.

Klove, H. & Matthews, C. G. (1967). Differential psychological performance in major motor, psychomotor and mixed seizure classification of known and unknown etiology. *Epilepsia* **9**: 117–28.

Koskiniemi, M. (1974). Psychological findings in progressive myoclonus epilepsy without Lafora bodies. *Epilepsia* **15**: 537–45.

Lindsay, J., Ounsted, C. & Richards, P. (1979). Long term outcome in children with temporal lobe seizures. III: psychiatric aspects in childhood and adult life. *Dev. Med. Child Neurol.* **21**: 630–36.

Loiseau, P., Pestre, M., Deartigues, J. F., *et al.* (1983). Long-term prognosis in two forms of childhood epilepsy: typical absence and epilepsy with Rolandic (centrotemporal) EEG foci. *Ann. Neurol.* **13**: 642–8.

McIntyre, M., Pritchard, P. B., III & Lombroso, C. T. (1976). Left and right temporal lobe epileptics: a controlled investigation of some psychological differences. *Epilepsia* **17**: 377–86.

Meldrum, B. S. (1983). Metabolic factors during prolonged seizures and their relation to nerve cell death. *Adv. Neurol.* **34**: 261–75.

Neugebauer, R., Paik, M., Nadel, E., *et al.* (1991). Association of stressful life events with seizure occurrence inpatients with epilepsy. *Epilepsia* **32** (suppl 3): 31.

Ounsted, C. & Lindsay, J. (1981). The long-term outcome of temporal lobe epilepsy in childhood.

In *Epilepsy and Psychiatry*, ed. E. H. Reynolds & M. R. Trimble, pp. 185–215. New York: Churchill Livingstone.

Ounsted, C. J. Lindsay, J. & Norman, R. (1966). Biologic factors in temporal lobe epilepsy. In *Clinics in Developmental Medicine*, No. 22. London: Heinemann.

Perales, M. (1999). Psychiatric management in epilepsy. Presented at the Via Christi Epilepsy Conference, Wichita, KS, 1999.

Reynolds, E. H. (1981). Biological factors in psychological disorders associated with epilepsy. In *Epilepsy and Psychiatry*, ed. E. H. Reynolds & M. R. Trimble, pp. 264–90. New York: Churchill Livingstone.

Rutter, M., Graham, P. & Yule, W. (1970). A neuropsychiatric study in childhood. In *Clinics in Developmental Medicine*, Vol. 25. London: Heinemann.

Schacter, S. C. (1996). The postictal state. Presented at the American Epilepsy Society Conference, 1996.

Sillanpaa, M. (1973). Medicosocial prognosis of children with epilepsy. *Acta Paediatr. Scand. suppl.* **237**: 6–104.

Stevens, J. R. & Hermann, B. P. (1981). Temporal lobe epilepsy, psychopathology and violence: the state of the evidence. *Neurology* **31**: 1127–32.

Stores, G. (1971). Cognitive function in children with epilepsy. *Dev. Med. Child Neurol.* **13**: 390–92.

Stores, G. (1977). Behavior disturbance and types of epilepsy in children attending ordinary school. In *Epilepsy, The Eighth International Symposium*, ed. J. K. Penry, pp. 245–9. New York: Raven Press.

Stores, G. (1978). School-children with epilepsy at risk for learning and behavior problems. *Dev. Med. Child Neurol.* **20**: 502–8.

Stores, G. (1981). Problems of learning and behavior in children with epilepsy. In *Epilepsy and Psychiatry*, ed. E. H. Reynolds & M. R. Trimble, pp. 33–48. New York: Churchill Livingstone.

Stores, G. (1987). Effects on learning of subclinical seizure discharges. In *Education and Epilepsy*, ed. A. P. Aldenkamp, W. C. J. Alpherts, H. Meinardi & G. Stores, pp. 14–21. Lissee: Swets & Zeitlinger.

Toidze, O. & Lomashvili, N. (1991). Clinical significance of the Rolandic and centrotemporal spikes in children with behavioral deviations. 19th International Epilepsy Congress. *Epilepsia* **32** (suppl 1): 15.

Trimble, M. R. (1988). Anticonvulsant drugs; mood and cognitive functions. In *Epilepsy, Behavior and Cognitive Function*, ed. M. R. Trimble & E. H. Reynolds, pp. 135–45. Chichester, UK: John Wiley & Sons.

Trimble, M. R. (1996). Postictal psychiatric symptoms. Presented at the American Epilepsy Society Conference, 1996.

Weisbrot, D. M. & Ettinger, A. B. (1998). Psychiatric aspects of pediatric epilepsy. *Primary Psychiatry* **June**: 51–67.

Weisbrot, D. & Ettinger, A. B. (2001). Psychiatric aspects of pediatric epilepsy. In *Psychiatric Issues in Epilepsy*, ed. A. B. Ettinger & A. M. Kanner, pp. 127–46. Philadelphia: Lippincott Williams & Wilkins.

Whitehouse, D. (1976). Behavior and learning problems in epileptic children. *Behav. Neuropsy-chiatry* **7**: 23–9.

Williams, D. T. & Mostofsky, D. I. (1982). Psychogenic seizures in childhood and adolescence. In *Pseudoseizures*, ed. T. L. Riley & A. Roy, pp. 169–84. Baltimore, MD: Williams & Wilkins.

Wolf, S. M., Forsythe, A., Sturnden, A. A., *et al.* (1981). Long-term effect of phenobarbital on cognitive function in children with febrile convulsions *Pediatrics* **68**: 820–23.

Zimmerman, F. T., Burgemeister, B. B. & Putnam, T. J. (1951). Intellectual and emotional makeup of the epileptic. *Arch. Neurol. Psychiatry* **65**: 545–56.

30

Overview: extrinsic factors

Many children with epilepsy have no behavioral problems, perform satisfactorily in school, and are socially well adjusted (Holmes, 1987). Some do have problems, however, and need help lest the social and behavioral problems become more handicapping than the seizures.

Emotional disturbances may be reactions to coping with both intrinsic and extrinsic causes, including the reactions of the family and others (Guerrant *et al.*, 1962). Medications may alter behavior and cognition, leading to feelings of lack of control and inadequate social and academic functioning (Weisbrot & Ettinger, 1998). Problems of interacting with others may be influenced by a low intelligence, language difficulties, specific learning disabilities, physical handicaps, family problems, school difficulties, and later vocational problems (Henricksen, 1977). The severity of the epilepsy rather than the condition itself appears to be the main determinant of psychosocial and social consequences (Avondet *et al.*, 1991). The basic approaches to such extrinsic disturbances include a combination of individual and family therapy, and medications to treat anxiety, depression, shame, embarrassment, and resentment.

The child

Epilepsy exists simultaneously as an individual medical disorder and as a family problem. The child must adapt to the epilepsy while developing a sense of self (Ziegler, 1981). Psychosocial problems in children with epilepsy may reflect the way they were brought up by their parents (Henricksen, 1977). A child has to find ways of adapting to the epilepsy while developing strategies for dealing with the family reactions. Some children may use their seizures as a way of controlling the family environment, which in turn, may result in the later development of non-epileptic seizures (Lambert & Robertson, 1999).

Self-concept

Children are less prepared to cope with the stresses of the epilepsy. Children with epilepsy are more dependent on others, whose attitudes shape personality development and social interactions.

Feeling different

The growing child with epilepsy may be treated differently from siblings in the family, and may often feel neglected, minimized, or rejected. The child gets the message that they are different (Svoboda, 1979).

Not being in control

At every age and at every stage of development, children battle to gain control over their lives. The unpredictability of seizures threatens the sense of control, leading to anxiety, depression, and low levels of self-esteem (Hartlage *et al.*, 1972; Stores & Piran, 1978; Ziegler, 1981; Hoare, 1984). Dependency is greater in children with epilepsy than in those with other disorders (Hartlage *et al.*, 1972; Lindsay *et al.*, 1979; Matthews *et al.*, 1982).

The patient is uncertain when the next loss of control will occur or what activity will be interrupted (Svoboda, 1979). The child faces rejection by those on whom the child must rely if consciousness is lost. The appearance of distress in people around them may often cause the child to develop a distorted impression of what happened (Holmes, 1987). The uncontrolled limb movements or loss of consciousness may lead to feelings of a lack of control and dependence (Weisbrot & Ettinger, 1998). Children may experience feelings of fear as the aura of an impending seizure begins to build up. The older child with tonic–clonic seizures may have difficulty understanding how one can be perfectly normal at one moment and in the middle of a seizure the next. Even the child with absence attacks may have difficulty grasping the idea of being out of touch for seconds and deny that the attack occurred (Vining, 1990).

Fear

A seizure may be fearsome to a young child. There may be a fear of returning to where the first seizure occurred, be it a classroom or a bed. The fear of dying during seizures may increase anxiety and dependence. When the child is old enough to understand what is happening, the seizure events become frightening, often distorted in the child's imagination. School-aged children worry about the seizures, medical procedures, medications, and the responses of others. Children want to know what caused the seizures (Austin, 1993; Austin *et al.*, 1993; Austin, 2001). An older child fears the social catastrophe of a seizure in public, seeking to conceal all aspects of the disorder that refuses to remain hidden (Svoboda, 1979).

Handicap

Children worry when they see handicapped children in public areas, fearing that they may turn out like them. Repeated attacks, examinations, and tests rapidly convince the child that they have a handicap (Austin, 2001).

Identity: disease concept

Miller (1978) writes that there are four independent scales that can be applied to a symptom to decide whether it demands attention: the degree of discomfort, of alarm, of disability, and of embarrassment. Most disorders rise high on one or two scales, whereas epilepsy, at one time or another, may be high on all scales. There are visible disabilities (e.g. cerebral palsy) and invisible, "surprise" disabilities (e.g. epileptic attack). People are more apt to accept disabilities that they are aware of, as they do not like being surprised.

Identity

The pressure to deal with reactions from peers who observe the seizures may lead to feelings of being different and thus rejected by others (Weisbrot & Ettinger, 1998). In adolescence, this negatively distorts the adolescent developmental basics of "Who am I?" (identity), "Where am I going?" (future) and "What am I doing here?" (status). Adolescents need peer acceptance. The epileptic teenager may not see hopeful answers. They may see an identity as damaged, perhaps incomplete, even possibly grotesque, and unwanted. Often, the adolescent imagines the attacks to be far worse than they really are. The future may seem bleak and limited (Svoboda, 1979).

The better the adolescent's seizure control, the less likely they are to discuss their epilepsy with others, i.e. a form of denial. Adolescents who are most normal neurologically are more negative about their social adjustment and the impact of the epilepsy on their families. Those who have had seizures in public appear to be better adapted than those who are fearful that someday it might actually happen.

Some adolescents with epilepsy begin to deny their epilepsy, such as by skipping medication. Seizure recurrence reinforces their poor self-concept as defenses are shattered. Some patients may become obsessed with their medicine and the adherence to a daily routine in order to avoid the attacks. A seizure breakthrough that occurs despite their best efforts is devastating (Svoboda, 1979).

Inferiority

Feelings of inferiority and insecurity may lead to withdrawal from social interactions, thus decreasing the chances of gaining social skills. Attitudes may be marked by negativity towards society, voiced with projection on to others for the child's own self-rejection. Society is more apt to reject the patient because of personality than because of epilepsy. If the depression becomes too great, adolescents may overdose on the medications or may drive recklessly, as if risking death (Svoboda, 1979).

Whose problem is it?

The child experiences being taken from doctor to doctor, from test to test, and from pill to pill, all in a futile search for cause and cure. Each doctor tends to talk to the parents before noticing the patient during the examination. The child is poked, prodded, pounded, and punctured. Then the physician turns their back and resumes talking with the parents. A child may decide that since the doctor pays attention to, talks with, and explains the problems to the parents, and since the parents are the ones who seem concerned about the medications, the seizure problem must be the parents' responsibility. Such children may know little about their epilepsy, leaving all up to their parents. Occasionally, teens may refuse, omit, or hide their pills in denial or may use the threat of a seizure to manipulate the parents (Svoboda, 1979). Doctors need to talk honestly with their young patients about their seizures, encouraging them to participate in the monitoring and care (Vining, 1990).

Learned helplessness

Individuals with intractable epilepsy who have learned that the occurrence of a seizure is beyond their control can develop a passive, helpless attitude towards many aspects of life. Then, as adults, if seizure surgery renders them seizure-free, the overall postoperative psychosocial adjustments may be more guarded, for such individuals may not have learned to depend on themselves. Two measures of learned helplessness, depression and a lack of resourcefulness, correlate with a poor psychosocial adjustment independent of the seizure outcome (McLachlan *et al.*, 1992).

Dependence versus independence

Part of the adolescent developmental crisis is the struggle between dependence and independence, the latter being the desired goal. If seizures are a chronic problem, the older child may not be able to cope with this struggle, retreating back to a childlike dependency, the so-called Peter Pan syndrome, rather than growing up to an overwhelming future. This is especially true if the seizures have been present since early childhood. If the seizures begin during the adolescent period, the patient is often able to make the transition to independence, although the trip may be a struggle (Svoboda, 1979).

The forever fourteen syndrome

Some individuals make it to the early adolescent stage of psychological development but seem to become stuck at the dependence versus independence stage, vacillating between dependency and rebellion well into adulthood (Svoboda, 1979).

Development

Perales (1999) noted that spurts, plateaus, and regressions mark normal psychological development. This is a major task for the growing child. The burden of epilepsy may be overwhelming to the child faced with the major challenge of maturation.

It is not just the seizure occurrences and the reactions of others that shape the child's behavior development; it is also the child's inherent temperament and the presence of other epilepsy-related language and learning problems that influence the child's behaviors. The total burden of management of the child's epilepsy and its complications may often be too heavy for the family to bear 24 hours a day. This may be especially prominent with younger children (Henriksen, 1988). The impact has to be considered in terms of the relevance to developing functions.

Infancy and toddler years

To develop autonomy and self-sufficiency, the child needs an environment that can allow increasing independence to emerge. When epilepsy emerges, a parental response of overprotection and overindulgence discourages normal development, deprives the child of feelings of competence, and fosters continued dependency. Children with chronic conditions often incorporate the disorder into their self-concept (Austin, 2001; Massie, 1985). Children with epilepsy at ages three to four years may be extremely difficult to handle. Their natural egocentricity, compiled with their parents' fear of inciting a seizure, can make them tyrannical monsters. They may display outbursts of temper, refuse to go to bed, or refuse to eat, and they are extremely difficult to handle if their demands are not fulfilled. This behavior begins early in life. Parents tend to be less firm when bringing up a handicapped child, trying to avoid anything that may precipitate a seizure or undesirable behavior. The child quickly senses this and becomes able to rule the parents and the home. The behavior problem can be greater than the seizure problem (Henricksen, 1977).

Childhood

Developmental tasks include becoming more independent and more involved with peers as part of developing social skills. Epilepsy can inhibit this in that negative experiences and exclusion by others cause withdrawal. Social development has also been related to parenting. The parents' restrictions of the child with epilepsy may inhibit the development of socialization opportunities. Children tend to be more dependent (Hartlage & Green, 1972). Maternal praise is related to the child's competence and positive affect. Conversely, intrusive and overcontrolling parenting behaviors are related to decreased child autonomy and decreased confidence (Hartlage et al., 1972; Austin et al., 1991).

Adolescence

The prime developmental task of adolescence is to consolidate one's identity. Major tasks include the achievement of independence, establishment of intimate relationships outside the family, and identification of a future vocation. The presence of a chronic condition such as epilepsy can interfere with the accomplishment of these developmental tasks, leading to a prolonged adolescence period (Strax, 1991). Children with epilepsy are more apt to be over-restricted and less experienced socially. This adds to the poor self-esteem and sense of being different (McCollum, 1981; Austin *et al.*, 1991). Even children with epilepsy newly diagnosed in adolescence feel different from others and fear being teased (Austin, 1993). Driving is restricted, further limiting independence and opportunities for social activities (Dean & Austin, 1996).

The parents

Studying the family dynamics becomes vital in understanding and helping the child. Perales (1999) emphasized the importance of family function. Seizures alter family functioning. This relates to the family size, care-taking demands, the frequency and severity of the seizures, and the family's financial and social status. Disruptions in the family life occur due to seizure unpredictability, changes in drug therapy, frequent physician visits, and mounting financial costs. Academic performance and behavior are affected. Adverse factors include marital conflicts, restricted activities, sibling difficulties, lack of social support, and loss of family cohesion. Parents may feel overwhelmed and feel a chronic fatigue, especially with children with nocturnal seizures.

Families of epileptic children with behavior difficulties display generally poorer functioning, less social support, and limited financial resources compared with families of well-functioning children. Divorce or separation is a strong predictor of behavior problems and depression (Hermann *et al.*, 1989; Weisbrot & Ettinger, 1998). Parental psychopathology, when present, correlates with psychiatric disturbances and dependency in epileptic children (Hoare & Kerley, 1991; Weisbrot & Ettinger, 1998).

In one study, although 42% of parents of epileptic children felt that neither they nor their child were disrupted by the onset of epilepsy, 33% perceived that their lives, rather than their child's, were disrupted. The majority of parents perceive their child as adapting well. Seizures of suspected but unproven cause rather than idiopathic epilepsy create greater suspense in parents. Children with seizure onset in adolescence and children with epilepsy plus additional handicaps adapt poorly (Oostrom *et al.*, 2001).

The diagnosis of epilepsy may promote family closeness and increase discussion in some. More agreement about the upbringing and management of the epileptic child emerges in parents. Family activities are altered. Outings tend to be restricted, especially if they risk the embarrassment of a seizure. Since the parents may not entrust their child to a babysitter, the family tends to stay at home. Often family members feel tied down (Svoboda, 1979).

Diagnosis: a grief reaction

Grass (1977) and the Federal Commission for the Control of Epilepsy and Its Consequences described the grief reaction of parents to the diagnosis of infantile spasms, which may apply to many types of epilepsy in children, based on the stages of a grief reaction to a loss, as explained by Ross & Peckham (1983). The stages include shock and denial, guilt and blame, bargaining and cure seeking, depression and withdrawal, and acceptance, in varied order. Determining the stage that the parent has reached can guide those working with them to help them move on to succeeding stages (Green & Solnit, 1964).

Shock and denial

The shock of the diagnosis is accompanied by the denial that it could possibly be epilepsy, not just by the parents but also by other relatives (Voeller & Rothenberg, 1973). This triggers fears and anxiety as well as feelings of inadequacy, leading to feelings that the child is especially vulnerable. The fear that the child will die, be brain damaged, be unable to learn, or be dependent on them into adulthood may emerge. The parents fear leaving the child alone (Henriksen, 1988). Anxieties relate to the seizures and management (including costs), reactions of others, needed lifestyle changes, and behavior challenges. As the child senses the parent is fearful of seizures, the child becomes fearful as well (Vining, 1990).

Most (73%) parents of epileptic children do not consider epilepsy a social stigma. They are more worried about their child's mind becoming weak (69%) and of having an uncertain future (52%). Their knowledge of epilepsy is poor, and they have mixed attitudes toward the child (Singhi *et al.*, 1991). Parents tend to expect their children with epilepsy to have more emotional problems and to be more unpredictable and highly strung (Long & Moore, 1979). Girls with epilepsy have more problems than boys. Family variables of decreased communication and consultation with medical personnel, increased family stress, and decreased extended family social support are associated with increased behavior problems (Austin *et al.*, 1991). School absenteeism is rarely related to seizure frequency but rather to the parents' failure to insist on attendance, often a symptom of overprotection (Ross & Peckham, 1983).

Families may not feel adequate to handle the challenges they envision of a child with epilepsy. They have to cope not only with the psychosocial stigma that haunts the disorder but also with what to disclose to others, including other parents, teachers, etc. They have to learn new vocabularies from special education and the mental health field (Austin, 1996). Parents come to the physician with concerns about present and future functioning, their own parenting adequacy, and about behavioral aspects and learning. The medical personnel respond by explaining the epilepsy classification name, the EEG results, how the medications are to be taken, and about blood levels.

Guilt and blame

Parents may come to think that somehow they were responsible for their child's epilepsy (Nhan, 1975). They worry about their ability to cope and about the financial responsibilities that will ensue, and they experience anger that fate has dealt this blow (Grass, 1977). The mother may feel that somehow she is to blame and therefore devote her time to trying to make it up to the child, even to the exclusion of other family members, including her spouse (Henriksen, 1988). The father may seek an intellectual pursuit for answers and to discover who is to blame. These two stages often give rise to a vulnerable child syndrome.

The parents often become angry because they do not know the cause or the future. They may focus their anger on the physician because of perceived insensitivity or because they feel the doctor is not working hard enough to find a cause, or they focus their anger on the school because they feel the school is not understanding or providing the right education or is being too restrictive (Vining, 1990).

Vulnerable child syndrome

A child who, in the parents' eyes, is felt to be fragile and vulnerable to harm because of a handicap or near-loss of an ability, a prior threatening experience, or resemblance to another family member who experienced medical problems is seen as needing to be protected from any further harm. The parent often appears overly concerned with trivial health matters and gives vivid recalls about previous concerns. The parent and child may have separation anxieties. Such a child often acts immature since the parents treat him or her like a younger child for fear that the child might grow up only to die young. Often, there is a history of school underachievement or phobia. The presentation may be modified by the nature of the insult and the recovery thereafter as well as the relationship between the child and parents and the relationships with the treating physician. The child's basic health and emotional personality are significant (Green & Solnit, 1964). Thus, the child ends up being overprotected, over-restricted, overindulged, and underdisciplined. When this emerges, family counseling is vital (Lerman, 1977; Henriksen, 1988). Prevention is preferable.

Excessive indulgence and permissiveness are admitted to by 80% of families with children who have epilepsy (Lerman, 1977). However, the same parents tend to be more dominant, restrictive, and strict with the epileptic child. Constant supervision is felt necessary by 32% of parents. Activities that are prohibited include swimming (28%), cycling (21%), and team sports (15%) (Long & Moore, 1979). School physicians may automatically bar the child from almost all school activities (Lerman, 1977), although the risks of injury from underprotection is less than the mental damage resulting from overprotection (Taylor, 1977).

Epilepsy in childhood is a major trigger of this vulnerability, when the parent has both good and bad feelings towards the child, which is normal. This often creates further fears of possible harm to the child. Parents need to be warned against overindulgence, permissiveness, and overprotection. The epileptic child should be brought up essentially as a healthy child with the same privileges and duties as demanded as others. Group therapy for parents and guidance of the child may be very helpful (Lerman, 1977).

Social outcasting

The child with epilepsy may be confined to the home with no friends and no one to talk about the seizures. The child feels rejected by school, friends and neighbors. Lack of normal social contacts means the child cannot learn to socialize. Thus, the child remains insecure, overdependent, emotionally immature, and socially inept when adulthood is reached (Lerman, 1977).

Family problems

The family may have difficulties coping with the illness of the child. Families of children with epilepsy have a distinct adjustment pattern different from families of children with other medical conditions, with a high risk for problems in family communication, cohesion, and integration (Ferrari *et al.*, 1982).

The mothers of children with secondarily generalized seizures show significantly more psychological stresses compared with those of mothers of children with idiopathic partial and primary generalized seizures. Improvement in seizure control does not mean the disappearance of psychosocial problems encountered in epileptic families. The families, especially mothers and spouses, show considerable psychologic distress (Kugoh & Hosokawa, 1991).

Marital stress

The majority (64%) of parents report that the child's epilepsy negatively affects their partners. Effects on the marital relationship are often described as either negative (44%) or positive (37%). The majority (63%) of parents report no parental disagreement with regard to their child, with each parent having equal say in decision-making (66%) (Eastman *et al.*, 1999).

Intractable seizures affect family life. The relationship between the parents is more stressful (80%). The time spent with the spouse is reduced significantly (50%). The time spent with their other children is diminished (50%). Parents express feelings of guilt because they focus most of their time and energies on their child with seizures, neglecting their other children (Lightstone *et al.*, 1993).

Bargaining and cure seeking

At this stage, families may seek spiritual comfort and guidance, looking for miracles of some sort. This may provide emotional relief and encouragement (Grass, 1977).

The parents go from doctor to doctor, from specialist to specialist, seeking a cure but often resulting only in interruptions and restarts in the care of the child. Any continuity of care is usually lost as the records are slow to reach the next physician. Eventually, some parents may turn to paramedical or non-medical healers offering unproven cures. The result is often a worsening of the seizure control and further discouragement.

If the seizures persist, the family begins to realize that they must deal with the ramifications of living with a chronic condition. The specter of a period of seizures hangs over the family. The uncertainty of when the next seizure will occur is a major social stress. The parents' adjustment includes understanding the illness, mastering treatments, trying to create a normal life for the child but adapting the family's routines to the condition, and negotiating with school and health professionals. Continued trips to the physician and pharmacy are inconvenient and expensive (Austin, 1996). Bonding with the child is often distorted. The child may be seen as a duty (born of guilt) or as an impediment (born of anger), although this is rarely voiced. Parental rejection leading to hostility or compensatory overprotection is seen, associated with psychosocial maladjustment in children with absence epilepsy (Lerman, 1977).

The incidence of child abuse is greatly increased in the handicapped population, with figures variously given as between 25% and 40%. Abuse may be physical, verbal, or sexual. Neglect is a form of abuse. Children with seizures, especially if other handicaps are also present, are especially prone to abuse and less able to defend themselves.

Depression and withdrawal

Families may go through a period of depression. The most common familial experience is a period of depression, which may be profound. Parents tend to become unable to interact normally with others and become withdrawn, much like the period of psychological mourning for a dead person. This depression may return for brief periods in the future but usually to a shorter and lesser degree (Grass, 1977). The family tends to accept the seizures as their fate and to begin missing appointments. They may refuse any new medicines or procedures, limiting care to that from a family physician, who will continue to supply the antiepileptic medications but often without monitoring the child. An occasional seizure is felt to be acceptable. In the extreme, parents may stop seeking medical care and try to withdraw the antiepileptic drugs, believing them to be ineffective in curing epilepsy. The parents may not wish to be seen in public with the child and thus may withdraw from society, staying home to care for the child. Intolerance of the child's behavior may be voiced, but the parents do not know how to manage the stigmatized child, the inattentive, disobedient child, or the overly energetic or clumsy child, often described as hyperactive (Svoboda, 1979).

The institutionalization cycle

Some parents may be so overwhelmed that they turn to a special school or institutional placement where experts reside. Even at such an institution, however, the child may not achieve hoped-for improvements, causing the parents to feel that they could achieve as much at home, thus recycling the whole process again. The authorities need to work with the parents on goals and updates and with provision of respite care opportunities (Svoboda, 1979).

Acceptance

The goal is acceptance of the situation by the family working together (Grass, 1977). Utilizing community supports, respite care facilities, and counseling can help this, as can a close cooperation with caring and concerned teachers (Holdsworth & Whitmore, 1974). Resolution of previous tensions may offer hope of better seizure control (Blumer & Levin, 1977). Beyond mere acceptance, it is important to look at the talents and skills of the child: determine not just what they cannot do but what they can do and how they can do better. In school, the emphasis should be on learning abilities, not just on learning disability. At home, the emphasis should be on accomplishments and good behaviors, not just on "You can't" and "You shouldn't."

The family

With appropriate seizure care approaches, a minority of children (39%) of autocratic parents continue to have seizures, whereas the majority of children (61%) of non-autocratic parents are seizure-free (Hauck, 1972). Families need to be encouraged to learn appropriate reactions to seizures and ways to promote independent living skills, to prevent their lives revolving around the family members with epilepsy (Thompson & Oxley, 1988).

Siblings

Siblings influence the child's reaction to the epilepsy. If they are jealous that the child gets too much attention, they are apt to develop behavior problems themselves. They may take out their resentment on their sibling by fighting or even ignoring them. Siblings may also feel guilty, for example feeling that they were playing too roughly with the child before the seizures began. The siblings need to be reassured that they did not cause the epilepsy. They may feel the need to protect their sibling, which can stifle normal interactions, or they may fear that epilepsy is contagious and they may get it or that they may have inherited the tendency (Vining, 1990).

Roles

An epileptic child may be categorized as the angelic child who can do no wrong, the scapegoat who is blamed for everything, or even the sick child for whom the rest of the family must provide care. The angel child struggles to achieve the level expected of them; the scapegoat begins to believe and act the role of the loser. In some families, there is the sick child, who everyone expects little of and takes care of as the burden to bear. Children with epilepsy often see themselves as imperfect and thus tend to grow towards dependency. Thus, roles that children may adopt can hurt more than help, as they constrict and stifle development.

Covert jealousy

Perales (1999) emphasizes that psychosocial adaptation to chronic illness affects siblings. Neglect of the healthy siblings may lead to jealousy and guilt in the rest of the family. Hostility and anger towards the afflicted child may emerge, which can alternate with periods of overindulgence. The child's siblings often appear to understand and help, although covertly they may be jealous of the extra attention the child with epilepsy receives. Sometimes, the siblings are teased about their epileptic brother or sister. Frequently, the siblings are given extra chores and responsibilities, while the epileptic child is given fewer duties (Svoboda, 1979).

Although children seldom voice their resentment that their brother or sister gets attention because of their epilepsy, they will often admit to it if questioned. They notice that mother shoulders the major burden and thus do not want to give her any extra work. They may feel guilty if they show any resentment of this interpreted favoritism. Such children tend either to grow up to work with individuals who have handicaps, or to avoid any such type of work, even forgoing dating and marriage for the fear that they too may have a handicapped child.

In one group counseling approach, the siblings of handicapped children were gathered together to discuss what it was like to have a handicapped brother or sister. The adult counselor leading the group posed a series of questions to the children, who were not allowed to respond until they were passed a seashell. Such questions included: "Who works the hardest in caring for your special brother or sister?," "What have you learned from your special brother or sister?," "What have you taught your special brother or sister?," and "Have you ever been jealous of your special brother or sister?" The answers were quite similar. Mother was credited with working the most in caring for the needs of the handicapped child. Jealousy was common for various reasons, including the extra attention, the jobs inherited by the siblings because the handicapped child could not do them, and the time the parents spent with the handicapped child (at the doctor's surgery or the hospital). None of the children wanted to exchange places with their special sibling, however, when it came to having the tests done, even if it meant receiving more attention.

School and society

A child with epilepsy needs to be in school as much as possible, not just to learn but to experience social interactions. The possibility of frequent absences from school may lead to difficulties maintaining academic performance (Weisbrot & Ettinger, 1998). The availability of longer-acting anticonvulsant drugs can help by avoiding the need for midday medication. A knowledgeable teacher can be a valuable part of the team monitoring the child's needs, progress, and performance (Svoboda, 1979). Academic achievements should be realistic and not just based on parent or teacher expectations. Underestimations of the child's potential (Weisbrot & Ettinger, 1998) may cause those concerned to be satisfied too easily with class performance (Green & Hartlage, 1971). In earlier grades, classmates may be sympathetic and supporting until they have had a chance to be told about seizures. At all ages, a sympathetic and knowledgeable teacher, especially one who has had seizures, can lead the entire class to understanding and acceptance. Some schools, anticipating future potential employment problems, begin a prevocational preparatory training in early adolescence and move on to vocational training, adapting the educational curriculum to the vocational needs, so that the child will be ready to be a working adult. Counseling is often a vital part of this approach (Svoboda, 1979).

REFERENCES

Austin, J. K. (1993). Concerns and fears of children with seizures. *Clin. Nurs. Pract. Epilepsy* **1**: 4–6.

Austin, J. K. (1996). A model of family adaptation to new-onset childhood epilepsy. *J. Neurosci. Nurs.* **28**: 82–92.

Austin, J. K. (2001). Psychosocial aspects of pediatric epilepsy. In *Psychatric Issues in Epilepsy*, ed. A. B. Ettinger & A. M. Kanner, pp. 319–32. Philadelphia: Lippincott Williams & Wilkins.

Austin, J. K., Dunn, D. W. & Levstek, D. A. (1993). First seizures: concerns and ends of parents and children. *Epilepsia* **34** (suppl 6): 24.

Austin, J., Risinger, M. W. & McNelis, A. (1991). Family, seizure and gender variables associated with child behavior problems. *Epilepsia* **32** (suppl 3): 29.

Avondet, M., Castelli, Y. & Scaramelli, A. (1991). Psychologic and social adjustment in adolescents with epilepsy. 19th International Epilepsy Congress. *Epilepsia* **32** (suppl 1): 43.

Blumer, D. & Levin, K. (1977). Psychiatric Complications in the epilepsies: current research and treatment. *McLean Hospital Journal*, Special Issue 15.

Dean, P. & Austin, J. K. (1996). Adolescent psychosocial issues in epilepsy. *Clin. Nurs. Pract. Epilepsy* **3**: 4–6.

Eastman, M., Ritter, F. J., Risse, G. L. & Frost, M. D. (1999). Impacts of child's epilepsy on the parents. *Epilepsia* **40** (suppl 7): 129.

Ferrari, M., Matthews, W. S. & Barabas, G. (1982). The family and the child with epilepsy. *Fam. Process* **22**: 53–9.

Grass, E. (1977). Infantile spasms. In *The Plan for Action on Epilepsy*, ed. Commission for the Control of Epilepsy and Its Consequences, Vol. 11, pp. 374–8. Bethesda, MD: National Institutes of Neurological and Communicative Disorders and Stroke.

Green, J. B. & Hartlage, L. C. (1971). Comparative performance of epileptic and non-epileptic children and adolescents. *Dis. Nerv. Syst.* **32**: 418–21.

Green, J. & Solnit, A. J. (1964). Reaction to the threatened loss of a child: a vulnerable child syndrome. *Pediatrics* **34**: 58–66.

Guerrant, J., Anderson, W. W., Fischer, A., *et al.* (1962). Personality in Epilepsy. Springfield, IL: Charles C. Thomas.

Hartlage, L. C. & Green, J. B. (1972). The relationship of parental attitudes to academic and social achievement in epileptic children. *Epilepsia* **13**: 21–6.

Hartlage, L. C., Green, J. B. & Offutt, L. (1972). Dependency in epileptic children. *Epilepsia* **13**: 27–30.

Hauck, C. (1972). Sociological aspects of epilepsy research. *Epilepsia* **13**: 79–85.

Henricksen, O. (1977). Behavior modification and rehabilitation of patients with epilepsy. In *Epilepsy, The Eighth International Symposium*, ed. J. K. Penry, pp. 225–34. New York: Raven Press.

Henriksen, L. (1988). Specific problems of children with epilepsy. *Epilepsia* **29** (suppl 3): 6–9.

Hermann, B. P., Whiteman, S. & Dell, J. (1989). Correlates of behavior problems and social competence in children with epilepsy, aged 6–11. In *Childhood Epilepsies: Neuropsychological, Psychosocial and Intervention Aspects*, ed. B. P. Hermann & M. Seidenberg, pp. 143–57. New York: John Wiley & Sons.

Hoare, P. (1984). Does illness foster dependency? A study of epileptic and diabetic children. *Dev. Med. Child Neurol.* **26**: 20–24.

Hoare, P. & Kerley, S. (1991). Psychosocial adjustment of children with chronic epilepsy and their families. *Dev. Med. Child Neurol.* **33**: 201–15.

Hodgman, C., McAnarney, R., Myers, G., *et al.* (1979). Emotional complications of adolescent grand mal epilepsy. *J. Pediatr.* **905**: 309–12.

Holdsworth, L. & Whitmore, K. (1974). A study of children with epilepsy attending ordinary school. I: their seizure patterns, progress and behavior in school. *Dev. Med. Child Neurol.* **16**: 746–58.

Holmes, G. L. (1987). Psychosocial factors in childhood epilepsy. In *Diagnosis and Management of Epilepsy in Children*, pp. 112–24. Philadelphia: W. B. Saunders.

Kugoh, K. & Hosokawa, K. (1991). Psychological aspects of patients with epilepsy and their family members. 19th International Epilepsy Congress. *Epilepsia* **32** (suppl 1): 43.

Lambert, M. V. & Robertson, M. M. (1999). Depression in epilepsy: etiology, phenomenology and treatment. *Epilepsia* **40** (suppl 10): 21–47.

Lerman, P. (1977). The concept of preventive rehabilitation in childhood epilepsy: a plea against overprotection and overindulgence. In *Epilepsy, the Eighth International Symposium*, ed. J. K. Penry, pp. 265–8. New York: Raven Press.

Lightstone, L., O'Dell, C., Moshe, S. & Shinnar, S. (1993). Social impact of intractable epilepsy in children on the family. *Epilepsia* **34** (suppl 6): 4.

Lindsay, J., Ounsted, C., & Richards, P. (1979). Longer-term outcome in children with temporal lobe seizures. III: psychiatric aspects in childhood and adult life. *Dev. Med. Child Neurol.* **21**: 630–36.

Long, C. G. & Moore, J. R. (1979). Parental expectations for their epileptic children. *J. Child Psychol. Psychiatry* **20**: 299–312.

Massie, R. K. (1985). The constant shadow: reflections on the life of a chronically ill child. In *Issues in the Care of Children with Chronic Illness*, ed. N. Hobbs & J. M. Perin, pp. 13–23. San Francisco: Josey-Bass.

Matthews, W. S., Barabas, G. & Ferrari, M. (1982). Emotional concomitants of childhood epilepsy. *Epilepsia* **23**: 672–81.

McCollum, A. T. (1981). *The Chronicailly Ill Child: A Guide for Parents and Professionals.* New Haven, CT: Yale University Press.

McLachlan, R. S., Chevaz, C. J., Derry, P. A., Blume, W. T. & Girvin, J. P. (1992). Learned helplessness is associated with poor psychosocial outcome after temporal lobectomy. *Epilepsia* **33** (suppl 3): 11.

Miller, J. (1978). Natural shocks. In *The Body in Question*, pp. 13–53. New York: Random House.

Nhan, N. (1975). *The Epileptic Child and His Family.* Leesburg, VA: National Children's Rehabilitation Center.

Oostrom, K. J., Schouten, A., Kruitwagen, C. J. J., Peter, A. C. B. & Jennekens-Schinkel, A. (2001). Parents' perception of adversity introduced by upheaval and uncertainty at the onset of childhood epilepsy. *Epilepsia* **42**: 1142–6.

Perales, M. (1999). Psychiatric management in epilepsy. Presented at the Via Christi Epilepsy Conference, Wichita, KS, 1999.

Ross, E. M. & Peckham, C. S. (1983). School children with epilepsy. In *Advances in Epileptology: XIVth Epielspy International Symposium*, ed. M. Parsonage, R. H. E. Grant, A. G. Craig, *et al.*, pp. 215–20. New York: Raven Press.

Singhi, P., Mukhopadhyay, K. & Singhi, S. (1991). Psychosocial stress, knowledge, beliefs and attitudes among parents of epileptic children. *Epilepsia* **32** (suppl 3): 849.

Strax, T. E. (1991). Psychological issues faced by adolescents and young adults with disabilities. *Pediatr. Ann.* **20**: 507–11.

Stores, G. & Piran, N. (1978). Dependency of different types in schoolchildren with epilepsy. *Psychol. Med.* **8**: 441–5.

Svoboda, W. B. (1979). Emotional and behavioral consequences of epilepsy. In *Learning About Epilepsy*, pp. 157–84. Baltimore, MD: University Park Press.

Taylor, D. C. (1977). Epilepsia and the sinister side of schizophrenia. *Dev. Med. Child Neurol.* **19**: 403–6.

Thompson, P. J. & Oxley, J. (1988). Socioeconomic accompaniments of severe epilepsy. *Epilepsia* **29** (suppl 1): 9–18.

Vining, E. P. G. (1990). The psychosocial impact of epilepsy in children and their family. *Int. Pediatr.* **5**: 186–8.

Voeller, K. & Rothenberg, M. (1973). Psychosocial aspects of the management of seizures in children. *Pediatrics* **51**: 1072–82.

Weisbrot, D. M. & Ettinger, A. B. (1998). Psychiatric aspects of Pediatric Epilepsy. *Prim Psychiatry* June pp. 51–67.

Ziegler, R. G. (1981). Impairments of control and competence in epileptic children and their families. *Epilepsia* **22**: 339–46.

31

Behavior problems: general

William Lennox advised us: "The burden of proof sits on anyone who contends that psychic symptoms in the absence of other epileptic symptoms is epilepsy."

Psychiatric challenges in seizure patients include personality disturbances, anger and aggressive reactions, depressions and suicidal reactions, hysterical behaviors, and psychotic disturbances. Children may have problems of immaturity, hyperactivity, temper, or acting-out episodes (Svoboda, 1979). In children, the emotional status may or may not relate to the age of seizure onset, the duration, the attack frequency, the EEG abnormality, or the extent of neuropsychological impairment (Berg et al., 1984). Family functioning variables are more influential in children with epilepsy (Hinton & Knights, 1969; Rutter et al., 1970; Whitehouse, 1971; Holdsworth & Whitmore, 1974; Cavazzuti, 1980; Weisbrot & Ettinger, 2001). The incidence of psychiatric disturbances at the time of seizure onset is between 24% and 45% (Papero et al., 1992; Austin et al., 1993; Dunn et al., 1997).

Children with epilepsy experience psychiatric disturbances four to five times more often than do children in control groups (Rutter et al., 1970; Henricksen, 1977). Comparing other medical conditions in childhood, the incidence of psychiatric problem is 31–48% in children with epilepsy, 21% in children with cardiac problems, 17% in children with diabetes, and 8.5% in controls (McDermott et al., 1995; Austin, 2001). If children are retarded and have epilepsy, the incidence of behavior problems is about 59% (Steffenburg et al., 1996). The incidence of behavior problems with complex partial epilepsy is twice that seen with other types of seizures (Guerrant et al., 1962; Rutter et al., 1970; Weisbrot & Ettinger, 2001).

Physicians who treat children with epilepsy will encounter patients with depression, anxiety, and a variety of behavior problems. Unrecognized, such problems lead to persistent emotional distress and affect academic, social, and emotional functions, and may result in later psychological maladjustments in adulthood (Weisbrot & Ettinger, 2001).

Factors

Factors that cause or influence psychopathology in epilepsy include neurobiologic variables, biologic variables, and psychosocial variables. Causes are usually multifactorial.

Neurobiological factors include the age of onset (especially if the onset occurs during critical periods of neurological development, such as during the formation of synaptic links), the type and frequency and duration of seizures, the etiology of the epilepsy, the degree of seizure control, the hemisphere of cerebral dysfunction, the ictal and interictal EEG, the drugs used, the seizure appearance, the neuropsychologic accompaniments, cerebral metabolism, and neurobehavioral and neurotransmitter aspects. The type of aura and the neuropsychological state at that time may be important (Hermann & Reill, 1981; Torta & Keller, 1999).

Biological factors include damage to areas related to psychologic functioning, emotional and cognitive side effects of the medications, either by interference with folate activity or by a direct action on neurotransmitters, and forced normalization. Medical aspects of this area also to be considered include monotherapy versus polytherapy, the total drug quantity, hormones and endocrine aspects, and cerebral and cerebellar metabolism (Torta & Keller, 1999).

Psychosocial factors include the chronicity, fear of seizures, and lifestyle changes caused by the seizures. Other factors include the individual's status (socioeconomic, educational, vocational), perceptions (stigma, discrimination), family influences (home environment, overprotection), legal limitations (such as driving), adjustment (to the seizures, lifestyle, vocational, financial), self-esteem, life event changes, and social support. Feelings of a lack of control over one's life are important. Environmental effects appear to be very potent. Factors increasing the risk for problems include work history, relationships, marriage, housing, social interactions, and finances (Torta & Keller, 1999).

The key predictors of problems include life event changes, adjustment to the environment, financial status, locus of control, and gender; financial status is the most significant. These are all causal or the result of the epilepsy problems. In children, the neuropsychologic problems may relate to the onset, duration, etiology, type, EEG, and control state. The psychologic status includes the family income and material support. Medical influences include monotherapy versus polytherapy, and the type and the number of antiepileptic drugs being used. Demographic factors include the age and gender. Other important aspects include social competence and behavior problems, which can be internalized or externalized. Thus, in the overall predictor listing, behavior factors include seizure control, marital status, and employment, whereas the social factors include seizure control, marriage, income, seizure duration, and possibly the age of onset and the seizure type (Hermann & Reill, 1981).

Stress triggers

Mattison (1993) reviewed the effects of stress on lowering the seizure threshold, noting that stress and sleep deprivation can both precipitate seizures. Sleep deprivation can increase the seizure discharge five- to ten-fold. Other triggers include missed medicine (82–84%), emotional stresses (57–58%), sleep deprivation (40–56%), physiologic states (28–37%), sensory stimuli (21–23%), alcohol (19–20%), menses (20–52%), fluid retention (11–14%), illness (9%), and other factors.

Emotional stressors in epilepsy include the unpredictability, which leads to feelings of a lack of control, anxiety, dependency, helplessness and poor self-esteem. The stress related to needing to deal with potential fear, horror, or other reactions of peers who observe the epilepsy leads to feelings of being different and being rejected by others. Another stress is the taking of medications that affect both behavior and cognition functions, potentially leading to feelings of a lack of control and both social and academic inadequacy. The stress of the fear of dying in a seizure leads to increased anxiety and dependence. The stress of frequent absences from school impairs school performance. The normal appearance between seizures leads to pressures to function completely normally. The underestimation by teachers of the child's intellectual potentials leads to poor self-esteem (Caplan *et al.*, 1997; Weisbrot & Ettinger, 2001).

Psychological precipitating factors

Reflex epilepsy is an almost immediate reaction to a stress. Stress may also alter the seizure threshold, leading to seizure development. Emotional stresses include fear or worry (59%), frustration (55%), anger (47%), stimulating experiences (46%), depression (25%), anticipation (20%), sudden stimuli (5%), boredom (6%), and happiness (3%) (Hermann & Reil, 1981; Weisbrot & Ettinger, 2001).

Complex partial epilepsies are most susceptible and generalized seizures least susceptible to such stimuli. Often, psychologic or classroom testing may inhibit or aggravate a discharge on the EEG. Attempts at correlating seizure frequency and occurrence with the stresses of day have not been successful, although seizures that occur at a certain time of day in children may be correlated with specific subjects in school or perhaps low points in blood levels of rapid-acting anticonvulsants. Switching the time of the subject may alter the seizure occurrence. Stressful interviews and acting out may show an occasional correlation between stress and the EEG. More often, a correlation is seen between stress, hyperventilation, and EEG. Anxiety can alter both the cardiac and brain activities. An increased discharge rate may be seen with suspense. Hyperventilation can be an stress reaction that the child is unaware of. Although hyperventilation is not ictal, both stress and novelty can produce hyperventilation, which in turn may activate focal, generalized, or myoclonic seizures. However, the aura of a seizure may trigger anxiety that can cause tachycardia and hyperventilation.

What may be stressful to the patient may not be seen as stressful to the physician. Stress may reduce medical compliance. Stress and emotions may result in insomnia, i.e. sleep deprivation, which can activate seizures. One factor may render a patient more susceptible to another factor. The feeling of stress without any physiological accompaniment may trigger seizures. Hospitalization, especially for monitoring, may reduce the environmental stresses of everyday life and thus result in fewer seizures. Elementary decision-making and simple psychosocial stresses may be sufficient to trigger seizures.

Effects of seizures on psychopathology

Trimble (1994) noted that a relationship between seizures and psychopathology is evident. Most antidepressants and many psychiatric drugs may produce seizures. Many anticonvulsants can produce psychiatric disorders, but some may help. Some antiepileptic drugs may be responsible for mood disturbances, but some may help. In some patients, psychiatric symptoms precede seizure onset, suggesting that underlying CNS disturbances rather than emotional reactions are largely responsible for behavioral difficulties in children. In other patients, external factors are most influential (Weisbrot & Ettinger, 2001). Electroshock therapy, postictal psychoses, and partial status epilepsy also indicate a link between psychopathology and seizures.

Patients presenting in a state of clouded consciousness may be mistaken as having a psychiatric condition when they actually are in complex partial status, with paranoid delusions, religious delusions, and other hallucinations. These usually relate to seizures involving the limbic system. Limbic system epilepsy is different from other forms of temporal lobe epilepsy. The mesial temporal lobe is markedly different genetically, cellularly, biochemically, and electrically from other paleocortex and the neocortex. This is especially true for the amygdala and hippocampus.

Trimble (1994) noted that in behaviors thought possibly to be seizure related, an EEG including sleep is important, especially including sleep stages 1 and 2, utilizing T1-2 as well as F7–8 electrodes. This will pick up about 80% of the seizure. Usually, the EEG picture is characteristic, but rarely the EEG may normalize. The problem is very rarely limited to just this area.

Biological antagonism

Various central neurotransmitter chemicals have been associated with epilepsy, including folic Acid, dopamine (Trimble, 1988), and GABA. Trimble noted that dopamine agonists produce psychotic tendencies and manifest anticonvulsant potentials, whereas dopamine antagonism is antipsychotic but produces an epileptic tendency. Is the expression of the disorder related to internal discharges from neo-cortical pathways, perhaps involving the limbic system with spread to the mesial forebrain?

Blumer (1994) noted that the mental changes in epilepsy might be secondary to inhibition. There is delayed appearance of at least a year or two after the onset of seizures. Persistence, exacerbation, or de novo appearance may occur after remission of seizures through anticonvulsants or through surgery. These may alternate with the presence of seizure activity (paradoxical normalization). There may be postictal emergence.

Controversial abnormal behaviors

Trimble (1994) noted that awareness and acceptance of the existence of psycho-pathology in a large number of epileptic patients are emerging. Psychiatric aspects of epilepsy include personality disorders, psychoses, depression, and anxiety disor-ders. Ictal-related psychopathology include prodromata, auras, postictal affective and psychotic states, and interictal psychopathology. The auras of a complex partial seizure closely resemble various psychiatric disorders, including panic disorders. Interictal psychopathology includes personality disorders, anxiety, affective disor-ders, impulse control, and psychoses, both paranoid and schizophrenic. Affective disorders are treatable yet cause a high morbidity. More effective anticonvulsants have resulted in fewer long-term neuropsychiatric sequelae. Patients with limbic lesions are more vulnerable. Although not all patients develop problems, some do because of impaired functions of the limbic system.

The division of psychiatric disorders of epilepsy into ictal and interictal types is convenient, but the distinction between the two is not always clear (Trimble, 1988). Blumer (1994) reported that at one epilepsy center, the psychiatric grouping included patients with an interictal dysphoria disorder (34%), with some other psychiatric disorder (9%), with non-epileptic seizures (21%), with only minor psychiatric disturbances (12%), or without psychiatric disturbances (22%). Many patients (65%) needed psychiatric treatment. Often, patients tend to present with multiple symptoms. Those with mood disorders and those with psychoses tend to be treated in a similar fashion.

Patients with behavioral changes presenting as a seizure prodrome are often males with developmental disabilities and frontal lobe onset of epilepsy. The prodrome begins at least ten minutes before the seizure and may last from ten minutes to 36 hours, until the seizure occurs. The symptoms include disinhibition, behavioral outbursts, extreme animation, and decreased cognitive acuity. This persists until the seizure occurrs. Some patients also have a history of behavioral problems distinct from the prodromal illness (Oderberg et al., 1999).

Presurgical psychological assessments of children with intractable epilepsy have shown that the main problems of preadolescents are an oppositional defiant disorder with attention difficulties. Rarely, an adjustment disorder with anxiety is seen. In young adolescents, a mixed attention deficit disorder and oppositional defiant disorder predominates, although occasionally an adjustment disorder with anxiety or organic personality disorder is diagnosed. In the 15–21 years age range, 50% have a personality disorder and 20% an adjustment disorder with depression. Conduct disorder is not commonly seen. Earlier intervention may diminish the progressive psychopathology (Sharp *et al.*, 1993).

Autism and autistic-like behaviors

Autism is a neurological development symptom complex characterized by early onset of deficits in verbal and non-verbal communication skills, social and communicative dysfunctions, and repetitive behaviors. Children may present with some of these symptoms, often as a frustration reaction to some other cause, such as a receptive language deficit. Often, these children are labeled as having autism when actually they are autistic (manifesting autism-like behaviors) for other reasons. Autistic behaviors in childhood epilepsy may be seen in Lennox–Gastaut syndrome, tuberous sclerosis with secondary generalized epilepsy, Rett's syndrome, and retardation or dementia. The category of acquired aphasia with epilepsy denotes the causal relationship to epilepsy. True childhood autism may or may not be associated with epilepsy. There seems to be no specific relation to the process of epilepsy (Onuma, 2000).

In autism, the self-documented increased frequency of seizures and abnormal EEG findings supports the concept of a neurobiological basis. The increased incidence of epilepsy in the autism spectrum ranges from a low of 7% to a high of 42%, the frequency seeming to increase with age. The first peak occurs in early childhood before age five and the second peak occurs in adolescence. To arrive at diagnosis of true autism, a language-processing disorder must be ruled out (Tuchman *et al.*, 1998).

The main risk factors for seizures in autism include low intelligence, especially if combined with a motor deficit, or a language dysfunction. In the latter group, an auditory agnosia is found in 41% of patients, often with a severe receptive and expressive language disorder. The prevalence of epilepsy with autism is more frequent in girls (Tuchman *et al.*, 1999).

No specific EEG findings are characteristic of the autism spectrum. Prolonged EEG studies, especially including overnight recordings, may show abnormalities (60%). Even those patients without seizures have abnormal EEGs (46%). In 65%, the spikes are localized to the temporal lobes, perhaps more on the left. Although data suggest that seizures in autistic-spectrum children are no more frequent than in the general population (nor is the management with antiepileptic drugs), the question remains whether the localization of the abnormalities to the temporal lobe is related causally to the language regression or contributes to the language dysfunction, as seen with Landau–Kleffner syndrome and epileptic status with spike-wave status in sleep syndromes (Tuchman *et al.*, 1999).

All children with an autism spectrum and with significant expressive and receptive language dysfunction or with a history suggestive of a significant regression in language skills should be considered for a prolonged EEG study that includes a significant amount of sleep recording. If epileptiform activity in the temporal area is found, one needs to consider a controlled trial of anticonvulsants or steroids (Tuchman *et al.*, 1999).

Personality and character disorders

The existence of personality and character disorders related to epilepsy, especially temporal lobe epilepsy, has been a subject of spirited debate for over a century (Weisbrot & Ettinger, 1998). Trimble (1993) noted that numerous interictal behavior traits have been attributed to patients with epilepsy. Various clusters have been put forth as the antitheses. Subgroups of temporal lobe epileptics may be more susceptible to certain personality traits. This may pertain especially to psychoses that may relate to limbic/medial basal temporal lobe discharges. Limbic stimulation may lead to a cluster of motor emotional behaviors rather than particular motor presentations of the neocortex. Personality disorders in patients with epilepsy may be due to underlying organic brain damage, probably involving the frontal or temporal lobe. An emotionally unstable personality is probably the most common personality disorders in epilepsy (Onuma, 2000).

Limbic-temporal lobe syndromes

Some specialists describe a temporal lobe seizure personality and some go so far as to try to specify a "left temporal lobe syndrome" and a "right temporal lobe syndrome." Kluver–Bucy syndrome and Gastaut–Geschwind syndrome may be related but opposite facets of a damaged, inhibited temporal lobe versus an ictal excitatory temporal lobe (Benson, 1979).

Kluver–Bucy syndrome

This syndrome is one of exploratory behavior, increased sexual appetite (hypersexuality), decreased aggressivity (placidity), and a continuous environmental exploration as the consequence of bilateral temporal ablation. This is linked with damage to the anterior temporal lobe. It may represent an inhibitory state. This has been demonstrated in animal studies.

Gastaut–Geschwind syndrome

This syndrome, linked with temporal lobe epilepsy, is one of deepened emotions, circumstantiality, religiosity, sexual concerns (hyposexuality), hypergraphia, and viscosity (stickiness). Attempts to replicate this have produced mixed results. The syndromes do suggest a limbic disturbance, although not exclusive. There is probably more than one focus. The limbic syndrome is an integrated system and not necessarily lateralized (Trimble, 1991).

Geschwind felt this presentation represented an interictal disturbance, not an ictal event or an epileptic phenomenon due to neuronal changes, drugs, or psychosocial effectors. The electrical discharge is actually a chemical disturbance and the cause may be the chemical effect, possibly a continuous kindling-like effect, not an electrical effect. The features are seen more commonly in individuals with temporal lobe epilepsy than in patient with other seizure types, but they may also be seen in patients with temporal lobe problems but without seizures. It is not a frontal lobe syndrome and it does not present with frontal lobe symptoms.

This is an organic brain syndrome thought to be related to the underlying neuronal activity related to temporal lobe epileptic abnormalities, although the neuronal substrate is unclear. Other aspects of temporal lobe epilepsy may be more relevant, such as antisocial behavior, neurotic problems, and non-epileptic seizures (Trimble, 1991). Four of the features, i.e. increased concerns with philosophic, moral, and religious issues, hypergraphia, hyposexuality, and irritability, have been referred to in the Geschwind epileptic personality. This may come on at any point after the seizure onset at any age. The symptoms appear to be acquired due to an organic insult and often are treated organically. The losses of bonding, of language, and of social skills are seen in many organic syndromes, leading to problems of social integration. These traits are subtle and are often not present unless elicited (Benson, 1979).

Interictal personality syndrome of Blumer

Blumer (1972) was among the first to describe an interictal personality syndrome including circumstantiality, altered sexuality, and altered mental functions. Circumstantiality involves motor, verbal, and writing functions. Motor acts are described as sticky or viscous. Verbal features are described as logorrhea and overinclusive. Writing is described as hypergraphia (excessive writing). Altered sexuality includes hyposexuality, sexual fetishes, homosexuality, and occasional perversions. Altered mental functions include cognitive and emotional aspects. Cognitive changes include religiosity, humorlessness, and cosmic concerns. Emotionality is often heightened, with intensified emotional responsiveness (Benson, 1979). In a small sample of adults, the dominant temporal lobe appeared to be associated with a sense of personal destiny, paranoia, humorlessness, and conscientiousness, whereas those with non-dominant temporal involvement were high in obsessionality, dependency, sadness, viscosity, circumstantiality, emotionality, hypermoralism, and sexual deviation (Bear & Fedio, 1977).

Common temporal syndrome symptoms

Obsessiveness, viscosity, paranoia, hypergraphia, circumstantiality, emotionality, anger, depression, and dependence are often mentioned. Patients with a limbic focus may show increased traits throughout, but especially hypergraphia, elation, guilt, and paranoia. Patients with left-sided foci may be increased slightly in self-rating scales. In depth electrode studies, all traits but especially humorlessness appear increased in frontal lobe epilepsy (Weisser, 1986). There is not a neat distribution of trait clusters among different epilepsy and control groups, although the traits tend to be more frequent in those with epilepsy (Csernansky et al., 1990).

Patients with complex partial seizures of temporal lobe origin are thought to be higher in manifestations of a sense of personal destiny, dependency, paranoia, and philosophical interests compared with those with generalized seizures (Hermann & Reil, 1981). Religiosity, humorlessness, and cosmic concerns have also been reported. Increased religious convictions is not a consistent feature, although allegedly is seen more often, with temporal lobe epilepsy, especially that involving the left temporal lobe (Csernansky et al., 1990). Religiosity, signifying the degree of religious fundamentalism, the type of religious beliefs, and the extent of participation in religious activity, is an obvious characteristic that occurs only rarely in patients with epilepsy. In screening patients with left, right, and non-temporal lobe seizures, no hyperreligiosity was seen (Pritchard, 1984; Tucker et al., 1985).

The left temporal lobe has also been linked with self-reported psychotic disorders, increased thought disorders, psychoses, and affect disturbances (Csernansky et al., 1990). Excessive moralism is seen with temporal-limbic foci, especially in males (Weisser, 1986). Humorlessness may be more frequent in left temporal lobe epilepsy, especially in patients with longer duration of refractory temporal lobe seizures.

Emotionality is often increased, with intensified emotional responsiveness, especially in females (Benson, 1979). Patients with seizure onset before age five show increased sadness (Weisser, 1986). Irritability, poor impulse control, and aggressiveness are also reported (Weisbrot & Ettiger, 1998). Aggression and hostility in epilepsy may be neuropsychologic or social factors, are seen most often in males, and are more likely in those with seizure onset before age ten. Other risk factors include premature interruption of formal schooling, lower intelligence, and a lower socioeconomic rating. At an epilepsy center, 5% of patients were found to manifest aggressive behavior. There may or may not be a link to temporal lobe seizures.

Circumstantiality of motor, verbal, and writing functions is reported to be more common with temporal-limbic foci (Benson, 1979; Weisser, 1986).

Circumstantiality is a characteristic of some patients who have insecurities in expressing their thoughts.

Hypergraphia is described as excessive writing (Benson, 1979). Written efforts are extensive and overly detailed. Hypergraphia is not characteristic in epilepsy, but when present it is most apt to be seen with temporal lobe foci (7–10%) (Hermann & Reil, 1981; Hermann et al., 1983; Hermann et al., 1985). Sometimes, the hypergraphic individual is the non-epileptic mother of the child with temporal lobe epilepsy, usually a mother who is anxious that she gets every fact to the medical clinic so that they may be able to find a cure.

Logorrhea refers to a tendency to speak incessantly and often overinclusively (Benson, 1979). The patient may be desperate to convey all facts. If interrupted, rather than picking up at the point of the interruption, the patient may begin all over again.

Altered sexuality, including hyposexuality, sexual fetishes, homosexuality, and occasionaly perversions (Benson, 1979) may be seen in both sexes (Weisser, 1986). This may be more common in left temporal lobe epilepsy, especially in patients with longer duration of refractory temporal lobe seizures.

Obsessiveness may be more common in left temporal lobe epilepsy, especially in patients with longer duration of refractory temporal lobe seizures.

Motor acts are described as sticky or viscous (Benson, 1979). Viscosity appears to be increased in the left temporal lobe group, perhaps related to some combination of linguistic impairment, social cohesion, mental slowness, or psychological dependency (Herman & Reil, 1981). It is characterized by a sticky and cohesive interpersonal style, with prolonged verbal contacts and an emotional need to seek and maintain contact with others. There may be language impairments, slowness of cognitive performance, psychological dependence, and a peculiar tendency to seek social cohesiveness (Torta & Keller, 1999).

Children

The existence of a personality syndrome in adults is debatable. There is even less evidence for its existence in children (Weisbrot & Ettinger, 2001). Personality stereotypes have also been ascribed to pediatric epilepsy patients, including beliefs that such children are more withdrawn, socially isolated, aggressive, tense, and unpredictable, as assumed by teachers, other children, and parents (Hartlage & Green, 1972; Stores, 1978; Weisbrot & Ettinger, 1998). These may play a major adverse role in a child's adjustment in school settings, with the emergence in some children of school avoidance or school refusal. Others develop panic attacks or anxiety in social settings related to embarrassment about seizures in school or other social settings (Weisbrot & Ettinger, 2001).

Seizure problems that begin in early childhood are more often associated with personality and character disorders, problems in getting along with others, aggressive acting-out behaviors, and hyperactivity. Destructive lesions of the temporal lobe may disrupt the interchange of information between the centers relating to emotions and those relating to sensory learning processes. Seizures may disrupt or overstimulate these centers and their connections. This disruption could result in new and changed associations (Svoboda, 1979).

In some older children with temporal lobe epilepsy, a peculiar type of vicious behavior develops. They become slow, circumstantial, and preservative in their speech, move on to new topics with great difficulties, and dislike interruption. They are similarly persistent, pedantic, and sticky in their motor and contact behavior. In adults, this is referred to as the epileptic personality, characteristic of temporal lobe epilepsies. At most, only one in six adults display this behavior (Bamberger & Matthess, 1959; Blumer & Levin, 1977).

Many patients with a temporal lobe seizure problem do not exhibit clear-cut signs of the various problems outlined. They may have overcome or suppressed the problem, or they may have been able to cope with the stresses that otherwise might have produced the problem. The emotional overreactions of the young child may mellow with maturation. Hyperactivity of early childhood may change into repetitive and persevering behavior by adolescence; sometimes, the change is toward more delinquent behavior. Temper outbursts in childhood often become rage reactions in adolescence, and may mellow to mere irritability in adulthood. Depression and suicidal tendencies become more common in later life (Svoboda, 1979).

Therapy

Personality traits as a whole are best referred for psychotherapy (Torta & Keller, 1999). Circumstantiality is usually treated with behavior modification and medication such as anticonvulsants, antidepressants, and antianxiety drugs. Cognitive interferences are treated with antipsychotic drugs and antianxiety drugs. Altered sexuality has been treated with anticonvulsants and epilepsy surgery (Benson, 1979). Unilateral anterior temporal lobectomy has eliminated marked irritability and global hyposexuality in some cases. Interictal episodic dyscontrol may respond to beta-blockers or behavioral oriented therapy. Some maladaptive personality traits (viscosity, hypergraphia) share characteristics seen in obsessive–compulsive disorders and thus may respond to serotonergic agents. These traits have psychopathological characteristics (e.g. perseverance, repetitiveness, compulsiveness) that are related to the spectrum of obsessive–compulsive disorders. Serotonergic agents such as selective serotonin reuptake inhibitors (SSRIs) may be beneficial if the characteristics are handicapping (Torta & Keller, 1999).

Seizures and seizure character traits

Adults and children with complex partial seizures of temporal lobe origin are thought to be prone to certain personality traits (Holmes, 1987). With children, cognitive, personality, and school problems are distributed equally between left and right temporal lobe foci (Camfield *et al.*, 1984).

Primary generalized seizures

In a study of children with primary generalized epilepsies, 54% were found to have psychiatric disorders (Caplan *et al.*, 1997). Early onset and poor seizure control are associated with the severity of illogical thinking in such children.

Absence seizures

Children with absence seizures may have greater difficulties in academic personal and behavior categories, especially with ongoing seizures. Poor sibling relationships, fewer social outings with peers, unwanted teen pregnancies, alcohol abuse, behavior problems reported by parents or teachers, and psychiatric as well as emotional difficulties, may present. School problems include below-average academic performance, repeating a grade, failing to graduate, and feeling left behind in school. Employment is less affected but there is a higher rate of unskilled labor and poor job satisfaction (Caplan *et al.*, 1997).

Juvenile myoclonic epilepsy

In children with juvenile myoclonic epilepsy (JME), reported traits include irresponsibility and impaired impulse control, neglect of duties, self-interest, emotional instability, exaggeration, inconsiderateness, quick temper, and distractibility. Self-induced sleep deprivation and poor compliance are common (Janz, 1959). There is a tendency to deny problems and conflicts. Such children may yield to temptations against better judgments (Bech *et al.*, 1976; Bech *et al.*, 1977). Higher rates of psychiatric disorders may be seen (Perini *et al.*, 1996; Vazquez *et al.*, 1993). These traits are also more common with adolescence. In past studies of personality traits, in individuals with juvenile myoclonic epilepsy and with psychomotor seizures, a higher degree of emotional weakness, emotional instability, and self-consciousness was said to exist compared with patients with generalized tonic–clonic seizures (Bech *et al.*, 1976; Bech *et al.*, 1977).

Frontal lobe seizures

Frontal dysfunction can alter personality, judgment, and executive function. Behavior problems such as an attention deficit/hyperactivity may be associated with orbital-frontal seizures (Powell *et al.*, 1997).

Temporal lobe seizures

There is no proven epileptic personality complex. Extremes of behavior can be accentuated in either direction. Some patients may be irritable and aggressive whereas others may become timid and apathetic. Psychoses, depression, paranoia, and personality disorders may be a negative pole of epilepsy-related behavior changes (Torta & Keller, 1999).

Complex partial seizures were once thought to be associated with global hypo-excitability or slowness, with cognitive deficits, depressed mood, and hyposexuality, but this has been doubted by a number of experts more recently. To this was added deepened emotional states, altered religious and sexual concerns, circumstantiality, and hypergraphia. The most common personality traits are viscosity, circumstantiality, hypergraphia, and, to a lesser degree, hyperreligiosity (Torta & Keller, 1999). Such trends are seen more often in certain types of learning and language problems that are associated with complex partial seizures.

Left and right temporal lobe tendencies

The two brain halves differ in their style of thought-processing. There may be significant differences in the related emotional behaviors. Each hemisphere may develop its own emotional reactions and behaviors, depending on that hemisphere's characteristic style of learning. The presentation may represent a combination of lateralized learning styles (auditory versus visual) and the reaction-responses of those interacting with the individual. Certain tendencies are reported more often depending on the laterality of the brain damage or seizure focus. A minority of children with seizures may display some of these tendencies. Often, such traits may reflect underlying differences and disabilities in learning and language styles that influence behavior development (Svoboda, 1979).

The left temporal lobe is involved more often than the right in epilepsy. Left temporal lobe seizures tend to appear at an earlier age than those on the right side. The left brain relates to language-processing. Misinterpretations may result in problems in interpersonal relationships as well as problems in the expression of the individual's own feelings. The individual is insecure in remembering and reporting, fearing the missing of some important detail. This can show up in excessive note-taking and overly detailed diaries. The distorted relationships between the emotional centers and the thinking centers that depend on verbal language processes may cause the patient to be overly aware of their feelings, consequently exaggerating them to others.

The right hemisphere handles non-verbal thinking. A child with a right temporal lobe seizure problem may have a more emotive disposition, which is displayed outwardly. Such displays include anger, sadness, elation, euphoria, talkativeness about trivia, a rigid tendency towards repeating the same behaviors, and a strict adherence to rules. Rarely, a child may desire strict punishment for anyone who disobeys the rules. The child may be more impulsive as the fragile emotions swing back and forth, often accompanied by acting-out behavior. This impulsivity may be directed outwards in aggressive behavior or inwards as depression.

Self-description

Patients with a left-sided disturbance may tend to overemphasize faults and minimize strengths and successes, thus tarnishing their image. Catastrophic reactions of anxiety and despair may appear when the patients is faced with a potential failure. Patients with a right-sided disturbance tend to minimize or deny proven socially unacceptable behaviors and documented aggressive acts and exaggerate valued qualities, as if trying to build a good image.

Orientation

Children with a left-sided disturbance tend to be described as more introspective, contemplative, and reflective, with intellectual ruminations. They feel that events influence their life and future. They tend to be repetitious. By contrast, the child with a right-sided disturbance tends to be more gregarious and impulsive. Emotions such as anger and sadness are externalized. Euphoria and elation may be seen. The child tends to be talkative about various subjects.

Reactions

The child with a left-sided disturbance expresses ideas verbally but tends to be excessively detailed in speech. By comparison, the child with a right-sided disturbance tends towards non-verbal acting out, with wide emotional swings. Aggressive acts are often denied.

Performance

In school work, the left-sided disturbance child tends to get stuck on details and may never finish the task. By comparison, children with a right-sided disturbance often rush through and may be done first but with many errors, as important details and small mistakes are overlooked.

A child with a left-sided problem may have an underlying yet undetected language disorder that can be brought out by stress. The child may be described as misunderstanding and feels misunderstood. Thus, the child may tend to depend on others to show them what to do, and may be especially anxious to be sure that others have understood what they are trying to express. By comparison, the child with a right-sided disturbance may be less adept at detecting and interpreting emotional cues correctly. They may miss out on visual body language cues and rush in to social interactions, only to be rejected.

Some of the presentations that are said to reflect a personality disorder of epilepsy display many of the features seen in individuals with underlying subtle language disabilities and lateralized learning disorders, which are very common in epilepsy.

Borderline personality

Borderline personalities are common in epilepsy. Such patients often have dissociative episodes and pseudoseizures. Many borderline patients are misdiagnosed.

In epilepsy centers, some 30% of patients with borderline personality disorders are misdiagnosed as epileptic (Trimble, 1991).

Socialization problems

Difficulties in social adjustment due to behavior problems are seen in 40% of patients with epilepsy (Pond, 1974). Low IQ and behavior problems influence social skills adversely. It is the teacher, not the parents, who rates the child as less socially competent should seizures occur (Mitchell *et al.*, 1993). In children with complex partial seizures, subtle language-processing problems may lead to misunderstandings, resulting in a tendency to avoid social contact. The child with a non-dominant focus may miss perceptual cues derived from body language cues, thus impulsively blundering into situations best avoided. Parental and school restrictions as well as the fearful child's avoidance may result in the child missing out on various curricular and extracurricular activities that are important to the development of socialization skills.

Escape to withdrawal

The child may appear shy and secretive, unwilling to participate in activities, for they may feel confused, overwhelmed, or threatened by social situations. Such children may act dull and dumb in order to avoid attention, decrease demands, and lessen expectations. Such a child needs a supportive explanation and ongoing encouragement with much reassurance.

Other disorders

Eating disorders and non-organized sleep disorders in epilepsy are uncommon. Such reports are probably due to chance combination (Onuma, 2000). However, sleep disorders, when actively searched for, are far more frequent than originally thought (see Chapter 18).

REFERENCES

Austin, J. K. (2001). Psychosocial aspects of pediatric epilepsy. In *Psychiatric Issues in Epilepsy*, ed. A. B. Ettinger & A. M. Kanner, pp. 319–32. Philadelphia: Lippincott Williams & Wilkins.

Austin, J. K., Dunn, D. W. & Levstek, D. A. (1993). First seizures: concerns and needs of parents and children. *Epilepsia* **34** (suppl 6): 24.

Bamberger, P. & Matthess, A. (1959). *Anfalle im Kindesalter.* Basel: Karger.

Bear, D. M. & Fedio, P. (1977). Quantitative analysis of interictal behavior in temporal lobe epilepsy. *Arch. Neurol.* **34**: 454–67.

Bech, P., Pedersen, K. K., Simonsen, N., *et al.* (1976). Personality in epilepsy. *Acta Neurol. Scand.* **54**: 348–58.

Bech, P., Pedersen, K. K., Simonsen, N., *et al.* (1977). Personality traits in epilepsy. In *Epilepsy: The Eighth International Symposium*, ed. J. K. Penry, 257–63. New York: Raven Press.

Benson, D. F. (1979). *Clinical Neurology and Neurosurgery Monographs: Aphasia, Alexia and Agraphia.* New York: Churchill Livingstone.

Berg, R. A., Bolter, C., Ch'ien, L. T., *et al.* (1983). Halstead Reitan and Luria-Nebraska comparison in children with chronic seizure disorders. *Clin. Neuropsychol.* **5**: 39.

Berg, R. A., Bolter, J. F., Ch'ien, L. T. & Cummings, J. (1984). A standardized assessment of emotionality in children suffering from epilepsy. *Int. J. Clin. Neuropsychol.* **4**: 277–84.

Blumer, D. (1972). Neuropsychiatric aspects of psychomotor and other forms of epilepsy in childhood. In *Comprehensive Management of Epilepsy in Infancy, Childhood and Adolescence*, ed. S. Livingston, pp. 486–97. Springfield, IL: Charles C. Thomas.

Blumer, D. (1994). Treatment of psychiatric illness in epilepsy patients. Presented at the American Epilepsy Society Conference, 1994.

Blumer, D. & Levin, K. (1977). Psychiatric complications in the epilepsies: current research and treatment. *McLean Hospital Journal*, Special Issue 15.

Camfield, P. R., Gates, R., Ronen, G., *et al.* (1984). Comparison of cognitive ability, personality profile and school success in epileptic children with pure right versus left temporal lobe EEG foci. *Ann. Neurol.* **15**: 122–6.

Caplan, R., Arbelle, S., Guthrie, D., *et al.* (1997). Formal thought disorder and psychopathology in pediatric primary generalized and complex partial epilepsy. *J. Am. Acad. Child Adolesc. Psychiatry* **36**: 1286–94.

Cavazzuti, G. B. (1980). Epidemiology of different types of epilepsy in school age children of Modena Italy. *Epilepsia* **21**: 57–62.

Csernansky, J. K., Leiderman, D. B., Mandabach, M., *et al.* (1990). Psychopathology and limbic epilepsy: relationships to seizure variables and neuropsychological function. *Epilepsia* **31**: 275–80.

Dunn, D. W., Austin, J. K. & Kuyster, G. A. (1997). Behavior problems in children with new-onset epilepsy. *Seizure* **6**: 283–7.

Guerrant, J., Anderson, W. W., Fischer, A., *et al.* (1962). *Personality in Epilepsy.* Springfield, IL: Charles C. Thomas.

Hartlage, C. C. & Green, J. B. (1972). The relation of parental attiudes to academic and social achievement in eplepitic children. *Epilepsia* **13**: 21–6.

Henricksen, O. (1977). Behavior modification and rehabilitation of patients with epilepsy. In *Epilepsy, The Eighth International Symposium*, ed. J. K. Penry, pp. 225–34. New York: Raven Press.

Hermann, B. P. & Reil, P. (1981). Interictal personality and behavioral traits in temporal lobe and generalized epilepsy. *Cortex* **17**: 125–8.

Hermann, B. P., Whitman, S. & Arnston, P. (1983). Hypergraphia in epilepsy: is there a specificity to temporal lobe epilepsy? *J. Neurol. Neurosurg. Psychiatry* **46**: 848–53.

Hermann, B. P., Whitman, S., Wyler, A. R., *et al.* (1985). The neurological, psychosocial and demographic correlates of hypergraphia in patients with epilepsy. *J. Neurol. Neurosurg. Psychiatry* **51**: 203–8.

Hinton, G. G. & Knights, R. M. (1969). Neurological and psychological characteristics of 100 children with seizures. In *Proceedings of the First Congress for the International Assoication of the Scientific Study of Mental Deficiency*, ed. B. Richard, pp. 361–5. London: Michael Jackson.

Holdsworth, L. & Whitemore, K. (1974). A study of children with epilepsy attending ordinary schools. I: their seizure patterns progress, and behavior in school. *Dev. Med. Child Neurol.* **16**: 746–66.

Holmes, G. L. (1987). Psychosocial factors in childhood epilepsy. In *Diagnosis and Management of Epilepsy in Children*, pp. 112–24. Philadelphia: W. B. Saunders.

Janz, D. (1959). *De Epilepsien*. Stuttgart: Georg Thieme.

Mattison, R. (1993). Positive diagnosis of non-epileptic events. Presented at the International Epilepsy Conference, Oslo, Norway, 1993.

McDermott, S., Mani, S. & Krishnaswami, S. (1995). A population-based analysis of specific behavior problems associated with childhood seizures. *J. Epilepsy* **8**: 110–18.

Mitchell, W., Scheier, L. M. & Baker, S. A. (1993). Long-term effects of psychosocial, cultural and medical risk factors on academic achievement and social competence in children and adolescence with epilepsy. *Epilepsia* **34** (suppl 6): 4.

Oderberg, A. D., Shantz, D. L. & Spitz, M. C. (1999). Behavioral changes as a prodrome in epilepsy. *Epilepsia* **40** (suppl 7): 220.

Onuma, T. (2000). Classification of psychiatric symptoms in patients with epilepsy. Proceedings of the 32nd Congress of Japan Epilepsy Society. *Epilepsia* **41** (suppl 9): 43–8.

Papero, P. H., Howe, D. W. & Reiss, D. (1992). Neuropsychological function and psychosocial deficits in adolescents with chronic neurological impairment. *J. Dev. Phys. Disabil.* **4**: 317–40.

Perini, G. I., Tosin, C., Carraro, C., *et al.* (1996). Interictal mood and personality disorders in temporal lobe epilepsy and juvenile myoclonic epilepsy. *J. Neurol. Neurosurg. Psychiatry* **61**: 601–5.

Pond, D. A. (1974). Epilepsy and personality disorders. In *Handbook of Clinical Neurology*, ed. B. Magnus & A. M. Lorentz, pp. 593–610. New York: Elsevier/North Holland.

Powell, A. L., Yudd, A., Zee, P., *et al.* (1997). Attention deficit hyperactivity disorder associated with orbit frontal epilepsy in a father and son. *Neuropsychiatry Neuropsychol. Behav. Neurol.* **10**: 151–4.

Pritchard, P. P., III (1984). Religiosity: an accompaniment of temporal lobe epilepsy? *Epilepsia* **25**: 646.

Rutter, M., Graham, P. & Yule, W. A. (1970). *A Neuropsychiatric Study of Children*. Philadelphia: J. B. Lippincott.

Sharp, G. B., Willliam, J., Griebel, M. L., *et al.* (1993). Patterns of psychopathology in children and adolescents evaluated for epilepsy surgery. *Epilepsia* **34** (suppl 6): 33.

Steffenburg, S., Gillberg, C. & Steffenburg, U. (1996). Psychiatric disorders in children and adolescents with mental retardation and active epilepsy. *Arch. Neurol.* **53**: 904–12.

Stores, G. (1978). School children with epilepsy at risk for learning and behavior problems. *Dev. Med. Child Neurol.* **20**: 502–8.

Svoboda, W. B. (1979). Emotional and behavior consequences of epilepsy. In *Learning About Epilepsy*, pp. 157–84. Baltimore, MD: University Park Press.

Torta, R. & Keller, R. (1999). Behavioral, psychotic and anxiety disorders in epilepsy: etiology, clinical features and therapeutic implications. *Epilepsia* **50** (suppl 10): 2–20.

Trimble, M. R. (1988). *Biologic Psychiatry*. New York: John Wiley & Sons.

Trimble, M. R. (1991). Interictal psychoses: risk factors. In *The Psychoses of Epilepsy*, pp. 136–49. New York: Raven Press.

Trimble, M. R. (1993). Interictal psychoses. Presented at the International Epilepsy Conference, Oslo, Norway, 1993.

Trimble, M. R. (1994). Psychiatric illness in epilepsy. Presented at the American Epilepsy Society Conference, 1994.

Tuchman, R., Jayakar, P., Yaylal, I., *et al.* (1998). Seizures and EEG findings in children with autism spectrum disorder. *CNS Spectr.* **3**: 61–70.

Tucker, D. M., Novelly, R. A. & Walker, P. J. (1985). Hyper-religiosity in TLE: failure to support the hypothesis. *Epilepsia* **26**: 539.

Vazquez, B., Devinsky, O., Luciano, D., *et al.* (1993). Juvenile myoclonic epilepsy: clinical features and factors related to misdiagnosis. *J. Epilepsy* **6**: 233–8.

Weisbrot, D. M. & Ettinger, A. B. (1998). Psychiatric aspects of Pediatric Epilepsy. *Primary Psychiatry* **June**: 51–67.

Weisbrot, D. & Ettinger, A. B. (2001). Psychiatric aspects of pediatric epilepsy. In *Psychiatric Issues in Epilepsy*, ed. A. B. Ettinger & A. M. Kanner, pp. 127–46. Philadelphia: Lippincott Williams & Wilkins.

Weisser, H. G. (1986). Selective amgydalohippocampectomy: indications, investigative techniques and results. *Adv. Techn. Stad. Neurosurg.* **13**: 39–133.

Whitehouse, D. (1971). Psychological and neurological correlates of seizure disorders. *Johns Hopkins Med. J.* **129**: 36–42.

32

Attention deficit disorders

Attention deficit disorders, with or without hyperactivity (ADD/ADDH, or ADHD), are a collection of similar behaviors caused by a wide variety of problems. Recognition of the cause is necessary to treat the problems effectively. Experts cannot agree on the cause, the diagnosis, the treatment, or the prevention. Some experts doubt their existence. The knowledge about the disorders remains speculative. It is unclear whether ADHD is at the far end of the continuum of normal behavior or whether it reflects a qualitatively different behavior syndrome. The symptoms have a CNS basis. There is some evidence of validity, but more study of this is needed (National Institutes of Health, 2000).

ADDs are frequent in children and adults with partial seizure disorders, but they may also occur in primary generalized epilepsy. ADD is seen in up to 48% of children with epilepsy, especially in boys (Holdsworth & Whitmore, 1974). Epileptic students show reduced alertness (Bennet-Levy & Stores, 1984).

Barry (1998) reviewed the treatment of attention disorders for the American Epilepsy Society Conference. Symptoms include a short attention span or distractibility, impulsive behavior, and poor frustration tolerance. Motor hyperactivity may be present. This may precede epilepsy. It occurs in one-third of children with epilepsy. ADD among patients with epilepsy can be confused with a dysphoria of epilepsy and can be mimicked by associated learning disabilities that interfere with auditory processing as well as by frequent absence seizures. Symptoms of ADD may be a side effect of antiepileptic drugs, especially in patients with retardation.

Attention deficit disorders

Definition

ADD comprises marked inattentiveness (undefined) and a lack of inhibition (impulsivity), often accompanied by restlessness (hyperactivity) present in two or more settings, of at least six months' duration, with onset before age seven years, and no indications for any major psychosis or other mental disorder, such as a mood disorder, anxiety, dissociative disorder, or personality disorder (Wolraich, 2001), that might account for the behaviors. The behavior should be atypical for the age and IQ of the child, often being described as maladaptive and inconsistent with the developmental level (National Institutes of Health, 2000). The World Health Organization stresses that the attention may be short in all situations, and the activity should be chaotic and not productive. Frostig (personal communication) notes that the child who can watch their favorite TV program for up half an hour does not have an attention deficit but rather has a selective attention.

ADD, with or without hyperactivity, is a syndrome of various etiologies that interfere with the child's coping with the environment. The etiologies may impair attention, resulting in an uninhibited, often overly active reaction to the distorted input (National Institutes of Health, 2000). Common associated problems include mood lability, stubbornness, bullying, poor response to discipline, and temper. The children often demonstrate low frustration tolerance and low self-esteem.

Incidence

The incidence of true ADD/ADDH is 0.2–0.5%, although in the USA 3–5% of school children are thought to have ADDH (Dunn *et al.*, 2000); school and community estimates often range much higher. Boys are about three times more likely than girls to be recognized as having ADDH (National Institutes of Health, 2000; Wolraich, 2001).

Subtypes

There are two subtypes: children with predominantly inattention and children with predominantly impulsivity–hyperactivity. The inattentive group may have other complications, including learning problems, verbal memory difficulties, depression, and anxiety. Referral tends to be delayed. This is seen more often in girls than in boys. There are fewer associations with oppositional defiant or conduct disorders (Solanto, 2000).

Related problems

Problems coexisting with ADHD include learning disabilities (20–30%), anxiety disorders (25%), depressive disorders (9–38%), and a conduct disorder/oppositional defiant disorder (50%) (Wolraich, 2001). Emotional lability and discipline problems are common. Other factors, such as illnesses, allergy, disability, and inadequate sleep, may be important.

Developmental presentation

The ADD infant is unable to sustain a focus for more than five to six seconds on a facial expression, presentation of a toy, or other interactive opportunity. The preschool child is unable to function and play appropriately and may appear immature, not wanting to engage in any activity long enough and not completing any activity. The short attention span and distractibility cause the child to miss important aspects of an object or situation. By school age and often into adolescence, the child has significant school and social problems, shifting activities and not completing tasks. Messiness and carelessness in schoolwork is noted. Tasks are started prematurely and without appropriate review of instructions, acting as if the child's mind is elsewhere and they are not listening. Organization is difficult. Activities that require concentration are disliked. Forgetfulness is prominent (American Academy of Pediatrics, 1996).

With ADHD, the infant is described as squirming frequently, with excessive climbing. Purposeful gestures or behaviors appear disorganized. Motor planning and sequencing is difficult, although these children enjoy gross motor activities. By early childhood, the picture is of a restless, excessively active, exploring child who cannot sit still, fidgets when watching TV, and is disruptive and grabbing. By adolescence, the child still fidgets, interrupts, bothers others, and is frequently in trouble, although the excessive activity may be replaced by a sense of restlessness (American Academy of Pediatrics, 1996).

Types by cause

ADHD is a resultant manifestation of diverse etiologies. ADD with or without hyperactivity is a disturbance of sensory input between the environment and the brain's processing of those sensations, manifest often as disturbed motor activities and deviant social interactions (Svoboda, 1979). Anything that interferes with the child's ability to handle environmental stimuli can result in a disturbed attention and often excessive activity. This can include a stressful environment, a neurosensory deficit of vision or hearing, or a learning problem, specific or global. Conditions that may be associated with ADHD-like behaviors can be subdivided into developmental, environmental, sensory impairments, neurologic, and psychogenic.

Developmental causes

There are normal variants to development. The child's basic temperament, i.e. constitutional activity, is a baseline. Some children are felt to be overly active when really they represent only a normal variant.

Environmental causes

The child who has trouble coping in a stressful environment is often active and fidgety. The inciting problem may be a threatening or changeable environment with which the child cannot cope, resulting in anxiety. Such environments produce behaviors including anxiety, anger, depression, and oppositional behavior. Placing the child in a school environment in which the child is too bright or of too low intelligence to be at ease often produces fidgeting and distractibility. These children are frustrated, threatened, or overwhelmed, and consequently respond with hyperkinetic behavior (Svoboda, 1975).

Neurogenic causes

Neurologic causes can be subdivided into brainstem-subcortical epileptic, and cortical.

Sensory causes

Problems such as hearing impairments and visual problems are often mistaken for ADD/ADHD. A hearing or visual problem that clouds or distorts incoming stimuli causes confusion and poses a threat to the child. Children with sensory impairments of vision or hearing may be inattentive but actually rely on alternate cues, often being distracted to these in a guarding manner.

Subcortical causes

If the problem is in the deeper brain areas that help deliver the incoming sensations to vital areas on the brain surface, and that also involve alertness and emotional reactions, three types of personalities may be seen: reticular-thalamic, frontal, and temporal-limbic forms.

In the reticular-thalamic type, the child appears restless but tries to perform the task. The hyperactivity is catching and everybody around becomes keyed up. Some children seem cheerful yet immature. They try, but they cannot control their behavior. They often chatter aloud. They take chances, although their coordination may be poor. There may be a family history of narcolepsy. This type of child responds well to a stimulant medication (Svoboda, 1975).

In the frontal form, the child is superficial and flits around with superficial relationships and aimless activity, not getting things done. They often lack the inhibition to control their impulsivity. Children with frontal lobe disturbances often seem placid and pleasant but inattentive, as they exhibit an aimless, unproductive energy, going from activity to activity. They persevere, doing the same things over and over again. They do not make social contacts or seem to interact with others. They may be rather clumsy. The EEG may show a frontal lobe abnormality. No drug works completely with this group, and psychiatric drugs may produce marked dullness. Behavioral approaches offer the most help (Svoboda, 1975).

In the temporal-limbic form, the child may seem overly aggressive and destructive, and the parents display minimal control. This may take on more of an aggressive, angry, or destructive nature. The behavior is unpredictable. The child may be difficult to manage. Seizures may be seen as a complication. The child with a left temporal lobe seizure problem is more often typically hyperactive, whereas the individual with a right temporal lobe seizure disorder may be more impulsive and aggressive in reactions. This hyperactivity is especially common with seizure onset in earlier childhood. Stimulants and tranquilizers are rarely of any benefit and may trigger seizures (Svoboda, 1975).

Cortical (cognitive and linguistic) causes

Cortical hyperactivity includes receptive learning and language disorders, the underplaced bright child, and the overplaced retarded child. Children with learning difficulties who are not placed properly may appear to be impulsive, active, or overly active as related to the frustrations of the struggle to learn. Learning struggles are often the cause, not the result, of an ADD.

Psychogenic causes

Psychogenic causes can be subdivided into those with a lack of internal control development and those with excessive demands on them. The lack of internal controls may be seen with defective parental controls, early childhood psychosis, or childhood variants of a bipolar disorder. If the child experiences excessive demands, one may see a situational hyperactivity or a neurotic form with many self-demands. A child with depression can seem hyperactive and inattentive with poor impulse control. About 25% of adults with bipolar disorders have a history of ADHD. The child who comes from a chaotic environment may have never developed the controls needed for life.

Evaluation

A child believed to have ADD/ADHD should be evaluated for possible language or learning problems or emotional disturbances, especially if symptoms suggest these are present. The family should be evaluated to determine the home situation (Dunn *et al.*, 2000). If there are episodes suggestive of seizures or some other medical condition, this should be pursued.

Diagnostics

There are no specific validated diagnostics for ADD. Questionnaires are subjective. School rating score sheets have proven to be of little value and need to be confirmed (Devinsky & Vazquez, 1993). The diagnosis is based on observations in a variety of situations and ruling out other causes (Jensen, 2000).

Electroencephalography

An EEG may be considered if there is any historical suggestion of possible seizures. Children with ADD/ADHD have an increased incidence of EEG abnormalities. Spikes have been found in 68.8%, but in many (46.6%) they are felt to be normal variants. Definite non-controversial EEG findings are seen in up to 30.1%, mainly focal and less often generalized. Bilateral spike-wave complexes are seen in 6.3% but appear rarely (73%). These are interpreted as representing a relatively inactive generalized type of discharge. Bilateral spike-wave complexes represent a cortico-reticular or generalized discharge and are found in 6% of all ADHD patients. In most patients, the occurrence is so infrequent as to not feel these are related to interrupted attention. Focal epileptiform activity is described in 23.9%, especially in the occipital or temporal areas, mainly left, but also in the central and frontal areas. The discharge occurrence is usually rare (33.3%) or frequent (28.6%) (Hughes et al., 2000).

The focal spiking found in about one-quarter of patients may represent an example of the clinical significance of interictal discharges, which can affect nearly all cerebral functions (Hughes et al., 2000) as related to transient cognitive impairments (Binnie et al., 1987; Kasteleijn-Nolste Trenite et al., 1987; Marston et al., 1993). Such patients may show cognitive improvements when placed on antiepileptic drugs (Kasteleijn-Nolste Trenite et al., 1987). Temporal (37.5%) and occipital (43.8%) spiking is seen most often. Left-sided discharges are often associated with errors of verbal tasks, while right-sided discharges are associated with errors of non-verbal or spatial tasks (Binnie et al., 1987; Hughes et al., 2000).

Other studies

The frontal lobe and basal ganglia are reported as being nearly 10% smaller in children with ADHD. Polymorphism in the dopamine D_4 receptor and transporter genes has been suggested (Hughes et al., 2000). In a SPECT study, 65% of patients with ADHD showed decreased perfusion in the frontal areas (Amen & Carmichael, 1997), the same areas that tend toward abnormal slow activities on quantitative EEG studies of ADHD (Charbot & Serfontein, 1996). This has been referred to as a "lazy frontal lobe" (Neidermeyer, 1990; Hughes et al., 2000).

Etiological theories

Reduced dopaminergic activity in the prefrontal-striatal circuitry pertaining to sensory input relates to attention, activity, and inhibition, with executive function deficits. Reduced norepinephrine activity in the prefrontal cortex and cingulate pertaining to executive function may produce deficits in inhibition. Brainstem norepinephrine activity may be diminished, possibly affecting alertness. Presynaptic dopamine activity appears to be impaired. Stimulants work by countering these deficits. Treatment data suggest a catecholamine hypothesis of ADHD, since nearly all medications effective in ADHD affect catecholamine transmissions of norepinephrine and dopamine (Schulz et al., 2000).

Therapy

No matter what the cause, the basic therapy of ADD is essentially one of behavior modification, parent–teacher counseling, provision of help for any medical or educational needs, and treating the aggravating problem.

If the child is treated with appropriate educational and behavioral approaches, the outlook is good; if treated primarily with drugs, the outlook is often for further problems, such as school underachievement and failure, delinquency, job failure, marriage failure, alcoholism, and substance abuse. Selling of stimulant drugs by patients, parents, and even teachers has been seen.

Attention deficit disorders of epilepsy

Children may exhibit ADD as a coincidental disorder but more commonly due to one of many factors associated with the epilepsy. Children with epilepsy are at risk for symptoms of ADHD. Children with epilepsy have poorer concentration and mental processing and are less alert than age-matched non-epileptic children (Dam, 1990). Alertness may be depressed in children with epilepsy (Stores, 1987).

Incidence

ADHD has been reported in 28.1–37% of children with epilepsy, 75% of these ADHD patients being boys (Stores *et al.*, 1978; Dunn *et al.*, 2000). Teachers report up to 48% as having ADD/ADHD (Holdsworth & Whitmore, 1974; Stores *et al.*, 1978; Baird *et al.*, 1980). The inattentive subtype is more frequent than the inattentive–hyperactive subtype. Impulsive behavior is seen in 39% of children with present or past epilepsy, compared with 11% of normal children (Dunn *et al.*, 2000). Teachers' ratings of attentiveness do not correlate well with other measures of attentiveness (Yule, 1980; Stores *et al.*, 1978) but may distinguish poor epileptic achievers from adequately achieving peers (Holdsworth & Whitmore, 1974; Yule, 1980). Inattention is seen in 20% of children with epilepsy with average school performance and 59% of epileptic children with below-average to retarded performance. Neuropsychological testing diagnoses 14–36% with ADHD. At least one symptom of ADHD is found in 77% of children with epilepsy. Severe overactivity and distractibility are seen in 8% (Dunn *et al.*, 2000).

Types

The epileptic factors determining the type of ADD most apt to be seen include the seizure type, drug reactions, epileptic anxiety, and seizure control "awakenings."

Epileptic etiologies

Deficits in sustained attention, characterized by general losing in visual continuous performance tasks, are felt to be unrelated to the type of epilepsy or type of EEG abnormality (Bruhn-Parsons & Parsons, 1977; Aldenkamp *et al.*, 1990). Attentiveness may vary with the EEG type of epilepsy and with the drug treatment (Stores *et al.*, 1978). Children with generalized seizure discharges are more apt to suffer from restlessness and inattentiveness. Children with focal seizure disorders are more at risk for specific learning disabilities and related attentional activity-like disturbances (Ounsted & Hutt, 1964). Examples of an ADD/ADHD state preceding seizures have been noted (Hughes *et al.*, 2000).

Generalized seizures

Generalized seizures, especially those with generalized spike-wave bursts on the EEG (in absence, atonic, and myoclonic seizures) are often seen in children who seem inattentive and impulsive. Abnormal spike-wave bursts interrupt attention. When the brief burst ends, the child may take off on a new action, thus seeming to be impulsive and overly active. A further increase in drug dosage may normalize the EEG and thus increase the attention abilities (Svoboda, 1979). Poor seizure control has been associated with hyperactivity in girls with incompletely controlled absence epilepsy (Dunn *et al.*, 2000).

Partial seizures

Children with epileptiform EEG abnormalities originating in the frontal lobe are more likely to be rated as having attention problems than those with non-frontal EEG abnormalities. They present more as the inattentive form rather than the combined form of ADHD. No differences between groups are found for impulsivity/hyperactivity. Key factors include polypharmacy but not seizure frequency or intellect (Sherman *et al.*, 2000). The development of inhibition skills may be faulty in some children.

If children with benign focal epilepsy of childhood have impairments of attention, the focus usually involves the right hemisphere (Dunn *et al.*, 2000).

Children with complex partial seizures may show up with ADHD (25%). In preschool children with complex partial epilepsy, up to two of every three may show some hyperactivity. The common syndrome may present with persistent hyperactivity, fidgetiness, short attention span, and a lack of normal inhibitions or fears. Aggressiveness and destructible behavior may often be seen, including severe temper outbursts. The mood is labile. This occurs most often in children with seizure onset before age five years, especially in boys. Intellectual development may be slowed. The behavior appears with or soon after the seizure onset and may lessen or be outgrown in puberty. Underlying brain damage may be present (Glaser, 1967; Ounsted *et al.*, 1968).

Impulsivity and distractibility may be seen, the type of which may relate to the laterality of the seizure. Children with left temporal seizures tend to be inattentive and overly active in noisy settings; children with right-sided seizures tend to be visually distractable. Children with frontal lobe discharges seem uninhibited and disorganized, with poor planning. A small group of children with left-sided seizures paradoxically seem to calm down in a noisy setting, suggesting an alerting response (Svoboda, 1979).

Epileptic-encephalopathy syndromes

Children with minor motor seizures may be inattentive and overly active, but this is part of their overall common problems of developmental delays and depressed IQ. Inattention is prominent in children with epileptic encephalopathy (Dunn *et al.*, 2000).

Subclinical discharges

Generalized seizure discharges, even though manifest as subclinical bursts, may interrupt attention and follow-through.

Attitudinal etiologies

Anxieties over the seizures transmitted to a young child by parents, peers, and teachers may cause an anxiety type of ADHD (Svoboda, 1979).

Drug reactions

Any seizure medication may cause (or relieve) attention problems or excessive activity. About one-third of children on phenobarbital may become hyperactive; about one in every six children calms down, especially if their problem is already hyperactivity. Phenytoin causes more of a nasty, attention-activity problem. Valproate may produce a delayed ADD/ADHD. Clonazepam is especially apt to cause behavior problems. Felbamate may also cause overactivity.

Seizure awakenings

A child who sits in class neither partaking in learning activities nor causing any problems may later be found to be having multiple absence seizures. An awakening occurs on anticonvulsant medication. Curiosity emerges, causing the child to investigate the seemingly new classroom environment. The teacher mistakenly blames the medication for distractibility and excess activity in investigating, not realizing that they are now seeing the normal self awakened. This may result in a series of medication changes being pursued.

Complications

Impairments of alertness, whether due to seizures or to other causes, may contribute to the underachievement of children with epilepsy (Reynolds, 1981). In addition, attention deficits may be due to seizure activity that is not controlled by medication or that may be occurring without any other clinical manifestations.

Causes

A combination of genetic and neuropsychological factors may cause ADD/ADHD (Dunn *et al.*, 2000). In the seizure patient, the environment, the deep brain processes, the early learning stages, and the intelligence may all contribute to hyperkinetic behavior, or the cause may be a mixture of problems, including environmental stresses. If the problem is primarily environmental, then the family often is found to be overly protective and overly indulgent; the child is often spoiled, anxious, and immature. If the child has a learning problem, the hyperactivity may appear primarily in school and homework situations (Svoboda, 1975).

Approaches

If the suspect ADD is of recent onset, it may be a reaction. If a child is suspected as having ADD/ADDH that begins after six years of age, it is probably something else. If the child can watch TV or quietly become involved in some other activity for up to 30 minutes, it is probably not an ADD problem. If the behavior is essentially limited to a specific situation or environment, the problem may be a reaction and not an underlying attention disorder. If the child has been placed on medication just before the behaviors emerged, the problem may be a medication reaction and the new drug may have to be reduced in dosage or changed to a different drug.

The evaluation for ADDH in epilepsy is essentially the same as ADDH without epilepsy once epileptic factors have been excluded.

Therapy

Effective therapy begins by diagnosing and treating the cause, the quality, and the target of the disturbance, not just the quantity of the disturbance. Any disability or handicap found in the evaluation needs to be treated appropriately. If the child is described as anxious or depressed, consider counseling. If there is a history of discipline or behavior problems such as aggressive or destructive behaviors or of disobedience and negativistic behavior, the child and family need referral for counseling and behavior modification. If there is a history of delusions, hallucinations, or incoherence suggestive of childhood psychoses, a referral to a child psychiatrist should be considered.

The approach of choice for ADD/ADDH, regardless of the cause of the hyperactivity, consists of counseling, modifying undesirable behaviors, and training in attending and inhibition. Some children may profit from medications used on a temporary basis and not as a substitute treatment. For some patients, a stimulant or similar medicine may reduce the activities and distractibility. Dietary manipulations, megadoses of vitamins, and other fads have not proven effective. With the preschool child, conservative approaches should be tried first, with behavioral approaches, parental support, and developing outlooks for the child's energy. In the school-age child, the same guidelines as in the preschool child are useful, but the teacher needs to be involved. The effectiveness of whatever approaches are used must be monitored. If the response is not working or if the behavioral excesses are intolerably high, short-term use of medication may be considered (Svoboda, 1975).

Many families do not have access to appropriate care. Families must often bear the costs of care. Often, a lack of integration of healthcare and educational systems in caring for ADHD children exists (Jensen, 2000). Some medical plan and third-party payers may not cover psychological approaches.

Adjusting antiepileptic medications

Attentional disorders can appear with antiepileptic drugs, especially barbiturates, benzodiazepam, and GABAergic drugs. Lamotrigine and gabapentin reactions can mimic ADD in children. ADD- and ADDH-like behavior may be the result of ictal, postictal, or interictal changes. Lesions may cause this (Devinsky & Vazquez, 1993). If attention deficits are due to antiepileptic therapy, it is more advisable to revise seizure therapies than add a stimulant drug.

Psychological intervention

There are a variety of non-drug approaches to ADDH. Psychological treatments depend upon the cooperation and interest of the child, the parents, and the teachers. Too often this is lacking. The child may have experienced years of failure and frustration. The parents may have become exasperated, guilty, or rejected. Teachers may feel helpless and seek to pass on the problems elsewhere (Taylor, 1985).

All ADHD children need behavioral approaches and all parents need counseling and guidance (Svoboda, 1975). Combining medication and psychosocial therapies may help the child with seizures, ADHD, and comorbid conditions (Dunn *et al.*, 2000).

Parent training

In parent training, the therapist works with the parents, focusing on assessing the problems and behavioral modification, using combinations of positive reinforcement for approved behaviors and either ignoring or punishing (including timeouts or loss of privileges) misbehaviors. School programs use a similar approach for these problems, with emphasis on providing structure and rapid feedback on a disruptive child (Dunn *et al.*, 2000).

Situational ADHD

If the child develops ADHD in certain situations or specific activities, environmental manipulation may be useful. The child needs to be removed from the irritating environment until successful training to tolerate this is accomplished (Taylor, 1985).

If the triggering activity is learning-related, an underlying learning disability may be the cause.

Contingency management

This approach can be applied to a wide range of problems and can be taught successfully to parents and teachers to reduce activity levels, to increase task behaviors, and to speed up the completion of academic tasks. Comparisons with drugs show that the drugs are more powerful and more consistent as agents of change (Taylor, 1985).

Self-control (cognitive) training

This approach seeks to increase the child's ability to regulate their own action and to teach problem-solving strategies. There is no good evidence that these approaches are of value in the setting where they are applied or that they can produce lasting effects.

Counseling

Counseling seeks to promote understanding and thus a change in the attitudes towards the child. The entire family should be involved. Reliance on drugs risks the idea that the child may attribute successes not to self-efforts but to the medication. This must be addressed. The parents need to be told that it is not their fault. Parent escape periods are often helpful. A firm, consistent, calm, quiet handling helps. The parents need to be taught to reward good behavior, not punish bad behavior. Regular routines until the child can learn to cope with change are important. This is incorporated into a behavior modification program.

Psychotherapy

Family therapy is relevant to the issues of attitudes towards the child and towards treatment. Family interactions are involved in the development of overactivity and inattentiveness in some cases. Whether these interactions can be modified is another question.

Multiple treatments

A multiple treatment approach for children with multiple difficulties is desirable but often not available or utilized. In the USA, the majority of children diagnosed as hyperactive receive drugs and only drugs as therapy. In Britain, drug treatment is seldom used.

Rational treatment must be guided by a thorough assessment and monitoring of the effects of intervention on the chosen target symptoms. Stimulants should be given a trial if the hyperactivity or inattention is severe enough to prevent the psychological approaches from working on their own. The purpose of medication is to facilitate psychological therapy. The key to any long-term maintenance of improvement is likely to be the child's own development of self-control, self-motivation, and a healthier self-esteem.

Pharmacologic intervention

The child with ADHD and epilepsy can be treated in the same way as the child with epilepsy. There has been a five-fold increase in the use of drugs to treat ADHD over the past decade. Stimulant medications are safe when used as prescribed, but they must be monitored carefully. There is no conclusive evidence that stimulant treatment leads to substance abuse, although reviews in the media report such. Combined treatments offer modest advantage over medication treatment alone. Medication treatments may yield improvement in social skills. Peers, teachers and, parents all rate children with ADHD as more likable when on medication (Jensen, 2000).

Stimulants

Stimulants are the first drug of choice for the treatment of ADHD, although the incidence of seizure activation is around 1% (Dunn *et al.*, 2000). Avoid insomnia by giving early dosages (Devinsky & Vazquez, 1993), and keep the doses low.

Improvements in academic performance, aggression, and social skills are seen with stimulants. The stimulant response rate is about 75% for the first drug and up to 90% if the first drug fails and a second drug is chosen (Adesman, 2001). In trial for a few weeks or months, stimulants reduce the severity of several problem behaviors and improve performance in laboratory tests of concentration and motor speed. It is not the effectiveness but rather the efficacy that is challenged. Drugs may be effective in up to 40% of hyperactive children in long-term treatment. By adolescence, some children outgrow the dependency on medications. Withdrawal should be gradual and done over atleast three weeks to avoid any rebound effect (Taylor, 1985). There is no difference in responsiveness to stimulant medication between the inattentive group and the ADHD group, but more children in the latter group are on medications, often at higher dosages (Schulz *et al.*, 2000).

The incidence of seizures precipitated by the use of a stimulant medication is accepted to be around 1%. Stimulants have been reported to lessen the frequency of absence and minor motor seizures by improving alertness. In the West Virginia University Pediatric Neurology Clinic, an average of three children yearly for ten years with a generalized seizure about two weeks after the beginning of a stimulant was noted. Behavior approaches were substituted for the medication and no further seizures occurred. Of interest was that generalized atypical spike-wave bursts did not reappear on follow-up EEGs, although focal dischargers were seen consistently.

Methylphenidate

Stimulants such as methylphenidate work by increasing levels of dopamine in the brain. Methylphenidate must be used only for children who do not improve sufficiently after intensive efforts to modify behavior. There is no contraindication to methylphenidate used to treat moderate to severe attention deficit disabilities. The long-term effects of methylphenidate are not yet known (Taylor, 1985). The *Physician's Desk Reference* states that methylphenidate may lower the convulsive threshold in epilepsy-prone patients, but this is debated. Some feel that the drug does not lower the seizure threshold when used in therapeutic doses (McBride *et al.*, 1986). Rarely, the drug may produce seizures. It may be safe with well-controlled seizures but may exacerbate uncontrolled seizures (Devinsky & Vazquez, 1993). Seizure-free patients rarely experience a breakthrough, but those in active seizures may have their seizures exacerbated. Methylphenidate may lower self-confidence and self-concept. It does not help with aggression, conduct problems, depression, or other types of learning problems. Such children may steal a little less but cheat more while on the drug.

Antidepressants

The tricyclics (such as imipramine, nortriptyline, and desipramine) may be useful, especially in children with combined ADHD and anxiety or depression, especially those with comorbid tics. The drugs are less effective for ADHD. Tricyclic antidepressants in low doses may be anti-hyperkinetic within hours, unlike their antidepressant effectiveness. However, the benefits may be lost after a year or so (Taylor, 1985). With some children, the initial benefits deteriorate after a few months to be replaced by unpleasantness. There is a concern for cardiac toxicity and, rarely, seizures (Adesman, 2001). Lowering of the seizure threshold may be seen, especially at higher doses (Dunn *et al.*, 2000). Sometimes, in patients who do respond the diagnosis is later found to be a depression.

Major tranquilizers

Major tranquilizers such as haloperidol may diminish restless behavior and improve laboratory tests of attention. Phenothiazines may decrease activity and help with some behavior problems, but they do not help and may impair cognitive behaviors. Thus, major tranquilizers are best reserved for more severe and refractory problems. In children with frontal lobe types of ADHD, the major tranquilizers may render the child overly sedated, inactive, and non-productive (Taylor, 1985). Sometimes the drugs are useful at low dosages as a supplement to another drug.

Other drugs

Other medications that may be useful include alpha-adrenergic agonists and antipsychotics. Clonidine and guanfacine may reduce hyperactivity but are less effective in improving attention (Dunn *et al.*, 2000). Clonidine, an alpha-2 agonist, may be useful in quite hyperactive or aggressive behavior, especially in patients with tics. This drug takes weeks to become effective. It does not seem to help attention; there are also cardiac risks. Bupropion (amfebutamone) may decrease hyperactivity and aggression and possibly improve cognitive performance but may decrease the seizure threshold and may exacerbate tics (Adesman, 2001). Bupropion (amfebutamone) at higher dosages may produce seizures in 1–5% of children.

Medications and combined treatment groups do equally well with respect to the ADHD core symptoms. Both do better than the behavioral treatment groups. Behavior treatment groups do better than untreated children. Children with ADHD and anxiety disorder respond as well to medications as children with only ADHD. Children in ADHD with anxiety in the combined treatment group do better than those in the medication-only group (Adesman, 2001).

Prognosis

About half of the children outgrow the syndrome, yet one-third to two-thirds continue to show some symptoms. The majority of children with ADHD by adulthood are working, yet their employment records are not as good as controls and they show a lower work status (Weiss, 1989).

Those with hyperactivity have lower self-esteem. Alcohol abuse is not more prevalent in children in prospective studies, even though retrospective studies have suggested such. Similarly, there are mixed reports regarding possible later drug abuse in adults who were treated for ADHD as children.

Hyperactivity in childhood may lead to adult antisocial personality disorders and antisocial behaviors in 10–55%. The outcome may be influenced adversely by a dysfunctional home. Hyperactivity with learning disabilities tends to result in social deviancy in adolescence.

Legal issues

In the USA, the treatment of children with ADHD has raised a number of legal issues, including medical malpractice and battery claims, especially when the parents are pressured to seek medications. Physicians have been charged with negligent misdiagnosis of ADHD and failure to obtain adequate informed consent for use, primarily by inadequate provision of information about side effects. Coercive use of medications by school systems in the absence of parental consent has raised issues of battery. Constitutional questions have arisen regarding limitations on parental rights to decline medical aid for their children as balanced against the state's interest in safeguarding the health and welfare of children. The children's own equal protection, due process, privacy rights, and their constitutional and statutory right to an education are also issues (Ouellette, 1991).

REFERENCES

Adesman, A. R. (2001). Treating ADHD: what are the options? *Contemp. Pediatr.* **May** (suppl): 11–19.

Aldenkamp, A. P., Alpherts, W. C. J., Dekker, M. J. A., *et al.* (1990). Neuropsychological aspects of learning disabilities in epilepsy. *Epilepsia* **31** (suppl 4): 9–20.

Amen, D. G. & Carmichael, B. D. (1997). High-resolution brain SPECT imaging in ADHD. *Ann. Clin. Psychiatry* **9**: 81–6.

American Academy of Pediatrics (1996). Hyperactive/impulse or inattentive behaviors. In *The Classification of Child and Adolescent Mental Diagnoses in Primary Care: Diagnostic and Statistical Manual for Primary Care (DSM-PC): Child and Adolescent Version*, ed. M. L. Wolraich, M. E. Felice & D. Drotar, p. 93. Elk Grove Village, IL: American Academy of Pediatrics.

Baird, H. W., John, E. R., Ahn, H., *et al.* (1980). Neurometric evaluation of epileptic children who do well and poorly in school. *Electroencephalogr. Clin. Neurophysiol.* **48**: 683–93.

Barry, J. (1998). Treatment of affective and attention deficit disorder. Presented at the American Epilepsy Society Conference, 1998.

Bennet-Levy, J. & Stores, G. (1984). The nature of cognitive dysfunction in school-children with epilepsy. *Acta Neurol. Scand.* **69** (suppl): 79–82.

Binnie, C. D., Kasteleijn-Nolst Trenite, D. G. A., Smit, A. M., *et al.* (1987). Interactions of epileptiform EEG discharges and cognition. *Epilepsy Res.* **1**: 239–43.

Bruhn-Parsons, A. T. & Parsons, O. A. (1977). Reaction time variability in epileptic and brain damaged patients. *Cortex* **13**: 373–84.

Dam, M. (1990). Children with epilepsy: the effect of seizures, syndromes and etiological factors on cognitive functioning. *Epilepsia* **31** (suppl 4): 26–9.

Devinsky, O. & Vazquez, B. (1993). Behavioral changes associated with epilepsy. *Neurol. Clin.* **11**: 127–49.

Dunn, D. W., Austin, J. K., Harezlak, J., *et al.* (2000). Attention deficit hyperactivity disorder and chronic epilepsy in childhood. *Epilepsia* **41** (suppl 7): 239.

Glaser, G. (1967). Limbic epilepsy in childhood *J. Nerv. Ment. Dis.* **141**: 392–7.

Holdsworth, L. & Whitmore, K. (1974). A study of children with epilepsy attending ordinary schools: their seizure patterns, progress and behavior in schools. *Dev. Med. Child Neurol.* **16**: 746–58.

Hughes, J. R., DeLeo, A. J. & Melyn, M. A. (2000). The electroencephalogram in attention deficit-hyperactivity disorder: emphasis on epileptiform discharges. *Epilepsy Behav.* **1**: 271–7.

Jensen, P. S. (2000). The National Institutes of Health Attention-Deficit/Hyperactivity Disorder Consensus Statement: implications for practitioners and scientists. *CNS Spectr.* **5**: 29–33.

Kasteleijn-Nolst Trenite, D. G. A., Riemersma, J. B. J., Binnie, C. D., *et al.* (1987). The influence of subclinical epileptiform EEG discharges on driving behavior. *Electroencephalogr. Clin. Neurophysiol.* **67**: 167–70.

Marston, D., Besag, F., Binnie, C. D., *et al.* (1993). Effects of transitory cognitive impairment on psychosocial functioning of clinical with epilepsy: a therapeutic trial. *Dev. Med. Child Neurol.* **3**: 574–81.

McBride, M. C., Wang, D. D. & Torres, C. F. (1986). Methylphenidate in therapeutic does not lower seizure threshold. *Ann. Neurol.* **20**: 428.

Niedermeyer, E. (1990). *Psychological, Psychiatric Aspects: The Epilepsies, Diagnosis and Management.* Baltimore, MD: Urban & Schwarzenberg.

National Institutes of Health (2000). National Institutes of Health Consensus Development Conference Statement: diagnosis and treatment of attention-deficit/hyperactivity disorder. *J. Am. Acad. Child Psychiatry* **39**: 182–92.

Ouellette, E. M. (1991). Legal issues in the treatment of children with attention deficit hyperactivity disorders. *J. Child Neurol.* **6** (suppl): 66–73.

Ounsted, C. & Hutt, S. J. (1964). The effects of attentive factors on bio-electric paroxysms in epileptic children. *Proc. R. Soc. Med.* **57**: 1178.

Ounsted, C., Lindsay, J. & Norman, R. (1968). *Biological Factors in Temporal Lobe Epilepsy.* London: Spastics Society and Heineman.

Reynolds, E. H. (1981). Biological factors in psychological disorders associated with epilepsy. In *Epilepsy and Psychiatry*, ed. E. H. Reynolds & M. R. Trimble, pp. 264–90. New York: Churchill Livingstone.

Schulz, K. P., Himelstein, J., Halperin, J. M., *et al.* (2000). Neurobiological models of attention deficit/hyperactivity disorder: a brief review of empirical evidence. *CNS Spectr.* **5**: 34–44.

Sherman, E. M. S., Armitage, L. L., Connolly, M. B., *et al.* (2000). Behaviors symptomatic of ADHD in pediatric epilepsy: relationship to frontal lobe epileptiform abnormalities and other neurologic predictors. *Epilepsia* **41** (suppl 7): 191.

Solanto, M. V. (2000). The predominantly inattentive subtype of attention-deficit/hyperactivity disorder. *CNS Spectr.* **5**: 45–51.

Stores, G. (1987). Effects on learning of "subclinical" seizure discharges. In *Education and Epilepsy*, ed. A. P. Aldenkamp, W. C. J. Alpherts, H. Meinardi & G. Stores, pp. 14–21. Lisse: Swets & Zeitlinger.

Stores, G., Hart, J. & Piran, N. (1978). Inattentiveness in schoolchildren with epilepsy. *Epilespia* **19**: 169–75.

Svoboda, W. B. (1975). The hyperkinetic syndrome. *W. V. Med. J.* **71**: 347–51.

Svoboda, W. B. (1979). Epilepsy and learning problems. In *Learning About Epilepsy*, pp. 186–200. Baltimore, MD: University Park Press.

Taylor, E. (1985). Syndromes of overactivity and attention deficit. In *Child and Adolescent Psychiatry: Modern Approaches*, ed. M. Rutter & L. Hersov, pp. 424–38. St Louis, MO: Mosby.

Weiss, G. (1989). Follow-up studies on outcome of hyperactive children. In *Child Neurolgoy and Developmental Disabilites*, ed. J. Grench, S. Harrel & P. Casaer, pp. 269–78. Baltimore, MD: Paul H. Brookes.

Wolraich, M. L. (2001). Diagnosing ADHD. *Contemp. Pediatr.* **May** (suppl): 3–10.

Yule, W. (1980). Educational achievement. In *Epilepsy and Behavior '79*, ed. B. M. Kulig, H. Meinardi & C. Stores, pp. 162–8. Lisse: Swets & Zeitlinger.

33

Anxiety disorders

Anxiety and epilepsy have been associated in the minds of people since antiquity (Scicutella, 2001). Not purely a mood, thought, or autonomic disorder, anxiety is a unique phenomenon in genesis and expression that needs multidisciplinary efforts to be understood (Goldstein & Harden, 2000).

Anxiety disorders include phobic disorders, anxiety states including panic disorders, generalized anxiety disorders, obsessive–compulsive disorders, and post-traumatic stress disorder (Trimble, 1988). Over half of adult patients in an epilepsy clinic have significant anxiety symptoms (Francis *et al.*, 1966; Ettinger *et al.*, 1998).

In children, anxiety in epilepsy is more difficult to recognize than disorders with more overt behavior difficulties such as ADHD or conduct disorders. When a child presents with anxiety symptoms, a family history of anxiety is not uncommon. At least one of every six children with epilepsy seen in an epilepsy clinic meets the criteria for anxiety (Ettinger *et al.*, 1998). An even higher number may experience fear and anxiety related to numerous factors, including fear of death, brain damage, or mental Retardation, and social phobias as a result of having seizures in public (Mittan & Locke, 1982). Sleep anxiety and seizure frequency appear to be related. Children with epilepsy have a higher rate of sleep disorders, particularly poor-quality sleep and anxieties about sleep (Ettinger *et al.*, 1998).

Parents have different anxieties to their children, leading them to be overprotective or overindulgent. Such fears may be transmitted to the children. It is as important to work with the parents of the anxious child as it is to work with the child (Weisbrot & Ettinger, 1998). Ictal fears offer a clue to their nature when associated with complex partial seizures.

The evolution of anxiety

Anxiety is the ultimate example of a phenomenon belonging to both psychological and neuropsychological domains. Anxiety is an outgrowth of the danger-sensing mechanisms. Anxiety and fear are closely related concepts. Often, the distinction between the two is vague (Goldstein & Harden, 2000).

Anxiety originates from faulty, distorted thought patterns contributing to symptom production. Patients with anxiety disorders overestimate the degree of danger and the probability of harm in a given situation while underestimating their abilities to cope with perceived threats. Patients with panic disorders can experience thoughts of loss of control and fear of dying that follow physiological sensations, such as palpitations, tachycardia, and lightheadedness (Caplan *et al.*, 1992; Goldstein & Harden, 2000).

The anatomy of anxiety

The amygdala is a key structure integrating intercepted stimuli, distributing processed afferent data to the multiple efferent system of the cortex, limbic system, basal ganglia, and hypothalamus, and brainstem, which produce the autonomic affective, cognitive, and endocrinologic components of the anxiety responses. Seizures, particularly those involving the limbic system, can hijack this system, giving rise to anxiety (Goldstein & Harden, 2000).

Anxieties of epilepsy

Anxiety episodes may present as auras, ictal episodes, postictal states, interictal behaviors, panic attacks, and non-epileptic events (Devinsky & Vazquez, 1993; Scicutella, 2001). The anxiety of epilepsy may be an anticipatory fear associated with the experiencing of an aura heralding a seizure, or the anxiety may occur without any warning of a seizure. It may be the ictal phenomenon of a simple partial seizure or it may be a preictal aura as part of a complex partial seizure. It may be a postictal event as an aftereffect of a seizure. It may be an interictal manifestation of the same underlying etiology as the primary seizure disorder. It may be an adverse consequence of the antiepileptic medication. It may be an adverse consequence of intrapsychic maladaptation to having epilepsy. It may be an adverse consequence of social malediction to having epilepsy. It may be an unrelated comorbid primary psychiatric disorder (Goldstein & Harden, 2000). In children, a situational anxiety may be related to the stress of a school, home, or peer activity, such stress possibly being related to an underlying language or learning behavior or prior adverse experience (Svoboda, 1979).

Anxiety disorders are reported in 5–32% of people with epilepsy, with an incidence of 13% in those with temporal lobe epilepsy (Hermann *et al.*, 2000). Generally, the incidence is thought to be about 15% in individuals with partial and generalized epilepsy, but in some areas of the world the incidence is 25%. In epilepsy units, an anxiety syndrome has been identified in 10.7–31.6%. Worry is present in 50% of patients. Panic reactions occur in 21% of epilepsy patients compared with 3% of controls. Phobias and obsession features with anxiety occur in 18% of temporal lobe epilepsy patients compared with about 2% of people without epilepsy (Scicutella, 2001).

Prodromal anxiety

Anxiety may emerge up to a week before a seizure, as seen with generalized tonic–clonic seizures. In temporal lobe epilepsy, fear and anxiety are localized to the anterior-medial temporal lobe or structures of the limbic system that produce symptoms of dread, fear, anguish, or despair. These episodes of anxiety are usually brief, lasting seconds to at most two minutes. These may be reported in teenagers or younger children (Scicutella, 2001). Fear and anxiety may be a prodrome in partial seizures in 10–15% of patients. Anteromedial temporal seizures and cingulate seizures may cause anything from a slight uneasiness and nervousness to intense emotions of fear and horror (Devinsky & Vazquez, 1993).

Anxiety aura

The onset of ictal fear is paroxysmal and the duration is usually 30 minutes to two hours (Devinsky & Vazquez, 1993). Fear is a common aura and may mimic panic attacks. Fear is reported as an aura in up to 15% of patients (Torta & Keller, 1999). Ictal fear may be seen as part of epileptic status lasting up to hours or even months. The incidence of ictal fear is about 3%, of neuroses around 16%, and of anxiety 15–25%.

Ictal anxiety

Sudden fear is the most common affective expression of a seizure, but often in children it may not be remembered and can only be inferred by the observer (Blumer & Levin, 1977). Seizure activity can produce symptoms and behaviors indistinguishable from a primary anxiety disorder. Fear is the most common ictal emotion reported in epilepsy (Robertson, 1996). It is seen with mesial-temporal structural lesions associated with intractable epilepsy. Ictal panics are briefer and have greater stereotypy than panic reactions (Young *et al.*, 1995; Goldstein & Harden, 2000).

Fear and anxiety are seen in simple partial seizures, anteromedial-temporal seizures, and cingulate seizures, all of which can cause symptoms from mild uneasiness to horror (Devinsky & Vazquez, 1993). In patients with non-seizure-related anxiety, 63.6% demonstrated abnormal ambulatory EEGs during a 24-hour period, of which 80% were felt to be epileptiform (Jabourian *et al.*, 1992). The discharges originate as temporal lobe EEG abnormalities, although parietal lobe foci may also be noted (Alemayehu *et al.*, 1995; Goldstein & Harden, 2000). Such panic reaction presentations respond well to anticonvulsants (McNamara & Fogel, 1990).

A similar phenomenon does not necessarily imply similar pathophysiology. There is a quite different pattern of benzodiazepine receptor binding potential in anxiety and somatoform disorder patients compared with epilepsy patients, suggesting divergent etiologic mechanisms (Tokunaga *et al.*, 1997; Goldstein & Harden, 2000).

Older adolescents and young adults with complex partial epilepsy may experience episodes of fear as an aural or an isolated ictal event. In a majority, but not all, there are associated video-EEG changes. Significant psychiatric problems including moderate to severe family discord and poor adoptive functioning may be found in 50% (Ficol *et al.*, 1984). Interictal anxiety must be distinguished from the occasional encountered sensation of fear that occurs as ictal symptoms (Weisbrot & Ettinger, 1998).

Postictal anxiety

Postictal fear and anxiety may last hours to days, sometimes even up to seven days post-seizure (Scicutella, 2001).

Interictal anxiety

Interictal periods of anxiety may be seen with both generalized and complex partial seizure syndromes. These periods are experienced as feelings of apprehension or manifest clinical anxiety syndromes such as panic disorders or generalized anxiety disorders (Scicutella, 2001). Interictal fear anxieties are reported by up to 66% of patients, especially in patients with partial seizures with limbic foci and in primarily generalized epilepsy. Two possible reasons include fear of seizure occurrence (seizure phobia) and issues surrounding the loss of control. Actual seizure phobias are rare. Problems related to a sense of loss of control can be profound in patients with epilepsy, potentially the source of discrete panic attacks or a persistent generalized anxiety disorder (McConnell & Duncan, 1998). These problems may be related to learned helplessness models of depression (Goldstein & Harden, 2000).

Postoperative anxiety

Patients with epilepsy commonly fear death and/or brain damage as a result of their seizures (Roth & Harper, 1962). In preoperative evaluations, depressive and anxiety disorders are most common (Krahn *et al.*, 1996). After epilepsy surgery, these emotions often dissipate about six weeks later, but new symptoms of anxiety or depression may develop. By three months postoperatively, anxiety symptoms have diminished whereas depressive states remain for months. Patients with a left hemisphere focus are most likely to experience such a persisting anxiety (Ring *et al.*, 1998).

Situational anxiety

Stressors of either physiologic or psychologic nature can lead to the occurrence of symptoms of anxiety, but it is not clear whether these can worsen seizure activity. The stresses of the unpredictability of epilepsy, reactions to and rejections by others, fear of dying, and fear of school embarrassment may all contribute to anxiety-induced lowering of the seizure threshold (Weisbrot & Ettinger, 2001). Stresses have been identified as a seizure precipitant by 54% of patients with complex partial epilepsy and 51% of those with generalized seizures. Negative events are more apt to trigger seizures. Significantly fewer seizures occur on low-stress days compared with high-stress days. In patients who identify stress as a precipitant, it is often found that the stress has led to sleep deprivation, medication non-compliance, or hyperventilation, which may be the seizure precipitant (Scicutella, 2001). School children may experience seizures that are time-linked to attending specific classes.

Some authors report that in at least 75% of adults with epilepsy, undesirable life events do not affect seizure frequency. There is no variance as per seizure type, gender, age of onset, or age when seizures recur (Neugebauer *et al.*, 1991b). There is a paradoxical relationship between very high seizure frequency and fewer anxiety symptoms. Whether this is a primary effect of the epilepsy syndrome or an adaptive psychological response to frequent repetitive traumatic events is not known. The effect of seizure focus laterality or of medication is also unknown (Goldstein & Harden, 2000).

Generalized anxiety

Generalized anxiety is characterized by excessive worry and uncontrollable concerns occurring daily for at least six months, with fatigue, reduced concentration, irritability, muscle tension, and sleep disturbances. Anxiety and panic can be seen with a variety of medical and neurologic conditions, including temporal lobe epilepsy (Scicutella, 2001).

Epileptic patients have a higher incidence of anxiety traits, especially those with a left temporal lobe EEG abnormality and with a briefer duration of symptomatic epilepsy (Spielberger, 1983; De Albuquerque & de Campos, 1993). A relatively high seizure frequency is associated with lower anxiety levels than a relatively low seizure frequency (Goldstein *et al.*, 1999; Goldstein & Harden, 2000).

Expressions of anxiety in epileptic patients include generalized anxiety disorder. The intrinsic neurochemical and neurophysiological changes related to anxiety appear to be associated with the seizure disorder or with anticonvulsant medication. General anxiety with constant worry and other personal issues occur independently of the epilepsy but are related to the loss of control. Fear of having seizures may become so disabling that it may lead to an agoraphobic state (Kanner *et al.*, 1993).

Panic disorders

Panic attacks occur more frequently in older children and adolescents than in younger children (Mattison, 1997; Weisbrot & Ettinger, 1998), although they are diagnosed most often between the ages of 20 and 30 years. In the epilepsy population, the incidence of panic attacks is about seven times that in the non-epileptic population (Scicutella, 2001).

Ictal panic attacks are briefer than the usual panic attacks and are without feelings of impending doom. The panic is more severe and there is not a prominent family history for panic attacks. Consciousness is maintained during the episode. Anticipatory anxiety is often seen. Non-epileptic panic attacks are more intense and last longer. There is a feeling of impending doom. A positive family history is often found (Kanner *et al.*, 1993; Scicutella, 2001).

Anxiety has been linked to temporal lobe dysfunction, but panic attacks have also been seen by subdural studies with partial seizures with a right parietal activity without mesiotemporal spread. Panic attacks have also been seen with adult-onset absence, juvenile myoclonic epilepsy, and frontal lobe epilepsy (Scicutella, 2001). The limbic system may be involved as a common denominator in complex partial epilepsy and in panic–depersonalization disorders. Patients with limbic seizures are more prone to develop intractable behavior disorders. In animals, stimuli to the amygdala and hippocampus can produce emotional responses such as anxiety-related reactions. Perhaps neuroplasticity processes such as neuronal hyperexcitability or modulation of GABA transmission may occur in structures involved in the control of fear-promoted reactions, such as the amygdala or periaqueductal gray matter, leading to the behavior changes (Depaulis *et al.* 1997).

Panic reactions may be confused with seizures (Mattison, 1997; Weisbrot & Ettinger, 1998). It is not uncommon for a patient to have an episode that is thought to be epileptic but that on video-EEG monitoring turns out to be a protective anxiety episode or a panic attack. Not all panic disorders are truly panic disorders. In the absence of generalization of seizure discharges, epileptic changes may not always be apparent on scalp EEGs, even during a seizure. In monitoring studies, the scalp EEGs may be normal when subdural electrodes show epileptiform activities. A clue to the epileptic etiology is the association of symptoms common to seizures, such as altered awareness or generalized convulsive activity, and epileptiform EEGs during an event (Weisbrot & Ettinger, 1998; Scicutella, 2001).

Obsessive–compulsive disorders

Since the end of the nineteenth century, an increased relationship of obsessive–compulsive disorder (OCD) and seizures has been noted, although histories of head injury are often present (Neugebauer *et al.*, 1991a). Symptoms for OCD can occur during different phases of seizures. Forced thinking can be an aura. Ictal states may manifest with compulsive acts and obsessive thoughts. The associations are rare and often limited to scattered case reports. There are occasional reports of children with OCD and seizures. In one child, a temporal lobectomy rendered the child seizure-free and removed a touching compulsion. A cingulectomy controlled compulsive hand movements and absence-like seizures in an 11-year-old (Caplan *et al.*, 1992; Levin & Duchowny, 1991; Kanner *et al.*, 1993; Eapen *et al.*, 1997; Scicutella, 2001).

Dissociative disorders and depersonalization disorders

Dual personalities have been reported in association with seizures and forced normalization (Devinsky & Vazquez, 1993).

Post-traumatic stress disorders

In post-traumatic stress disorder, the individual experiences, witnesses, or is confronted by events that physically threaten one's self or others, resulting in a response of intense fear, helplessness, or horror. Later, this is experienced through at least two reminders, including recurrent, intrusive, distressing recollections or distressing dreams, flashbacks, or intense psychological distresses at the exposure to events that symbolize or resemble the original traumatic event. There may be a physiological reactivity to cues that symbolize or resemble the traumatic event. Such events may include, for example, being the victim of a natural calamity, of kidnapping, of sexual abuse, or of cultic involvement (Pitman, 1997).

Avoidance criteria include any two of the avoidance of associated thoughts and feelings or of associated activities or situations, the inability to recall important aspects of the trauma, marked diminished interest in significant activities, feelings of detachment or estrangement from others, restricted range of affect (numbing), and a sense of a foreshortened future. Arousal criteria, of which at least two need to be present, include insomnia, irritability, outbursts of anger, difficulties in concentration, hypervigilance, and exaggerated startle responses. These must be of at least one month's duration; the result is clinically significant stressor impairment (Pitman, 1997). Some studies have suggested that neurotransmitter changes are associated with this syndrome as a result rather than the cause of the original experience.

A significant number of patients seen in one epilepsy center presented with a history of a highly dysfunctional family or cultic involvement, with physical, verbal, and at times sexual abuse. The patients often had to be removed from the family. Such children often presented with symptoms of anxiety and related conditions resembling a post-traumatic stress syndrome that was not previously recognized.

Non-epileptic seizures as a result of post-traumatic stress

Children, especially but not exclusively adolescents, may develop non-epileptic seizures as a response to stress. One type of pseudoseizure is triggered by a flashback to a prior trauma, resulting in acting out. Often, but not invariably, this is related to sexual abuse. Non-epileptic events may be part of a chronic post-traumatic stress disorder. This tends to be a resistant form. The history of a prior trauma does not in itself exclude the possibility of epilepsy. Non-epileptic events are a form of communication, i.e. a cry for help, that needs to be understood.

The background level of abuse in a control population of psychiatric patients is 32% compared with 5–10% in the "normal" population. In the UK, 5–10% of children are abused and 25% have long-term pathology as a result.

Non-epileptic seizure-like episodes seen with post-traumatic stress disorder generally fall into one of four categories, namely disassociation (as a survival technique), acting out flashbacks (tantrums), avoidance behavior (as a distraction), or abreactive (showing of strong emotion in reliving the previous traumatic episode). The resultant manifestations can be subdivided into episodes that mimic seizures (76%), episodes that resemble tantrums (42%), and abreactive episodes (82%), the latter referring to episodes of unreactivit, with thrashing, gasping, pelvic thrusting, gagging, or vomiting. Sometimes the child stares or swoons, occasionally with a minor tremor noted.

Generally in children with post-traumatic stress, the syndrome may present with a variety of other symptoms. There may be a history of flashbacks and recurrent nightmares. There may be recurring episodes of anxiety. The child may demonstrate severe distress or nervousness in certain situations. They may not be able to let go of the memories. There is both behavioral and cognitive avoidance of remembering. There may be rumination on the trauma, i.e. the "Why did I survive?" question.

There are several other courses of post-traumatic stress disorder. In children, underlying causes include school (30%), adolescence (24%), a traumatic experience (19%), or a regressive affection (8%). There may be multiple stresses (14%). The etiology is unclear in 5% of patients.

School may cause problems of overexpectation. In adolescence, there may be overprotectiveness. Traumatic experiences include loss, rape, and incest. Problems of affection are usually associated with an inability to handle such feelings.

There is a long list of chemical and biological abnormal responses to post-traumatic stress disorder, including sleep changes, P300 responses to target stimuli, and changes in the hippocampal volume (Pitman, 1997).

Some parents of children with intractable epilepsy may develop the symptoms of post-traumatic stress syndrome due to the stresses of coming to terms with the child's illness and obtaining appropriate services (Robin et al., 1992). Families who have been involved in cultic activities and then "deprogrammed" through counseling may be found to exhibit post-traumatic stress disorders. Sometimes, these may present at an epilepsy center as non-epileptic seizures.

Conclusions

The existence of marriage and family problems is increased with non-epileptic seizures. The non-epileptic event population is quite heterogeneous. Such patients often have high levels of depression and low self-esteem. The family functioning is important in both diagnosis and therapy. Marital partnerships and extended family must often be considered.

Therapy

Epileptic children and their families need frank and repeated discussion to address both appropriate and irrational fears about epilepsy. Peer support groups can be helpful. When symptoms of anxiety do not respond rapidly to psychosocial and behavioral interventions, the use of psychotropic medication may be considered as adjunct therapy. SSRI and tricyclic antidepressants may be helpful for anxiety. Benzodiazepines are useful in adults and have anticonvulsant properties. For intense panic or disabling anxiety, lorazepam and clonazepam may be useful as primary or adjunctive therapy. Withdrawal seizures may result from abrupt discontinuation of these agents, and patients and their caregivers should be warned of this (Weisbrot & Ettinger, 1998).

Enzyme-inducing anticonvulsants lower the serum concentrations of other drugs metabolized in the liver, including most psychotropic drugs. SSRI antidepressants, such as fluoxetine, sertraline, fluvoxamine, and paroxetine, inhibit cytochrome P450 and thus may inhibit anticonvulsant metabolism. This can increase levels of drugs such as phenytoin. Citalopram does not have a metabolic effect. Paroxetine inhibits the CB2 enzyme and thus has no anticonvulsant interactions. Protein binding is also seen with SSRIs (Scicutella, 2001).

Imipramine is effective for panic disorders, but it can produce seizures in a minority of patients (0.3–0.6%) (Scicutella, 2001). SSRIs are effective for both panic disorders and OCD and are less epileptogenic than other antidepressants. Paroxetine has a seizure incidence of 0.1%. Monoamine oxidase inhibitors are helpful for panic reactions and are among the least proconvulsive of the antidepressants; however, they can potentiate the activity of CNS depressants (Scicutella, 2001).

Benzodiazepines can treat both seizures and anxiety, although they may be less well tolerated than other drugs. Patients with or without a history of seizures are at risk for withdrawal seizures if these drugs are discontinued abruptly, and thus the drugs should be tapered slowly (Weisbrot & Ettinger, 1998). Clonazepam and alprazolam have been shown to be effective for anxiety. Shorter-acting agents should be avoided because of the chances of rebound anxiety episodes. Abrupt discontinuation of any of these drugs can cause withdrawal symptoms, including anxiety, insomnia, and autonomic hyperactivity. Valproate has been reported to improve symptoms in panic disorders. Carbamazepine has been effective in OCD, with mixed efficacy in panic disorders. Oxycarbazepine may also help (Scicutella, 2001).

Behavior approaches such as hypnosis, biofeedback, and muscle relaxation have been used to reduce anxiety symptoms. Cognitive behavioral approaches may help adults with phobias or patients with temporal lobe epilepsy and OCD, with a 50% reduction in the ritualistic mannerisms. Psychoeducational methods can help patients to deal with their illnesses and reduce anxiety (Scicutella, 2001).

Escapism, forgetfulness, and fugue states

Rowan & Rosenbaum (1991) have reviewed ictal amnesia and fugue states, noting that drugs, recurrent seizures, depression, and active CNS degeneration can impair memory.

Episodic memory loss

Recurrent paroxysmal memory disturbances without alterations of consciousness and with related EEG disturbances may be epileptic. These are brief but usually recurrent. There may or may not be a retrograde memory loss. Benign epileptiform transients of sleep (BETS) must be differentiated. Bilateral amygdalar and hippocampal involvement is necessary to produce a memory loss; unilateral involvement is not enough. Although rare, this can be seen in children around 11 years of age, with right temporal spikes, the episode lasting ten minutes. The major criterion for an ictal memory loss is that an epileptic seizure should have occurred immediately before or after the event. The duration of memory loss is usually up to 60 minutes. This is repetitive. The patient must have at least one other associated criterion, including EEG abnormalities, confusion, past history of seizures, and/or positive drug response (Rowan & Rosenbaum, 1991).

Psychogenic fugues

Psychogenic fugues may be associated with a retrograde amnesia without any anterograde amnesia. There may be a preceding stress that may be trivial (Rowan & Rosenbaum, 1991).

Purposeful forgetting

Memory problems may be claimed as part of malingering, but this is purposeful forgetting, usually seen in adults. An older child may try this but usually has been coached by an adult for devious purposes. Some may claim forgetfulness for an act, but this proves to be a form of denial. The individual has amnesia limited only to the event. Adults may use this to avoid criminal prosecution. A child caught in a forbidden act may deny such an event happened (Rowan & Rosenbaum, 1991).

Epileptic fugues

This is a twilight state that can occur in a variety of seizures:

Absence status

In absence status, amnesia may correlate with a stupor and confusion. The patient may seem slowed and variable in responses. It is doubtful that it occurs with a clear sensorium (Rowan & Rosenbaum, 1991).

Complex partial epileptic status

There is severe anterograde and retrograde amnesia, although the anterograde amnesia may resolve. A brief hippocampal distorted memory may be involved. Most epileptic amnesias are postictal sequelae of subtle seizures. Ictal amnesias are rare and are bitemporal in involvement (Rowan & Rosenbaum, 1991).

Memory impairment leading to decreased alertness and distractibility may be seen with a slow EEG picture with spiking. This may be part of a non-convulsive status or may be non-ictal, as a metabolic disturbance. The stress may be post-traumatic or may lead to a loss of any anxiety, as with a psychiatric amnesia. One must also consider malingering or pseudoseizures. If the episode is prolonged for hours, a transient ischemic attack must be considered in an older person or a young person with a blood dyscrasia. If the associated EEG is epileptic, the activity is most often ictal.

Postictal confusion

After a seizure, a severe confusional state may last for days to weeks. An epileptic encephalopathy may exist, with a prolonged epileptic confusion lasting one to two weeks. The EEG may be slowed. The etiology of the seizures is usually acquired. Often, mild imaging abnormalities are found. Such patients are often of below-average intelligence. Usually, there are multifocal structural abnormalities involving the brain.

Seizures may appear with amnesia as the main presentation, but other seizure symptoms may also be present. It is hard to differentiate what is ictal and what is postictal in a prolonged postictal confusion. True postictal confusion is not responsive to an anticonvulsant load; it gradually resolves independently of therapy (Rowan & Rosenbaum, 1991).

Self-evoked seizures

Up to 5% of seizures may be evoked seizures. Such attacks may be auditory-, sensory-, movement-, visual-, or visceral-induced. Primary attacks are those with a deliberate alteration of seizure activity, as with self-induction. Secondary attacks are those with an unintended alteration of seizure activity as a result of chance exposure.

Some children and also a few adults will induce their own seizures. Such individuals often have seizures that can be precipitated easily by, for example, deep breathing or flashing lights. The seizure can be intrinsically pleasurable or can be used to manipulate the environment. Some adults and children may try to stimulate their seizures to get out of an anxiety-producing situation or to manipulate sympathy from another individual.

It is not enough just to ignore the behavior; rather, it is important to determine why the patient seeks such a manipulative behavior and to work with that. Occasionally, people injure themselves in a self-induced seizure. Some patients will utilize medication omissions in the same manner, to purposefully trigger seizures. If the result is status epilepticus, the results could be fatal.

REFERENCES

Alemayehu, S., Bergey, G., Barry, E., *et al.* (1995). Panic attacks as ictal manifestations of parietal lobe seizures. *Epilepsia* **36**: 824–30.

Blumer, D. & Levin, K. (1977). Psychiatric complications in the epilepsies: current research and treatment. In *Proceedings of the Conference on Psychiatric Disorders in Epilepsy, McLean Hospital Journal*, Special Issue 15.

Caplan, R., Guthrie, D., Shields, W. D., *et al.* (1992). Formal thought disorder in pediatric complex partial seizure disorders. *J Child Psychol. Psychiatry* **33**: 1399–1412.

De Albuquerque, M. D. & de Campos, C. J. R. (1993). Epilepsy and anxiety. *Arq. Neuropsiquiatr.* **51**: 313–18.

Depaulis, A., Helfer, V., Deransart, C., *et al.* (1997). Anxiogenic like consequences in animal models of complex partial seizures. *Neurosci. Biobehav. Rev.* **21**: 767–74.

Devinsky, O. & Vazquez, B. (1993). Behavioral changes associated with epilepsy. *Neurol. Clin.* **11**: 127–49.

Eapen V., Champion, L. & Zeitlin, H. (1997). Tourette syndrome, epilepsy and emotional disorder, a case of triple comorbidity. *Psychol. Rep.* **81**: 1239–43.

Ettinger, A. B., Wisbrot, D. M., Nolan, E. E., *et al.* (1998). Symptoms of depression and anxiety in pediatric epilepsy patients. *Epilepsia* **39**: 595–9.

Ficol, M., Ramani, V. & Herron, C. (1984). Episodic fear in epilepsy. *Epilepsia* **25**: 669–70.

Francis, S., Weisbrot D. M., Jandorf, L., *et al.* (1966). Anxiety in epilepsy. *Epilepsia* **37**: 3.

Goldstein, M. A. & Harden, C. L. (2000). Epilepsy and anxiety. *Epilepsy Behav.* **1**: 228–34.

Goldstein, M. A., Harden, C. L., Ravdin, L. D., *et al.* (1999). Does anxiety in epilepsy patients decrease with increasing seizure frequency? *Epilepsia* **40** (suppl 7): 60–61.

Hermann, B. P., Seidenberg, M. & Bell, B. (2000). Psychiatric comorbidity in chronic epilepsy: identification, consequences, and treatment of major depression. *Epilepsia* **41** (suppl 2): 31–41.

Jabourian, A. P., Erlich, M., Desvignes, C., *et al.* (1992). Panic attacks and 24-hour ambulatory EEG monitoring. *Ann. Med. Psychol. (Paris)* **150**: 240–44.

Kanner, A. M., Mirris, H. H., Stagno, S., *et al.* (1993). Remission of an obsessive compulsive disorder following a right temporal lobectomy. *Neuropsychiatry Neuropsychol. Behav. Neurol.* **6**: 126–9.

Krahn, L. E., Ruimmans, T. A. & Peterson, G. C. (1996). Psychiatric implications of surgical treatment of epilepsy. *Mayo Clin. Proc.* **71**: 1201–4.

Levin, B. K., & Duchowny, M. (1991). Childhood obsessive-compulsive disorders and cingulate epilepsy. *Biol. Psychiatry* **30**: 1049–55.

Mattison, R. (1997). Separation anxiety disorder and anxiety in children. In *Comprehensive Textbook of Psychiatry*, ed. H. I. Kaplan & B. J. Sadock, pp. 2345–51. Baltimore, MD: Williams & Wilkins.

McConnell, H. W. & Duncan, D. (1998). Treatment of psychiatric comorbidity in epilepsy. In *Psychiatric Comorbidity in Epilepsy*, ed. H. W. McConnell & P. J. Snyder, pp. 245–362. Washington, DC: American Psychiatric Press.

McNamara, M. & Fogel, B. (1990). Anticonvulsant responsive panic attacks with temporal lobe EEG abnormalities. *J. Neuropsychiatry* **2**: 193–6.

Mittan, R. J. & Locke, G. E. (1982). Fear of seizures: epilepsy's forgotten problem. *Urban Health* **40**: 38–9.

Neugebauer, R., Johnson, J. & Hornig, C. (1991a). Epidemiologic study of obsessive compulsive disorder and seizures: the "temporal lobe personality" considered. *Epilespia* **32** (suppl 3): 39.

Neugebauer, R., Palk, M., Nadel, E., *et al.* (1991b). Association of stressful life events with seizure occurrence in patients with epilepsy. *Epilepsia* **32** (suppl 3): 31.

Pitman, R. K. (1997). Overview of biological themes in PTSD. In *Psychobiology of Posttraumatic Stress Disorder*, ed. R. Yehuda & A. C. McFarlane. *Ann. N. Y. Acad. Sci.* **821**: 1–9.

Ring, H. A., Moriarty, J. & Trimble, M. R. (1998). A prospective study of the early postsurgical psychiatric associations of epilepsy surgery. *J. Neurol. Neurosurg. Psychiatry* **64**: 601–4.

Robertson, M. (1996). Epilepsy and anxiety. In *Psychiatric Literature.* Vol. 6, p. 1015. New York: Sanofi Winthrop.

Robin, M., Frost, M., Ritter, F. J., *et al.* (1992). Posttraumatic stress disorder in families of children with intractable epilepsy. *Epilespia* **33** (suppl 3): **8**.

Roth, M. & Harper, M. (1962). Temporal lobe epilepsy and phobic anxiety, depersonalization syndrome. Part II: practical and theoretical considerations. *Compr. Psychiatry* **3**: 215–26.

Rowan, M. & Rosenbaum, D. H. (1991). Ictal amnesia and fugue states. In *Advances in Neurology*, ed. D. B. Smith, D. M. Treiman & M. R. Trimble, Vol. 55, pp. 357–68. New York: Raven Press.

Scicutella, A. (2001). Anxiety disorders in epilepsy. In *Psychiatric Issues in Epilepsy*, ed. A. B. Ettinger & A. M. Kanner, pp. 95–110. Philadelphia: Lippincott Williams & Wilkins.

Spielberger, C. D. (1983). *Manual for the State-Trait Anxiety Inventory.* Palo Alto, CA: Consultant Psychologist Press.

Svoboda, W. B. (1979). Emotional and behavioral consequences of epilepsy. *In Learning About Epilepsy*, pp. 157–84. Baltimore, MD: University Park Press.

Tokunaga, M., Ida, I., Higuchi, T., *et al.* (1997). Alterations of benzodiazepine receptor binding potential in anxiety and somatoform disorders measured by ^{123}I-SPECT. *Radiat. Med.* **15**: 163–9.

Torta, R. & Keller, R. (1999). Behavioral, psychotic, and anxiety disorders in epilepsy: etiology, clinical features, and therapeutic implications. *Epilepsia* **40** (suppl 10): 2–20.

Trimble, M. (1988). *Biological Psychiatry.* New York: John Wiley & Sons.

Weisbrot, D. M. & Ettinger, A. B. (1998). Psychiatric aspects of Pediatric Epilepsy. *Primary Psychiatry* **June**: 51–67.

Weisbrot, D. & Ettinger, A. B. (2001). Psychiatric aspects of pediatric epilepsy. In *Psychiatric Issues in Epilepsy*, ed. A. B. Ettinger & A. M. Kanner, pp. 127–46. Philadelphia: Lippincott Williams & Wilkins.

Young, G. B., Chandrara, P. C., Blume, W. T., *et al.* (1995). Mesial temporal lobe seizures presenting as anxiety disorders. *J. Neuropsychiatry Clin. Neurosci.* **7**: 352–7.

34

Mood disorders

Hippocrates felt that melancholiacs become epileptics and epileptics become melancholic. What is spoken of now as mood disorders of epilepsy was once envisioned as an epileptic personality described as languid, spiritless, unsociable in any period of life, sleepless, and subject to many horrid dreams (Kanner & Balabanov, 2002).

Mood disorders include major depression, bipolar disorder, dysthymic disorders, and a double depression state. Major depression usually begins in late adolescence but has been diagnosed as early as four years of age. A bipolar disorder may vary as to the age of appearance. In children and younger teens, both mania and deep depression may present simultaneously, whereas in older adolescents, the more typical cycle between mania and deep depression is noted. A dysthymic disorder is a chronic, persistent, mild depression that begins in early childhood and lasts for decades. A double depression is seen in individuals who alternate between a dysthymic disorder and a major depression.

In epilepsy, there are three types of mood disorder, ictal, peri-ictal, and interictal. Peri-ictal disorders include the cluster of affective systems that may precede or follow a seizure by hours to days. Ictal disorders represent seizures presenting with affective symptoms. There is an interictal dysphoric disorder with an intermittent course, including depressive mood, lack of energy, pain, and insomnia. The affective symptoms include irritability, euphoria, fear, and anxiety (Barry *et al.*, 2001).

Depression

Depression is often unrecognized and undertreated in patients with epilepsy, especially children. There is often a delay in the diagnosis and remediation of depression disorders of epilepsy of a year or more, unrelated to the severity of the disorder (Kanner & Balabanov, 2002).

Symptoms

The dysphorias of epilepsy may be brief, non-precipitated mood changes of rapid onset and termination without any alteration of consciousness. These may recur in a fairly regular manner independent of any seizures (Kanner & Balabanov, 2002).

Individuals with epilepsy present with complaints of dysphoria (25%) such as depression, irritability or euphoria, pain (20%), or anxiety or fears (12–15%). Other complaints include a lack of energy, insomnia, or suicidal tendencies. Rarely, hallucinatory or psychotic symptoms (2%) may occur. The moods may be paroxysmal or labile, waxing and waning over hours to days. Patients tend to minimize symptoms, fearing a psychiatric stigma or feeling that this is part of the epileptic process. Physicians may overlook the diagnosis or fear adverse reactions to antidepressant therapy (Kanner & Balabanov, 2002).

Incidence

In the general population, mood disorders are prevalent in 6–17% (Hermann *et al.*, 2000). Around 3% of normal people, especially women, experience significant depression (Hauser & Hesdorffer, 2000). About 4.9% of the general population experiences a bipolar disorder and 3.3% a dysthymic disorder (Barry *et al.*, 2001). In a lifetime, 17% of the general population experiences a major depression (Hauser & Hesdorffer, 2000).

The prevalence of depressive disorders in people with epilepsy is not known (Kanner & Balabanov, 2002). The incidence of mood disorders is probably in the range 29–37% (Barry *et al.*, 2001). In a lifetime, the incidence is more in the range 44–63% (Onuma, 2000). Within the epilepsy population, 32% of people have a major depression history and 25% have a minor depression history (Hermann *et al.*, 2000). Reports of feeling depressed have been found in up to 80% of patients with epilepsy (Currie *et al.*, 1971; Blumer & Zielinski, 1988; Kanner & Balabanov, 2002). Atypical depressions are the most common (Kanner & Balabanov, 2002).

Suicide attempts, including deliberate self-harm, in the epileptic population are at least four to five times that seen in the general population. In patients with temporal lobe epilepsy, suicide attempts occur up to 25 times more frequently (Zielinski, 1974; Hawton *et al.*, 1980; Barraclough, 1981; Trimble, 1988; Harris & Barraclough, 1997; Weisbrot & Ettinger, 1998; Barry *et al.*, 2001). Risk factors for suicide include previous history of deliberate self-harm, family history of suicide, stressful life events, poor morale, stigma, and psychiatric disorders, especially alcohol and drug abuse, depression, psychosis, and personality disorders (Harris & Barclough, 1997; Robertson, 1997).

Depression in its various forms is a psychiatric comorbidity that is under-recognized and undertreated in chronic epilepsy. Only 55% of primary care patients with depression are identified, and only 11% receive medication. From 38–43% up to 60–67% of patients with depression are untreated (Hermann *et al.*, 2000).

Types of epileptic depression ˎ

Mood disturbances are fairly common. Depressive episodes may occur predominantly as preictal, ictal, postictal and interictal, but postoperative depressions also occur. Differentiation may be difficult in patients with frequent seizures (Lambert & Robertson, 1999).

Pre-epilepsy depression

About 16% of patients with epilepsy, especially those with complex partial seizures, may experience a bout of depression before the seizure disorder emerges (Hauser & Hesdorffer, 2000). Depression and epilepsy may have common pathogenic mechanisms (Kanner & Balabanov, 2002).

Preictal depression

Behavioral premonitory symptoms of irritability, depression, fears, elation, and anger preceding partial seizures by 30 minutes are seen in 20–33% of patients (Blumer, 1991), persisting from from ten minutes to three days in a waxing and waning course (Blanchet & Frommer, 1986). The low mood may represent a symptom of subclinical seizure activity or of physiologic or biologic processes involved in initiation of both lowered mood and seizures.

Ictal depression

Depression presenting as abrupt, out-of-context feelings ranging from mild fear or sadness to profound hopelessness and despair may be a part of the seizure symptom. This is seen in about 1% of patients, and in up to 10% of complex partial epilepsy patients (Devinsky et al., 1994). Complex hallucinations may occur. Some patients report suicidal urges and attempts, which may persist for hours to a few days. Often, seizures are poorly controlled (Blumer, 1991; Kanner & Balabanov, 2002). An ictal depression of prolonged duration may represent underlying subclinical seizure activity (Weil, 1959; Williams, 1956).

Postictal depression

Symptoms of depression during the postictal period are relatively frequent in patients with poorly controlled partial seizure disorders. This usually lasts a day or two, although it may last up to a week and may be recurrent (Kanner & Balabanov, 2002). Such symptoms may be the persistence of an ictal depression or may be part of a separate entity (Blumer, 1992). Postictal depression is seen especially with complex partial epilepsy and may be worse than the seizure disorder itself (Blumer, 1992). The postictal depression may be the consequences of inhibitory mechanisms involved in the termination of seizures (Blumer, 1991; Devinsky et al., 1994).

Interictal depression

Interictal depression is more common (11–50%) and often more severe than peri-ictal depression (Standage & Fenton, 1975; Kogeorgos *et al.*, 1982; Mendez *et al.*, 1986; Mendez *et al.*, 1993; Barry *et al.*, 2001), especially in patients with severe, frequent seizures (Lambert & Robertson, 1999). The depression appears to be endogenous, with sudden onset, marked fluctuations, and abrupt cessation. It may be accompanied by agitation and impulsive suicidal behavior. Neurotic traits are less prominent and psychotic traits are more common (Betts, 1981; Mendez *et al.*, 1986; Mendez *et al.*, 1993; Lambert & Robertson, 1999). Between major attacks, a tendency towards dysthymia with irritability and humorlessness may be seen.

There are different subtypes of interictal depression. An atypical presentation of interictal depression is relatively frequent (Kanner & Balabanov, 2002). Brief labile depressive symptoms lasting from half a day to several days may recur up to several times a month. Paroxysmal irritability and euphoric moods lasting hours may occur. A labile affect presenting with fear and anxiety or depression may also be reported. Patients with a large number of intense dysphoric symptoms may be at increased suicide risk (Blumer, 1991). The cause of these symptoms may be complex partial seizures, anticonvulsants such as barbiturates and vigabatrin, or psychosocial factors (Lambert & Robertson, 1999). These symptoms are seen especially with right or bitemporal limbic discharges (Blumer, 1991; Devinsky *et al.*, 1994).

Medication-related depressions

About 12% of patients with epilepsy experience episodes of depressed mood related to increasing or changing antiepileptic drugs (especially phenobarbital or pheny-toin) or rarely with neuroleptic therapy. Symptoms emerge gradually, often with slowing and suicidal ideations. Reduction of the anticonvulsant dosage and/or insti-tution of a neuroleptic may be considered. Carbamazepine and valproate treatment has been helpful. In 37% of patients, depression persists and has to be treated. Treat-ment with an antidepressant is usually needed for at least two weeks (Sarzhevskiy, 1998).

Postoperative depression

A self-limited mild to severe depression may emerge after a temporal lobectomy when seizure control is gained. Postoperative lessening of excitatory activity and relative predominance of inhibition may predispose to the emergence of dysphoric, affective, and psychotic disorders. Mood instability with anxiety appears in the ini-tial six weeks postoperatively, lasting for several months before fading. A depression emerges at about two months, persisting for at least three months. Patients with a prior history of depression are at greater risk. Depression is more apt to be seen with a right-sided operation (75%). A bipolar affective disorder has also been seen (Ring *et al.*, 1998; Lambert & Robertson, 1999).

A reactive depression may also be seen. The epilepsy can be a crutch: after surgery, adjusting to life without seizures may be difficult. This is seen in about 6%. The epilepsy may have served as an excuse for failures in personal, social, and occupational areas. Without the excuse, the patient may become depressed. Postoperative counseling may be important (Thompson, 1991; Usiskin, 1995).

Types of epilepsy

The incidence of depression and anxiety is much higher in patients with partial seizures, especially of left temporal lobe etiology (Barry *et al.*, 2001), although some authors have found no relationship to the lateralization, gender, or frequency of seizures (Piazza & Canger, 2001).

Generalized epilepsies

Individuals with juvenile myoclonic epilepsy, and their relatives, may experience a mild to moderate depression with lack of insight and denial (Murray *et al.*, 1994; Lambert & Robertson, 1999; Rey *et al.*, 2000).

Partial epilepsies

Depression is far more frequent in patients with uncontrolled seizures of the frontal or temporal lobes involving the limbic system (Kanner & Balabanov, 2002; Gilliam *et al.*, 2000).

In patients with complex partial epilepsy, especially with more frequent attacks (Lambert & Robertson, 1999), 20–30% are or will become depressed. This rises to 62–87% if the seizures are intractable, with up to 51% experiencing depressive episodes; which are often recurrent. Suicidal ideas are noted in 47% (Currie *et al.*, 1971; Blumer & Zielinski, 1988; Blumer, 1992; Kanner & Balabanov, 2002). Males with left-sided foci appear to be especially prone (Lambert & Robertson, 1999).

A frontal lobe dysfunction also has been associated with depression. Complex partial epilepsy may compromise frontal lobe function. A bilateral reduction in inferior frontal metabolism is seen, even in patients with well-located temporal lobe foci with a primary or secondary depression of any origin (Bromfield *et al.*, 1990). A concomitant dysfunction of mesial-temporal structures has also been suggested. Hippocampal atrophy with mesiotemporal sclerosis may be seen with major depressions.

Depression, like anxiety and perhaps hypomania, is more often seen with left-sided foci, although either side may be involved (Heilman *et al.*, 1975; Devinsky *et al.*, 1994; Lambert & Robertson, 1999; Barry *et al.*, 2001; Piazza & Canger, 2001). Functional neuroimaging studies with PET and SPECT have shown lower metabolism and blood flow in the left hemisphere than in the right hemisphere in patients with partial epilepsy and a history of interictal depression (Kanner & Balabanov, 2002). In some patients with progressively controlled temporal lobe epilepsy, a variety of recurrent episodes of affective disorders that are almost indistinguishable from pure episodes of mood disorders may appear. These are associated with right (80%) or bilateral (20%) foci (Frangos & Alexandrakou, 1991; Lambert & Robertson, 1999).

Modifying factors

Depression is affected by gender, age, introversion, pharmacology, polytherapy, and a longer duration of epilepsy (Ratti *et al.*, 1998).

Etiology

The etiology of depression in chronic epilepsy is not known, but it appears to be multifactorial, with both endogenous and exogenous contributions (Hermann *et al.*, 2000).

Endogenous factors

Depressed patients exhibit fewer neurotic traits and more psychotic symptoms, such as paranoia, delusions, and persecutory auditory hallucinations. Women report depression more often than men (Standage & Fenton, 1975; Altshuler *et al.*, 1990; Strauss *et al.*, 1992; Ratti *et al.*, 1998; Lambert & Robertson, 1999). There may be an increased incidence of left-handedness (Altshuler *et al.*, 1990; Indaco *et al.*, 1992; Lambert & Robertson, 1999). Depression may occur more often with structural lesions (Taylor, 1972; Koch-Weser *et al.*, 1988), although this is debated (Mendez *et al.*, 1986; Mendez *et al.*, 1993; Hermann & Whitman, 1989; Lambert & Robertson, 1999). A family history is seen in more than 50% of patients (Robertson, 1998; Kanner & Balabanov, 2002). Depression and psychiatric problems are more apt to occur in individuals with lower intelligences or learning disabilities (Deb & Hunter, 1991; Lambert & Robertson, 1999).

There appears to be no relationship to the onset age or duration of the epilepsy (Lambert & Robertson, 1999). The incidence rises proportionally to the seizure frequency, although some authors have suggested a decrease in frequency before the onset of the depressive illness. In some patients, depression may be a reactive process to epilepsy. Predictors of depression include increased perceived stigma, poor social support, increased stressful events, poor adjustment, and poor control (Kanner & Balabanov, 2002).

Depression is more common in patients treated with polytherapy, especially with barbiturates, phenytoin, and vigabatrin (Lambert & Robertson, 1999; Mendez *et al.*, 1993; Fiordelli *et al.*, 1993). Drugs such as phenobarbital and phenytoin may cause depressive suicidal ideations at any age (Pratt *et al.*, 1984; Brent *et al.*, 1987; Smith & Collins, 1987; Barabas & Matthews, 1988; Hermann & Wyler, 1989). In high-risk patients, other drugs should replace antiepileptic drugs that cause dysthymic states (Weisbrot & Ettinger, 1998). Primidone, tiagabine, vigabatrin, felbamate, and topiramate frequently cause symptoms of depression. Even anticonvulsants with mood-stabilizing properties such as carbamazepine and valproate can occasionally cause depressive episodes (Kanner & Balabanov, 2002). Withdrawal of antiepileptic drugs, especially benzodiazepines and barbiturates, may result in depression (Dodrill *et al.*, 1984; Kendrick *et al.*, 1993). Antiepileptic drugs may cause depression by decreasing folate levels. Folates are important in methylation in the nervous system (Vickrey *et al.*, 1992). Methylation reactions are involved with neurotransmitters and monoamines implicated in the etiology of affective disorders (Lambert & Robertson, 1999).

Antidepressants may increase the risk of seizures, perhaps due to inhibition of serotonin reuptake at the synaptic cleft. Tricyclic antidepressants, SSRIs, and neuroleptics can cause seizures. Tricycles increase spike activity in animal studies (Hauser & Hesdorffer, 2000). Depression with its neurochemical correlates may make the brain more vulnerable to seizures.

Neurometabolic changes

Epilepsy and depression share common pathogenic mechanisms mediated by decreased serotonergic, noradrenergic, dopaminergic, and GABAergic activity, especially as related to depressed frontal lobe activity. Carbamazepine, lamotrigine, zonisamide, valproic acid, and vigabatrin all increase both norepinephrine and 5-hydroxytryptamine levels (Meldrum, 1991; Kanner & Balabanov, 2002).

Exogenous factors

Factors that may contribute to the development of depression include lack of social acceptance, poor adjustment to the disorder, the need to significantly alter lifestyles, irrational fears about self-injury or dying (Mittan, 1986; Mittan, 1987; Kanner & Balabanov, 2002), and socioeconomic limitations (Dodrill *et al.*, 1984).

Childhood depression

Depression is often overlooked in children, for children may deny symptoms and parents appear more focused on the epilepsy than on the mood (Weisbrot & Ettinger, 1998).

Clinical

Symptoms include a dropping school performance, withdrawal from friends, and loss of pleasure from previous enjoyable activities (Weisbrot & Ettinger, 1998). A negative attitude towards the epilepsy, dissatisfaction with family relationships, and a feeling of a lack of control over one's own life and destiny are clues (Glauser, 1999). Even with significant depression, the child may show only irritability.

Incidence

Depression, often unrecognized in children and adolescence, occurs in about 23–26% of children with epilepsy, and 9% of epileptic children show depressive tendencies (Ettinger & Perrine, 1996; Dunn *et al.*, 1997; Weisbrot & Ettinger, 1998), which is four times greater than in controls (Ronald & Duman, 1999; Hauser & Hesdorffer, 2000; Kanner & Balabanov, 2002). Major depression, rare in preschool children, occurs in 2% of children and 5% of adolescents with epilepsy. About 23% of adolescents with epilepsy have symptoms of depression (Dunn *et al.*, 1997). It is more common in girls at this age (Kashani *et al.*, 1987). In follow-up, 53% of epileptic females and 12% of epileptic males were depressed. Depression is a frequent cause of pediatric suicide attempts (Brent *et al.*, 1987; Weisbrot & Ettinger, 1998).

Ages of depression

The state of sadness that defines depression in adults presents somewhat differently in children. Children are involved in different psychosocial developmental stages at different ages. Depression, when present, may show up in different presentations at different ages.

Infancy

Infants develop attachment through gratification. The loss of such may result in displaced attachments, distancing and apathy, a devaluing of the self, and anger. The child's accomplishments may be a means of gaining family acceptance, and affection needs to be earned. The infant may present with a failure to thrive or an apathetic withdrawal. The young child who develops seizures may find that the focus is more on the seizure aspects and thus find it hard to get affection for other aspects.

Childhood

Children may place excessive demands upon themselves. If depression ensues, sadness may not always be evidenced or even complained of. There may be paradoxical behaviors and psychosomatic symptoms. Both passive and active reactions are seen.

The child may set high standards. Toddlers may present with aggressive and opposi- tional behaviors. The school-aged child may present with inattention, hyperactivity, school problems, or social withdrawal. Often, the diagnosis is missed or misinter- preted. The child's performance efforts may be impeded by the epilepsy and its consequences. Variables relating to this include the child's attitude towards having seizures, the family relationships, negative coping, the ability to talk out feelings, acting out, and a powerful loss of control; the child's attitude, acting out, and loss of control are particularly important (Dunn, 1996).

Adolescence

By adolescence, there may be identity confusions and impaired self-image. Conflicts emerge in initiative versus apathy, dependence versus independence, acting out ver- sus escapism, and affection-seeking versus self-condemnation. Clinically, one may see wide mood swings, low self-esteem, attacks on the parent, indecisiveness, dissat- isfaction, affection-seeking, fantasy retreat, oversensitivity, self-condemnation, and acting-out behaviors. The teenager may present with somatic complaints, acting- out behaviors, conduct disorders, substance abuse, or more obvious depression. The adolescent with epilepsy is already caught up in the battle of dependence versus in- dependence and often has developed a low-self esteem. Almost half of adolescents with complex partial epilepsy display moderate depression symptoms (Macniak, 1999).

Factors

Family attitudes towards the epilepsy, feelings of shame, fear, and embarrassment, the experience of social rejection, and parental insecurities may be depressing to the child (Lambert & Robertson, 1999). Parents may expect their child with epilepsy to have more emotional problems (Long & Moore, 1979). Social isolation and school difficulties accentuate the feelings of low worth (Robertson, 1998).

Diagnosis

Medical staff (Mayou & Hawton, 1986) and general practitioners (Roberts, 1995) overlook roughly half of all cases of childhood depression. The low moods tend to be pervasive and long-lasting. Drug intoxication with antiepileptics, especially phenytoin, may mimic depression (Betts, 1981).

In diagnosing depression in children, the depression should be of at least two weeks' duration, and manifest by sadness, self-deprecation, inability to have fun, and a low self-image. There are at least two to four associated features, including excessive or deficient activity, aggressiveness, reduced interest, impaired school- work, somatic complaints, sleep or appetite disturbances, or even a death fixation. Depression may occur in boys and girls equally, although by adolescence it is seen more often in girls (67%). Childhood depression is often misdiagnosed as anxiety (10%), ADHD (10%), a conduct disorder (42%), an eating disorder (33%), oppositional behavior, separation anxiety, a socialization problem, or psychotic behavior. Teenage depression may be reactive and situation, or bipolar in presentation. It is important to look for psychosocial factors at all ages (Barry *et al.*, 2001).

Assessment and interventions should be directed toward the attitudes, feelings, and family communication (Dunn, 1996). The diagnosis is reduced to a good history and wise interpretations of the symptoms. It is helpful to know whether there is any family history of depression: depressed parents tend to have depressed children.

At any age there is no diagnostic test, laboratory study, or neuropsychologic means of diagnosing depression or any related dysphorias. The WISC IQ test may show performance depression more than verbal depression. The dexamethasone suppression test shows a 40–70% failure rate, especially if the individual is on anticonvulsants. This may show up with postictal depression as well as an interictal depression (Blumer, 1991).

EEG

There is no typical EEG change with depression. If known epileptic symptoms and behaviors occur together, then the child may be epileptic. It is very rare for a child with pure behaviors to be epileptic. Stereotypic behaviors suggest seizures (Blumer, 1991). A child with EEG paroxysms but no seizures and with school problems may respond to an anticonvulsant, since subclinical discharges may be interfering with processing; similarly, subclinical discharges theoretically contribute to behavioral outbursts. A negative EEG suggests a psychiatric disorder, especially if there is no history of any brain insult. However, there are cases in which depth electrodes are epileptiform-positive and surface electrodes are negative.

Outlook

An earlier onset of depression is associated with a worse prognosis and more frequent recurrences. If not treated, there may be resolution with recurrences or there may be chronic depression, resulting in the child becoming an underachieving loner with delinquency. Development of personality, social interactions, and sexuality are often distorted. Substance abuse is common. Depressed teens may attempt suicide; this may be an impulse or a planned escape. The act may be a means of getting attention or a way of escaping a seemingly insurmountable situation. Girls attempt suicide more often, but boys are more successful.

Therapy

Define the treatment plan to patients with epilepsy and depression, considering all options and recommending that which is best for the individual patient. Consider drug interactions. Although seizure cessation is the undisputed goal of epilepsy treatment, the findings are that depression and adverse medication effects may be correlated more closely with health outcomes than seizure frequency or severity in patients with uncontrolled seizures (Viikinsalo *et al.*, 2000).

Anticonvulsant optimization

Treatment begins by optimizing seizure control. The cause may be an anticonvulsant-related depression, especially if barbiturates are being used. Avoid polypharmacy if possible. Check folate levels. The seizures and epilepsy syndrome should be re-evaluated and treated with the most appropriate anticonvulsant, preferably as monotherapy. In polypharmacy, reduction of anticonvulsants can result in significant decreases in anxiety and depression scores three to six months later (Barry *et al.*, 2001). Valproate, carbamazepine, and lamotrigine should be considered as first-line antiepileptics; whenever possible, barbiturates, phenytoin, and vigabatrin should be avoided. Depression may result from the discontinuation of an antiepileptic with psychotropic properties in patients with an underlying unipolar depression (Kanner & Balabanov, 2002). Priority should be given to attaining optimal control. Remission of seizures is often accompanied by an improvement in psychosocial functioning (Jacoby, 1992).

Therapy in older adolescents and adults

Treatment approaches include psychotherapy, rationalization of antiepileptic drug medication, antidepressant treatment, and ECT (Lambert & Robertson, 1999). Lithium and ECT may be used in depressed or bipolar epileptic patients.

Psychologic therapy

Depressive reactions should be treated with supportive therapy, counseling (Usiskin, 1995), and rehabilitation (Thompson, 1991). Depressive reactions should not be treated medically unless they are prolonged and atypical, because such episodes may become protracted if treated with antidepressants or tranquilizers (Betts, 1981). More severe reactions may require specialized psychotherapy, such as cognitive behavioral therapy. An intervention procedure to alter attributional style towards optimism has been developed for patients with epilepsy, which may ameliorate depression (Gehlert, 1994). Psychotherapy can increase coping skills, which improves mild depressive illness and anxiety and also reduces seizure frequency (Gillham, 1990). Patient support groups provide fellow suffers with emotional support and help patients to overcome feelings of hopelessness, rejection, and isolation by significantly modifying depression and dysthymia in outpatients with epilepsy (Becu *et al.*, 1993). Support groups and/or psychotherapy are not sufficient to treat depressive patients; antidepressants are often necessary for treating depressive illnesses in patients with severe epilepsy (Lambert & Robertson, 1999).

Antidepressant usage

All antidepressants are effective for treatment of depression in patients with epilepsy, with variable rates of adverse events (Lambert & Robertson, 1999). The major classes of antidepressants include the tricyclics and related mono-, bi-, tetra-, and hetero-cyclics, the monoamine oxidase inhibitors, and the SSRIs (Pisani *et al.*, 1999). The latter appear to be relatively safe in patients with epilepsy, as the incidence of seizures in patients taking these drugs is well below 1% (Barry *et al.*, 2001). Drug-resistant depression in epileptic patients may be augmented by a tricyclic at low dosage (Favale *et al.*, 1995; Prediville & Gale, 1993). Drugs such as fluoxetine, paroxetine, and sertraline, which increase serotonergic transmission, are less convulsant or even more anticonvulsant than others (Pisani *et al.*, 1999). Doxepine, trazodone, desipramine, and fluoxetine may reduce seizure frequency (Favale *et al.*, 1995; Kanner & Balabanov, 2002). Of the older antidepressants, trazodone is felt to have the lowest epileptogenic potential, even at toxic dosages (Lambert & Robertson, 1999).

Antidepressants should be introduced at a low dosage and increased slowly, with regard to other antiepileptic medications being used, especially those that are metabolized hepatically (Kanner & Balabanov, 2002; Lambert & Robertson, 1999). Antidepressants are too often prescribed in subtherapeutic doses (Keller *et al.*, 1986). Medications known to reduce the seizure threshold should be avoided. Monitor drug levels closely, especially if hepatically active antiepileptic agents are used. Some anticonvulsants and antidepressants may potentiate each other. Seizures tend to occur early in treatment or after dose increases, especially if increased rapidly. If seizures do occur, the patient should be changed to an antidepressant with a lower seizure risk. The antidepressant should be continued for least four months after complete clinical recovery to reduce the chance of relapse (Prien & Kupfer, 1986; Lambert & Robertson, 1999).

Psychiatric comorbidity is not unusual after anterior-temporal lobectomy, most often presenting as a mood lability or frank depressive episode. Symptoms can be identified in the initial six weeks and may be brought out by steroids used to alleviate postsurgical edema. The patients should be forewarned of this. With a prior history of developmental disabilities, sertraline at low doses (250–500 mg/day in adults; lower doses in children) is often sufficient to prevent symptoms occurring; patients should be maintained on this regimen for three to six months (Kanner & Balabanov, 2002).

At least 60–70% of acute major depressive episodes will respond to antidepressant treatment at a modest dosage (Blumer & Zielinski, 1988; Klerman, 1990). Early treatment intervention reduces the duration of the episode by almost 50% (Kupfer *et al.*, 1989).

Vagal nerve stimulation

Vagal nerve stimulation has been said to have a response rate of 40% for a 50% reduction in the depression severity. It may affect mood-regulating neurotransmitter systems such as serotonin, norepinephrine, GABA, and glutamate (Barry *et al.*, 2001).

Electroconvulsive therapy

Electroshock therapy is not contraindicated in epilepsy (Kanner & Balabanov, 2002). ECT raises the seizure threshold by 25–200% and facilitates GABA neurotransmission. The criteria for the use of ECT in patients with comorbid epilepsy and a psychiatric disorder are no different to those for patients without epilepsy. Anticonvulsants should be continued while ECT is being administered (Barry *et al.*, 2001).

Therapy in children

In depression, there are several guiding principles. At each age, the needs of the child with epilepsy are different and must be addressed. The child is either normal or in need to some degree in each of the areas of need. Education and behavioral management are similar. In behavior management, approaches are aimed at helping the child to learn to behave. In education, the teacher expects a specific behavior response to occur in their teaching. Drugs for behavior cover up the problems during the crisis periods but rob the child of the needed opportunity to learn how to deal with such problems. Such learning is an essential developmental advance. A child who has not developed such a behavioral skill may regress to a childish way of dealing with similar problems when experienced in adulthood (Brent *et al.*, 1987).

In infants, the therapeutic focus is often on parenting and on crisis intervention psychotherapy without drugs. The toddler is treated similarly, with play therapy, parent and family counseling, and the use of Head Start preschool programs. In the past, minor tranquilizers were also utilized.

In the school-age child, the therapy emphasis is on parent counseling, family therapy, and play therapy, with involvement of the school. The teenager is often placed in both individual and group therapy, with family therapy also being used. Tricyclics have been used in the past, but the efficacy of them has been questioned. For some depressions in older children and teens, fluoxetine has been used. The proper choice of antiepileptic drugs is important to avoid those that may provoke depression and to select those that may help. Psychiatric drugs are never a substitute for therapy.

Treatment of childhood depression should include parent and teacher involvement in addition to directing attention to the child. Psychotherapy, including family therapy and individual sessions for the child, should be considered. Cognitive behavioral approaches and interpersonal therapy may be useful with adolescents. Interventions in the school environment such as reducing academic pressures may be crucial. A child psychiatrist may consider prescribing antidepressant medication. In-patient psychiatric evaluation may be required if there are suicidal ideations or attempts, dangerous behaviors, or severe side effects from previous medications. Psychoeducation of patients and family is critical (Weisbrot & Ettinger, 1998).

In children, antidepressant usage is still under evaluation but should be considered for moderate to severe cases (Barry *et al.*, 2001). The placebo response rate is high. In children, tricyclic antidepressants (amitryptyline, imipramine, desipramine, doxepin) are often used initially, although their effectiveness is questioned. The tricyclics have been associated with sudden cardiac deaths in prepubertal children. Doxepine has a lower risk for seizures of the tricyclics. SSRIs have now become first-line antidepressants. Fluoxetine, paroxetine, and sertraline are tolerated well in children and are relatively low risk for producing seizures (0.1–0.5%). Some children become disinhibited with fluoxetine. Bupropion (amfebutamone) and other drugs are being considered for use in children. There are excessive concerns regarding the lowering of the seizure threshold. Amoxapine and bupropion (amfebutamone) carry a higher potential for seizures. The morbidity of untreated depression may be far greater than the risk of a potentiated seizure. Monoamine oxidase inhibitors are used infrequently in the pediatric population because of the side effects, although they carry a low risk of seizure induction and some may have anticonvulsant properties (Weisbrot & Ettinger, 1998).

Bipolar disorders

In the epileptic population, 9.8% of patients have been diagnosed with bipolar disorder compared with 1.5% in the general population. Up to 20% of individuals with temporal lobe epilepsy may meet the criteria for a bipolar disorder; The incidence in the general population is 1.5%. Bipolar disorders often go recognized.

Clinical

The presentation may be one of isolated manic or extreme elation episodes or of a more typical bipolar history. Manic episodes are thought to be rare (Kudo *et al.*, 2001).

Isolated manic episodes

Periodic dysphoria is reported to appear with sudden onset and a short duration in patients with epilepsy. Many patients display dependent, immature, childish behavior. Childish and capricious personalities have been seen in patients with frontal lobe discharges and with awakening epilepsies, such as juvenile myoclonic epilepsy. An epileptic dysphoria has been described, which appears interictally and suddenly, lasting for hours to a few days, with a variety of affective symptoms. Manic states may appear during ictal or postictal epileptic events and after increased epileptic activity or seizure suppression by antiepileptic drugs.

Temporal lobe epilepsy is reported to be a major cause of organic (secondary) mania. Brief fluctuating mood disturbances and epileptic dysphoria are not rare in patients with epilepsy. The epileptic zones involve the frontal and temporal lobe, which plays an important role in the mood episodes of the majority of patients with epilepsy. Secondary mania may be caused by a disturbance between the limbic system and deep midline hemisphere structures, including the basal ganglia, thalamus, hypothalamus, and midbrain, or a disturbance between the limbic or limbic-related areas, such as the orbital-frontal and baso-temporal cortex, the head of the caudate and thalamus, and the frontal lobe.

The clinical features of the interictal manic episodes of an epilepsy group of adults are different from those in the bipolar group. The manic episodes of the epilepsy group appear to be heterogeneous in their causal factors. There is no family history of a mood disorder. Episodic mania may develop secondarily after injury of the temporal and frontal lobes. Symptoms are almost the same in the postictal manic state and the interictal manic episodes in patients having both. Interictal manic episodes otherwise have no causative factors and no postictal mania. Emotional deficits, depressed abnormal IQ, brain damage, epilepsy, and mania may overlap in causes.

Cyclic manic-depressive disorder

Bipolar disorders may be seen, but manic-depressive symptoms can occur at the time of a cluster of seizures. Rarely, a patient may be elated rather than depressed. Such events are usually independent of the surroundings, unprovoked, and inappropriate. Interictal manic-depressive episodes may also be seen.

Patients with complex partial epilepsy may experience an increased lifetime prevalence of manic-depressive episodes. Left-lateralized seizures are significantly more associated with manic-depressive episodes (Lopez-Rodriguez et al., 1999). Often, there is a bipolarity between excitement and depression. Other symptoms reported include violence, hallucinations, lability of mood, alterations with normality, sudden mood changes, depression, and psychoses. Sudden mood changes are the most common form; these may be extreme in some patients. The depression itself is often transient and may have some psychotic traits, including paranoia. Subtle interictal personality traits may be seen. The psychoses may be heterogenous as a group, with changing presentation and variability in pathology (Blumer et al.,

1991). The manic episodes and the depressive states are usually less severe than those of isolated episodes. Rapid cycling of manic and depressive episodes is seen in 62% of patients with epilepsy who also have brief emotional and affective deficits, which is more than four times that seen with bipolar patients.

Cause

Mental changes in epilepsy may be secondary to neural inhibition. There is a delayed appearance after the onset of the seizures of at least one to two years, but more often a decade or so. There is a persistence, exacerbation, or de novo appearance after the remission of seizures either pharmacologically or surgically. There may be an alternation of manic-depressive episodes and the presence of seizure activity (paradoxical normalization/alternating psychosis versus uncontrolled seizures). This may emerge postictally (Blumer, 1991).

In the interictal phase, the structures involved in the ictal discharge are still not normal (Blumer, 1991). Seizures may release an exogenous opioid, which can act as a "euphorogen," to which epileptic patients become more dependent. The seizure mechanisms may contribute to periodic withdrawals.

PET scans show a similar hypo metabolism to hypermetabolism cycling, with a background of global hypometabolism. Patients with more hypermetabolic temporal lobes are more apt to respond to carbamazepine therapy. Those with hypometabolic temporal and frontal lobes do not respond well to medication, especially carbamazepine. Anterior frontal hypometabolism parallels the severity of the depression. (This is also seen in obsessive–compulsive patients.)

Treatment

Carbamazepine, gabapentin, lamotrigine, topiramate, and tiagabine are more effective in bipolar disorders, especially in the manic effective and the depressive phases, than in unipolar depressive disorders. Carbamazepine is an effective antidepressant in patients with epilepsy and a good prophylactic in the control of manic-depressive illnesses (Emrich et al., 1985; Fenwick, 1992), as are valproate, lamotrigine, and gabapentin (Calabrese et al., 1996; Walden et al., 1996; Ryback et al., 1997; Schaffer & Schaffer, 1997; Sporn & Sachs, 1997). These drugs have replaced lithium as first-line treatment in bipolar affective disorders (Barry et al., 2001). Zonisamide and oxcarbazepine have shown mood-stabilization effects in early studies (Harden, 2002).

Lithium does not show special adverse effects in patients with epilepsy (Shukla et al., 1988; Lyketsos et al., 1993), although seizures have been reported at therapeutic and at toxic dosages. EEG abnormalities may be seen (Schou et al., 1979; Spring, 1980; Simard et al., 1989; Wharton, 1969).

Childhood bipolar disorders

In older adolescents bipolar disorders may cycle between mania and deep depression, whereas in younger teens and children both symptoms may be experienced at the same time. Often, the child is misdiagnosed as having ADHD, the existing mood disorder being neglected (Wozniak *et al.*, 2001). Childhood onset of bipolar disorder may account for a significant number of child psychiatry referrals (Weller *et al.*, 1986; Faedda *et al.*, 1995; Geller & Luby, 1997). Bipolar disorder has been estimated to occur at a rate of about 0.6–1% (Carlson & Abbott, 1995). The onset is usually (75%) in the preschool years, when the child is about 4.5 years of age.

Clinical

Children with bipolar disorder are atypical in presentation by adult standards. Irritability is the major impaired mood state (92%). Impaired levels of euphoria or elation (giddy, goofy, high moods) may be seen (17%), but these are less impairing than the irritable mood. Irritability and euphoria are present for more than three-quarters of the day for more days than not (Weller *et al.*, 1995; Wozniak *et al.*, 2001).

Depressive irritability

The depressive type of irritability is characterized by an unhappy, hard-to-please, child with cranky moods. It is more severe and is more pervasive than age-appropriate irritability. Depressive irritability is more likely to be associated with expression of self-hatred, low self-esteem, and self-destructive statements and actions (Wozniak *et al.*, 2001).

The irritability of mania is much more hostile, vicious, and attacking in quality. There are also dysphoric, explosive episodes, which occur usually daily without much precipitation. These explosions can last for an hour or more. During these rages, the child may be hard to calm down and often lashes out physically at those around them, with kicking, hitting, biting, spitting, swearing, and hostile comments. Parents "walk on the edge," fearing precipitation of these unpredictable outbursts (Wozniak *et al.*, 2001).

Euphoria

The history of euphoric moods may be elicited by inquiring for giddy, goofy, hyper-excited, or silly states with laughing fits. These are often described as immature, clowning behavior. Children may experience grandiose ideas but parents often describe these as "cute," often laughing them off (Wozniak *et al.*, 2001).

Parents may describe a grandiose defiance. With a bipolar disorder, there almost universally is a comorbid oppositional defiant disorder in a very severe form. Such children are often labeled as having an attitude problem and inspire anger in adults, for the child feels that they know better than them (Wozniak *et al.*, 2001).

With manic episodes in children, 90% have at least one depressive episode and 84% have a depressive episode overlap in time with the manic state, presenting in a mixed state. The child switches unpredictably in and out of depression, irritable mania with expressions, and euphoric silly mania throughout the day, almost daily, much like a rapid-cycling state. Thus, childhood mania is an abnormal mood that presents almost daily during most of the day for a majority of the time. The children also show mood reactivity. The parents, clinicians, and teachers may see different facets of the child, mirroring the situation (Wozniak *et al.*, 2001).

Diagnostic confusion

A marked majority (79–98%) of children who prove to have bipolarity have previously been thought to have ADHD. The commonality of talkativeness, distractibility, and hyperactivity/agitation contributes to the confusion, leading to inappropriate use of stimulant or anti-ADHD antidepressants, which can exacerbate the mania. Manic children generally have greater psychopathology and poorer functioning. ADHD screening scales do not distinguish between the two entities. ADHD criteria do not include a mood component. If the chief complaint or presenting symptom is severe moodiness, then a mood disorder should be considered. In this group of children, there appears to be a high incidence of learning disabilities and educational needs (Wozniak *et al.*, 2001).

In a study of boys referred with ADHD, 12% were found in follow-up to exhibit mania. Four years later, an additional 12% had developed mania (Farone *et al.*, 1997). The rates of oppositional defiant disorder, conduct disorder, major depression, and anxiety disorders are higher in this group than in boys who did not develop mania. By adolescence, the rate of euphoria increases as irritability and the explosive outbursts continue. The course is more chronic. The mixed presentation persists. By the later part of adolescence, the cyclic nature evolves. ADHD-like features persist in 60% of patients (Wozniak *et al.*, 2001).

In children with a bipolar disorder with mania, there is often a family history of a major depressive disorder and bipolar disorders not seen in non-manic ADHD children. Nearly all relatives with bipolar disorder also have ADHD features. The combination of bipolar disorder with ADHD-like features seen in first-degree relatives suggests a distinct genetic subtype (Farone *et al.*, 1997).

Manic-depressive variant

Some children will present with a characteristic picture of transient irregular outbursts of aggressive, destructive behaviors directed at a person or object lasting minutes to hours, usually precipitated by insignificant events. Between these storms, the child is passive and often seems pleasant and well-behaved. Hyperactivity with chronic, tense, rapid speech and rapid shifts of interests without grandiosity, delusions, or hallucinations may be seen in some. There may be a history of impaired interpersonal relationships, sleep disturbances, bed-wetting, and other problems, such as learning disabilities. The child has a chronic temporal difficulty and may have exhibited personality problems. Such children are quite capable of developing personal and affective bonds with others, but their relationships are seriously troubled due to the erratic explosive unpredictable behavior. Some children exhibit EEG abnormalities (Davies, 1979).

The child may come from a dysfunctional family. There may be family members with manic-depressive problems or similar episodic dyscontrol affective storms. Depression, suicide, and alcoholism may be found. There may be a significant history for similar affects. The family history may reveal serious sibling disturbances or a negative attitude towards the child associated with a parental remorse born of the guilt of producing the child or at least the child's problems. The child has a self-deprecating self-image as a "bad person" (Davies, 1979).

Other comorbid conditions

Children with bipolar disorders are often diagnosed as having ADHD, but they are also apt to be diagnosed as having conduct disorders, anxiety disorders, and substance abuse disorders. There are two types of conduct/antisocial personality disorders in relatives of children with conduct disorders and mania: those with mania and those without mania. It is suggested that bipolar disorders are highly comorbid with anxiety disorders, with 52% of patients having both. There are multiple anxiety disorders in 56% of patients. Thus, children with mania should be screened routinely for bipolar disorders. Juvenile-onset mania may be a particular risk for substance abuse disorders.

Treatment

Treatment begins with awareness and recognition. Therapy is based on family and individual counseling, psychotherapy, and medication. For children with childhood bipolar disease, mood stabilizers are used frequently, with significant improvement in the symptoms of mania. Lithium carbonate, carbamazepine, valproate, and lithium carbonate have been used. Atypical antipsychotic drugs, such as resperidone, have been used. Antidepressants and stimulants do not lead to improvement in mania. Lithium carbonate and carbamazepine at higher doses (with blood levels monitored closely) produce greater clinical improvement. The response is slow, requiring follow-up and dose adjustments over a year or more. The relapse rate is high.

Atypical antipsychotics have been used as alternative treatment. In many (82%) patients taking risperidone, improvements in both manic and aggressive symptoms occur relatively quickly, over about two months. Resperidone has been effective in managing aggressive children with conduct disorder. Olanzapine monotherapy produces significant improvements in both mania and depression and is well tolerated. For symptoms of ADHD, depression, or anxiety, once the symptoms of mania are controlled, medications may be sequenced cautiously, for this may exacerbate the mood instability.

REFERENCES

Altshuler, L. L., Devinsky, O., Post, R. M., *et al.* (1990). Depression, anxiety, and temporal lobe epilepsy. Laterality of focus and symptoms. *Arch. Neurol.* **47**: 284–8.

Barabas, G. & Matthews, W. (1988). Barbiturate anticonvulsants as a cause of severe depression. *Pediatrics* **82**: 284–5.

Barraclough, B. (1981). Suicide and epilepsy. In *Epilepsy and Psychiatry*, ed. F. H. Reynolds & M. R. Trimble, pp. 72–6. Edinburgh: Churchill Livingstone.

Barry, J., Lembke, A. & Huynh, N. (2001). Affective disorders in epilepsy. In *Psychiatric Issues in Epilepsy*, ed. A. B. Ettinger & A. M. Kanner, pp. 45–72. Philadelphia: Lippincott Williams & Wilkins.

Becu, M., Becti, N., Manzur, G., *et al.* (1993). Self-help epilepsy groups: an evaluation of effect on depression and schizophrenia. *Epilepsia* **34**: 841–55.

Betts, T. A. (1981). Depression, anxiety and epilepsy. In *Epilepsy and Psychiatry*, ed. E. H. Reynolds & M. R. Trimble, pp. 60–71. Edinburgh: Churchill Livingstone.

Blanchet, P. & Frommer, G. P. (1986). Mood change preceding epileptic seizures. *J. Nerv. Ment. Dis.* **174**: 471–6.

Blumer, D. (1991). Epilepsy and disorders of mood. In *Neurobehavioral Problems in Epilepsy*, ed. D. B. Smith, D. M. Treiman & M. R. Trimble, pp. 185–95. New York: Raven Press.

Blumer, D. (1992). Postictal depression: significance for the neurobehavioral disorder of epilepsy. *J. Epilepsy* **5**: 214–19.

Blumer, D. & Zielinski, J. (1988). Pharmacologic treatment or psychiatric disorders associated with epilepsy. *J. Epilepsy* **1**: 135–50.

Brent, D. A., Crumrine, P. K., Varma, R. R., *et al.* (1987). Phenobarbital treatment and major depressive disorder in children with epilepsy. *Pediatrics* **80**: 909–17.

Bromfield, E. B., Altshuler, L. & Leidermann, D. B. (1990). Cerebral metabolism and depression in patients with complex partial seizures. *Epilepsia* **31**: 625.

Calabrese, J. R., Fatemi, S. H. & Woyshville, M. J. (1996). Antidepressant effects of lamotrigine in rapid cycling bipolar disorder. *Am. J. Psychiatry* **153**: 1236.

Carlson, G. A. & Abbott, S. F. (1995). Mood disorders and suicide. In *Comprehensive Textbook of Psychiatry*, ed. H. I. Kaplan & B. J. Sadock, pp. 2367–91. Baltimore, MD: Williams & Wilkins.

Currie, S., Heathfield, K. & Henson, R. (1971). Clinical course and prognosis of temporal lobe epilepsy: a survey of 666 patients. *Brain* **94**: 173–90.

Davies, R. E. (1979). Manic depressive variant syndrome of childhood: a preliminary report. *Am. J. Psychiatry* **136**: 702–6.

Deb, S. & Hunter, D. (1991). Psychopathology of people with mental handicap and epilepsy. II: psychiatric illness. *Br. J. Psychiatry* **159**: 826–30.

Devinsky, O., Kelley, K., Yacubian, E. M. T., *et al.* (1994). Postictal behavior: a clinical and subdural electroencephalographic study. *Arch. Neurol.* **51**: 254–9.

Dodrill, C. B., Breyer, D. N., Diamond, M. B., *et al.* (1984). Psychosocial problems among adults with epilepsy. *Epilepsia* **25**: 168–75.

Dunn, D. W. (1996). Factors related to depression in adolescents with epilepsy. Presented at the American Epilepsy Society Conference, 1996.

Dunn, D. W., Austin J. K. & Huyster, G. A. (1997). Behavior problems in children with new-onset epilepsy. *Seizure* **6**: 283–7.

Emrich, M., Dose, M. & von Zerssen, D. (1985). The use of sodium valproate, carbamazepine and oxcarbazepine in patients with affective disorders. *J. Affect. Disord.* **8**: 243–50.

Ettinger, A. B. & Perrine, K. (1996). Psychiatric/psychosocial issues in epilepsy. In *Epilepsy Update*, ed. J. French, W. D. Shields, T. T. Sutula & B. W. Braxton, pp. 13–24. Norwalk, CT: GEM Communications.

Faedda, G., Baldessarini, R., Suppes, T., *et al.* (1995). Pediatric-onset bipolar disorder: a neglected clinical and public health problem. *Harv. Rev. Psychiatry* **3**: 171–95.

Farone, S. V., Biederman, J., Mennin, D., *et al.* (1997). Attention deficit hyperactivity disorder with bipolar disorder: a familial subtype? *J. Am. Acad. Child Adolesc. Psychiatry* **36**: 1378–87, 1387–90.

Favale, E., Rubino, V., Mainardi, P., *et al.* (1995). The anticonvulsant effect of fluoxetine in humans. *Neurology* **45**: 1925–7.

Fenwick, P. B. C. (1992). Antiepileptic drugs and their psychotropic effects. *Epilepsia* **33** (suppl 6): 533–6.

Fiordelli, E., Beghi, E., Bogliun, G., *et al.* (1993). Epilepsy and pscyhaitric disutrbance. A cross-sectional study. *Br. J. Psychiatry* **163**: 446–50.

Frangos, E. & Alexandrakou, P. (1991). Temporal lobe epilepsy and affective disorders. 19th International Epilepsy Congress. *Epilepsia* **32** (suppl 1): 51.

Gehlert, S. (1994). Perceptions of control in adults with epilepsy. *Epilepsia* **35**: 81–8.

Geller, B. & Luby, J. (1997). Child and adolescent bipolar disorder: a review of the past 10 years. *J. Am. Acad. Child Adolesc. Psychiatry* **36**: 1168–76.

Gillham, R. A. (1990). Refractory epilepsy: an evaluation of psychological methods in outpatient management. *Epilepsia* **31**: 427–32.

Gilliam, F., Maton, B., Martin, R. C., *et al.* (2000). Extent of 1H spectroscopic abnormalities independently predicts mood status and quality of life in temporal lobe epilepsy. *Epilepsia* **41** (suppl 7): 54.

Glauser, T. A. (1999). Topiramate. *Epilepsia* **40** (suppl 5): 71–80.

Harden, C. L. (2002). The co-morbidity of depression and epilepsy, epidemiology, etiology and treatment, *Neurology* **59** (suppl 4): 48–55.

Harris, E. C. & Barraclough, B. (1997). Suicide as an outcome for mental disorders: a meta-analysis. *Br. J. Psychiatry* **170**: 205–28.

Hauser, W. A. & Hesdorffer, D. C. (2000). Psychosis, depression and epilepsy: epidemiologic considerations. In *Psychiatric Issues in Epilepsy: A Practical Guide to Diagnosis and Treatment*, ed. A. B. Ettinger & A. M. Kanno, pp. 7–17. Philadelphia: Lippincott Williams & Wilkins.

Hawton, K., Fagg, J. & Marsack, P. (1980). Association between epilepsy and attempted suicide. *J. Neurol. Neuosurg. Psychiatry* **43**: 168–70.

Heilman, K. M., Scholes, R. & Watson, R. T. (1975). Auditory affective agnosia: disturbed comprehension of affective speech. *J. Neurol. Neurosurg. Psychiatry* **38**: 69–71.

Hermann, B. P. & Whitman, S. (1989). Psychosocial predictors of interictal depression. *J. Epilepsy* **2**: 231–7.

Hermann, B. P. & Wyler, A. R. (1989). Depression, locus of control, and the effects of epilepsy surgery. *Epilepsia* **30**: 332–8.

Hermann, B. P., Seidenberg, M. & Bell, B. (2000). Psychiatric comorbidity in chronic epilepsy: identification, consequences, and treatment of major depression. *Epilepsia* **41** (suppl 2): 31–41.

Indaco, A., Carrieri, P. B., Nappi, C., *et al.* (1992). Interictal depression in epilepsy. *Epilepsy Res.* **12**: 45–50.

Jacoby, A. (1992). Epilepsy and the quality of everyday life: findings from a study of people with well-controlled epilepsy. *Soc. Sci. Med.* **42**: 657–66.

Kanner, A. M. & Balabanov, A. (2002). Depression and epilepsy: how closely related are they? *Neurology* **58** (suppl 5): 27–39.

Kashani, J. H., Carson, G. A., Beck, N. C., *et al.* (1987). Depression, depressive symptoms and depressed mood among a community sample of adolescents *Am. J. Psych.* **144**: 931–4.

Keller, M. B., Lavori, P. W., Klerman, G. L., *et al.* (1986). Low levels and lack of predictors of somatotherapy and psychotherapy received by depressed patients. *Arch. Gen. Psychiatry* **43**: 458–68.

Kendrick, A. M., Duncan, J. S. & Trimble, M. R. (1993). Effects of discontinuation of individual antiepileptic drugs on mood. *Hum. Psychopharmacol.* **8**: 263–70.

Klerman, G. L. (1990). Treatment of recurrent unipolar major depressive disorder: commentary on the Pittsburgh Study. *Arch. Gen. Psychiatry* **47**: 1158–61.

Koch-Weser, M., Garron, D. C., Gilley, D. W., *et al.* (1988). Prevalence of psychological disorders after surgical treatment of seizures *Arch. Neurol.* **45**: 1308–11.

Kogeorgos, J., Fonagy, P. & Scott, D. F. (1982). Psychiatric symptom patterns of chronic epileptics attending a neurological clinic: a controlled investigation. *Br. J. Psychiatry* **140**: 236–43.

Kudo, T., Ishida, S., Kubota, H., *et al.* (2001). Manic episode in epilepsy and bipolar disorder: a comparative analysis of 13 patients. *Epilespia* **42**: 1036–42.

Kupfer, D. J., Frank, E. & Perel, J. M. (1989). The advantage of early treatment intervention in recurrent depression. *Arch. Gen. Psychiatry* **46**: 771–5.

Lambert, M. V. & Robertson, M. M. (1999). Depression in epilepsy: etiology, phenomenology and treatment. *Epilepsia* **40** (suppl 10): 21–47.

Long, C. G. & Moore, J. R. (1979). Parental expectations for their epileptic children. *J. Child Psychol. Psychiatry* **20**: 299–312.

Lopez-Rodriguez, F., Altshuler, L. & Kay, J. (1999). Depression and laterality of epileptogenic region in patients with medically-refractory temporal lobe epilepsy. *Epilepsia* **40** (suppl 7): 60.

Lyketsos, C. G., Stoline, A. M., Longstreet, P., *et al.* (1993). Mania in temporal lobe epilepsy. *Neuropsychiatry Neuropsychol. Behav. Neurol.* **6**: 19–25.

Macniak, J. (1999). Studies on depression disorders in temporal lobe epilepsy in adolescents. 23rd International Epilepsy Congress. *Epilepsia* **40** (suppl 2): 274.

Mayou, R. & Hawton, K. (1986). Psychiatric disorder in the general hospital. *Br. J. Psychiatry* 149: 172–90.

Meldrum, B. S. (1991). Neurochemical substrates of ictal behavior. In *Neurobehavioral problems in epilepsy*, ed. D. B. Smith & D. M. Treiman, Vol. 55, pp. 35–45. New York: Raven Press.

Mendez, M. F., Cummings, J. L. & Benson, D. F. (1986). Depression in epilepsy: significance and phenomenology. *Arch. Neurol.* **43**: 766–70.

Mendez, M. F., Doss, R. C., Taylor, J. L., *et al.* (1993). Depression in epilepsy: relationship to seizures and anticonvulsant therapy. *J. Nen. Ment. Dis.* **181**: 444–7.

Mittan, R. (1986). Fear of seizures. In *Psychopathology in Epilepsy: Social Dimensions*, ed. S. Whitman & B. P. Hermann, pp. 90–121. New York: Oxford University Press.

Mittan, R. (1987). The influence of seizure–related variables upon patients' fears of death and brain damage. *Epilepsia* **28**: 540.

Murray, R. E., Abou-Khalil, B. & Griner, L. (1994). Evidence for familial association of psychiatric disorders and epilepsy. Biol. Psychiatry **36**: 428–9.

Onuma, T. (2000). Classification of psychiatric symptoms in patients with epilepsy. Proceedings of the 32nd Congress of Japan Epilepsy Society. *Epilepsia* **41** (suppl 9): 43–8.

Piazza, A. & Canger, R. (2001). Depression and anxiety in patients with epilepsy. In *Epilespia and Learning Disabilities*, ed. G. F. Ayala, M. Elia, C. M. Cornaggia & M. R. Trimble. *Epilepsia* **42**: 29–31.

Pisani, F., Spina, E. & Oteri, G. (1999). Antidepressant drugs and seizure susceptibility: from in vitro data to clinical practice. *Epilepsia* **30** (suppl 10): 38–56.

Pratt, J. A., Jenner, P., Johnson, A. L., *et al.* (1984). Anticonvulsant drugs alter plasma tryptophan concentrations in epileptic patients: implications for antiepileptic action and mental function. *J. Neurol. Neurosurg. Psychiatry* **47**: 1131–3.

Prediville, S. & Gale, K. (1993). Anticonvulsant effect of fluoxetine on focally evoked limbic motor seizures in rats. *Epilepsia* **34**: 381–4.

Prien, R. F. & Kupfer, D. J. (1986). Continuation drug therapy for major depressive episodes: how long should it be maintained? *Am. J. Psychiatry* **143**: 18–23.

Ratti, M. T., Raffacle, M., Galimberti, C. A., *et al.* (1998). Depressed mood in people with epilepsy. 3rd European Congress of Epilepsy. *Epilepsia* **39** (suppl): 122.

Rey, G., Carrazana, E., Garaycoa, G., *et. al.* (2000). Affective disorders in juvenile myoclonic epielspy: a prospective study. *Epilepsia* **41** (suppl 7): 236.

Ring, H. A., Moriarty, J. & Trimble, M. R. (1998). A prospective study of the early postsurgical psychiatric associations of epilepsy surgery. *J. Neurol. Neurosurg. Psychiatry* **64**: 601–4.

Roberts, A. (1995). The use of antidepressant drugs in general practice. *Prescriber* **5**: 35–53.

Robertson, M. M. (1997). Depression in neurological disorders. In *Depression and Physical Illness*, ed. M. M. Robertson & C. L. E. Katona, pp. 305–40. Chichester, UK: John Wiley & Sons.

Robertson, M. M. (1998). Mood disorders associated with epilepsy. In *Psychiatric Comorbidity in Epilepsy. Basic Mechanisms, Diagnosis, and Treatment*, ed. H. W. McConnell & P. J. Sander, pp. 132–67. Washington, DC: American Psychiatric Press.

Ronald, S. & Duman, R. (1999). The neurochemistry of mood disorders: preclinical studies. In *Neurobiology of Mental Illness*, ed. D. S. Charney, E. J. Nesler & B. S. Bunney, pp. 333–48. New York: Oxford University Press.

Ryback, R. S., Brodsky, L. & Munasilfi, F. (1997). Gabapentin in bipolar disorder. *J. Neuropsych. Clin. Neurosci.* **9**: 301.

Sarzhevskiy, S. (1998). Peculiarities of depression owing to drug treatment in epilepsy. 3rd European Congress of Epileptology. *Epilepsia* **39** (suppl 2): 123.

Schaffer, C. B. & Schaffer, L. C. (1997). Gabapentin in the treatment of bipolar disorder. *Am. J. Psychiatry* **154**: 291–2.

Schou, M., Amdisen, A. & Trap-Jensen, J. (1979). Lithium poisoning. *Am. J. Psychiatry* **125**: 520–27.

Shukla, S., Mukherjee, S. & Decina, P. (1988). Lithium in the treatment of bipolar disorders associated with epilepsy: an open study. *J. Clin. Psychopharmacol.* **8**: 201–4.

Simard, M., Gumbiner, B., Lee, A., *et al.* (1989). Lithium carbonate intoxication: a case report and review of the literature. *Arch. Intern. Med.* **194**: 36–46.

Smith, D. B. & Collins, J. B. (1987). Behavioral effects of carbamazepine, phenobarbital, phenytoin and primidone. *Epilepsia* **28**: 598.

Sporn, J. & Sachs, G. (1997). The anticonvulsant lamotrigine in treatment resistant manic-depressive illness. *J. Clin. Psychopharmacol.* **17**: 185–9.

Spring, G. K. (1980). EEG observations in confirming neurotoxicity. *Am. J. Psychiatry* **136**: 1099–100.

Standage, K. F. & Fenton, G. W. (1975). *Psychiatric symptom profiles of patients with epilepsy:* a controlled investigation. *Psychol. Med.* **5**: 152–60.

Strauss, E, Wada, J. & Moll, A. (1992). Depression in male and female subjects with complex partial seizures. *Arch. Neurol.* **49**: 391–2.

Taylor, D. C. (1972). Mental state and temporal lobe epilepsy: a correlative account of 100 patients treated surgically. *Epilepsia* **13**: 727–65.

Thompson, P. J. (1991). Memory function in patients with epilepsy. In *Neurobehavioral Problems in Epilepsy. Advances in Neurology*, ed. D. Smith, D. Treiman & M. R. Trimble, Vol. 55, pp. 369–84. New York: Raven Press.

Trimble, M. R. (1988). *Biological Psychiatry.* New York: John Wiley & Sons.

Usiskin, S. (1995). Counseling in epilepsy. In *Epilepsy*, 2nd edn, ed. A. Hopkins, S. Shorvon & G. Cascino, pp. 565–71. London: Chapman & Hall.

Vickrey, B. G., Hays, R. D., Graber, J., *et al.* (1992). A health-related quality of life instrument for patients evaluated for epilepsy surgery. *Med. Care* **30**: 299–319.

Viikinsalo, M., Sawrie, S., Kuzniecky, R., *et al.* (2000). Depression and medication toxicity but not seizure frequency of severity predict health outcomes in refractory epilepsy. *Epilepsia* **41** (suppl 7): 174.

Walden, J., Hesslinger, B., van-Calker, D., *et al.* (1996). Addition of lamotrigine to valproate may enhance efficacy in the treatment of bipolar affective disorder. *Pharmacopsychiatry* **29**: 193–5.

Weil, A. A. (1959). Ictal emotions occurring in temporal lobe dysfunction. *Arch. Neurol.* **1**: 87–97.

Weisbrot, D. M. & Ettinger, A. B. (1998). Psychiatric aspects of pediatric epilepsy. *Primary Psychiatry* **June**: 51–67.

Weller, E., Weller, R. & Fristad, M. (1995). Bipolar disorder in children: misdiagnosis, under diagnosis and future directions. *J. Am. Acad. Child Adolesc. Psychiatry* **34**: 709–14.

Weller, R. A., Weller, E. B., Tucker, S. G., *et al.* (1986). Mania in prepubertal children: has it been underdiagnosed? *J. Affect. Disord.* **11**: 151–4.

Wharton, R. N. (1969). Grand mal seizures with lithium treatment. *Am. J. Psychiatry* **125**: 152.

Williams, D. (1956). The structure of emotions reflected in epileptic experiences. *Brain* **79**: 29–67.

Wozniak, J., Biederman, J. & Richards, J. A. (2001). Diagnostic and therapeutic dilemmas in the management of pediatric-onset bipolar disorder. *J. Clin. Psychiatry* **62** (suppl 14): 10–15.

Zielinski, J. J. (1974). Epilepsy and mortality rate and cause of death. *Epilepsia* **15**: 191–201.

35

Disruptive behavior problems

Behavior disorders occur in 28.6% of children with uncomplicated seizures and in 58.3% of children with seizures and other brain dysfunctions, according to parent and teacher reports (Dunn & Austin, 1998). Children struggling with the problem of epilepsy often display acting-out behaviors. They may seem moody or they may display erratic, variable, unpredictable behaviors. Some children seem irritable, exhibiting angry outbursts of temper. Their attention spans may seem shortened. Some children are anxious and jittery, with hyperactive behavior.

Rebellious, resentful attitude

The child, especially in adolescence, may try to escape from the parents' overly restrictive demands through rebellion. Some children may be so discouraged that they lash out angrily. Some may try to blame others for rejecting them because of the seizures. They seem angry, hostile, and aggressive. The school record may be one of absenteeism. Some may develop frank antisocial and delinquent behavior. Such children need intensive guidance and counseling so that they may finally accept the epilepsy and develop a better self-concept and therefore move ahead.

Impulse-control problems

Over the years, impulse-control problems have emerged with a variety of names, including episodic dyscontrol syndrome, intermittent explosive disorder, and "rage" reactions. Impulse-control problems may be seen in personality disorders, with cerebral damage as with seizure activity, structural loss, antiepileptic drugs, and social deprivation.

The possibility of an ictal basis for aggressive symptoms as part of the interictal period, in which aggressive behavior may follow one or more serial unrecognized seizures, is debated. Undetected episodic impairments of higher function due to minimal seizures may also account for aggressive behavior (Ferguson *et al.*, 1980). Language and learning disabilities, often associated with temporal lobe dysfunctions, may result in aggressive behavior as a frustration response.

Seizure types

Aggression has been reported to be one of the most common characteristics of patients with temporal lobe seizures (Fenwick, 1981) and patients undergoing an anterior temporal lobectomy. In this group, 5% present with destructive and assaultive behavior (Rodin, 1973). Complex partial seizures suggest underlying brain dysfunction, often involving the limbic system. Underlying brain damage may contribute to both seizures and behavioral disturbances, including violence (Holmes, 1987).

Children with temporal lobe foci are more aggressive than those with other seizure types (Nuffield, 1961). Aggressive behavior and rage outbursts may be seen in about 7%, especially with early onset of seizures, often in the first year of life. There is no relationship to the seizure frequency (Sillinpaa, 1973). Such children have a higher incidence of diagnosed ADHD. Often, they come from chaotic homes (Caplan et al., 1997; Dunn & Austin, 1998). They tend to have problems with behavior and social competence (Hermann et al., 1980; Hermann et al., 1981). Habitually aggressive adolescents have a much higher incidence of complex partial seizures (6%) (Lewis, 1976; Lewis et al., 1981). By late adolescence and adulthood, patients with chronic complex partial epilepsy may show personality changes with aggressiveness (Sillinpaa, 1973).

Seizure-related aggression

Aggression is an offensive act with intent to harm. Violence is damage not necessarily associated with any intent to do harm (Trieman, 1986). There are four types of peri-ictal aggression: preictal or prodromal, ictal (primary or reactive), postictal, and interictal. Ictal aggression, well-directed, does occur although it is rare. Most often, this is part of ictal confusion. The environmental setting modifies ictal behaviors. Aggressive behaviors are seen during a seizure in 37% of children; interictal aggression is seen in 56% (Glaser, 1967). Some children may display aggressive behavior during a seizure. Postictal aggressive behavior is seen rarely, primarily in adults, and usually as part of a postictal psychosis (Delgado-Escueta et al., 1981; Gerad et al., 1998; Niedermeyer, 1990; Weisbrot & Ettinger, 1998).

Preictal aggression

Aggressive symptoms may be a seizure prodrome, occurring minutes, hours, or, rarely, days before a seizure, presenting as a predictable change in behavior, such as irritably, anxiety, or aggression (Fenwick, 1981; Blanchet & Frommer, 1986).

Ictal aggression

Ictal aggressive acts against inanimate objects or people are seen with complex partial seizures. All ictal aggressive acts are sudden, without evidence of planning, lasting an average of half a minute (Fenwick, 1981). Automatisms are too short-lived and fragmentary to be directed, coordinated acts of violence, as shown in studies of adults (Delgado-Escueta *et al.*, 1981). Primary ictal aggression may exist as excitatory neurologic behaviors. Secondary ictal aggression may be a reaction to a noxious stimulation or an inhibition release (Trieman, 1986). Ictal aggression emerges especially in late adolescence and in adults. Usually, the aggression of seizures is not directed. Rarely, if ever, is it accompanied by directed, purposeful aggression towards a person (Rodin, 1973). Aggressive activities during seizures may be harmful if another person gets in the way. EEG recordings during spontaneous ictal aggressive behavior may show spike and slow activity in the amygdala and hippocampus. The attack begins as menacing activities or hostile posturing (Saint-Hilaire *et al.*, 1980).

Directed acts of violence or severe bodily assaults are not epileptic seizures. Ictal aggression can usually be differentiated from non-epileptic aggression, which is goal-directed and usually of longer duration with the patient being aware throughout (Delgado-Escueta *et al.*, 1981).

Postictal aggression

Resistive violence may occur at the end of a seizure, i.e. postictal, or as a defensive violence. Usually, the individual is confused and the violent acts are not goal-directed. Violence can also be a part of a postictal psychosis (23%) (Trieman, 1986; Kanemoto *et al.*, 1999; Schacter, 2001).

Interictal aggression

Interictal aggression, often impulsive, may be seen in up to 56% of individuals with complex partial seizures. Catastrophic rage episodes are seen in 36% of children with temporal lobe epilepsy. These episodes are more often associated with a history of head injury or cerebral infection, with seizure onset before age one year. Other factors include a disordered home, loss of the mother, and a psychosis or chronic neurosis in one or both parents. There is no relationship to the seizure frequency. In adults thought to have symptomatic epilepsy, 4.8% have a history of assaultive and destructive behavior. This is seen especially in young men of below-average intelligence who have a history of predating behavior difficulties (Rodin, 1973; Hermann *et al.*, 1980). Violent behaviors are seen most often with early onset of seizures and a history of chronic behavior difficulties. Violent epileptic patients are more apt to be mentally impaired compared with non-violent patients. (Mendez *et al.*, 1993; Schacter, 2001). No relationship to any specific EEG abnormalities or scan findings or a history of psychosis is noted (Herzberg & Fenwick, 1988; Schacter, 2001).

Episodic irritability

In children, episodic irritability is manifest by outbursts of temper or rage with verbally or physically abusive behavior. These outbursts of abusive behavior with a characteristic build-up, peak, and subsequent calm may be described erroneously as "seizures." Such behaviors appear to be particularly characteristic for complex partial seizures. A nasty or even vicious mood may persist for up to a few days but appears to be regretted afterwards. This is in contrast to the exceptionally good-natured behavior sometimes combined with a very religious attitude that prevails with many patients. The parents may refer to a "Jekyll and Hyde" personality in their child (Gastaut *et al.*, 1955; Szondi, 1963; Blumer, 1967). Up to 75% of children with this presentation show increased emotional irritability. Outbursts of rage may occur in one-third, indicating a link to the episodic dyscontrol syndrome (Blumer, 1967; Glaser, 1967; Ounsted *et al.*, 1968).

Episodic dyscontrol syndrome

Episodic dyscontrol, sometimes called an intermittent explosive disorder or rage reactions, is seen in children and adults who may display episodic violent behavior but do not otherwise have an aggressive personality. The temper escalates over minutes and is greatly out of proportion to the provocation, if any (Fenwick, 1981). This probably represents the more severe form of episodic irritability. These rage reactions often occur in the presence of people who are emotionally important to the patient, and usually last 20–30 minutes. The patient seems unable to terminate the rage. Afterwards, the patient is often remorseful, regretful, or embarrassed, for they understand that their behavior has been excessive (Bach-y-Rita *et al.*, 1971; Maletzky, 1973).

Rage outbursts classified as aggressive are seen in 7% of people with temporal lobe epilepsy. Discharges in the limbic structures are postulated to play a role (Fenwick, 1981; Schacter, 2001). Ictal aggressiveness may either be well localized in the temporal limbic system or may be diffuse, spreading beyond the temporal portion of the limbic system. There is a complex behavioral organization in which restraint is not a provocative element (Saint-Hilaire *et al.*, 1980). Most of the time, episodic dyscontrol is not epilepsy but rather a form of episodic irritability. In individuals with epilepsy, it may be considered as part of the interictal dysphoria. In people without seizures, this is not epilepsy, but the two entities may have similar anatomic correlates. This disorder may respond to anticonvulsant therapy. Without clinical evidence of epilepsy, one cannot properly diagnose epilepsy.

Episodic dyscontrol episodes are often seen with damage or dysfunction of the frontal lobe structures. There appears to be an impairment of normal social and emotional inhibitory mechanisms. There are often concomitant neurotic deficits. Aggressive or violent behavior may also be seen with the use of certain medications, including antiepileptic drugs. Reducing the dose of sedative drugs may be reasonable. Violent behavior may be part of a psychosis. Street drugs may also trigger such behavior.

Childhood rage reactions

A rage reaction is a sudden outburst of aggressive rage precipitated by a rather minor frustration. This entity is far more apt to be seen in males. The syndrome may be developmental or acquired. The acquired form may follow head injury (0.5%) or may appear with complex partial seizures (20%) (Maletzky, 1973).

The presentation is of frequent episodes of intense rage, often triggered by trivial irritations. The rages are accompanied by verbal or physical violence. The speech may be explosive, with a tendency towards obscene and profane content. The physical violence may be of biting, gouging, kicking, spitting, or multiple stabbing. This is often followed by remorse, in which the child may seem contrite, ashamed, forgetful, and confused. Some children are not bothered by the behavior, and others may overtly deny the problem. The patient may appear docile and submissive between the attacks, providing that there are no other behavior problems (Svoboda, 1979). Such children often come from a poor socioeconomic background. There may be a history of accidents and injuries due to the aggressive behavior.

There is often a history of temper tantrums in infancy or early childhood. There may be a history of a perinatal brain insult, convulsions in infancy, or preceding head trauma. Childhood rage reactions are seen in temporal lobe seizure problems of early onset, often following a brain insult or after an excessively prolonged seizure. In some children, the seizures may be multifocal or complex partial, and especially involving the right temporal lobe (Kaufman et al., 1999). In patients with a history of a significant head trauma, the child may previously have been well behaved; symptoms may follow the head trauma months to a few years later. In some children, there may be a past history of belligerence. In incarcerated teens, with definite or probably epilepsy, 89% have a history of brain trauma or perinatal difficulties. Paranoid ideation and allocations may be present and contribute to violent acts (Lewis, 1976).

The child may have a temper problem during the preadolescent years. In adolescence, formidable explosive rages emerge. Later, persistent or episodic schizophrenic-like symptoms may be noted. In adulthood, the individual appears to outgrow the rages but smoldering depression with a suicide risk may remain (Svoboda, 1979). Alcoholism is prominent in adulthood in such patients. A small amount of alcohol may trigger an attack and may lead to a drunken state.

Rage reactions are not seizures. They may occur in people who do not have seizures and in whom normal EEGs are found. However, rage outbursts are seen in up to 36% of children with chronic temporal lobe seizures (Ounsted *et al.*, 1968). Seizure problems beginning in early childhood are more often associated with personality and character disorders, problems in getting along with others, aggressive acting-out behaviors, and hyperactivity. The problem is especially apt to occur in children who have suffered a brain insult, such as encephalitis, and who subsequently develop seizures. An impulse control problem may also emerge, which can expand to violent rage reactions towards family members and objects (Kaufman *et al.*, 1999). Rage reactions to minor frustrations may be due to a slowed and incomplete ability to cope with and adapt to stresses. The child reacts without inhibition. The child's reaction is a primitive, immature response rather than a more mature effort to adapt.

The problem of rage reactions may relate to brain damage involving the temporal and adjacent underneath portions of the frontal lobe as well as more central portions relating to emotions. Children with intractable partial epilepsy and aggressive behavior have been studied with FDG-PET scanning and psychodevelopmental assessment (Juhasz *et al.*, 2001). The aggressive children showed developmental delay and, occasionally, autistic symptoms. Reduced metabolism of glucose is seen in the bilateral prefrontal and temporal neocortices in children with epilepsy and aggressive behavior, suggesting a widespread dysfunction of cortical regions that normally exert an inhibitory effect.

Children with epilepsy have an increased rate of cognitive and behavioral problems, pervasive developmental delays, and aggression, which are often related to poor seizure control. Aggression is found to be associated with early-onset temporal lobe epilepsy, suggesting that seizures interfering with the developing brain might play a role in facilitating aggressive behavior. Certain anticonvulsants may induce aggressive behavior despite providing improved seizure control. The mechanism of this paradoxical behavior effect is poorly understood (Juhasz *et al.*, 2001).

Pathogenesis

Violence in epilepsy, especially in patients with temporal lobe epilepsy, is often thought to be due to other neurologic or psychiatric deficits rather than to the epilepsy. However, five basic questions arise: What is the aggression due to? Is it an ictal event? Does ictal aggression exist? If so, why? How can this be determined (Trieman, 1986)?

The limbic system is involved either as the main organizer of aggressive behavior or as a coordinator of interaction function in the integration of subjective emotional and aggressive behavior. The hippocampus may be the specific structure responsible for interactional behaviors. The anatomic substratum of aggression in the limbic system perhaps relates to the norepinephrine pathways or a non-specific precursor, such as levodopa (Saint-Hilaire *et al.*, 1980).

The source of aggressive behavior appears to be the amygdala, the para-amygdala, and perhaps the contramesial thalamus. The amygdala may manifest a higher level of electrophysiological excitability in episodically violent epileptic patients (Gastaut *et al.*, 1955; Szondi, 1963; Blumer, 1967). Amygdaloid stimulation may produce fear without aggression. With increasing stimulation, patients respond with a decrease in the frequency of aggressive behavior reported. Unilateral or bilateral amygdalar lesions reduce or abolish aggressive outbursts.

Diagnosis

Any abnormal, non-provoked stereotypic behaviors that occur symptom-independent of the environment (although the environment may modify) may be part of a seizure. Such behaviors are usually associated with impaired consciousness, with partial to complete amnesia for the event. There is an abrupt cessation or progressive clearing after the event. Primitive, non-organized behaviors coexist with hypersynchronous cortical discharges. The behavior is accompanied by a typical EEG change, usually detectable by scalp EEG leads although occasionally showing up only on depth leads. There is a stereotyped consistency to the morphology, localization, and presentation of the electrographic event.

Only 10% of alleged ictal violence is verified. These acts include defensive ictal violence, which are most often postictal, i.e. emerging after the seizure onset, as a resistive automatism. Violent automatisms are non-directive, defensive, brief, and often postictal. Ictal violent aggression tends to be stereotypic, simple, and non-sustained, and never occurs with a sequence of purposeful movements.

Epilepsy violence has been questioned. This is defined as an aggressive act during a seizure and usually occurs at the onset of a seizure. The initial symptoms may be forgotten in the seizures. True violence with seizures is usually brief, lasting less than half a minute. The aggression is stereotyped and unconstrained, and does not consist of a consecutive series of movements. The outburst is not preplanned or redirected and is usually defensive in nature. To diagnose epilepsy violence, the diagnosis of epilepsy must be proven and the presence of epileptic automatisms documented. Video monitoring is needed for this. The aggression must be characteristic of the habitual seizures. It still depends on the judgment of the neurology specialists (Delgado-Escueta *et al.*, 1981; Trieman, 1986).

If an individual is felt to exhibit an aggressive episode, a detailed history and neuropsychiatric evaluation must be taken. The target behavior is identified and data collection is set up. If this is a new onset of aggression, a medical etiology must be sought and either treated or ruled out. If the patient is on medication, a change in the dosage or the drug(s) may reduce the problem.

Treatment

Behavioral approaches

Behavior intervention and consoling is always indicated for both the patient and the family. Pharmacological agents may reduce the frequency and severity of the attacks. The rages do not respond to anticonvulsant medications. Tranquilizers may partially suppress the aggression, but these drugs may aggravate the seizures, slow down learning, and inhibit the development of necessary coping skills. Behavior modification is the desired therapy. The rages of childhood tend to mature to mere episodes of irritability by adulthood (Kaufman *et al.*, 1999).

Once diagnosed, a given maladaptive behavior can be treated by reducing the antecedent behaviors that tend to elicit the aggressive response, rewarding the patient for performance of an alternative desirable behavior, or reducing the amount of positive reinforcement the patient receives for performing the aggressive target behavior. Commonly, individuals who resort to violence lack non-violent conflict-resolution approaches and thus need to be taught acceptable alternatives. The most successful behavioral modification occurs in an in-patient or group home setting. Unstructured time should be minimized. Staff need to be educated in respect to what constitutes reinforcement and non-reinforcement of behavior. It is highly important that there is a consistency across all shifts. The patient family must be aware of the behavior plan.

Comprehensive therapy should include preventive and remedial help for both cognitive function and personality development, provided appropriate re-education strategies can be devised to offset these deficits (Stores, 1971).

Psychopharmacology

If the problem is moderate to severe, behavior approaches may be less successful, especially in early stages, and medication as adjunctive therapy is often needed. The first step is to optimize the anticonvulsant medication. Then a psychopharmacologic agent may be added.

Anticonvulsants such as carbamazepine have been used for agitation and episodic dyscontrol (Lewin & Summers, 1992; Stone *et al.*, 1986). Valproate may be useful (Davis *et al.*, 2000; Fenwick, 1997), as may gabapentin and lorazepam (Schacter, 2001). Some of the newer anticonvulsants such as tiagabine may control both seizures and psychiatric symptoms. Barbiturates may paradoxically accentuate the attacks and should probably be discontinued (Kaufman *et al.*, 1999). Clozapine may reduce aggressive and violent actions in psychoses and self-mutilation behaviors (Chengappa *et al.*, 1999), but it may produce dose-related seizures in 3–5% of patients. Minimal therapeutic levels are not as crucial. For acute episodes, lorazepam may be useful. For chronic use, clonazepam may been tried; in some patients, this produces depression, sedation, or occasionally behavior problems. There is a lowered seizure threshold during withdrawal.

Antidepressants may work occasionally (Schacter, 2001). SSRIs such as fluoxetine have a long half-life. Paroxetine may be the best SSRI to use in combination with antiepileptic medications. Tranquilizers such as haloperidol, thioridazine, and risperidone may be used, but these bear the risk of sedation, tardive dyskinesias, and, rarely, seizures. Clonidine, which has an antiadrenergic effect, has been used in children and adults with aggression. Other medications have also been used, including benzodiazepines and propranolol. No agent has been developed specifically for the treatment of aggression. All psychopharmacologic agents used successfully for aggressive behavior may cause exacerbation of aggression in some cases. The phenothiazines, haloperidol, and stimulants may accentuate the problem.

Conduct and oppositional disorders

Children with simple epilepsy do not seem to have an increased risk for oppositional defiant or conduct disorders. There is no relationship between antisocial conduct disorders and temporal lobe epilepsy. With intractable seizures or additional CNS damage, the risks may be increased. Children, especially males, with epilepsy and frontal dysfunction or mental retardation may be at special risk for disruptive behaviors (Fenwick, 1981; Dunn & Austin, 1998). Antisocial behavior and related behavior disorders in epilepsy are seen in 18.5% of patients, which is more than twice that expected (Dunn & Austin, 1998).

Oppositional-defiant disorder

Oppositional-defiant disorder (ODD) is the term used for angry, irritating, hard-to-discipline children who stress the adults of this world. The disorder is differentiated from a conduct disorder by the absence of serious violation of the rules of society. The disorder must have persisted for at least six months and must include significant impairments, such as temper tantrums, anger, vindictiveness, refusal to obey, annoyance of others, and blaming others for their own mistakes. Developmentally, ODD may be an early manifestation of a conduct disorder (Dunn & Austin, 1998).

Oppositional behavior is seen in 28.1% of children with epilepsy, two to four times the incidence in controls (2–15%). In children with chronic epilepsy, 14% of parents and teachers report disobedience as a major problem, and 5% of parents and 4% of teachers report at least one of the symptoms consistent with a conduct disorder. Slightly more than 12% of school children with epilepsy meet the criteria for ODD.

In this group, 18% show high-risk scores for aggression and 10% show delinquent behaviors (Caplan *et al.*, 1997; Dunn & Austin 1998; Henry *et al.*, 1997).

Conduct disorder

Conduct disorder is a more severe behavior problem than ODD, involving serious violations of the rules of society. Such acts include aggression (fighting, use of a weapon, sexual assault, cruelty to people or animals), destroying property, lying, theft, truancy, and running away. The problem must be present for at least six months to a year. It may begin before or after ten years of age. Conduct disorder is usually divided into childhood-onset and adolescent-onset subtype.

Children with epilepsy may show a higher incidence of conduct disorders and other behavior abnormalities, although such disorders are frequent in the non-epileptic population (Pond & Bidwell, 1954; Cavazutti, 1980). Slightly more than 12% of children with epilepsy meet the criteria for a conduct disorder, compared with 5–15% of boys and 2–9% of girls in the non-epileptic population (Dunn & Austin, 1998).

Children with complex partial epilepsy have high rates of conduct disorders and other behavior abnormalities. There may be a debated relationship between rage attacks and the subsequent development of antisocial features in adulthood. This may relate to underlying brain insults, known risk factors for psychiatric problems such as rage attacks and acting-act behaviors that may also be the cause of seizure-like behaviors (Keating, 1961; Hermann *et al.*, 1981; Lindsay, 1981; Weisbrot & Ettinger, 1998).

Risk factors

Risk factors are multiple. The etiology of ODD and conduct disorders seems to involve a combination of genetic, social, and environmental factors. No significant differences in attention, aggression, or delinquency have been substantiated. Poor seizure control is associated with aggression and delinquency. Infantile spasms may be followed by hyperactivity in 15% of patients. There is a relatively low incidence of disruptive behaviors but a high prevalence of autistic disorders that usually precludes the diagnosis of ADHD, ODD, or conduct disorder (Dunn & Austin, 1998).

ODD and ADD often have a history of a dysfunctional, chaotic home. Aggression and cruel behavior in girls with epilepsy may stem from divorced or separated parents. Such factors also predict depressed, withdrawn, and ODD behaviors but not delinquent or aggressive behaviors in boys with epilepsy. Counseling must involve the entire family, not just the child (Dunn & Austin, 1998).

Antiepileptic medications may contribute to behavior problems. Usually this occurs within the first five to six months of treatment. Barbiturates may be associated with adverse behavioral reactions. The newer anticonvulsants show fewer adverse effects on behavior and cognition, although topiramate has caused a decrease in attention. Increases in hyperactivity, aggression, and oppositional behavior after starting gabapentin may be seen in children with epilepsy with pre-existing behavior or learning problems. Vigabatrin has caused hyperactivity and aggressiveness in children. If a relationship between the drug and the behavior is suspected, then a change in medication, especially to a medication unlike the inciting drug, may be most effective (Dunn & Austin, 1998).

Diagnosis

Screens and standardized questionnaires are effective in screening for behavior disturbances. Once specific behavioral problems have been identified, more focused questionnaires can be used. Questionnaires may be biased as they reflect the parents' and teachers' interpretations and own emotions in targeting children's behaviors. Screening results must be confirmed. If school problems that are not explained clearly and fully by behavior problems are found, formal psychologic assessments with measures of intelligence and academic achievement should be used to check for contributing problems that need treatment (Dunn & Austin, 1998).

Therapy

Psychosocial therapies are essential for children with seizures and ODD or conduct disorders, with medications such as antiepileptic drugs, stimulants, antidepressants, and antipsychotic agents useful as adjuvant treatment for severe presentations (Dunn & Austin, 1998).

Parent management training is effective in ODD and conduct disorders. The therapist works with the parents, focusing on assessment of problems and behavioral modification, using combinations of positive reinforcement for approved behaviors and either ignoring or punishing (including timeouts and loss of privileges) misbehaviors. School programs use a similar approach for these problems, with emphasis on providing structure and rapid feedback on a disruptive child (Dunn & Austin, 1998).

Cognitive behavior techniques may be effective in ODD and conduct disorders. The child is instructed to address distorted perceptions and use problem-solving techniques. Social skills training is used to correct disrupted interpersonal relationships (Dunn & Austin, 1998).

Drug treatment of ODD and conduct disorder should be considered only as an adjunct to behavior treatments. Methylphenidate hydrochloride may help with antisocial behaviors if ADHD is also present, since the risks of this drug precipitating a seizure are very low. Anticonvulsants such as carbamazepine have not been shown to be any more effective than placebo. Valproic acid has shown effectiveness in reducing explosive outbursts in teenagers. Lamotrigine has reduced self-injurious behaviors in retarded teenagers and shown improvements or worsening of irritability and behavior (Dunn & Austin, 1998).

REFERENCES

Bach-y-Rita, G., Lion, J. R., Climent, C. E., *et al.* (1971). Episodic dyscontrol: a study of 103 violent patients. *Am. J. Psychiatry* **127**: 1473–8.

Blanchet, P. & Frommer, G. P. (1986). Mood changes preceding epileptic seizures. *J. Nerv. Ment. Dis.* **174**: 471–6.

Blumer, D. (1967). The temporal lobes and paroxysmal behavior disorders. *Z. Psychiol.* **51**: 273–85.

Caplan, R., Arbelle, S., Guthrie, D., *et al.* (1997). Formal thought disorder and psychopathology in pediatry primary generalized and complex partial epilepsy. *J. Am. Acad. Child Adolesc. Psychiatry* **36**: 1286–94.

Cavazzuti, G. B. (1980). Epidemiology of different types of epilepsy in school age children of Modena Italy. *Epilepsia* **21**: 57–62.

Chengappa, K. N., Ebeling, T., Kang, J. S., *et al.* (1999). Clozapine reduced severe self-mutilation and aggression in psychotic patients with borderline personality disorder. *J. Clin. Psychiatry* **60**: 477–84.

Davis, L. L., Ryan, W., Adinof, B., *et al.* (2000). Comprehensive review of the psychiatric uses of valproate. *J. Clin. Psychopharmacol.* **20** (suppl 10): 1–17.

Delgado-Escueta, A. V., Mattsen, R. H., King, L., *et al.* (1981). Special Report: the nature of aggression during epileptic seizures. *N. Engl. J. Med.* **305**: 711–16.

Dunn, D. W. & Austin, J. K. (1998). Behavioral aspects of pediatric epilepsy. In *Psychiatric Issues in Epilepsy*, ed. A. B. Ettinger & P. B. Hermann, pp. New York: Lippincott Williams & Wilkins.

Fenwick, P. (1981). EEG studies. In *Epilepsy and Psychiatry*, ed. E. M. Reynolds & M. R. Trimble, pp. 42–63. New York: Churchill Livingstone.

Fenwick, P. (1997). Episodic dyscontrol. In *Epilepsy: A Comprehensive Review Textbook*, ed. J. Engle & T. A. Pedley, pp. 2767–74. Philadelphia: Lippincott-Raven.

Ferguson, S. M., Ryaport, M. & Corrie, W. S. (1980). Mechanisms of aggressive behavior in patients with temporal-limbic epilepsy. In *Advances in Epileptology, The Xth Epilepsy International Symposium*, ed. J. A. Wada & J. K. Penry, p. 527. New York: Raven Press.

Gastaut, H., Morin, G. & Lesevre, N. (1955). Etude du comportement des epileptiques sychomotoeurs dans l'intervalle de leurs crises. *Ann. Med. Psychol.* 1–27.

Gerad, M. E., Spitz, M. C., Towbin, J. A., *et al.* (1998). Subacute post-ictal aggression. *Neurology* **50**: 384–8.

Glaser, G. (1967). Limbic epilepsy in childhood. *J. Nerv. Ment. Dis.* **141**: 392–7.

Henry, A. S., Berkovic, S. F., Wrennall, J. A., *et al.* (1997). Temporal lobe epilepsy in childhood: clinical, EGG and neuroimaging findings and syndrome classification in a cohort with new-onset seizures. *Neurology* **49**: 960–63.

Hermann, B. P., Black, R. B. & Chabria, S. (1981). Behavioral problems and social competence in children with epilepsy. *Epilepsia* **22**: 703–10.

Hermann, B. P., Schartz, M. S., Whitman, S., *et al.* (1980). Aggression and epilepsy: seizure-type comparisons and high risk variables *Epilespia* **22**: 691–8.

Herzberg, J. & Fenwick, P. B. C. (1988). The etiology of aggression in temporal-lobi epilepsy. *Br. J. Psychiatry* **153**: 50–5.

Holmes, G. L. (1987). Psychosocial factors in childhood epilepsy. In *Diagnosis and Management of Epilepsy in Children*, pp. 112–24. Philadelphia: W. B. Saunders.

Juhasz, C., Behen, M. E., Muzik, O., *et al.* (2001). Bilateral prefrontal temporal neocortical hypometabolism in children with epilepsy and aggression. *Epilespia* **42**: 991–1001.

Kanemoto, K., Kawasaki, J. & Mori, E. (1999). Violence and epilepsy: a close relation between violence and post-ictal psychosis. *Epilespia* **40**: 107–9.

Kaufman, K. R., Kugler, S. L., Sachdeo, R. C., *et al.* (1999). Tiagabine in the management of post-encephalitic epilepsy and impulse control disorders. *Epilespia* **40** (suppl 7): 57.

Keating, L. E. (1961). Epilepsy and behavior disorder in school children. *J. Ment. Sci.* **107**: 161–80.

Lewin, J. & Sumners, D. (1992). Successful treatment of episodic dyscontrol with carbamazepine. *Br. J. Psychiatry* **161**: 261–2.

Lewis, D. O. (1976). Delinquency, psychomotor epileptic symptoms and paranoid ideation: a triad. *Am. J. Psychiatry* **133**: 1395–8.

Lewis, D. O., Pincus, J., Shanok, S., *et al.* (1981). Psychomotor epilepsy and violence in a group of incarcerated adolescent boys. *Am. J. Psychiatry* **139**: 882–7.

Lindsay, J. (1981). The long-term outcome of temporal lobe epilepsy in childhood. In *Epilepsy and Psychiatry*, ed. E. H. Reynolds & M. R. Trimble, pp. 185–215. London: Churchill Livingstone.

Maletzky, B. M. (1973). The episodic dyscontrol syndrome. *Dis. Nerv. Syst.* **34**: 180–84.

Mendez, M. F., Doss, R. C. & Taylor, J. L. (1993). Interictal violence in epilepsy: relationships to behavior and seizure variables. *J. Nerv. Ment. Dis.* **181**: 566–9.

Neidermeyer, E. (1990). Psychological-psychiatric aspects. In *The Epilepsies, Diagnosis and Management*, pp. 213–81. Baltimore, MD: Urban & Schwarzenberg.

Nuffield, E. J. A. (1961). Neuro-physiology and behavior disorders in epileptic children. *J. Ment. Sci.* **107**: 438–58.

Ounsted, C., Lindsay, J. & Norman, R. (1968). *Biological Factors in Temporal Lobe Epilepsy*. London: Spastics Society and Heinemann.

Pond, D. A. & Bidwell, B. H. (1954). Management of behavior disorders in epileptic children. *Br. Med. J.* **11**: 1520.

Rodin, E. A. (1973). Psychomotor epilepsy and aggressive behavior. *Arch. Gen. Psychiatry* **28**: 210–13.

Saint-Hilaire, J. M., Gilbert, M., Bouvbier, G., *et al.* (1980). Epilepsy and aggression: two cases with depth electrode studies. In *Epilepsy Updated: Causes and Treatment*, ed. P. Robb, pp. 145–75 Chicago: Year Book Medical Publishers.

Schacter, S. C. (2001). Aggressive behavior in epilepsy. In *Psychiatric Issues in Epilepsy*, ed. A. B. Ettinger & A. M. Kanner, pp. 201–14. Philadelphia: Lippincott Williams & Wilkins.

Sillinpaa, M. (1973). Medico-social prognosis of children with epilepsy. *Acta Paediatr. Scand. Suppl.* **237**: 6–104.

Stone, J. L., McDaniel, K. D., Hughes, J. R., *et al.* (1986). Episodic dyscontrol disorders and paroxysmal EEG abnormalities: successful treatment with carbamazepine. *Biol. Psychiatry* **21**: 208–12.

Stores, G. (1971). Cognitive function in children with epilepsy. *Dev. Med. Child Neurol.* **13**: 390–92.

Svoboda, W. B. (1979). Emotional and behavioral consequences of epilepsy. In *Learning About Epilepsy*, pp. 157–84. Baltimore, MD: University Park Press.

Szondi, L. (1963). *Schicksalsanalytische Therapie*. Bern: Hans Huber.

Trieman, D. M. (1986). Epilepsy and violence: medical and legal issues. *Epilepsia* **27**: 77–104.

Weisbrot, D. M. & Ettinger, A. B. (1998). Psychiatric aspects of pediatric epilepsy. *Primary Psychiatry* **June**: 51–67.

36

Psychoses of epilepsy

Psychosis is a condition characterized by delusions, hallucinations, and disorganized speech and behavior (American Psychiatric Association, 1994). Psychoses due to epilepsy differ from non-epileptic psychoses. Psychoses may be ictal, postictal or interictal; the latter may be subdivided into episodic and chronic ongoing. Treatment-related psychoses include postoperative psychosis, anticonvulsant-induced psychosis, and the entities of alternating psychosis and forced normalization.

Psychotic disorders are increased in incidence among patients with epilepsy, especially those with complex partial seizures. A schizophreniform disorder occurs in up to 9.25% of epilepsy patients. Psychosis is a rare phenomenon in children yet significantly increased in epileptic children compared with the normal population. Sporadic cases of psychoses have been reported in children with complex partial seizures, manifest by prominent automatisms, especially when from the left temporal lobe, perhaps of medial-temporal origin. Often, these psychoses are associated with a cerebral abnormality or mental retardation (Dunn, 1998; Lindsay et al., 1979b; Weisbrot & Ettinger, 1998).

Thought disorders

Children with complex partial seizures exhibit an excess of illogical thought patterns, even to the point of psychotic proportions, as compared with children with primarily generalized epilepsy. In both groups, the existence of such problems exceeds that in the non-epileptic population. Children with complex partial epilepsy are prone to display more illogical thought patterns, hallucinations, and delusions compared with children with primary generalized seizures. Complex partial epilepsy patients lack the loose associations or negative signs, such as apathy and flat affect, that are typical for schizophrenia. When psychotic symptoms are present, they tend to be stereotyped (Caplan et al., 1991; Caplan et al., 1997). The most severe presentation is that of schizophrenia-like psychoses. Thought disorders are associated with EEG evidence of frontal-temporal involvement, as well as verbal, performance, and global cognitive dysfunction (Caplan et al., 2000). In a study that followed children with epilepsy into adulthood, it was found that a hallucinatory delusional state or other psychotic symptom may develop after discontinuation of antiepileptics. Patients with hallucinations tended to have earlier onset of seizures as well as psychoses. No differences in seizure frequency or medication used were noted (Kubagawa *et al.*, 1997).

Psychoses

A schizophrenia-like psychosis with epilepsy, especially with a left temporal focus, may appear ten to 20 years after the onset, often in childhood, of uncontrollable epileptic seizures. These take the form of postictal psychoses, intermittent episodic psychosis, alternating psychoses, or chronic, schizophrenia-like psychoses lasting more than several years. A psychosis may follow temporal lobe surgery (Hauser & Hersdorffer, 2001; Jablinski *et al.*, 1992). Episodic psychoses of epilepsy may be classified as acute, transient psychoses and chronic, schizophrenia-like psychoses, which might be included as a persistent delusional psychotic disorder (Onuma, 2000).

Seizures that tend to envolve into a psychosis often begin in early adolescence. These patients tend to have complex partial seizures, most often from the left temporal area, perhaps involving the mesial-basilar area, presenting with automatism, with a tendency towards secondary generalization. The typical age of seizure onset is in early adolescence; the psychosis emerges 11–15 years later. This is more common in females than in males. The incidence of left-handedness is increased in this group. The psychosis frequently presents as a schizophrenia-like or paranoid type of presentation. Structural lesions may be found on investigation. Seizures may diminish in frequency during psychoses (Trimble, 1988; Trimble, 1991). The seeds of seizure psychoses appear to be planted in childhood, to emerge by young adulthood, for reasons not yet understood.

Epilepsy types

The incidence of psychosis is very high in patients with temporal lobe epilepsy (14%) and is high in patients with idiopathic generalized epilepsy (3.3%). In a 30-year follow-up, up to 10% of children with temporal lobe epilepsy will develop a psychosis by adulthood, compared with a general population incidence of around 0.8%. This is true especially if the seizures continue into adulthood. The child with epilepsy is at risk of developing schizophrenia (Hermann & Whitman, 1984; Onuma, 2000; Hauser & Hersdorffer, 2001). The psychoses seen with complex partial epilepsy tend to be more chronic, with more prominence of hallucinations, delusions, and bad temper. These symptoms tend to occur more with frequently occuring seizures. With the generalized group, the patient seems more perplexed, with a variety of other psychotic symptoms often being noted, with a lower frequency and a more characteristic relationship to epileptic discharges. The onset of both types is in mid-adolescence to young adulthood (Sengoku *et al.*, 1997).

Risk factors

Possible risk factors include onset of epilepsy before age 20 (Taylor, 1975), often around puberty, duration of more than ten years, female gender (Hermann, 1979; Roberts *et al.*, 1990), left-handedness (Hermann, 1979; Kristensen & Sindrup, 1978), relative absence of febrile convulsions (Umbricht *et al.*, 1995), history of complex partial seizures (Sander *et al.*, 1991; Savard *et al.*, 1991; Stevens, 1991; Taylor, 1975), history of seizure clustering (Umbricht *et al.*, 1995), temporal lobe seizure focus, especially left-sided (Flor-Henry, 1968; Sherwin, 1981; Sherwin *et al.*, 1982; Trimble, 1988) or bilateral (Umbricht *et al.*, 1995), with secondary generalization (Torta & Keller, 1999), abnormal tissue (Savard *et al.*, 1991), such as gangliogliomas in early developmental stages and focal neuropathological lesions (Kristensen & Sindrup, 1978; Taylor, 1975), social deterioration, antiepileptic drug and polytherapy, especially at high doses (Cummings & Trimble, 1995; Devinsky *et al.*, 1995). There may be a mediobasal-temporal localization related to the auras (Torta & Keller, 1999). The average age of seizure onset is shortly before the beginning of puberty, whereas the corresponding age of onset for patients with postictal psychoses is at the end of adolescence (Trimble, 1991). In one study the median age for presenting with psychoses was 34 years, after a median period of 25.1 years of seizure duration (Hermann & Whitman, 1984).

Clusters of intractable seizures can be much more detrimental if they occur before or during adolescence, when some systems, e.g. the prefrontal cortex, are reaching functional maturity (Umbricht *et al.*, 1995). This may relate to remarkable changes in both physiological activity and synaptic structures in the hippocampus and amygdala. At this time, high-frequency neuron discharges, like those of epilepsy, normally occur from restricted areas of the amygdala, hippocampus, hypothalamus, and other limbic nuclei during pulsatile endocrine release, estrus, ovulation, and copulation (Kawakami *et al.*, 1970; Stevens, 1991).

Epileptiform psychoses

Epileptic psychoses can be classified as peri-ictal (ictal and postictal), which are usually of short duration, and interictal, which are usually prolonged (Torta & Keller, 1999). Psychotic disorders are classified as ictal if they are an expression of the seizure activity, postictal if they occur within seven days of a seizure or seizure cluster, and interictal if they occur independently of seizures (Kanner, 2000).

Ictal psychoses

An ictal psychosis is an expression of the seizure activity (Kanner, 2000). An acute psychotic episode may be an extension of the ictal perception (an aura) or may be prolonged and often misdiagnosed. An ictal psychosis may be an expression of a non-convulsive status epilepticus, such as simple and complex partial status, and also absence status (Umbricht *et al.*, 1995; Hauser & Hesdorffer, 2001). In a simple partial status, a scalp electrode may not detect the ictal pattern. An EEG is needed to confirm the ictal psychosis (Devinsky *et al.*, 1995). Brief psychotic episodes in epilepsy frequently end in a clinical convulsion (Torta & Keller, 1999). The onset of ictal psychoses is later than that of other types of epileptic psychoses, and the course is more benign. Negative psychiatric symptoms are seen rarely. Associated thought disorders are infrequent. Affect is not lost. These episodes respond to pharmacotherapy with a neuroleptic mediation (Kanner, 2000).

Postictal psychoses

Postictal psychoses occur in about 6–11% of people with epilepsy, representing 25% of psychotic episodes seen in patients with chronic epilepsy of about ten to 25 years' duration. Within one to seven days of a cluster of generalized tonic–clonic seizures or a complex partial seizure, such as after video-EEG-monitoring (10%), the patient, most often a male with chronic, bilateral, independent temporal (80%) or frontal (20%) seizures after a relative lucid period, develops an affect-laden delusional psychosis, a mixed manic-depressive psychosis, or bizarre thought disorder, often grandiose and religious in content, with hallucinations, memory disturbances, and fears. This may last for days to weeks and then cease, without recurrence. This is not associated with ongoing ictal discharging with a disorganized slowing seen even with depth recordings. The episode is self-limited, and tends to remit within days to weeks. Only 10% of patients develop a chronic psychoses or a cognitive disorder. In these patients, a paranoid state may recur frequently, sometimes without any preceding seizure. Mood alterations incur a high suicidal risk when present, but these remit spontaneously. There may be a history of depression. The seizures are most often found to be due to abnormal brain tissue. Unilateral hippocampal mossy fiber sprouting and bilateral asymmetric neuronal loss is seen in episodic postictal psychosis (Mathern *et al.*, 1995). The condition responds rapidly to temporary use of an antipsychotic drug in combination with a neuroleptic, or sometimes to benzodiazepines, started at the first sign, which is often insomnia. A low dosage of risperidone may be used for three to five days. The rapid responsiveness to neuroleptic medications suggests a possible relationship to alterations in dopaminergic function (Devinsky & Pacia, 1994; Devinsky *et al.*, 1995; Kanemoto *et al.*, 1996; Kanner *et al.*, 1996; Kanner, 2000; Lancman *et al.*, 1994; Onuma, 1997; So *et al.*, 1990; Torta & Keller, 1999; Unbricht *et al.*, 1995).

Although infrequent, children are more apt to exhibit a stereotypic picture following a seizure. They may be amnestic to the actual content of the hallucinations.

Peri-ictal auditory or visual hallucinations may be frightening but recognized as not real (Weisbrot & Ettinger, 1998).

Interictal psychoses

An interictal psychosis occurs independent of seizures (Kanner, 2000). Interictal psychoses are generally described as schizophreniform as they do not meet the usual *Diagnostic and Statistical Manual of Mental Disorders* (DSM) criteria for schizophrenia (Hauser & Hesdorffer, 2001). Children with schizophreniform psychoses typically are able to describe the content of their auditory hallucinations and may not be upset by the experience (Weisbrot & Ettinger, 1998).

Interictal psychoses of epilepsy can show up in various ways. They may be schizophrenic-like. These appear to be related to complex partial epilepsy in the left hemisphere, especially involving the left temporal lobe. Schizophrenia itself may show mainly left-sided medial-temporal activities on scans (Trimble, 1993). In children with complex partial epilepsy, left temporal lobe impairment, and interictal schizophrenia-like psychoses, the affect remains intact without the negative signs of schizophrenia (Caplan *et al.*, 1991; Caplan *et al.*, 1997).

Episodic psychoses with epilepsy

Some patients with chronic uncontrolled temporal or frontal partial seizures may develop episodes of psychosis after a decade or two. These are of acute or subacute onset and last several months, but they are not related in time to the seizures. Patients with episodic psychoses show perceptual changes, alternations in consciousness, and a poor memory for events, with a return to normal baseline of function between episodes. Episodic psychoses are usually associated with epilepsy. Non-episodic chronic psychoses of epilepsy may be due to coalescence of the epileptic partial epilepsy, drug toxicity, or simply a coincidence of psychoses and epilepsy occurring together (Rayport & Ferguson, 1998).

Clinical

Episodic psychoses of epilepsy occur predominantly in adults with temporal limbic epilepsy or in those with partial seizures that propagate to the temporal limbic structures from other lobes (Rayport & Ferguson, 1998). The onset of the episodic psychoses usually occurs ten to 20 years after the seizure onset, which was usually in childhood (Onuma, 1997). Patients present with prominent paranoid delusions, often with auditory hallucinations, with a significant affective component, such as anxiety, irritability, or fear. Social withdrawal and flattening of the affect is not highly evident, as the patient retains interpersonal contact, without incoherent thoughts and speech. These episodes tend to be recurrent, last days to weeks, and are often paralleled by an increased seizure frequency. These brief psychoses remit spontaneously. Although full recovery occurs, with repeated episodes, a chronic, schizophrenia-like psychosis may emerge. The prognosis is poor (Onuma, 1997; Rayport & Ferguson, 1998).

These events are not related to structural cerebral changes. Rather, they may relate to focal subclinical seizure discharges, as shown by depth electrode demonstration of polyspike and spike-wave discharges in the amygdala, hippocampal, and septal areas, seen only during the psychotic episodes and not recorded on scalp leads (Mendez & Grau, 1991). Psychiatric evaluation and psychotherapy may be of use, with a goal towards compliance in antiepileptic drug therapy. The treatment begins with a re-assessment of antiepileptic therapy with updated antiepileptic drug levels. Epileptic psychoses usually end when the seizures are reduced to a low frequency or are controlled (Rayport & Ferguson, 1998)

Generalized epilepsy and psychoses

Some patients with psychoses and epilepsy have infrequent generalized convulsions seizures that began about the same time or even earlier than the onset of the psychosis. The seizures occur every few years. The psychotic symptoms often emerge in adolescence or early adulthood, presenting similar pictures of schizoaffective disorders with a borderline personality. The patients often manifest emotional instability with a depressive mood and occasional self-injuries or attempted suicide. Paranoid delusions are often seen. The EEG shows generalized epileptiform abnormalities. These psychoses may be classified as atypical (Onuma, 1997).

Chronic schizophreniform psychoses with epilepsy
Combinations of schizophreniform psychoses and seizures

True schizophrenia and temporal lobe epilepsy can occur concomitantly, but often the schizophrenia begins before the temporal lobe seizures (Trimble, 1993). Some epileptic patients have symptoms that are indistinguishable from schizophrenia, with emotional withdrawal, poor affect, and poor interpersonal contact. Thoughts and speech are incoherent. Seizures are infrequent. The onset of psychosis may have preceded the onset of the epilepsy. Antipsychotic drugs may trigger both the schizophrenia and the epilepsy (Onuma, 1997). In children with complex partial epilepsy, left temporal lobe impairment, and interictal schizophrenia-like psychoses, the affect remains intact without the negative signs of schizophrenia (Caplan et al., 1991; Caplan et al., 1997).

There is no specific neuropathic lesion for schizophrenia. The findings are diffuse, perhaps with gliosis. This is most severe in the midline. The pathologic findings are of an atypical frontal lobe, with many changes in the temporal lobe and amygdala and atrophy in the basal ganglia and the dorsomedial nucleus of the thalamus. Some patients' brains are found to have gray-matter nodules (16–20%) and perivascular gliosis. The ventricles are enlarged in 10–20% of patients. The dopamine hypothesis in schizophrenia is that there is kindling by a pharmacologic effective drug. An increase of dopamine receptors in the basal ganglia and the amygdala in schizophrenia is found (Trimble, 1997).

Chronic epileptiform schizophreniform psychoses

The incidence of a schizophrenia-like psychosis in epilepsy, especially temporal lobe epilepsy, is 3–8%. It is found in 10% of children growing up with temporal lobe epilepsy. The entity of schizophrenia-like psychoses of epilepsy is a heterogeneous group of chronic, persistent psychoses that differ clinically from schizophrenia by the presence of a paranoid or schizophrenia-like psychosis with a preponderance of purely delusional states, preservation of warm affect and personality, and predominance of visual more than auditory hallucinations. Religious and mystical content are common. Such patients can maintain their affect and functioning, unlike patients with true schizophrenia, and affect may be increased. Family and social behavior are unimpaired. These patients may be friendly and superficially appropriate. Less common may be formal thought disorders and negative symptoms, a relatively rare familial schizophrenia or schizoid premorbid personality, and a generally more favorable outcome. Patients describe symptoms in a detached manner. The history is most important. The premorbid personality is normal. Epilepsy comes first, followed by the psychoses, even when the seizures are well controlled. Patients with this syndrome do not deteriorate, and they retain their usefulness and function (Trimble, 1993; Torta & Keller, 1999).

PET and MRI studies show a dominant hemisphere hypometabolism, especially involving the temporal lobe white matter if there are hallucinations (Trimble, 1993). Patients with a left-sided temporal epileptic lesion are at increased risk for developing a schizophrenic psychosis. Many of these people are left-handed, possibly due to an early childhood epilepsy-induced functioning shift (Sherwin, 1981; Sherwin et al., 1982; Torta & Keller, 1999). This does not appear to be a primary thought disorder but may represent a language disturbance, as related to thought disorders and emotional symbolism (Trimble, 1993; Rayport & Ferguson, 1998). The management of patients with chronic psychoses may require neuroleptic drugs such as fluphenazine, perphenazine, or resperidone (Rayport & Ferguson, 1998). Seizure control does not lead to remission of the psychosis, even with surgery, although some improvement in the psychoses may be seen.

Post-temporal resection psychosis

De novo psychoses may be seen in about 7% of patients following an anterior temporal lobectomy (Taylor, 1975; Jensen & Vaemet, 1977; Trimble, 1992; Matsuura, 1997). The incidence is 3.7% in patients who were psychiatrically normal before surgery but is 11.8% in patients who were not psychiatrically intact before surgery (Rayport & Ferguson, 2001). This is seen especially in patients who do not become seizure free postoperatively (Mace & Trimble, 1981; Manchanda et al., 1993; Leinonen et al., 1994; Hauser & Hesdorffer, 2001). The patient may be normal for half to one year following temporal lobectomy before the psychotic symptoms of a paranoid nature emerge. The disorder is seen more often with a later seizure onset, which manifests as an unreality or déjà vu feeling rather than an epigastric aura; this is often associated with bilateral symptomatic epilepsy (Stevens, 1990). This may be due to an errant regeneration associated with a pathologic reorganization of deafferented projection sites in the remaining brain. This process may be related to a possible abnormal enhancement of brain dopamine. Possibly this is a kindling mechanism or a syndrome of subcortical neurotransmitter imbalance (Carlsson & Carlsson, 1990). Synaptic changes may be due to aberrant reinnervations after temporal lobectomy (Trimble, 1991; Matsuura, 1997).

Risk factors for postoperative psychosis include surgery after age 30 years (Glosser et al., 2000), a family history of psychosis (Mace & Trimble, 1981), right-hemispheric foci (Manchanda et al., 1993; Kanemoto et al., 1996; Leinonen et al., 1994), hamartomas and cortical dysplasias of the temporal lobe (Taylor, 1975; Andermann et al., 1999), and benign foreign tissue lesions. There is a favorable response of postlobectomy psychosis to low doses of neuroleptics (Flor-Henry, 1968; Stevens, 1990). A history of psychosis is not a contraindication to epilepsy surgery. Surgically controlled seizures do not alter the course or severity of a psychosis that is already present (Reutens et al., 1977).

Forced normalization (alternating psychosis)

The alternative psychosis is a separate category in which the onset of a paranoid psychotic state with clear consciousness follows the suppression of seizure activity and relative EEG normalization (Kanner, 2000). The psychosis presents as a behavior disturbance of acute or subacute onset, characterized by a psychosis with a thought disorder, a significant mood change, anxiety, depersonalization, or hysteria (Krishnamoorthy & Trimble, 1999). Consciousness is not clouded. A richness of affective symptoms is characteristic (Gibbs, 1951; Kanner, 2000; Pakalnis et al., 1987; Sander et al., 1991). In some patients, there is a relationship between the control of seizures and the emergence of a psychosis, and vice versa. The incidence is probably 1% or less (Schmitz, 1966). Such psychoses may occur with generalized or partial epilepsies of 15 years' or more duration (Kanemoto et al., 1996). Absence seizures may also be associated with psychotic presentations in 15.3% of patients, with forced normalization seen in 7.8%. The only other significant problem seen in these patients is that often they are not well integrated socially (Trimble, 1998).

Some children exhibit misbehavior (rather than a psychosis) or uncontrolled seizures. In children, control with drugs such as phenobarbital may lead to a dramatic deterioration in behavior. The child may have active seizures, which are often complex partial but may be generalized seizures. When the seizures are active, there are no behavior problems; when the seizures are controlled by a variety of medications, the behavior is unmanagable and at times even described as bizarre. Such children often acquire a long list of behaviors triggered by otherwise effective medications. One mother called this an "either–or syndrome": either her son had seizures or he was intolerable. Parents of children with epilepsy may report the occurrence of dysphoric symptoms, including increased irritability, mood liability, and overt symptoms of depression preceding their child's seizures, only for these symptoms to disappear the day of the ictus. This may be an expression of an "alternative psychopathology," although of milder severity, which occurs frequently (Blanchet & Frommer, 1986; Kanner, 2000).

Patients who are more susceptible to forced normalization/alternative psychoses include those with chronic epilepsy, most often focal epilepsy of the limbic site, with a previous predisposition to develop behavioral disorders (Krishnamoorthy & Trimble, 1999). Normalization psychoses may be seen with almost every anticonvulsant potent enough to suppress seizures, including ethosuximide, phenacetylurea, phenytoin, primidone, valproate, carbamazepine, and vigabatrin (Gibbs, 1951; Kanner, 2000; Pakalnis et al., 1987; Sander et al., 1991; Sander & Duncan, 1996). With the newer antiepileptic drugs, forced normalization and alternative psychoses are most often seen with GABAergic substances, such as vigabatrin and topiramate, in both children and adults (Trimble, 1991). Clinical features include schizophrenia-like psychoses and autistic withdrawal (Amir & Gross Tsur, 1994).

The mechanism for forced normalization is not known. The alternating psychoses may relate to a modification of neurochemical balance or seizure-related electrical brain activity (Hauser & Hersdorffer, 2001). There may be a biologic antagonism between seizures and psychoses, or continuing epileptic status in the limbic system, or a propagation of epileptiform discharges along unusual pathways. The reticular activating system and its interactions with hippocampal structures may play a role. Anticonvulsants may influence underlying metabolic processes or increase activation, leading to sleep withdrawal and psychoses, reactions of the healthy parts of the brain against the epileptic focus. With forced normalization, the epilepsy appears to be active but subcortical and restricted, whereas inhibitory processes are active. The inhibition leads to insomnia, hypervigilance, and dysphoria. At this point, the condition can easily become a psychosis, especially if there is a history of past psychoses, a premorbid personality for such, or a lack of social competence (Wolf, 1984; Wolf, 1991; Krishnamoorthy & Trimble, 1999).

There appears to be an antagonistic relationship between seizures and psychoses. Antiepileptic drugs serve to control epilepsy but may worsen schizophrenia, whereas drugs such as the phenothiazines do the opposite. Antiepileptic drugs that increase GABA levels are associated with the development of a psychopathologic state in up to 10% of patients, characterized by mood changes, agitation, and even psychotic symptoms of a paranoid nature (Coyle, 1996; Krishnamoorthy & Trimble, 1999).

In people with epilepsy, with the emergence of the psychotic state, the scalp EEG spiking is reduced by more than 50%, if not normalized, usually with a complete cessation of seizures for at least one week (Krishnamoorthy & Trimble, 1999). However, subdural EEG leads show epileptic discharges in the temporal limbic structures, suggesting that there is only a drop in cortical voltage or suppression that accompanies seizure activity in the depth (Rayport & Ferguson, 2001).

Early control of prepsychotic dysphorias may prevent the forced normalization. The treatment is to reduce or discontinue the antiepileptic drug until overt seizures recur, allowing a remission of the psychotic symptoms. A rapid tapering under video-EEG monitoring has been considered. Treatment is by transient use of a neuroleptic mediation. ECT or pentylenetetrazol may be used to induce seizures if necessary. With the recurrence and remission of psychotic symptoms, antiepileptic drugs should be reintroduced slowly (Kanner, 2000; Ried & Mothersill, 1998).

Antiepileptic drug-induced psychoses

Psychoses are a rare complication of all conventional antiepileptic drugs (Trimble, 1998). Often, there are biologic and genetic predispositions. Forced normalization is seen with ethosuximide in 2% of children and 8% of adults (Wolf, 1991). Schizophrenia-like psychoses are seen with phenytoin (Perlo & Schwab, 1969) at intoxicating serum levels (McDanal & Bolman, 1975), as well as with phenobarbital and primidone (Rivinus, 1982). Psychoses have been reported as a side effect of the newer antiepileptic drugs, such as vigabatrin (Sander et al., 1991), lamotrigine, topiramate, levetiracetam (Kanner, 2000), felbamate (McConnell et al., 1996), tiagabine, and zonisamide. Psychotic disorders can follow the discontinuation of antiepileptic drugs, especially those with mood-stabilizing properties, such as carbamazepine, phenytoin, valproic acid, and, especially, benzodiazepines, manifest by anxiety, depression, and psychosis (Kanner, 2000; Ketter et al., 1994; Schmitz, 1966; Sironi et al., 1979).

The newer antiepileptic agents have been reported to produce psychoses and affective disorders. With vigabatrin, psychiatric complications are seen in 3.4–7% of patients, which is almost the same as the incidence in the population with epilepsy in general. Problems are more apt to be seen in patients with severe intractable epilepsy, for reasons that are still unclear (Sander & Duncan, 1996). There is a decrease in specific binding in the left hemisphere basal ganglia, which may lead to psychoses in vulnerable patients (Ring et al., 1994). Risk factors include more severe epilepsies, especially complex partial epilepsy, patients with which often exhibit GABAergic cortical-subcortical alteration favorable for the appearance of the psychoses after introduction of vigabatrin (Thomas et al., 1996; Torta et al., 1993).

Similar psychoses have been seen with topiramate (Luef & Bauer, 1996; Theodore *et al.*, 1995), felbamate (McConnell *et al.*, 1996), and tiagabine (Schmitz *et al.*, 1966).

In patients with chronic epilepsy, the incidence of anticonvulsant drug-triggered psychosis is 5%, and that of affective disorder is 10–15%. It is not clear whether any particular chemical class of drugs is interlined with forced normalization, although some studies suggest that GABAergic drugs may be particularly involved (Krishnamoorthy & Trimble, 1999). This is rare post-surgically and is usually associated with a lesion. Successful cessation of seizures does not protect the patient against any other symptoms that may become active. It is not at all uncommon for behaviors to become worse when seizures become controlled (Trimble, 1994).

Pathogenesis of epileptic psychoses

Limbic system epilepsy is different from other forms of temporal lobe epilepsy. The mesial-temporal lobe is markedly different genetically, cellularly, biochemically, and electrically from other paleocortex and neocortex. This is especially so for the amygdala and hippocampus, which are common sites of pathology in epilepsy. The medial limbic system is linked closely to dopaminergic areas of the brain, an area of study in schizophrenia research.

Schizophrenia may be a neurodevelopment disorder of the hippocampal formation and its association with the entorhinal cortex. Disordered neural communication, perhaps a maldevelopment, of the normal circuitry underlies psychosis and schizophrenia (Weinberger & Berman, 1996). Cerebral lesions increase the susceptibility to psychoses (Davison & Bagley, 1969; Taylor, 1975; Torta & Keller, 1999). Perinatal lesions of the temporal frontal area appear common with psychoses (Roberts *et al.*, 1990; Bolwig, 1994). Microscopic abnormalities are also common (Ben Ary & Repressa, 1990; Mathern *et al.*, 1995). Temporolimbic dysfunction, particularly hyperfunction in the temporal limbic system in the dominant left hemisphere, appears to arise at the time of the psychotic state in epileptic psychosis, especially with hallucinations (Jibiki *et al.*, 1993; Conlon *et al.*, 1995). Circulation may be reduced in the left medial-temporal region (Gallhofer *et al.*, 1985; Marshall *et al.*, 1993).

The psychosis relates to the epileptogenic focus. Patients with frontobasal (temporal anterior) foci are prone to paranoia, whereas patients with temporal lobe foci are particularly depressed and patients with sagittal-line foci present with predominantly expansive, hypomanic behaviors, as determined by EEG monitoring (Psatta *et al.*, 1991; Torta & Keller, 1999).

The exact relationship between a seizure and a psychosis is unclear. With schizophrenia, the normal prefrontal recruitment is lacking. The frontal activation is reduced and other cortex recruitment is deficient. The left inferior frontal gyrus is deficient, whereas the hippocampus may be overly active. The frontal component shows the clearest divergence from temporal lobe epilepsy, in which the frontal area is hypoactive and the hippocampal area is overly active (Weinberger & Berman, 1996).

The psychoses of epilepsy appear to be related to overactivity in the mesolimbic system, with secondary activations of various cortical areas depending on the symptoms. Frontobasal, mediofrontal, and prefrontal areas appear to be especially involved. Abnormalities of dopamine activity with periodic excesses are noted, possibly against a low baseline, which may relate to receptor abnormalities. Dopamine agonists produce psychotic tendencies and show anticonvulsant activities. Dopamine antagonists are antipsychotic and epileptogenic. GABA also appears to be involved (Trimble, 1988; Torta & Keller, 1999).

Traditional antipsychotic drugs inhibit dopamine activity not only in the mesolimbic system but elsewhere, which contributes to their side effects. The older drugs, such as the phenothiazines, block dopaminergic receptors in the mesolimbic structures, but elsewhere such blocking impairs movements and cognition. Newer drugs bind less vigorously to the receptors but still block sufficient dopamine to ease symptoms in the mesolimbic receptor sites without inhibiting pathways in other areas in the cortex (Bernsweig *et al.*, 2002).

Diagnosis

There are numerous cases of patients with clouded consciousness being mistaken as being in a psychiatric state when actually it is complex partial status. This can present with paranoid delusions, religious delusions, and other hallucinations. These symptoms almost always relate to seizures originating in the limbic system. An EEG including sleep as well as wake recordings, using T1–2 and F7–8 electrodes, may help to differentiate the problem. Anticonvulsant blood levels should be checked for excesses or deficiencies. The folic acid level should be measured. An MRI should be obtained to rule out a small ganglioglioma or harmatomas, which may be multiple (Taylor, 1972; Bruton *et al.*, 1994). If video-EEG shows a single ictal focus, then surgery may be considered (Kanner, 2000).

Prognosis

Unlike schizophrenia, with the psychoses of epilepsy there is an absence of negative symptoms, better premorbid function, and rare deterioration of the personality (Toone *et al.*, 1982). There are two types of presentation: episodic psychosis of epilepsy and chronic or non-episodic psychoses of epilepsy. The episodic form is seen primarily in patients with temporal lobe epilepsy and is linked closely to the status of the seizure control; the episodes last a few days to several weeks. The non-progressive form, which has a more guarded prognosis, is more prolonged and non-episodic. A mixture of both types may be seen (Kanner, 2000).

Treatment

The primary treatment of postoperative psychosis with epilepsy is optimal seizure control. If an episode occurs and persists for a protracted period, then a neuroleptic drug may be necessary (Kanner, 2000).

Pharmacological treatment

With antipsychotic drugs, there is always the risk of lowering the seizure threshold or inducing seizures de novo; this is seen in about 1% of cases (Devinsky & Pacia, 1994). Antipsychotic drugs are best used with an antiepileptic drug, particularly valproate or lamotrigine (Weisbrot & Ettinger, 1998). The risk is higher with certain drugs, in patients with a history of epilepsy, in patients with abnormal EEG recordings, in patients with a history of a CNS disorder, with rapid titration of the neuroleptic dosage, with high dosages, and with concomitant use of other drugs that lower the seizure threshold (Kanner, 2000; McConnell & Duncan, 1998).

Antipsychotic drugs with a lower seizure risk include haloperidol, molindone, fluphenazine, perphenazine, trifluoperazine (McConnell & Duncan, 1998), and risperidone (Kanner, 2000). The newer atypical antipsychotic agents such as risperidone and olanzaprine appear to carry a very low risk of inducing seizures (Trimble, 1991). Risperidone and olanzapine are more favored in pediatric patients. Weight gain is seen with the use of these drugs. Clonazepam has an approximately 3–4% risk of inducing seizures. Haloperidol has a lower risk of inducing seizures than the phenothiazines (Weisbrot & Ettinger, 1998).

Most neuroleptics produce EEG changes with slowing of the background at high dosages. Some of these drugs can cause paroxysmal EEG changes in the form of interictal sharp waves and spikes, but these are not predictive of seizure occurrence. Severe disorganization of the EEG recording is more likely to predict seizure occurrence (Kanner, 2000; Toth & Frankenberg, 1994).

Hepatic enzyme induction by many antiepileptic drugs, such as carbamazepine, phenytoin, phenobarbital, and primidone, may increase the clearance rate of most neuroleptics, reducing the neuroleptic effectiveness. Discontinuation of such an antiepileptic may cause the neuroleptic levels to raise, resulting in extrapyramidal adverse events. Such drug interactions must therefore be reviewed carefully (Kanner, 2000; McConnell & Duncan, 1998).

Electroshock treatment

Electroshock treatment is not contraindicated in adults with severe psychoses with epilepsy, although it is known to increase the seizure threshold. Such treatment is antipsychotic, antidepressant, and antimanic. Anticonvulsants are with held in the morning before treatment but otherwise are kept at baseline doses (Kanner, 2000). ECT has not been considered for use in children.

Surgery

After a temporal lobectomy, some patients with episodic psychotic states are improved mentally, suggesting that deep epileptic discharges might have been the cause of their psychotic states (Sengoku *et al.*, 1997). Early surgical intervention for patients whose seizures are resistant to medication control may prevent the emergence of epileptic psychoses in adulthood. Early lesional surgery for those with demonstrated lesions associated with an epileptic focus may prevent later development of psychoses.

REFERENCES

American Psychiatric Association (1994). *Diagnostic and Statistical Manual of Mental Disorders (DSM IV)*. Washington, DC: American Psychiatric Association.

Amir, N. & Gross Tsur, V. (1994). Paradoxical normalization in childhood epilepsia. *Epilepsia* 35: 1060–64.

Andermann, L. F., Savard, G., Meencke, H. J., *et al.* (1999). Psychosis after resection of ganglioglioma or DNET: evidence for an association. *Epilepsia* 40: 83–7.

Ben Ary, Y. & Repressa, A. (1990). Brief seizure episodes induce long-term potentiation and mossy fibre sprouting in the hippocampus. *Trends Neurosci.* 13: 312–19.

Bernsweig, D., Stern, E. & Lieberman, J. (2002). The brain. *Newsweek*, March 1, 2002.

Blanchet, P. & Frommer, G. P. (1986). Mood change preceding epileptic seizures. *J. Nerv. Ment. Dis.* 174: 471–6.

Bolwig, T. G. (1994). Seizures in therapy of psychoses. *Neuropsychiatry* 9: 79.

Bruton, C. J., Stevens, J. & Frith, C. D. (1994). Epilepsy, psychosis and schizophrenia: clinical and neuropathologic correlations. *Neurology* 44: 32–42.

Caplan, R., Arbelle, S., Guthrie, D., *et al.* (1997). Formal thought disorder and psychopathology in pediatric primary generalized and complex partial epilepsy *J. Am. Acad. Child Adolesc. Psychiatry* 36: 1286–94.

Caplan, R., Guthrie, D. & Siddarth, P. (2000) Thought disorders in complex partial seizures and petit mal. *Epilespia* 41 (suppl 7): 88.

Caplan, R., Shields, W. D., Mori, L., *et al.* (1991). Middle childhood onset of interictal psychosis. *J. Am. Acad. Child Adolesc. Psychiatry* 30: 893–6.

Carlsson, M. & Carlsson, A. (1990). Schizophrenia: a subcortical neurotransmitter imbalance syndrome? *Schizophr. Bull.* 16: 425–32.

Conlon, P., Trimble, M. R. & Rogers, D. (1995). A study of epileptic psychosis using magnetic resonance imaging. *Br. J. Psychiatry* 156: 231–5.

Coyle, J. T. (1996). The glutaminergic dysfunction hypothesis of schizoprhenia. *Harv. Rev. Psychiatry* **3**: 241–3.

Cummings, J. L. & Trimble, M. R. (1995). *Concise Guide of Neuropsychiatry and Behavioral Neurology.* Washington, DC: American Psychiatric Association.

Davison, K. & Bagley, C. R. (1969). Schizophrenia-like psychoses associated with organic disorders of the central nervous system: a review of the literature. *Br. J. Psychiatry* **4**: 113–83.

Devinsky, O., Abramson, H., Alper, K., *et al.* (1995). Postictal psychosis: a case control series of 20 patients and 150 controls. *Epilepsy Res.* **20**: 247–53.

Devinsky, O. & Pacia, S. V. (1994). Seizures during clozapine therapy. *J. Clin. Psychiatry* **55**: 153–6.

Dunn, D. W. (1998). Behavioral aspects of pediatric epilepsy. In *Psychiatry In Epilepsy: A Practical Approach to Diagnosis and Management,* ed. A. B. Ettinger & B. P. Hermann. New York: Symposium Proceedings.

Flor-Henry, P. (1968). Psychosis and temporal lobe epilepsy: a controlled investigation. *Epilepsia* **10**: 353–95.

Gallhofer, B., Trimble, M. R. & Frackowiak, R. (1985). A study of cerebral flow and metabolism in epileptic psychosis using positron emission tomography and oxygen. *J. Neurol. Neuorsurg. Psychiatry* **48**: 201–6.

Gibbs, F. A. (1951). Ictal and non-ictal psychiatric disorders in temporal lobe epilepsy. *J. Nerv. Ment. Dis.* **113**: 522–8.

Glosser, G., Zwil, A. S., Glosser, D. S., *et al.* (2000). Psychiatric aspects of temporal lobe epilepsy before and after anterior temporal lobectomy. *J. Neurol. Neurosurg. Psychiatry* **68**: 53–8.

Hauser, W. A. & Hesdorffer, D. C. (2001). Psychoses, depression and epilepsy: epidemiological considerations. In *Psychiatric Issues in Epilepsy,* ed. A. B. Ettinger & A. M. Kanner, pp. 187–9. Philadelphia: Lippincott Williams & Wilkins.

Hermann, B. P. (1979). Psychopathology in epilepsy and learned helplessness. *Med. Hypotheses* **5**: 723–9.

Hermann, B. P. & Whitman, S. (1984). Behavior and personality correlates of epilepsy: a review. Methological critique and conceptual model. *Psychol. Bull.* **95**: 456–97.

Jablinsky, A., Sartorius, N., Ernberg, G., *et al.* (1992). Schizophrenia: manifestations, incidence and course in different cultures. A World Health Organization ten country study. *Psychol. Med. (suppl)* **20**: 1–97.

Jensen, I. & Vaemet, K. (1977). Temporal lobe epilepsy: follow-up investigation of 74 temporal lobe resected patients. *Acta Neurochir.* **37**: 173–200.

Jibiki, I., Maeda, T., Kubota, T. & Yamaguchi, N. (1993). 123 I-IMP SPECT brain imaging in epiletic psychosis: a study of two cases of temporal lobe epilepsy with schizophrenia-like syndrome. *Neuropsychobiology* **28**: 207–11.

Kanemoto, K., Kawasaki, J. & Kawai, J. (1996). Postictal psychosis: a comparison with acute interictal and chronic psychoses. *Epilepsia* **37**: 551–6.

Kanner, A. M. (2000). Psychosis of epilepsy: a neurologist's perspective. *Epilepsy Behav.* **1**: 219–27.

Kanner, A. M., Stagno, S., Kotagal, P., *et al.* (1996). Postictal psychiatric events during prolonged video-electroencephalographic monitoring studies. *Arch. Neurol.* **53**: 258–63.

Kawakami, M., Terasawa, E. & Ibuki, T. (1970). Changes in multiple unit activity over the brain during the estrous cycle. *Neuroendocrinology* **6**: 30–48.

Ketter, T. A., Malow, B. A., Flamini, R., *et al.* (1994). Anticonvulsant withdrawal: emergent psychopathology. *Neurology* **44**: 55–61.

Krishnamoorthy, E. S. & Trimble, M. R. (1999). Forced normalization: clinical and therapeutic relevance. *Epilepsia* **40** (suppl 10): 57–64.

Kristensen, O. & Sindrup, E. H. (1978). Psychomotor epilepsy and psychosis. I: physical aspects. *Acta Neurol. Scand.* **57**: 361–9.

Kubagawa, T., Furusho, U. J. & Maruyama, H. (1997). Study of psychiatric symptoms after discontinuation of antiepileptic drugs. Proceedings of the 30th Congress of Japan Epilepsy Society. *Epilepsia* **38** (suppl 6): 26–31.

Lancman, M. E., Craven, W. J., Asconape, J. J., *et al.* (1994). Clinical management of recurrent postictal psychosis. *J. Epilepsy* **7**: 47–51.

Leinonen, E., Tuunainen, A. & Lepola, U. (1994). Postoperative psychoses in epileptic patients after temporal lobectomy. *Acta Neurol. Scand.* **90**: 394–9.

Lindsay, J., Ounsted, C. & Richards, P. (1979a). Long-term outcome in childrenn with temporal lobe seizures. II: marriage, parenthood and sexual differences. *Dev. Med. Child Neurol.* **21**: 433–40.

Lindsay, J., Ounsted, C. & Richards, P. (1979b). Long-term outcome in children with temporal lobe seizures. I: social outcome and childhood factors. *Dev. Med. Child Neurol.* **21**: 630–36.

Luef, G. & Bauer, G. (1996). Topiramate in drug-resistant partial and generalized epilepsies. *Epilepsia* **37**: 69–73.

Mace, C. J. & Trimble, M. R. (1981). Psychosis following temporal lobe surgery: a report of 6 cases. *J. Neurol. Neurosurg. Psychiatry* **64**: 639–44.

Manchanda, R., Miller, H. & McLachlan, R. S. (1993). Postictal psychosis after right temporal lobectomy. *J. Neurosurg. Psychiatry* **66**: 277–9.

Manchanda, R., Schaefer, B., McLachlan, R. S., *et al.* (1996). Psychiatric disorders in candidates for surgery for epilepsy. *J. Neurol. Neurosurg. Psychiatry* **61**: 82–9.

Marshall, E. J., Syed, G. M. S., Fenwick, P. B. C., *et al.* (1993). A pilot study using single photon emission computerized tomography. *Br. J. Psychiatry* **163**: 32–6.

Mathern, G. W., Pretorius, J. K., Babb, T. L., *et al.* (1995). Unilateral hippocampal mossy fiber sprouting and bilateral asymmetric neuronal loss with episodic postictal psychosis. *J. Neurosurg* **82**: 228–33.

Matsuura, M. (1997). Psychoses of epilepsy with special reference to anterior temporal lobectomy. Proceedings of the 30th Congress of the Japan Epilepsy Society. *Epilepsia* **38** (suppl 6): 32–4.

McConnell, H. & Duncan, D. (1998). Treatment of psychiatric comorbidity in epilepsy. In *Psychiatric Comorbidity in Epilepsy: Basic Mechanisms, Diagnosis, and Treatment*, ed. H. McConnell & P. J. Snyder. Washington, DC: American Psychiatric Press.

McConnell, H., Snyder, P. J., Duffy, J. D., *et al.* (1996). Neuropsychiatric side effects related to treatment with felbamate. *J. Neuropsychiatry Clin. Neurosci.* **8**: 341–6.

McDanal, C. E. & Bolman, W. M. (1975). Delayed idiosyncratic psychosis with diphenylhydantoin. *JAMA* **231**: 1063.

Mendez, M. F. & Grau, R. (1991). The postictal psychosis of epilepsy: investigation in two patients. *Int. J. Psychiatry Med.* **21**: 85–92.

Onuma, T. (1997). Paranoid-hallucinatory state in patients with epilepsy: historical perspective in Japan. Proceedings of the 30th Congress of the Japan Epilepsy Society. *Epilepsia* **38** (suppl 6): 17–21.

Onuma, T. (2000). Classification of psychiatric symptoms in patients with epilepsy. Proceedings of 32nd Congress of Japan Epilepsy Society. *Epilepsia* **41** (suppl 9): 43–8.

Pakalnis, A., Drake, J. K., & Kellum, J. B. (1987). Forced normalization: acute psychosis after seizure control in seven patients. *Arch. Neurol.* **44**: 289–92.

Perlo, V. P. & Schwab, R. S. (1969). Unrecognized Dilantin intoxication. In *Modern Neurology*, ed. S. Locke, pp. 589–97. Boston: Little, Brown.

Psatta, D. M., Tudorache, B., Matei, M., *et al.* (1991). Cerebral dysfunction revealed by EEG mapping in the schizoform epileptic psychosis. *Rom. J. Neurol. Psychiatry* **29**: 81–98.

Rayport, M. & Ferguson, S. M. (1998). Psychoses of epilepsy. In *Psychiatric Aspects of Epilepsy: A Practial Guide to Diagnosis and Treatment*, ed. A. B. Ettinger & A. M. Kanner, Baltimore, MD: Lippincott Wiliams & Wilkins.

Rayport, M. & Ferguson, S. M. (2001). Psychoses of epilepsy, an integrated approach. In *Psychiatric Issues in Epilepsy*, ed. A. B. Ettinger & A. M. Kanner, pp. 730–94. Philadelphia: Lippincott Williams & Wilkins.

Reutens, D. C., Savard, G., Andermann, F., *et al.* (1977). Results of surgical treatment in temporal lobe epilepsy with chronic psychosis. *Brain* **120**: 1929–36.

Ried, S. & Mothersill, I. W. (1998). Forced normalization: the clinical neurologist's view. In *Forced Normalization and Alternative Psychoses of Epilepsy*, ed. M. R. Trimble & B. Schmitz, pp. 77–94. Petersfield, UK: Wrightson Biomedical.

Ring, H. A., Trimble, M. R., Costa, D. C., *et al.* (1994). Striatal dopamine receptor binding in epileptic psychoses. *Biol. Psychiatry* **356**: 375–80.

Rivinus, T. M. (1982). Psychiatric effects of the anticonvulsant regimens. *J. Clin. Psychopharmacol.* **2**: 165–92.

Roberts, G. W., Done, D. J. & Crow, T. J. (1990). A "mock-up" of schizophrenia: temporal lobe epilepsy and schizophrenia-like psychosis. *Biol. Psychiatry* **28**: 127–43.

Sander, J. W. & Duncan, J. S. (1996). Vigabatrin. In *The Treatment of Epilepsy*, ed. S. Shorvon, F. Dreifuss, D. Fish & D. Thomas, pp. 491–9. Oxford: Blackwell Science.

Sander, J. W., Hart, Y. M., Trimble, M. R., *et al.* (1991). Vigabatrin and psychosis. *J. Neurol. Neurosurg. Psychiatry* **54**: 435–9.

Savard, G., Andermann, F., Olivier, A., *et al.* (1991). Postictal psychoses after partial complex seizures: a multiple case study. *Epilepsia* **31**: 225–31.

Schmitz, B. (1966). *Psychiatrische Symptoms bei Epielspie – welchen Effect haben Antiepileptika?*, pp. 24–7. German League Against Epilepsy.

Sengoku, A., Toichi, M. & Murai, T. (1997). Comparison of psychotic states in patients with idiopathic generalized epilepsy and temporal lobe epilepsy. Proceedings of the 30th Congress of the Japan Epiepsy Society. *Epilepsia* **38** (suppl 6): 22–5.

Sherwin, I. (1981). Psychosis associated with epilepsy: significance of the laterality of the epileptogenic lesion. *J. Neurol. Neurosurg. Psychiatry* **44**: 83–5.

Sherwin, I., Perin-Magnon, J., Bancaud, J., *et al.* (1982). Prevalence of psychosis in epilepsy as a function of laterality of epileptogenic lesion. *Arch. Neurol.* **39**: 621–5.

Sironi, V. A., Franzini, A., Ravaghati, L., *et al.* (1979). Interictal psychoses in temporal lobe epilepsy during withdrawal of anticonvulsant therapy. *J. Neurol. Neurosurg. Psychiatry* **42**: 724–30.

So, H. K., Svard, G., Andermann, F., *et al.* (1990). Acute postictal psychosis, a stereo EEG study. *Epilepsia* **31**: 188–93.

Stevens, J. R. (1990). Psychiatric consequences of temporal lobectomy for intractable seizures: a 20–30 year follow-up of 14 cases. *Psychol. Med.* **20**: 529–65.

Stevens, J. R. (1991). Psychosis and the temporal lobe. In *Advances in Neurology*, ed. D. Smith, D. Treiman & M. Trimble, Vol. 55, pp. 79–96. New York: Raven Press.

Taylor, D. C. (1972). Mental state and temporal lobe epilepsy: a correlative account of 100 patients treated surgically. *Epilepsia* **13**: 727–65.

Taylor, D. C. (1975). Factors influencing the occurrence of schizophrenia-like psychoses in patients with temporal lobe epilepsy *Psychol. Med.* **56**: 249–65.

Theodore, W. H., Albert, P., Stertz, B., *et al.* (1995). Felbamate monotherapy: implications for antiepileptic drug development. *Epilepsia* **36**: 105–10.

Thomas, L., Trimble, M. & Schmitz, B. (1996). Vigabatrin and behaviour disorders: a retrospective survey. *Epilepsy Res.* **25**: 21–7.

Toone, B. K., Garralda, M. E. & Ron, M. A. (1982). The psychosis of epilepsy and the functional psychosis: a clinical and phenomenological comparison. *Br. J. Psychiatry* **141**: 256–61.

Torta, R. & Keller, R. (1999). Behavioral, psychotic and anxiety disorders in epilepsy: etiology, clinical features and therapeutic implications. *Epilepsia* **50** (suppl 10): 2–20.

Torta, R., Monaco, F., Bergamasco, L., *et al.* (1993). Lack of adverse cognitive effects of vigabatrin in epileptic patients: neuropsychology and neuropsychological evaluation. *Ital J. Neurol. Sci. Suppl.* **14**: 110.

Toth, P. & Frankenburg, F. R. (1994). Clozapine and seizures: a review. *Can. J. Psychiatry* **39**: 236–8.

Trimble, M. R. (1988). *Biological Psychiatry.* New York: John Wiley & Sons.

Trimble, M. R. (1991). Treatment of epileptic psychosis. In *The Psychoses of Epilepsy*, ed. M. R. Trimble, pp. 150–63. New York: Raven Press.

Trimble, M. R. (1992). Behavior changes following temporal lobectomy, with special reference to psychosis. *J. Neurol. Neurosurg. Psychiatry* **55**: 89–91.

Trimble, M. R. (1993). Interictal psychoses. Presented at the International Epilepsy Conference, Oslo, Norway, 1993.

Trimble, M. R. (1994). The effects of seizures on psychopathology. Presented at Psychiatric Aspects of Epilepsy: New Directions in the 1990s, Vancouver.

Trimble, M. R. (1997). Psychiatric profiles and patterns of cerebral blood flow in focal epilepsy: interactions between depression, obsessionality, and perfusion related to the laterality of the epilepsy. *J. Neurol. Neurosurg. Psychiatry* **62**: 458–63.

Trimble, M. R. (1998). Forced normalization and the role of anticonvulsants. In *Forced Normalization*, ed. M. R. Trimble & B. Schmitz, pp. 169–78. Petersfield: Wrintgson Biomedical.

Umbricht, D., Degreef, G., Barr, W. B., *et al.* (1995). Postictal and chronic psychoses in patients with temporal lobe epilepsy. *Am. J. Psychiatry* **152**: 224–30.

Weinberger, D. & Berman, K. (1996). Prefrontal function in schizophrenia: confounds and controversies. *Philos. Trans. R. Soc. Lond. B Biol. Sci.* **351**: 1495–1503.

Weisbrot, D. M. & Ettinger, A. B. (1998). Psychiatric aspects of pediatric epilepsy. *Prim. Psychiatry* **June**: 51–67.

Wolf, P. (1984). The clinical syndromes of forced normalization. *Folia Psychiatr. Neurol. Jpn.* **38**: 187–92.

Wolf, P. (1991). Acute behavioral symptomatology at disappearance of epileptiform EEG abnormality: paradoxical or "forced normalization." In *Advances in Neurology*, ed. D. Smith, D. Treiman & M. Trimble, Vol. 55, pp. 127–42. New York: Raven Press.

37

Non-epileptic events

About 18% of children, including adolescents, with new seizures are found to have pseudoseizures (Golden *et al.*, 1985; Pakalnis *et al.*, 1999; Lancman *et al.*, 2002; Lelliott & Fenwick, 1999). These events have been called non-epileptic events or episodes, non-epileptic seizures, pseudoseizures, hysterical seizures, conversion convulsions, and "fake" seizures (Gross, 1983; Gumnit & Gates, 1986; Riley & Roy, 1982; Trimble, 1981).

In conversion reactions, adults often present with a loss of function, whereas children tend to present with pain, pseudoseizures, or syncope. In children, the incidence of a conversion reaction is at least 1–2% and perhaps as high as 5% (Robins & O'Neal, 1953; Hersov, 1985; Hinman, 1958; Goodyer, 1981). Such reactions occur three times more often in adolescents than in younger children. Children often present with anxiety and psychological problems, whereas adults may present with a "la belle indifference" affect (Dubowitz & Hersov, 1976; Malony, 1980; Goodyer, 1981).

Non-epileptic seizures are one of the most common conversion symptoms in childhood. They appear in children with and without epileptic seizures. They may involve subconscious reactions to a past or present stress, or the intentional production of symptoms either to achieve a goal (Mills & Lipian, 1997; Weisbrot & Ettinger, 1998). When a child experiences both epilepsy and non-epileptic events, the parents may find the decision to seek mental health help difficult, especially if there is a history of brain injury.

Definition

Non-epileptic seizures are clinical events that resemble epileptic attacks but are not associated with physiologic CNS changes. Non-epileptic seizures are subdivided into physiologic events that resemble seizures such as fainting episodes, cardio-circulatory disturbances, and gastrointestinal problems, and psychologic events of various types, such as conversion reactions, panic attacks, factitious disorders, and malingering.

Frequency

About 10–20% of children referred for refectory epilepsy are found to have non-epileptic events, of which 44% have pure non-epileptic events and the remainder have mixed non-epileptic and epileptic seizures. Preadolescents tend to present with repetitive, stereotyped behaviors, whereas adolescents present more with pseudoepileptic seizures (Williamson & Spencer, 1986).

Epidemiology

Gender

By adolescence, similar to in the adult population, 65–74% of patients with non-epileptic episodes are girls (Holmes *et al.*, 1980; Leonard & George, 1999; Pakalnis *et al.*, 1999; Williams & Grant, 2000; Lancman *et al.*, 2002). The incidence is more equal in boys and girls in younger children (Williams, 2000).

Age

Occurrence of non-epileptic seizures before age five and after age 55 is rare (Holmes *et al.*, 1980; Lancman *et al.*, 2002). Of childhood non-epileptic seizures, 32–46% appear prepubertally and 54–68% appear in adolescence (Pakalnis *et al.*, 1999; Leonard & George, 1999; Williams & Grant, 2000). Generally, there are two peaks of the occurrence of non-epileptic seizures: in late adolescence, from 19 to 22 years, and in early adulthood, from 25 to 35 years (Lancman *et al.*, 1994; Lancman *et al.*, 2002).

Family

Children with non-epileptic seizures usually live with immediate or extended family members, with few requiring institutional care. About 40% are the firstborn child (Williams & Grant, 2000). A family history of epilepsy is found in 37.6% of patients with psychogenic non-epileptic seizures. (Guberman, 1982; Lancman *et al.*, 1994; Lancman *et al.*, 2002).

Health status

The children are usually healthy (25%) or experience only minor health problems (60%), with no prior neurologic history (52%). A small number (15%) may experience major physical conditions that alter their lives. A history of epileptic seizures (22%) or severe head injuries (15%) may be noted (Williams & Grant, 2000). In adolescents with non-epileptic seizures, there may be a positive neurologic history (21%), such as meningitis or arachnoid cysts, but this does not seem to increase the incidence of non-epileptic seizures (Lancman *et al.*, 2002).

Development

Development is often normal (74%), although some patients experience delayed development (13%), speech delays (13%), or a below-average to borderline intelligence (Lancman *et al.*, 2002). About half are in regular education, yet learning problems (40%) and retardation (12%) are found. With the onset of non-epileptic seizures, school attendance often decreases (34%) (Williams & Grant, 2000).

Behavior history

Children with non-epileptic seizures do not have the severe psychiatric and personality disorders seen in adults. Nearly half have no psychiatric diagnosis. The others bear diagnoses of ADDH, oppositional defiant or conduct disorders (19%), an affect disorder (19%), or both. A significant family history of psychiatric disorders, mood disorders, impulsive control addictions, and antisocial behaviors may be found (Williams & Grant, 2000).

Clinical

Children with non-epileptic seizures often present with unresponsiveness, fainting, tremor, or thrashing of all extremities, or occasionally lateralized movements (Hempel, 2000). Younger children may have an increased frequency of staring episodes, which are not controlled by medication. The non-epileptic seizures may be provoked or shortened by suggestions. Evidence of secondary gain may be found (Carmant *et al.*, 1993).

Precipitants

Stresses are often elicited by a good history in 78% of patients. At least one stress is found in 34% of patients, and multiple stresses are found in the rest (Williams & Grant, 2000). An obvious stress may provoke seizures readily, but other precipitants may not be readily apparent. The seizures emerge under stressful circumstances, with the apparent primary gain being anxiety alleviation. There may be secondary gains, such as getting attention, being excused from school or a task, achieving a reward, obtaining financial compensation, or escaping an intolerable social situation. Non-epileptic seizures are produced unintentionally, representing either the repression of an unacceptable emotion or dissociation from distressing experiences. Major stressors for children include family, school, relationships, traumatic experience, and parental illness.

Family

In children, family stresses include conflicts such as parent–child conflicts (45%), history of parental illness, death, divorce or separation (35%), marital discord

(30%), high parent or child expectations (25%), parental psychopathology (10%), and parental alcoholism. (10%) (Hempel, 2000).

School

School stresses are found in at least 30% of patients with school difficulties (70%), of below-average intelligence (44%) (Hempel, 2000), and with learning disabilities (Silver, 1982). Overexpectation often exists.

Relationships

Relationships are important, especially in teens, where identified stresses include peer relationship problems (45%), various adolescent stresses (24%), regressive affections (8%), sexual stressors (10%), grief (Hempel, 2000), forced separation from family members, and moving to a new home.

Traumatic experiences

Traumatic experiences (19%) include loss, rape, and incest (Goodwin *et al.*, 1979; Gross, 1979; Hempel, 2000): The common history of sexual or physical abuse in non-epileptic seizures in adults is reported less frequently (6%) in children and adolescents with non-epileptic seizures (Wyllie *et al.*, 1991; Alper *et al.*, 1993). Over half deny any history of sexual abuse, but it is estimated that up to 31% have been sexually abused and 15% have been physically abused (Williams & Grant, 2000). Other dissociative phenomena are common. The sexually abused child may attempt a physical and/or mental escape, such as suicide or conversion. The altering of consciousness is an attempt to escape reality. Other family members tend to keep the abuse secret out of shame or fearing retaliation, disturbance of the family equilibrium, or loss of financial support. The family may have incompatible sexual attitudes. Daughters and mothers may be estranged. The families tend to be isolated from other social systems (Trimble, 1981; Riley & Roy, 1982; Gross, 1983; Gumnit & Gates, 1986).

Illness

Parental medical problems may be associated with non-epileptic events in a child. Children with chronic uncontrolled epileptic seizures may develop additional non-epileptic seizures under stress (Holmes *et al.*, 1980; Onuma, 2000). Non-epileptic seizures typically may occur in later adolescence following childhood-onset seizures, usually with a few years' interval. A long history of uncontrolled seizures and use of multiple antiepileptic drugs can produce considerable stress and possible cognitive dysfunction, which may be responsible for the underlying psychopathology (Onuma, 2000). When chronic childhood seizures are controlled, the child may develop pseudoseizures as an excuse for the epilepsy-related problems that remain.

Other precipitants

Multiple stresses may be found in 14% of patients. In about 5% of children, there is no clear relationship to any stress. In adolescence, there may be overprotectiveness. Problems of affection are usually associated with an inability to handle this (Hempel, 2000).

Presentation

Non-epileptic presentations fall into four broad categories: seizure mimics, tantrum-like behaviors (44%), unresponsiveness (26%), and motionless staring. The episodes tend to represent escape, manipulative behaviors, or a flashback to a disturbing prior experience. Clinical characteristics are similar in children and adults (Lancman *et al.*, 1994; Lancman *et al.*, 2002).

Imitative

Patients may present with episodes that mimic seizure behaviors, having learned the behaviors by observing a friend or family member with epilepsy, or from cinema or television dramas, often with a secondary gain subconsciously in mind. Children may respond like they imagine the seizures appear.

Dissociation

The individual may fade out of association when experiencing a stressful environment or recollection. These are gradual in onset and in resolution and appear to be dissociative escape mechanisms as a survival technique. In some patients, there may be fine tremors. In others, there is only a motionless stare.

Tantrum-like behavior

Tantrum like behaviors, with violent, disorganized, incoordinated motor activity, appear to be an expression of the inner feelings of the patient to a stress or recollection, suggesting an underlying anger. These are acting-out flashbacks.

Avoidance-distractive reaction

Abreactive flashbacks may represent recall of a previous traumatic event and a retreat to a type of protective behavior in an attempt to render the person less vulnerable, i.e. more distasteful to the attacker. The latter episodes are episodes of unreactivity, with thrashing, gasping, pelvic thrusting, gagging, or vomiting.

Considerations

Suspect episodes may be truly epileptic events, perhaps triggered by emotions, or they may be non-epileptic events. Non-epileptic events may be physiologic reactions or emotional (psychologic) reactions misinterpreted as epileptic. Individuals may present with a mixture of epileptic and non-epileptic episodes. In addition, a child's episodes may be created by others, such as in Munchausen's syndrome by proxy (Gates *et al.*, 1991; Besag, 1999; Ritter & Kotagai, 2000). Given abnormal behaviors that might be epileptic, one must first try to determine whether this is an epileptic or a non-epileptic event. If non-epileptic, is it a physiologic or a psychologic reaction?

Psychogenic and self-stimulated seizures

Spells that seem to be brought on by strong emotions can be divided into pseudoseizures and psychogenic, true seizures. Rarely, seizures can be brought on by focused thinking involving cortical systems or by strong emotions involving the limbic system. Anxiety may produce hyperventilation, which in turn can activate absence attacks. The reverse may be seen in which the aura of a complex partial seizure may lead to anxiety-produced hyperventilation.

Physiologic events

Seizure mimics should be considered in three aspects: the seizures they resemble, the child's age, and the type of physiologic episodes that mimic seizures.

Seizure-like episodes

Non-epileptic events are widely variable and often are bizarre. During the attack, non-epileptic events may not show much change, and the child may appear normal. Drug levels are unrelated to or even elevated with non-epileptic events. Non-epileptic events are often atypical, occur only with an audience and only in the wake state, are inducible, are time-limited, and are sometimes able to be terminated. Prolonged events lasting five to 14 minutes plus, and that are not benefited by anticonvulsant medication, are suspect. The events provide secondary gain. During the episode the patient may be unresponsive, but afterwards they can recall what was occurring during the event if they are willing to do so. Findings of histrionic characteristics and transient neurological soft findings are suggestive but must be verified.

Generalized motor-like events

Generalized tonic–clonic attacks with jerk–relax movements are stereotypic, without recall for the event. With non-epileptic spells that mimic tonic–clonic seizures, the tonic phase occurs infrequently, incontinence is rare, and the movement is more a to-and-fro effort. Recall may be present and sometimes can be elicited in children (Williamson & Spencer, 1986).

Stares

Staring spells may be daydreaming or an escape from boring or stressful tasks. An EEG is necessary to diffrentiate between absence and non-epileptic event stares. A regular EEG in the fasting drowsy state, with five minutes of hyperventilation, preferably performed twice during the recording, is worth four hours of video-EEG monitoring. With simple or partial complex epileptic stare, video-EEG monitoring may not always show epileptiform features. Spells lasting minutes to hours with varying manifestations are suspect. Even in proven absence seizures, 20% of patients may be found to also have non-epileptic events.

Confusion with automatisms

Episodes thought to be complex partial seizures may include episodic behavior disorders, sleep disturbances, migraines, or a variety of metabolic impairments that impair consciousness. The circumstances of the event are important. There may be violent behavior, but, especially if directed, this is rarely epileptic.

Atypical events

Epilepsy and non-epileptic events may occur together. The episodes may fail to conform to a physiologic patterns. Fixed, dilated pupils unreactive to light suggest epilepsy. Non-epileptic seizures tend to manifest as characteristic movements and bizarre behaviors. Crying and shouting are often seen. Dyssynergy between sides, to and fro movements, and pelvic thrusting usually indicate non-epileptic events, although frontal lobe seizures may also show this. Self-injury, incontinence, and postictal confusion or somnolence are unusual (Mostofsky & Williams, 1982; Williamson & Spencer, 1986).

Age of the child

Duchowny (1995) emphasized that in children with suspicious spells, the physician must consider a wide range of symptoms and the anxieties of the parents. Rather than psychogenic seizures, infants experience events that look like seizures, which often terrify the parents. In young children, non-epileptic seizures are more apt to be physiologic events. Impaired children may exhibit paroxysmal non-epileptic events (30–60%), which may be misdiagnosed and treated as epilepsy. Some children have both epileptic and non-epileptic events. Startles, head drops, brief jerks, and repetitive self-stimulatory or stereotyped behaviors are the most common behaviors misdiagnosed as epileptic (Ritter & Kotagai, 2000). Children with ADD who fail to stay on task may be misdiagnosed as having absence epilepsy (North *et al.*, 1990). Older children and adolescents may present with a wide assortment of behaviors, ranging from motionless stares and swoons to convulsive activity (Weisbrot & Ettinger, 1998).

Physiologic mimics

Cardiac and circulatory episodes, gastrointestinal attacks, metabolic disorders, non-epileptic neurologic episodes such as movement disorders, and sleep disorders may all be mistaken for seizures.

Psychodynamics

Epilepsy places a child at substantial risk for social and school problems compared with siblings and peers, often leading to the development of a variety of emotional and behavioral disorders as well as pseudoseizures. Non-epileptic events reduce conflict anxiety by keeping the conflict out of awareness while still allowing it to be expressed symbolically. Secondary gains may be evidenced, such as avoiding noxious activities or getting support from the environment (Mostofsky & Williams, 1982).

Caplan (1995) emphasized that non-epileptic events of an emotional origin in children differ from those seen in adults. Pediatric pseudoseizures are a cry for help with emotional difficulties. These pseudoseizures are then reinforced by increased attention. Without appropriate intervention, the child's emotional difficulties go unsolved and a crippling viscous cycle ensues, fostering marked maladaptive behaviors. Children with non-epileptic seizures often have problems expressing negative feelings of anger, resentment, shame, or embarrassment. Such expressions are not heard or heeded. The child feels powerless, channeling the increased tension into body functions. The child is very passive to the point of being apathetic about the seizures, referring all questions about the seizures to the parents.

The family

Children may seek the avenue of regression at times of stress. Developing children normally struggle with issues of separation and individualization from their parents. The presence of seizures may foster a tendency towards regression in this emotional maturation. Caplan (1995) observed that parents tend to tread a fine line between overprotectiveness and overnormalization (neglect). Some parents pay more attention to children when the seizures are not controlled. Other parents, expecting a given level of academic and social functioning from the child, may become inappropriately punitive and harsh in insisting that this level be maintained. In children who have learning disabilities, parents may not recognize or may deny that the child has the problem (Mostofsky & Williams, 1982).

The diagnosis depends on observing the fine interplay between the child and the parents regarding the child's personality characteristics and poor problem-solving techniques, parental problems, child and parental responses to epilepsy, secondary gain or emotional advantages derived from the non-epileptic events, and the exclusion of the possibility of abuse. Relationships between the child's difficulties and the parents' responses are important. Parental psychopathology affects the parental coping with the child's epileptic seizures. Problems include the presence or absence of abusive behavior, marital discord, parental control, and the promotion of seizure-related secondary gain to get attention. The interaction between the child's problems and the parental response, such as with learning difficulties and social difficulties, as well as the child's responses to parental separation/divorce and the possibility of sexual abuse may provide clues (Mostofsky & Williams, 1982).

Diagnosis

Unclassifiable epilepsy tends to be non-epileptic (Oostrom *et al.*, 2001). When children with suspected seizures are video monitored, 23.6% are found to have non-epileptic events, which may be recorded in 20%. Of those experiencing non-epileptic events, 20.8% also have epilepsy (Ritter & Kotagai, 2000).

The diagnosis of non-epileptic seizures is often within one year of the onset in children (79%), but in adults there is often a delay of three to four years before the attacks are identified properly as non-epileptic events (Alper *et al.*, 1993; Alper *et al.*, 1995; Wyllie *et al.*, 1984). Delayed diagnosis may lead to unwarranted exposure to antiepileptic drugs and their risks, interfering with daily activities, creating school absences, and labeling the child as "sick" (Lancman *et al.*, 1994). Daily to weekly episodes may occur (84%). About 63% are on anticonvulsants. Often, the child presents with recent onset and a high frequency of seizures before the diagnosis, sometimes with a dramatic increase before admission (Williams & Grant, 2000). A videotape of the event, if available, may be revealing.

Non-epileptic seizures should be considered in all children with refractory epilepsy, especially if the seizures are frequent, are atypical, show no response to appropriate medications, or are not correlated closely with definitely abnormal EEG findings. Supporting clues include a history of family dysfunction, academic problems, and the possibility of secondary gain. The medications in some cases increase the frequency of non-epileptic seizures (Ritter & Kotagai, 2000). A family history of similar episodes or related disorders is very helpful.

Clinical phenomena commonly used to differentiate non-epileptic seizures from true seizures include tongue biting, self-injury, and incontinence (Gates *et al.*, 1991; Weisbrot & Ettinger, 1998). Movements commonly considered to be functional, such as pelvic thrusting, unusual vocalizations, thrashing movements, and the absence of a postictal confusional state, may occur in epileptic seizures, particularly those of frontal lobe origin (Leis *et al.*, 1992; Saygi *et al.*, 1992; Weisbrot & Ettinger, 1998). Patients may embellish upon poorly identified genuine epileptic syndromes (Weisbrot & Ettinger, 1998).

The three most commonly used means of identification are electrophysiological testing, determination of serum Prolactin levels, and neuropsychological assessment (Brunquell, 1995).

Electroencephalography

The diagnosis is clinical. EEG recordings can be misleading, since a normal EEG does not exclude epilepsy and epileptiform activity does not exclude the diagnosis. An abnormal EEG is not always diagnostic of epilepsy and may be misleading, resulting in unnecessary medication and its associated toxicity. The interictal EEG is normal in some patients with true seizures and abnormal in patients with coexistent seizures. Interictal abnormalities or epileptiform abnormalities neither confirm nor exclude non-epileptic seizures (Weisbrot & Ettinger, 1998). Epileptiform discharges (spikes, spike waves) occur in 2.2–5.0% of routine EEGs in healthy children who do not have epilepsy (Ziven & Ajmone-Marsan, 1968; Ritter & Kotagai, 2000). Between 16% and 46% of children with benign Rolandic spikes do not manifest clinical seizures (Smith & Kellaway, 1964; Beaussart, 1972). The diagnosis can be suspected but not proven by the absence of changes on the ictal EEG. The reliance on clinical presentation is thus necessary for accurate diagnosis.

Video-EEG monitoring

Withdrawal of medications for video-EEG monitoring studies usually worsens epilepsy but may improve pseudoseizures (Williamson & Spencer, 1986). Video monitoring with the identified stressors being utilized during the testing is the only way to make the diagnosis. About 29% of patients can describe what they must do to make a seizure occur. This includes tension (65%), depression (65%), anger (50%), excitement (40%), fatigue (48%), and boredom (33%). Children are often able to predict seizures, and some (17%) can evoke seizures on request. Stress seizures are often related to the home (four-fold), school (nearly two-fold), or miscellaneous transient stresses (two-fold), compared with the normal reported incidence of such stresses in children. About 18–25% of patients can induce seizures.

Video-EEG monitoring can accurately determine the diagnosis in 90% of patients if the event in question is recorded. Identifying videotaped seizures without the accompanying EEG show that only 71–73% of episodes can be identified correctly as either epileptic or non-epileptic. Ictal events, seen in 55% of patients, are suggested by rhythmic slowing, suppression of activity, and electrodecremental responses. In a study of patients with frequent attacks, i.e. more than ten a day, when monitored for two to three days, 55% had no events, 34% had motor behaviors, 14% had staring, and 18% had true seizures. Failed EEG monitoring is suggestive but not conclusive of a non-epileptic event (Wyllie *et al.*, 1991; Alper *et al.*, 1993; Alper *et al.*, 1995; Weisbrot & Ettinger, 1998). In some situations, an obvious stressor may provoke non-epileptic seizures, but this may not be readily apparent. With non-epileptic seizures, the EEG during the seizure is normal, with no postictal slowing (Mostofsky & Williams, 1982).

Less severe partial epileptic seizures, especially those that are not associated with altered awareness, may be too focal or too deep to have an obvious correlate on scalp-recorded EEGs. Muscle artifacts, caused by clinical motor activity associated with generalized convulsive seizures or some frontal seizures, may obscure EEG activity (Leis *et al.*, 1992; Weisbrot & Ettinger, 1998). Ictal EEGs are abnormal in only 11% of scalp recordings with simple partial seizures (Brunquell, 1995).

Sometimes, induction of seizure-like episodes may be necessitated. Verbal encouragement is often helpful in bringing on an attack. Ancillary diagnostic maneuvers include suggestion (show us how you do it), reward, saline injection, and peri-ictal prolactin to differentiate between generalized seizures and non-seizures.

Provocatory testing

Provocatory testing sensitivity is high. The diagnosis depends on provoking objective responses, not subjective feelings. The rate of correct classification is at least 93% (Cohen & Suter, 1982). Use of intravenous saline placebo "spell-induction" may be helpful but does not conclusively distinguish epileptic seizures from non-epileptic seizures (Wyllie *et al.*, 1984).

Prolactin testing

Prolactin testing shows documented elevations of the hormone following a seizure involving the limbic system, peaking within 15–20 minutes and returning to baseline about one hour postictally. The expected rise may be inhibited by prolactin feedback, which may be depleted by repeated, prolonged, or status seizures. Prolactin rises significantly following generalized tonic–clonic seizures, partial seizures with secondary generalization, and complex partial seizures associated with automatisms or posturing. Prolactin does not rise with absence, myoclonic, or akinetic seizures, most simple partial seizures, or complex partial seizures without motor involvement (Laxer *et al.*, 1985; Wyllie *et al.*, 1984). Prolactin determinations are best used as a cue rather than a replacement for provocatory monitoring (Brunquell, 1995).

Other diagnostic approaches

Duchowny (1995) noted that neuroimaging and other laboratory studies are rarely helpful. Concurrent electrocardiogram monitoring may be useful in cardiac arrhythmias. Neuropsychometric testing has a limited role in establishing the diagnosis of non-epileptic seizures, as it assists in the delineation of comorbid disorders, such as depression, ADD, and learning disabilities, that may require individual treatment (Brunquell, 1995).

The final diagnosis depends on recording typical spells that are not accompanied by any significant EEG changes but that may be associated with other demonstrable causes (if physiologic) or related to specific psychologic findings. A non-recording of any spell does not make any diagnosis except that a spell was not recorded. The final impression is a clinical judgment.

Underlying psychiatric problems

Non-epileptic seizures are outward signs of an underling psychiatric problem. To diagnose the episodes as non-epileptic is an obligation to pursue the underlying problem so that appropriate help can be provided.

Adolescents may be found to have undifferentiated somatoform disorders, somatization disorders, malingering, panic disorders, hypochondriasis, depersonalization, psychotic disorders, associated disorders not otherwise specified, or posttraumatic stress. Before age 12, these psychogenic etiologies, with the exception of reinforced behavior patterns and Munchausen's syndrome by proxy, are rare (Ritter & Kotagai, 2000).

Anxiety and affect disorders

Affective and anxiety disorders are common. Depression occurs commonly (73%). Anxiety disorders include acute stress disorders, post-traumatic stress disorders, and panic disorders. A significant number of children have a non-supportive family environment, often with severe family psychopathology, such as a recent divorce or separation. About 6% of children with non-epileptic seizures have been sexually abused. In studies acute stressful situations precipitated all episodes of non-epileptic seizures (Leonard & George, 1999; Pakalnis et al., 1999).

Panic reactions may present, with worry about further attacks and their significance. Trembling, cardiac irregularities, dyspnea, dizziness, depersonalization, paresthesias, and fears of dying often accompany these attacks (Gates et al., 1991). Mahowald (1995) noted that nocturnal panic events might present with bad dreams (54%) and intrusive thoughts and images when trying to sleep, especially with a post-traumatic stress disorder.

Phobic anxiety reactions may show clear presenting symptoms at the onset that may be protracted and disabling. Often, this follows a traumatic event such as bereavement. The seizures emerge abruptly. Depersonalization is common, often presenting with fear and drowsiness. There is no aphasia or clear evidence of a clouded consciousness. Memory distortions are frequent. The attacks tend to increase in frequency and to terminate gradually. Often, there are other unrelated neurologic traits (Trimble, 1981; Riley & Roy, 1982; Gross, 1983; Gumnit & Gates, 1986).

Attention-seeking behavior

Behaviors thought to be epilepsy may arise as symptoms of secondary gain. There is a model for the symptom. The children do not seem concerned about the symptom. The symptoms do not occur with sufficient regularity to suggest a conversion disorder. Such children are most often multiply handicapped (Hempel, 2000). The children may learn subconsciously to produce seizure-like episodes that result in secondary gain from the environment. These are learned behaviors, often paradoxically reinforced by the parents or others. A simple, direct behavior-modification program is the most reasonable approach to this disorder (Ritter & Kotagai, 2000).

Conversion reactions

Conversion seizures are the most common form of psychogenic non-epileptic seizures seen in children and adolescents (Mostofsky & Williams, 1982). The children are unaware of the intentional nature of the symptoms and of the reasons for producing them. The underlying sources of conflict may be varied, including separation anxiety, parental conflicts, learning disabilities, other causes of poor academic performance, unresolved grief, and poor peer relationships (Renken, 1987). A history of sexual abuse is found (Betts & Boden, 1992) at least three times more often in children with non-epileptic seizures than in children without seizures (Brunquell, 1995). Non-epileptic seizures, utilizing the defense mechanisms of repression and dissociation (Bowman, 1993), may represent expressions of hidden negative feelings or conflicts (Weisbrot & Ettinger, 1998).

Dissociative disorders

Dissociative disorders include fugue states and depersonalization. In a dissociative disorder, there is a disruption of the usual integrated functions of consciousness, memory, identity, and perception of the environment. Fugue states are an amnesic-like departure from one's usual activities, during which new behaviors emerge. After the episode, the person can remember events before but not during the fugue. This is a feeling of detachment from one's self (Gates et al., 1991). Mahowald (1995) observed that bizarre, potentially injurious psychogenic dissociative symptoms might arise prominently or exclusively in the sleep period but at times when the patient is shown to be awake by polysomnography.

Intermittent explosive disorder

Rage reactions may be misdiagnosed as seizures because they occur more often in individuals with complex partial seizures. Characteristically, there are discrete episodes of loss of control of aggressive impulses, resulting in serious assault or destruction of property. The behavior is grossly out of proportion to any precipitating psychosocial stressors. There is an absence of signs of generalized impulsivity or aggressiveness between episodes. This disorder is encountered most commonly in children and adolescents who have organic brain dysfunction, including epilepsy. Conduct disorders in children and adolescents are often found. Rage reactions may be specifically responsive to pharmacologic intervention (Mostofsky & Williams, 1982).

Intentionally produced or feigned seizures

Malingering, factitious disorders, and Munchausen's syndrome are intentionally produced symptoms motivated by external incentives, such as avoidance of responsibilities (Alper *et al.*, 1995; Mills & Lipian, 1997; Weisbrot & Ettinger, 1998). Factitious disorders are more common in parents who induce genuine seizures in their children (Munchausen's syndrome by proxy), such as by smothering or by giving medication. They are rarely a cause of non-epileptic seizures in children (Weisbrot & Ettinger, 1998).

Malingering

In malingering, there is the intentional production of symptoms, the patient being motivated by secondary gain, such as avoiding responsibility, obtaining compensation, or attempting mitigating circumstances (Gates *et al.*, 1991). Seizures are feigned consciously and voluntarily in pursuit of a goal that, when known, is obviously recognizable with an understanding of the individual's circumstances. Such goals include avoiding schoolwork or military services, obtaining financial compensation, evading criminal persecution, and obtaining drugs (Mostofsky & Williams, 1982).

Factitious seizures

In factitious disorders, the patient produces a plausible and dramatic history of symptoms to play the sick role and seek hospitalization (Gates *et al.*, 1991). This has been called Munchausen's syndrome. Some patients present with non-epileptic seizures characterized by physical or psychological symptoms produced by the patient and under the patient's voluntary control. This is a diagnosis of exclusion. A factitious disorder may coexist with a neurologic disorder. When in doubt, it is usually best to give the patient the benefit of the doubt and interpret to the child and family the plausibility of an unconscious mechanism. This may be a face-saving mechanism allowing the establishment of a therapeutic alliance. If this does not work, a more confrontational stance may be justified (Mostofsky & Williams, 1982).

Munchausen's syndrome

In Munchausen's syndrome by proxy, the adult is the perpetrator; the child only experiences the problem. This is a form of child abuse in which the parent fabricates the symptoms or causes an illness in the child, leading to extensive and unnecessary medical evaluation. This can be very hard to detect and is probably underreported. It may be fatal. The parent, usually the mother, is the historian, giving a story of the child having experienced a life-threatening illness. The story most commonly involves symptoms including bleeding, seizures, reduced consciousness, apnea, diarrhea, vomiting, fever, and rash. Fictitious epilepsy may be seen in a medical setting, in which a caregiver deliberately creates the impression of a non-epileptic child experiencing seizures (Bye & Nunan, 1992). Signs of Munchausen's syndrome or fictitious epilepsy include frequent seizures that disappear in the parent's absence, aberrant historical features, such as generalized tonic–clonic attacks followed by immediate return of normal behavior, other siblings with unexplained brain damage or sudden infant death syndrome, and a lack of appropriate concern (Dreifuss & Gates, 2000).

The diagnostic clues are of a recurrent, unexplained or persistent illness in which symptoms or signs do not correspond and the child is said to have an uncommon disorder. If not diagnosed, the death rate may be as high as 10% in patients and in their siblings. Further history suggests that up to 10% of the mothers themselves had Munchausen's syndrome and may have experienced child abuse. Family dysfunction such as separation or divorce, parental absence, or parental neglect are common, and there is an increased occurrence in military families. The child is repeatedly reported to have spells or episodes of some type despite the most excellent care by various centers. Often, the mother saves the child during such a spell, for example if the child has recurrent seizures. The child may seem postictal at times, but no neurologic or medical abnormalities are found. If sent home, the child may be brought back with recurrences until finally the child is hospitalized or placed on antiepileptic drugs based on the history, only for the child to experience further spells despite medication. There is often a history of going from doctor to doctor to doctor (Dreifuss & Gates, 2000).

The mother, often having had nursing training (25%), presents as being extremely attentive to her child and often joins in care as if part of the healthcare team. The mother may be seen to produce apnea spells by placing a pillow over the child's face or to induce coma by giving intravenous injections of barbiturates. There may be an excess of unexplained deaths in the child's siblings. Such children do well if separated from their mothers. Seizures occur only when the mother is with the child in the epilepsy unit and tend to occur under bizarre circumstances, often being reported by the mother just after the monitoring electrodes have been removed (Dreifuss & Gates, 2000).

The diagnosis is difficult. Video monitoring may be useful and occasionally may catch the mother in the act. The management of the problem is equally difficult. There must be proof, as a confrontation must be avoided so that the mother does not sign the child out of the hospital and flee. The mother is a risk for suicide so a member of the team should remain with her. The parent must receive psychotherapy, and the child (and siblings) must be placed in protective fostering. Eventually, the child is usually returned to the family (Dreifuss & Gates, 2000).

Svengauli syndrome

Svengauli syndrome is a variant of Munchausen's syndrome in which a member of the opposite sex influences the patient to experience a variety of symptoms that cannot be verified by any tests. The symptoms may not be bothersome to the patient. The patient is often relatively passive and easily manipulated, often with a domineering spouse who may have a healthcare professional background. One individual influences and the other experiences through compliance in this essentially adult syndrome (Dreifuss & Gates, 2000).

The therapy approach to non-epileptic events is to encourage the young person to control the attacks without confronting them with the diagnosis. Counseling is important. Munchausen's syndrome by proxy is managed by working with the parents to address the underlying problems in their relationships with the child. Adolescents and preadolescents may respond to simple confrontation. The management of the pseudoseizures depends on both the classification of the attacks and the context in which they occur. A high success rate can be achieved by using a rational management approach (Besag, 1999).

Psychoses

Another subgroup is the child with psychoses (Brunquell, 1995). The peculiar behaviors seen in such children may be misdiagnosed as a complex partial seizure, especially if the EEG is misinterpreted. Physicians must remember that the presence of an abnormal EEG is more frequent in children and needs to be correlated with the symptoms.

Somatoform disorder

Somatoform disorders include the presence of physical symptoms that are suggestive but not the result of a medical condition but rather are the direct effects of substance abuse or other mental disorders, including panic disorders. About one-quarter of patients with a conversion presentation have evidence of general medical causes (Gates et al., 1991). There are no organic findings to explain the symptoms, and evidence may emerge to suggest a linkage to psychologic factors. A somatoform disorder may coexist with a true neurologic disorder. Unlike a factitious disorder, the problem is not under voluntary control. The patient is not aware of any purposeful production of symptoms nor intentional law of normal function (Mostofsky & Williams, 1982).

Somatization disorder (Briquet's syndrome)

This is a chronic fluctuating disorder that often begins during childhood or adolescence. It is characterized by recurrent and multiple somatic complaints for which medical attention is sought. No physical illness is found. Anxiety and depressive features are common. Later, alcohol and substance abuse and antisocial behaviors are often found. This is most common in adolescent and young adult women. It may include the presence of conversion seizures. The personality is often described as histrionic (Mostofsky & Williams, 1982).

Therapy

Studies of people with non-epileptic events reveal that 60% have been misdiagnosed as epileptic and 69% have been treated unsuccessfully with antiepileptic medications.

Disclosure

Therapy begins with the presentation of the diagnosis to the family after reviewing the recorded events to be sure these are typical. The family need to realize that these events are not epileptic seizures but rather are a stress reaction type of seizure. Possible triggers need to be determined. The family needs to be convinced that the spells can be controlled by behavioral approaches and that these are available. Thus, the future looks better and the patient and their family can learn to overcome the spells and realize need to that they do not live with the anxieties of dealing with epilepsy. It is important to use the term "non-epileptic seizures" and the family must be made to realize that they are not to blame. Treatment should be initiated as soon as possible (Ho *et al.*, 2000; Kanner *et al.*, 2001).

If the family accepts the possibility of a psychologic process, they should be encouraged to elaborate on their reasons. If the family adamantly refutes the possibility of a psychologic cause, then a neuropsychologic and neuropsychiatric evaluation is suggested to rule out that possibility. If the parents are adamant about certainty of an organic or epileptic process triggering the spells, and the evaluation has erred in the evaluation, then the diagnostic process is reviewed with the patient and family (Kanner *et al.*, 2001). The family may seek second opinions, which may be facilitated, but continued searching should be discouraged.

Therapeutic approaches

The commonest diagnoses are oppositional-defiant disorder, impulse-control disorder, psychoses, anxiety, and depression. Other problems include somatoform problems, reinforced behaviors, dissociative disorders, and purposeful behaviors of malingering or factitious diseases (Mostofsky & Williams, 1982; Hempel, 2000). A majority (74%) are followed up with out-patient mental health care, but some

(12%) patients require in-patient care. At discharge, anticonvulsants may be reduced in 17% of patients; psychotropic medication may be added in 17% (Williams &
Grant, 2000).

The diagnosis is challenging. A psychological assessment can be perceived as invasive and threatening, especially to patients and families who have limited awareness
of psychological issues. The families will need psychological support. A holistic
approach addressing family, peers, and school is important. At each stage of the
program, resistance should be anticipated in both the child and their family (Ho
et al., 2000).

Cause-related therapy

A variety of emotional disorders may be found, or may be envisioned as developing,
in children, especially adolescents, who present with non-epileptic events. Often,
there is a history of a dysfunctional family, so the therapy must include the family as
well as the child. Frequently, school struggles and failures are found, thus academic
help may be needed (Mostofsky & Williams, 1982; Hempel, 2000). Reinforced
behavior patterns may be seen (Gates *et al.*, 1991).

Escape efforts

Some patients find that seizures help them to avoid unpleasant situations or gain
extra attention and benefits, so they augment this by imitating seizures that they
have seen or experienced. The seizures become an advantage rather than a liability.
This can be of conscious or subconscious origin. The precipitant and results must
be identified, and the patient and family must want to change. They need to learn
acceptable alternatives to handling the precipitants (Trimble, 1981; Riley & Roy,
1982; Gross, 1983; Gumnit & Gates, 1986).

Anxiety-induced episodes

Children often have a milder form of anxiety as a trigger, for which therapy may be
most effective (Duchowny, 1995). Younger age of onset of pseudoseizures confers
a better prognosis (Guberman, 1982). Teaching the child alternative ways to express negative feelings and reducing attention to the episodes and their associated
secondary gain are recommended treatment strategies (Caplan & Gillberg, 1997;
Weisbrot & Ettinger, 1998). The major challenge is the family and any functional
problems that exist; thus, effective family therapy is of great importance. It may be
that the child is the symptom and the family is the problem.

School struggles

Children, especially teenagers, may develop non-epileptic seizures due to their
need to escape from difficult situations related to learning struggles, often unrecognized and therefore untreated. Such pseudoseizures symbolize the child's feelings

of helplessness and damage, providing an acceptable outlook for their frustration and anger, for which they cannot be held accountable. Such children need help not only for the learning problems but also in improving coping skills (Silver, 1983).

Psychologic intervention

Psychologic intervention begins by identifying issues and means to relieve anxiety. More appropriate expression of emotions needs to be developed to help the child and parents cope better with stress and change. Children need to learn to express their feelings. They do not understand direct confrontations or interpretations. The symptoms must be placed in the family context. Children with affect problems tend to ignore emotions and thus need to become aware of appropriate emotional expression. Children with behavior problems need to focus on the precipitating symptoms and develop more appropriate methods to relieve the symptoms (Ho *et al.*, 2000).

Cognitive approaches initially strive to help the child recall factors in a safe environment to help them recover from painful experiences. The child needs to learn the association between the stresses and the physical symptoms. The child then needs to learn better ways to express negative feelings. Attention to the episodes and secondary gains should be reduced (Caplan & Gillberg, 1997).

Task-oriented psychotherapy can be useful, but for children who obtain strong secondary gain, are poorly motivated, or are of low intelligence, behavior modification measures may be preferable (Ramani, 1993). Conditioning techniques, including denial of reward, a penalty program, a relief-avoidance program, a punishment program, an overt or covert reward program, habituations, or extinction, can be effective. Psychodynamic approaches include a psychoanalytically oriented program, identifying emotional triggers, and learning how to deal with them; this often requires a fairly sophisticated family and child. Desensitization may be effective in some situations (Mostofsky & Williams, 1982).

Relaxation techniques and biofeedback may be useful for children with underlying anxiety. Graded exposure may be necessary for patients grounded in phobia. Strategic family therapy is often necessary when the non-epileptic events are the consequence of interfamilial conflict. Psychiatric illnesses such as anxiety disorders, depression, and psychosis should be formally addressed (Brunquell, 1995).

Home and school general approaches

Suggested behavioral intervention for children with non-epileptic seizures begins with affirming the disability and normalizing the role of the environment, regardless of the etiology. This includes addressing the role of the environment and endorsing behavioral recommendations. The child is taught appropriate coping strategies.

Suggesting that the attacks are not real has been found to be counterproductive. Coping behaviors may include relaxation and pleasant imagery. The child should be taught more appropriate responses in situations that would normally provoke seizures. The parents need to be helped to see that the approaches are meant to directly treat the seizure activity (Kuhn *et al.*, 1995).

Immediate caregivers need guidelines to encourage independent functioning. This ensures against secondary gain from the seizure activity and encourages the child to use their newly developed anticonvulsant coping behaviors. As the child develops the skills, the parents need to decrease their efforts to manage the seizures. This means eliminating discussions at home about seizures and reinforcing main-tenance of normal daily activities, such as daily school attendance and completing homework assignments. When the child warns by of a seizure coming on, the par-ents respond, "You know what to do." Teachers and other supervising adults need to respond in a similar manner. Teachers and other pertinent school personnel need to review and coordinate approaches with the parents.

Family therapy

The dysfunctional family needs help to help the patient. The structure is a short-term problem often. The prognosis is dependent on prevention. The existence of marriage and family problems is common with children with non-epileptic seizures. Depression and low self-esteem are found frequently. The family functioning is important in diagnosis and in therapy. Marital partnerships and extended family must often be considered. Childhood non-epileptic seizures need a family or friend model. Often, the seizure begins after an accident.

Psychopharmacology

Specific psychopharmacologic drugs along with psychotherapy, may be used tem-porarily for specific types of non-epileptic seizure causes. Neuroleptics lower the seizure threshold, so it is wise to begin at low dosage and make increases slowly, as needed. In younger children, some drugs paradoxically exacerbate some conditions, such as depression (Mostofsky & Williams, 1982).

Prognosis

The prognosis of non-epileptic seizures in children and adolescents is better than in adults, especially if the symptoms are detected early and the duration of the disorder is short (Wyllie *et al.*, 1991). Adolescents may accept and cope with the diagnosis. Some seek calmly to learn how to handle the stressor and keep up in school. They often find it helpful when parents are present during and immediately after the episode. They need to have the episode explained by the physician and know that the symptoms are being taken seriously. Explanations connecting the stressors and symptoms decrease their anxieties (Lach & Peltz, 2000).

Parents experience both positive and negative emotions. They may experience shame because they feel they cannot discuss the diagnosis with friends and family members who may not understand. Parents need to talk about their own anxiety about the child's episodes and to be helped to handle future episodes (Lach & Peltz, 2000).

Outcome

Generally, the prognosis is more favorable in children, with 78% of children becoming asymptomatic compared with 40–50% of adults. Children are to epilepsy centers much earlier than adults. By three years post-diagnosis, 81% of children are symptom-free, compared with 40% of adults (Brunquell, 1995).

Predictors of favorable outcome include female gender, achieving an independent lifestyle, receiving formal psychotherapy, and the absence of coexisting epilepsy (Lancman *et al.*, 1994). The prognosis is worse in people with pre-existing psychiatric difficulties (Bowman, 1993). Non-epileptic event patients with personality disorders are difficult to manage, less compliant with follow-up, and experience poor outcomes (Drake *et al.*, 1992).

REFERENCES

Alper, K., Devinsky, O., Perrine, K., *et al.* (1993). Nonepileptic seizures and childhood sexual and physical abuse. *Neurology* **43**: 1950–53.

Alper, K., Devinksy, O., Perrine, K., *et al.* (1995). Psychiatric classification of non-conversion nonepileptic seizures. *Arch. Neurol.* **562**: 199–201.

Beaussart, M. (1972). Benign epilepsy of childhood with Rolandic (centrotemporal) paroxysmal foci. A clinical entity: study of 221 cases. *Epilespia* **13**: 795–811.

Besag, F. M. (1999). Classification and management of pseudoseizures in children. *Epilespia* **40** (suppl 7): 59.

Betts, T. & Boden S. (1992). Diagnosis, management and prognosis of a group of 128 patients with nonepileptic attack disorder. Part II: previous childhood sexual abuse in the etiology of these disorders. *Seizure* **1**: 27–32.

Bowman, E. S. (1993). Etiology and clinical course of pseudoseizures relationship to trauma, depression and dissociation. *Psychosomatics* **34**: 333–42.

Brunquell, P. J. (1995). Psychogenic seizures in children. *Int. Pediatr.* **10** (suppl): 47–54.

Caplan, R. (1995). Psychiatric aspects of psychogenic seizures in childhood. Presented at the American Epilepsy Society Conference, 1995.

Caplan, R. & Gillberg, C. (1997). Child psychiatric disorders. In *Epilepsy: A Comprehensive Textbook*, ed. J. Engle & T. A. Pedley, pp. 2125–39. Philadelphia: Lippincott-Raven.

Caplan, R., Arbelle, S., Guthrie, D., *et al.* (1997). Formal thought disorder and psychopathology ion pediatric primary generalized and complex partial epilepsy. *J. Am. Acad. Child Adolesc. Psychiatry* **36**: 1286–94.

Carmant, L., Kramer, U., Riviello, J., Jr, *et al.* (1993). Pseudoseizures presenting at the young age of six years in two children. *Epilespia* **34** (suppl 6): 99.

Cohen, R. J. & Suter, C. (1982). Hysterical seizures: suggestion as a provacative EEG test. *Ann. Neurol.* **11**: 391–5.

Drake, M. E., Pakalnis, A. & Phillips, B. B. (1992). Neuropsychological and psychiatric correlates of intractable pseudoseizures. *Seizures* **1**: 11–14.

Dreifuss, F. E. & Gates, J. R. (2000). Munchausen syndrome by proxy and Svengali syndrome. In *Non-Epileptic Seizures*, ed. J. R. Gates & A. J. Rowan, 2nd edn, pp. 237–44. Boston: Heinemann.

Dubowitz, V. & Hersov, L. (1976). Management of children with non-organic (hysterical) disorders of motor function. *Dev. Med. Child Neurol.* **18**: 358–68.

Duchowny, M. S. (1995). Psychogenic seizures in the pre-addescent child. Presented at the American Epilepsy Society Conference, 1995.

Gates, J. R., Luciano, D. & Devinsky, O. (1991). The classification and treatment of nonepileptic events In *Epilepsy and Behavior*, ed. O. Devinsky & W. Theodore, pp. 251–63. New York: Wiley-Liss.

Golden, N., Bennett, H. S., Pollack, M. A., *et al.* (1985). Seizures in adolescence: a review of patients admitted to an adolescent service. *J. Adolesc. Health Care* **6**: 25–7.

Goodwin, J., Simms, M. & Bvergman, R. (1979). Hysterical seizures: a sequel to incest. *Am. J. Orthopsychiatry* **49**: 698–703.

Goodyer, I. (1981). Hysterical conversion relations in childhood. *J. Child Psychol. Psychiatry* **22**: 179–88.

Gross, M. (1979). Incestuous rape: a cause for hysterical seizures in four adolescent girls. *Am. J. Orthopsychiatry* **49**: 704–8.

Gross, M. (1983). Hysterical seizures: a sequel of incest. In *Pseudoepilepsy*, ed. M. Gross, pp. 119–28. Lexington, MA: Lexington Books.

Guberman, A. (1982). Psychogenic pseudoseizures in non-epileptic patients. *Am. J. Psychiatry* **27**: 401–4.

Gumnit, R. J. & Gates, J. R. (1986). Psychogenic seizures. *Epilespia* **27** (suppl 2): 124–9.

Hempel, A. (2000). Cognitive features and predisposing factors in children with psychotogenic seizures. In *Non-Epileptic Seizures*, ed. J. R. Gates & A. J. Rowan, 2nd edn pp. 185–96. Boston, MA: Butterworth Heinemann.

Hersov, L. (1985). Emotional disorders. In *Children and Adolescent Psychiatry*, ed. M. Rutter & L. Hersov, pp. 373–5. London: Blackwell Scientific.

Hinman A. (1958) Conversion reactions in childhood. *J. Dis. Child* **95**: 420–45.

Ho, A. M. W., Ransby, M. J., Farrell, K., *et al.* (2000). Psychological assessment and treatment of non-epileptic seizures and related symptoms in children and adolescents: study. In *Non-Epileptic Seizures*, ed. J. R. Gates & A. J. Rowan, 2nd edn, pp. 207–36. Boston, MA: Butterworth Heinemann.

Holmes, G. L. Sackellares, J. C., McKiernan, J., *et al.* (1980). Evaluation of childhood seizures using EEG telemetry and video-tape monitoring. *J. Pediatr.* **97**: 554–8.

Kanner, A. M., Palac, S. M., Lancman, M. E., *et al.* (2001). Treatment of psychogenic pseudo-seizures: what to do after we have reached the diagnosis? In *Psychiatric Issues in Epilepsy*, ed. A. B. Ettinger & A. M. Kanner, pp. 379–90. Philadelphia: Lippincott Williams & Wilkins.

Kuhn, B. R., Allen, K. D. & Shriver, M. D. (1995). Behavioral management of children's seizure activity. *Clin. Pediatr.* **34**: 570–75.

Lach, L. M. & Peltz, L. (2000). Adolescents' and parents' perception of non-epileptic seizures: a retrospective and qualitative glance. In *Non-Epileptic Seizures*, ed. J. R. Gates & A. J. Rowan, 2nd edn, pp. 227–36. Boston, MA: Heinemann.

Lancman, M. E., Asconape, J. J., Graves, S., *et al.* (1994). Psychogenic seizures in children: long-term analysis of 43 cases. *J. Child Neurol.* **9**: 404–7.

Lancman, M. E., Lambrakis, C. C. & Steinhardt, M. J. (2002). Psychogenic pseudoseizures: a general overview. In *Psychiatric Issues in Epilepsy*, ed. A. B. Ettinger & M. Kanner, pp. 341–54. Philadelphia: Lippincott Williams & Wilkins.

Laxer, K. D., Mullooly, J. P. & Howell, B. (1985). Prolactin changes after seizures classified by EEG monitoring. *Neurology* **35**: 31–5.

Leis, A. A., Ross, M. A. & Summers, A. K. (1992). Psychogenic seizures: ictal characteristics and diagnostic pitfalls. *Neurology* **42**: 95–9.

Lelliott, P. T. & Fenwick, P. (1999). Cerebral pathology in pseudoseizures. *Acta Neurol. Scand.* **83**: 129–32.

Leonard, E. L. & George, R. M. (1999). Internalizing psychopathology relating to nonepileptic seizures in a hospitalized EEG monitored pediatric population. *Epilespia* **40** (suppl 7): 121.

Mahowald, M. W. (1995). Paroxysmal sleep disorders in childhood. Presented at the American Epilepsy Society Conference, 1995.

Malony, M. J. (1980). Diagnosing hysterical conversion reactions in children. *J. Pediatr.* **97**: 1016–20.

Mills, M. J. & Lipian, M. S. (1997). Malingering. In *Comprehensive Textbook of Psychiatry*, ed. H. I. Kaplan & B. J. Sadock, pp. 1614–22. Baltimore, MD: Williams & Wilkins.

Mostofsky, D. I. & Williams, D. T. (1982). Psychogenic seizures in childhood and adolescents. In *Pseudoseizures*, ed. T. L. Riley & A. Roy, pp. 169–84. Baltimore, MD: Williams & Wilkins.

North, K. N., Ouvrier, R. A. & Nugent, M. (1990). Pseudoseizures caused by hyperventilation resembling absence epilepsy. *J. Child Neurol.* **5**: 288–94.

Onuma, T. (2000). Classification of psychiatric symptoms in patients with epilepsy. Proceedings of 32nd Congress of Japan Epilepsy Society. *Epilespia* **41** (suppl 9): 43–8.

Oostrom, K. J., Schouten, A., Kruitwagen, C. J. J., *et al.* (2001). Parents' perception of adversity introduced by upheaval and uncertainty at the onset of childhood epilepsy. *Epilespia* **42**: 1142–6.

Pakalnis, A. O., Paolicicchi, J. M. & Gilles, E. E. (1999). Neuropsychiatric aspects of psychogenic status epilepticus in children. *Epilespia* **40** (suppl 7): 117.

Ramani, V. (1993). Review of psychiatric treatment strategies in nonepileptic seizures. In *Nonepileptic Seizures*, ed. A. J. Rowan & J. R. Gates, pp. 259–66. Boston, MA: Butterworth Heinemann.

Renken, B. (1987). Pseudoseizures in children and adolescents. In *The Somatizing Child*, ed. E. G. Shapiro & A. A. Rosenfeld, pp. 115–31. New York: Springer-Verlag.

Riley, R. L. & Roy, A. (1982). *Pseudoseizures*. Baltimore, MD: Williams & Wilkins.

Ritter, F. J. & Kotagai, P. (2000). Non-epileptic seizures in children. In *Non-Epileptic Seizures*, ed. J. R. Gates & A. J. Rowan, 2nd edn, pp. 95–112. Boston, MA: Butterworth Heinemann.

Robins, E. & O'Neal, P. (1953). Clinical features of hysteria in children. In *The Nervous Child*, pp. 246–71.

Saygi, S., Katz, A., Marks, D. A., *et al.* (1992). Frontal lobe partial seizures and psychogenic seizures: comparison of clinical and ictal charateristics. *Neurology* **42**: 1274–7.

Silver, L. B. (1982). Conversion disorder with pseudoseizures in adolescence: a stress reaction to unrecognized and untreated learning disabilities. *J. Am. Acad. Child Psychiatry* **21**: 508–12.

Silver, L. B. (1983). Conversion disorder in pseudoseizures in adolescence: a stress reaction in unrecognized and untreated learning disabilities. In *Pseudoepilepsy*, ed. M. Gross, pp. 109–18. Lexington, MA: Lexington Books.

Smith, J. M. B. & Kellaway, P. (1964). Central (Rolandic) foci in children: an analysis of 200 cases. *Electroencephalogr. Clin. Neurophysiol.* **17**: 460.

Trimble, M. R. (1981). Hysteria and other non-epileptic convulsions. In *Epilepsy and Psychiatry*, ed. E. H. Reynolds, & M. R. Trimble, pp. 92–112. New York: Churchill Livingstone.

Weisbrot, D. M. & Ettinger, A. B. (1998). Psychiatric aspects of Pediatric Epilepsy. *Primary Psychiatry* **June**: 51–67.

Williams, J. & Grant, M. L. (2000). Characteristics of pediatric non-epileptic seizure patients: retrospective study. In *Non-Epileptic Seizures*, ed. J. R. Gates & A. J. Rowan, 2nd edn, pp. 197–206. Boston, MA: Butterworth Heinemann.

Williamson, P. D. & Spencer, S. S. (1986). Clinical and EEG features of complex partial seizures of extratemporal origin. *Epilespia* **27** (suppl 20): 46–63.

Wyllie, E., Friedman, D., Luders, H., *et al.* (1991). Outcome of psychogenic seizures in children and adolescents compared with adults. *Neurology* **41**: 742–4.

Wyllie, E., Luders, H., MacMilllan, J., *et al.* (1984). Serum prolactin levels after epileptic seizures. *Neurology* **34**: 1601–4.

Ziven, L. & Ajmone-Marsan, C. (1968). Incidence and prognostic significance of "epileptiform" activity in the EEG of nonepileptic subjects. *Brain* **91**: 751–8.

38

Possible treatment issues

Any therapy, be it drug, surgery, or other approaches, can produce adverse effects in a minority as well as benefits in a majority of patients. The goal is to choose the right therapy for the individual in terms of benefit and tolerance.

Antiepileptic drugs

Antiepileptic medications can produce side effects alone or in combinations with other drugs. In monotherapy, the side effects of the drugs can be noted (Herranz *et al.*, 1988). Any antiepileptic drug may produce emotional problems, especially in young, elderly, and or brain-damaged patients. Milder forms of the behaviors are transient, fading after two to three weeks. More severe and persistent problems may be accentuations of previous tendencies brought out by the drug or may be a pre-existing problem that is later blamed on the drug. The rates of these effects are highly variable (Weisbrot & Ettinger, 1998).

Problems can range from inattention, hyperactivity, or depression to a major psychotic reaction, seen in 1% of patients. Psychiatric reactions are not simply idiosyncratic but depend on the drug's anticonvulsant strength and the patient's genetic and biological psychiatric predisposition. The principal three types of complications are toxic (3%), metabolic (3%), and allergic (1%) (Schmitz, 1999; Vaintrub, 1998). Brain-damaged and retarded children are more susceptible to the adverse behaviors of antiepileptic drugs (Schain, 1983).

The risks for reactions relate to the severity of the epilepsy, polytherapy, rapid drug titration, high dosage, forced normalization, drug withdrawal, and folate deficiency. Antiepileptic drugs may be deleterious to patients who already have behavioral problems (Holmes, 1987). Patients with previous psychiatric problems or a family predisposition are prone to behavioral side effects (Schmitz, 1999; Vaintrub, 1998). At higher levels of the older anticonvulsants, the tendency towards non-epileptic seizures is increased in patients who are functionally impaired and who are less able to cope with the challenges of life.

Folic acid deficiency

Vitamin B6 (pyridoxine) and folic acid have been implicated in cognitive and behavior complications of epilepsy. Both vitamins may be significantly depressed in individuals with mental changes. Depression of either or both vitamins may be seen without any symptoms in about a third of patients (Reynolds *et al.*, 1966).

Pyridoxine derivatives facilitate the conversion of glutamic acid to glutamate. An excess of glutamic acid or a deficiency of glutamate contributes to seizures. A pyridoxine deficiency is found more often in individuals with a multiple personality presentation. Mental disturbances occur twice as frequently with a pyridoxine deficiency as with a folate deficiency (Reynolds *et al.*, 1966).

Folate is associated with affect disorders and depression more than anxiety. A folic acid deficiency can produce a drop in intelligence, depression, psychoses, and a variety of behavior disorders in children and adults, adversely affecting alertness, motivation, mood, cognition, and sociability (Trimble *et al.*, 1980; Lambert & Robertson, 1999). Reduced folate levels are found with most antiepileptics, especially with polytherapy. It occurs commonly with liver-enzyme-inducing antiepileptics, such as phenobarbital, primidone, and phenytoin (Lambert & Robertson, 1999). Folate levels may be decreased in 11–15% of patients on anticonvulsants, and up to 50% of those on phenobarbital or phenytoin (Reynolds *et al.*, 1966).

Folic acid plays a role in mediating a variety of neurotransmitter metabolism pathways (Trimble *et al.*, 1980). Folate deficiency may increase the seizure tendency. A severe deficiency can precipitate epilepsy. Folates block GABA presynaptic inhibition (Reynolds *et al.*, 1966). Folates are important in methylation reactions (Vickery *et al.*, 1992) involved with neurotransmitters and monoamines implicated in the etiology of affective disorders (Lambert & Robertson, 1999). Affective disorders respond more to the correction of a folate deficiency than to correction of a pyridoxine deficiency. Schizophrenic and depressed non-epileptic patients who are deficient in folic acid show an improvement in both depression and schizophrenia with correction of the deficiency (Reynolds *et al.*, 1966).

Older antiepileptics

The older antiepileptics have been in use for decades and thus have gathered a long list of side effects, especially behavioral. The fears of a behavior reaction have tended to influence teachers and caregivers to look for such behaviors. The existence of such behaviors has been mostly subjective on diagnosis, made by biased observers, dividing the world of medicine into the deniers and the claimers. With these drugs, knowledge is largely empirical and anecdotal (Schmitz, 1999).

Long-term treatment of children with antiepileptic drugs in the therapeutic range leads to the appearance of side effects in 50%, necessitating treatment modification in 18% and withdrawal in 7%. Side effects are seen in 31% of children on antiepileptic drugs and in 17–22% on monotherapy. The order of occurrence of drugs producing side effects, from greatest to least, is phenytoin, phenobarbital, carbamazepine, valproate, and primidone. Intolerable side effects are related to high drug dosages, both transient and permanent (Herranz *et al.*, 1988).

Every antiepileptic drug has occasionally triggered adverse behavior effects. Every drug has produced psychotropic benefits in some patients, and certain antiepileptics are becoming as valuable for their benefits on behavior as on seizures. Carbamazepine and valproate are valuable in the treatment of psychiatric patients with affective disorders and in the management of episodic dyscontrol (Schmitz, 1999).

Barbiturates and primidone

The barbiturates show minor tranquilizing benefits but are not considered to be helpful for psychiatric conditions (Stores, 1975) and appear more apt to produce behavior problems. They are best avoided whenever possible in children of school age (Stores, 1976). Barbiturates may produce aggression, destructiveness (Stores, 1975), depression, and withdrawal symptoms. In children on barbiturates, ADHD behaviors (Brent *et al.*, 1987) and hyperactivity or agitation may be seen. Impulsive and distractable behavior may emerge, even when seizures are controlled (Thorn, 1975; Wolf & Forsythe, 1978), especially if a coexisting tendency is already present (Kinsbourne & Kaplan, 1979). Depression may occur in adolescents with a personal or family history of affect disorders, or on higher dosages or polytherapy (Brent *et al.*, 1987; Perrine & Congett, 1994; Robertson *et al.*, 1987; Schmitz, 1999). Suicidal ideations (47%) may emerge (Brent, 1986; Robertson *et al.*, 1987). Irritability (Camfield *et al.*, 1979; Ferrari *et al.*, 1983) and conduct disorders (Corbett *et al.*, 1985; Trimble & Reynolds, 1976) may appear. The excitatory side effects of barbiturates disappear in half of the patients with an increase in the dosage (Herranz *et al.*, 1988).

Metharbital, mephobarbital, and primidone are thought to be better tolerated (Barlow, 1978). With metharbital and mephobarbital, the active components are the derived phenobarbital, with levels that are erratic and often subtherapeutic. Neither seizure protection nor behavior reactions are seen. Some children on mephobarbital for subclinical seizures become distractable, loud, and boisterous, with a deterioration in attention (Gadow, 1982). A significant portion of primidone becomes phenobarbital, with all of its adverse effects seen.

Phenobarbital

Phenobarbital is cheap, simple, and safe. Children who are developmentally disabled appear more at risk for behavior reactions, such as depression, sedation, paradoxical hyperactivity, and behavior agitation, when placed on phenobarbital (Stores, 1975; Brent *et al.*, 1987; Stagno, 1993; Favale *et al.*, 1995).

Parents and teachers note behavioral problems in children on phenobarbital (Vining *et al.*, 1987). The incidence of behavior problems at up to 42% or higher is about twice that seen with placebos (20%) (Camfield *et al.*, 1979; Trimble, 1983). Side effects include irritability (24%), restless sleep (24%), hyperactivity (22%), insomnia (11%), aggressiveness (2%), drowsiness (7%) (Herranz *et al.*, 1988), excitement, tantrums, tearfulness, and disobedience (Stores, 1975; Thorn, 1975; Jeavons, 1977; Ozdirim *et al.*, 1978; Stores, 1981; Theodore & Porter, 1983; Trimble, 1983; Holmes, 1987). These side effects do not necessarily relate to the drug concentration (Trimble, 1983). The behavior problems may arise anew or may be an aggravation of a prior behavior (Stores, 1975; Wolf & Forsythe, 1978). Reduction of the dose levels of phenobarbital may lead to improvements in anxiety, fatigue, aggression, and depression but not sedation or other behaviors after months (Trimble, 1980; Trimble, 1982).

Behavior problems may emerge fully at about six to nine weeks after starting the drug, unrelated to blood levels. At therapeutic levels, the problem then appears greater than at one year. About 33% of patients show behavioral deterioration and 8% show definite behavioral improvements on phenobarbital at controlled levels (Trimble, 1983). Discontinuing the barbiturate causes the behavior to disappear in 73% (Trimble, 1983).

Hyperactivity, unrelated to drug concentrations, is estimated to occur in 18–50% (Vining, 1990). Excitatory side effects may appear at lower dosages. This usually does not diminish over time, although milder forms of this behavior are transient and fade after two or three weeks. More severe and persistent hyperactive, like emotional behaviors, may be accentuations of previous tendencies brought out by the drug or may be a pre-existing problem that is later blamed on the drug (Herranz *et al.*, 1988; Kulig, 1980).

In young children, behavioral changes, seen in 9%, may include increased fussiness and characteristic sleep disturbances, such as difficulty in falling asleep, early awakening, and daytime irritability. These occur even at lower therapeutic dosages (Camfield *et al.*, 1979; Holdsworth & Whitmore, 1974; Trimble, 1983).

Phenobarbital can cause depression (40%), including suicidal ideation, as well as mood shifts at all ages, especially in adolescence. Risk factors include a family history of a major affect disorder in first-degree relatives (Barabas & Matthews, 1988; Brent, 1986; Brent *et al.*, 1987; Ettinger *et al.*, 1998; Ettinger & Steinberg, 2001; Hermann *et al.*, 1981; Herranz *et al.*, 1988; Kanner & Balabanov, 2002; Smith *et al.*, 1994; Trimble, 1982). Children are described as being unable to stop repeated activities, unhappy, disobedient, excitable, and anxious, with multiple somatic complaints and difficulties in making friends (Vining *et al.*, 1987). This is not dose-related, although a reduction in the dose may lead to an improvement in anxiety and other neurotic disorders after a few months (Stores, 1975; Trimble, 1982; Trimble, 1983).

Withdrawal of a barbiturate may also result in depression (Kendrick *et al.*, 1993; Lambert & Robertson, 1999).

There is no relationship between the phenobarbital blood level and conduct disorders (Trimble, 1983), although rating scales may suggest a worsening at higher doses (Ozdirim *et al.*, 1978; Theodore & Porter, 1983). Psychiatric illnesses and personality changes have been reported, especially with higher drug levels (Reynolds & Travers, 1974). An acute confusional state may be seen (Stores, 1975). Acute psychotic reactions with bizarre behaviors, hallucinations, and a distorted sense of reality have been noted (Vining, 1990). Phenobarbital toxicity may accentuate the patient's tendency towards pseudoseizures (Trimble, 1980; Trimble, 1982).

Primidone

Primidone was originally thought to benefit children by reducing neurotic behaviors and improving moods (Louiseau *et al.*, 1983; Trimble, 1983; Herranz *et al.*, 1988), aggression, destructiveness, and self-mutilation, especially in mentally retarded patients (Trimble, 1983). At higher doses, primidone produces similar problems to phenobarbital. Side effects are seen in 22–29%, including hyperactivity (8%), irritability (8%), drowsiness (5%), sleep restlessness (4%), aggressiveness, (4%), and fatigue (1%) (Herranz *et al.*, 1988). Anxiety and depression may occur (Trimble, 1982; Kanner & Balabanov, 2002). Behavior may deteriorate (Dreifuss, 1983). Tendencies towards hyperactivity or impulsive behavior may be aggravated (Kinsbourne & Caplan, 1979). Personality deterioration, with mood swings, confusional state, and even paranoid psychosis has been reported, especially at higher drug levels (Stores, 1975; Rodin *et al.*, 1976; Theodore & Porter, 1983). High drug levels may lead to development of non-epileptic seizures (Trimble, 1982).

Phenytoin

Phenytoin is used frequently in children, despite the fact that it can cause restlessness, irritability, mental slowing, and depression. This drug is probably best avoided whenever possible in children of school age (Stores, 1976), since it may be the worst tolerated of the older drugs (Herranz *et al.*, 1988). Phenytoin may benefit those with anxiety (McDanal & Bolman, 1975; Schmitz, 1999), with both positive and negative effects reported (Pratt *et al.*, 1984).

In children, excitation behavioral disorders are seen with phenytoin, especially at higher plasma levels. Behavioral side effects, seen in 16%, include irritability (5%), restless sleep (5%), hyperactivity (3%), fatigue (2%), drowsiness (2%), and insomnia (2%) (Herranz *et al.*, 1988). Other problems reported include anxiety, aggression, and depression (Stores, 1976; Rivinus, 1982). At higher levels, children have more neurotic presentations, suggesting that phenytoin and carbamazepine tend to have somewhat opposing effects. The hyperactivity of phenytoin may be combined with irritability. Teenage girls may be distraught over the cosmetic changes of the drug, such as coarsening of facial features, overgrowth of the gums, and hirsutism. If the phenytoin is tapered over weeks rather than months, increased irritability may be noted.

Phenytoin is associated with other psychiatric conditions, including conversion symptoms, tactile and visual hallucinations, somatic delusions, and schizophrenic psychoses, especially at higher serum levels (McDanal & Bolman, 1975; Schmitz, 1999). Phenytoin may cause a paradoxical excited delirium (Ferrari *et al.*, 1983). At normal therapeutic ranges, insidious changes in personality may be seen (Stores, 1981), which become more prominent at higher drug levels. Some of these changes may relate to a folate deficiency (Stores, 1975). Folate levels are also significantly lower in children on phenytoin who are rated as neurotic or depressed (Trimble & Cull, 1990; Trimble, 2001). Phenytoin toxicity has been associated with a greater tendency for pseudoseizures.

Carbamazepine

Carbamazepine is well-tolerated antiepileptic drug (Herranz *et al.*, 1988) with behavior benefits in children with and without epilepsy. Improvements in anxiety, aggressiveness, depression, behavior, school performance, family relationships, adaptation to the environment, and interpersonal relationships are noted, although some retarded children paradoxically are more aggressive. In epilepsy, carbamazepine has been helpful in treating impulsive control disorders, borderline personality problems, antisocial and apathetic behaviors, aggression, and dyscontrol syndromes (Sonnen *et al.*, 1975; Stores, 1975; Pratt *et al.*, 1984; Smith *et al.*, 1994).

Carbamazepine is related chemically to the tricyclic tantidepressants (Dalby, 1975; Drake & Peruzzi, 1986). The drug has antimanic and antidepressant effects (Vining, 1990), with mood-stabilizing and impulse control benefits (Friedman *et al.*, 1992). Improvements in mood are reported in 90% of children taking carbamazepine (Herranz *et al.*, 1988). Carbamazepine, like valproate, is prophylactic in the control of manic-depressive illnesses (Lambert & Robertson, 1999). Whereas barbiturates and phenytoin reduce plasma free tryptophan, carbamazepine increases the levels, influencing serotonin turnover, which may relate to its psychotropic benefits (Pratt *et al.*, 1984). Carbamazepine and valproate paradoxically may cause depressive episodes (4%) (Trimble, 1982) or mania (Kanner & Balabanov, 2002). In children, there is no association with neurotic-like behaviors (Trimble, 1982). The suicidal ideation rate in children on carbamazepine is 4%.

Carbamazepine may produce adverse behavior reactions in 10% of patients (Friedman *et al.*, 1992) especially in children (Weisbrot & Ettinger, 1998). In children, behavioral effects are seen in 31%, including drowsiness (11%), restless sleep, irritability (5%), fatigue (3%), and hyperactivity (3%) (Herranz *et al.*, 1988). Slowed thinking, drowsiness, and aggressiveness occur in 17%. Side effects appear, although 85% of patients with complex partial epilepsy experience improved seizure control and 40% show improved school performance and alertness (Silverstein *et al.*, 1982a; Silverstein *et al.*, 1982b). Side effects may be intermittent, corresponding with fluctuations in plasma levels, especially with polytherapy (Herranz *et al.*, 1988). This has been overcome greatly by using longer-acting formulations. In about 3.5% of patients on carbamazepine, acute adverse behavioral affects appear, some of which are dramatic and alarming. These effects include extreme irritability, developmental regression, agitation, obsessive thoughts, auditory hallucinations, combativeness, incoherent behavior, feeling spaced out, straining to think, personality changes, insomnia, feeling detached, aggressive physical outbursts, hyperactivity, anger, and paranoia (Silverstein *et al.*, 1982a; Silverstein *et al.*, 1982b).

A rare psychiatric syndrome related to carbamazepine-induced hyponatremia is psychosis with polydipsia (Schmitz, 1999; Schimitz & Trimble, 1995). Rare psychotic behaviors with emotional explosiveness and confusion may be seen, especially in brain-damaged individuals. In 3.5% of children, early problems of agitation, psychotic behavior, and delirium at therapeutic levels are seen, especially in handicapped children. Slow reintroduction of the drug allows tolerance in 71% (Silverstein *et al.*, 1982a; Silverstein *et al.*, 1982b). Children with cerebral atrophy may be especially prone to such reactions (Stores, 1975).

Valproate

Valproate has been linked with both benefits and adverse reactions in behavior problems (Pratt *et al.*, 1984). Psychotropic benefits have been reported with valproate, although not to the degree seen with carbamazepine. Valproic acid has been useful for bipolar affective disorders, agitation, mood disorders, irritably, and aggressive or self-injurious behaviors (Freeman *et al.*, 2002; Post *et al.*, 1996; Small *et al.*, 1991; Stoll *et al.*, 1994). Valproic acid shows mood-stabilizing and antimanic benefits (Schmitz, 1999), especially when used in combination with lithium (Herranz *et al.*, 1982). Autistic behaviors tend to improve with valproate-induced seizure control (Sherard *et al.*, 1980).

In children, behavior problems occur in 17% (Weisbrot & Ettinger, 1998), including drowsiness (5%), irritability (5%), hyperactivity (3–5%), aggressiveness (2–9%), sadness and depression (2%), fatigue (2%), agitation, and anxiety, especially at higher drug levels (Herranz *et al.*, 1982; Trimble, 1982; Trimble, 1983; Herranz *et al.*, 1988). Up to 8% of children on valproate display belligerent behaviors or experience hallucinations. These are seen particularly in children on polytherapy with other protein-binding antiepileptics. Valproate reduces protein binding, leading to increased CNS free levels and toxic effects of other drug being taken. Discontinuing concurrent drugs such as phenobarbital may reduce adverse symptoms.

About 5% of patients develop emotional upsets, hyperactivity, and/or aggressiveness soon after the initiation of the drug. Excitation (overstimulation) may appear (Herranz et al., 1988). Valproate may induce or worsen hyperactivity and aggressive behaviors (Wolf et al., 1984). The adverse effects on activity tend to worsen over time (Kulig, 1980), and in some patients may emerge after months to a year on the drug.

Succinimide

Ethosuximide was thought initially to be free of significant behavior reactions (Hartlage et al., 1980) and possibly to benefit anxiety (Trimble, 1997). Rarely, irritability and unruly behavior occur, including confusion, excessive activity, euphoria, depression, sleep disturbances, hostility, aggressiveness, and depression (Stores, 1975; Landolt, 1958; Stagno, 1993; Wolf et al., 1984).

Adolescents and young adults on ethosuximide may develop psychotic episodes. This is seen rarely in children (Perrine & Congett, 1994; Stagno, 1993). Often, there is a history of prior psychiatric disturbances. The psychoses show up as delusions, hallucinations, anxiety, depression, or depersonalization (Browne et al., 1974). In some patients, this may be a forced normalization phenomenon (Trimble, 1982) or an alternating psychosis (Trimble, 1998), seen in 2% of children (Schmidt, 1992) and 8% of adults (Wolf et al., 1984; Schmitz, 1999), resulting in paradoxical behavioral abnormality (Landolt, 1958; Wolf, 1991).

Benzodiazepines

Benzodiazepines have both positive and negative behavioral effects. Benefits include antianxiety and sedative qualities, with minor tranquilizing benefits (Stores, 1975), but side effects include withdrawal syndromes, disinhibition (Schmitz, 1999), and unwanted behaviors. The reported range of side effects is 13–91%. Giving benzodiazepines with a barbiturate accentuates the problems (Holmes, 1987). Benzodiazepines can produce irritability, hyperactivity (10%) (Ettinger & Steinberg, 2001), aggression, conduct disorder, poor concentration, anxiety, depression, hostility (Theodore & Porter, 1983; Trimble, 1997), and behavioral disturbances, including irritability, disobedience, and antisocial activity (Holmes, 1987). Withdrawal, especially if rapid, may produce depression, delirium, or psychosis (Rivinus, 1982; Kendrick et al., 1993; Lambert & Robertson, 1999; Ettinger & Steinberg, 2001).

Clonazepam

Clonazepam impairs intellect, attention, concentration, and behavior in children (Dreifuss, 1983; Trimble & Cull, 1990). Aggressive behaviors may improve (Trimble, 1983). Behavior problems seen in up to 50% include irritability, aggressiveness, excitability, inattention, antisocial behavior, temperamental behavior, violence, disobedience, nosiness, and difficulties in discipline. Pre-existing hyperactivity may be worsened (Bensch *et al.*, 1977; Dreifuss, 1983; Theodore & Porter, 1983; Trimble, 1983). Situational hostility and disinhibition may occur (Stores, 1975).

Nitrazepam

Nitrazepam has been of benefit to children with myoclonic seizures and especially infantile myoclonic spasms. When the seizures are controlled, behavior improves. Children who, prior to their seizures, are not mentally retarded improve dramatically in the number of academic errors present when the seizures are controlled. In those who are retarded, behavior improvement is not paralleled by academic improvement (Mayeux *et al.*, 1980). Problems with behavior effects and drowsiness have been reported (Stores, 1975).

Clobazam

Clobazam may improve or impair behavior (Farrell *et al.*, 1984; Trimble & Cull, 1990). About 10% of children treated with clobazam experience non-specific behavioral changes that require discontinuation of medication. In some children with developmental disabilities, a sudden change in behavior, with marked hyperactivity and uncontrollable behavior, may be seen ten to 50 days after beginning the medication, even if the drug response is good. Younger children with refractory epilepsy and pervasive developmental disabilities seem at risk for catastrophic behavioral deterioration when treated with clobazam (Sheth *et al.*, 1992). Rarely, psychotic episodes may appear (Trimble, 1983).

New drugs

The initial trails of newer drugs have been predominantly in adults, so behavior problems have been noted more often in adults than in children. Psychiatric problems appear to be increased significantly with the use of GABAergic substances, such as vigabatrin, tiagabine, and topiramate (Trimble, 1997), which may frequently cause depression (Kanner & Balabanov, 2002). Forced normalization or alternate psychosis has been reported with all of the newer drugs, but especially with the more powerful substances such as vigabatrin and topiramate (Schmitz, 1999; Trimble, 1998).

Felbamate

Felbamate is a use-dependent sodium channel blocker and inhibitor of glutamate neurotransmission. Felbamate shows stimulant action, which may be beneficial or negative, depending on persisting psychopathology. Benefits include increased alertness, improved attention, and enhanced concentration. Problems of anorexia, insomnia, agitation, anxiety, mania, psychoses, and behavior disturbances have been seen, especially in retarded patients (Ettinger & Steinberg, 2001; King, 1994; Schmitz, 1999). Felbamate may cause depression (Kanner & Balabanov, 2002).

Psychoses are rare, being reported in 0.2% (Ketter *et al.*, 1994; Rogers *et al.*, 1993). Felbamate use is restricted greatly by its associations with fatal hepatitis and aplastic anemia.

Gabapentin

Gabapentin is more apt to help than harm behavior in both epileptic and non-epileptic individuals, especially women. Gabapentin is an antianxiety and possibly antidepressant drug (Schmitz, 1999). Psychiatrists have used gabapentin in the treatment of behavior dyscontrol (Ryback *et al.*, 1997; Weisbrot & Ettinger, 1998), anxiety states (Pollack *et al.*, 1998), social phobia, self-injurious behaviors (McManaman & Tam, 1999), depression (Schmitz, 1999), and bipolar disorders (Sander *et al.*, 1991; Ring *et al.*, 1998; Lambert & Robertson, 1999), including both the manic (Ryback & Ryback, 1995; Schaffer & Schaeffer, 1997; McElroy *et al.*, 1997; Knoll *et al.*, 1998) and the depressive (Ghaemi *et al.*, 1997; Young & Robb, 1997) phases.

Rarely, gabapentin has shown negative psychotropic effects in children. Gabapentin may produce somnolence, personality changes, emotional lability, hostility, irritability, hyperactivity, agitation, aggressiveness, thought disorders, and hyperactivity in both normal and developmentally disabled children (Ettinger & Steinberg, 2001; Lee *et al.*, 1995; Nemeroff *et al.*, 1995; Tallian *et al.*, 1996; Wolf *et al.*, 1995; Barry, 1998). Rare cases of aggressive behavior in children have been reported, associated with a hyperkinetic aggressive presentation (Lee *et al.*, 1995; Schmitz, 1996; Tallian *et al.*, 1996; Wolf *et al.*, 1995).

Lamotrigine

Lamotrigine inhibits presynaptic voltage-dependent sodium channels, leading to a decreased release of the excitatory amino acids glutamate and aspartate. It has a reputation as a positive psychotropic drug that improves mood, emotions, and cognition, unrelated to seizure control (Ettinger *et al.*, 1998). Handicapped patients on lamotrigine may become more alert and demanding. Improvements in energy, alertness, temper, fatigue, and worry have been noted (Brodie *et al.*, 1995; Meador *et al.*, 2001).

In patients on lamotrigine, especially mentally retarded individuals, both behavioral improvements and severe behavioral deterioration have been demonstrated (Beran & Gibson, 1998). Behavior disorders (3.5%), mood disorders (2%), and psychoses (nearly 1%) are reported (Kanner *et al.*, 2000). Sleepiness, confusion, and abnormal thinking have been noted. In children, lamotrigine can cause ADHD symptoms, with hyperactivity and sometimes irritability. It has been associated with unprovoked aggression (11%), agitation, and banging, slamming, attacking, or other behavior reactions, (25%), often within one month of beginning therapy (Beran & Gibson, 1998; Dodrill *et al.*, 1998). Occasional patients respond to psychiatric intervention. A neuropsychiatric history may be a risk factor for lamotrigine (Kanner *et al.*, 2000).

The antidepressant effects of lamotrigine have been established, with a resultant sense of wellbeing, increased happiness, and a sense of being in control (Kasumakar & Yatham, 1997; Schmitz, 1999). Lamotrigine is an effective bipolar affective disorder agent (Sporn & Sachs, 1997; Lambert & Robertson, 1999; Kanner *et al.*, 2000). Lamotrigine can cause insomnia and, rarely, a psychosis, the latter presenting as a hypomania. This occurs in 6% of patients on monotherapy (Fitton & Goa, 1995; Schmitz, 1999).

Levetiracetam

In adults, adverse side effects of levetiracetam, which occur in at least 5% of patients, include drowsiness (21%). In children, the most common side effects are drowsiness and mood changes/depression (Wilner, 2002). Behavioral symptoms, reported in 13%, include agitation, hostility, anxiety, apathy, emotional lability, depersonalization, mood changes including depression (10%), aggression/irritability (9%), and, rarely, psychotic symptoms (0.7%) and suicidal behavior (0.2%) early in the therapy (Harden, 2001; Mandelbaum *et al.*, 2001). Children and adolescents may develop an acute psychosis within days to months of drug initiation, with both visual and auditory hallucinations. Agitation, hyperreligiosity, and persecutory delusions may be seen. All these effects improve dramatically with a decrease in dosage or withdrawal of the drug. Risk factors may include cognitive deficits and prior mild behavior problems. The drug is best initiated slowly and cautiously, dose adjustments being made according to the tolerance (Kossoff *et al.*, 2002).

Oxcarbamazepine

Mood ratings show a significant increase in feelings, clear-headedness, and speed of thought, especially with higher doses of oxcarbamazepine in the first week (Curran *et al.*, 1991).

Progabide

Progabide has produced transient alternations of mental states. In one study, a patient with a prior psychiatric disorder history developed hallucinations, fears, and paranoid ideation. Other patients became disinhibited, with overt aggressiveness and social withdrawal (Gutierrez *et al.*, 1984).

Sulthiame

Sulthiame may benefit disturbed epileptic patients, particularly those with aggressiveness and motor excitement (Stores, 1975). Patients tend to experience an improvement in their sense of wellbeing. In some (20%), problems of sedation, apathy, and depression appear (Trimble, 1980), as may personality changes and behavior abnormalities (Ettinger & Steinberg, 2001). Rarely, acute confusional episodes are seen as a toxic manifestation (Stores, 1975).

Stiripentol

Stiripentol may have a positive psychotropic effect if used with carbamazepine, in reducing the level of the toxic epoxide metabolite metabolized from the carbanazepine (Loiseau *et al.*, 1988).

Tiagabine

Tiagabine is a GABA reuptake inhibitor. It may produce a paradoxical provocation of non-convulsive status, which should be checked by EEG if behavior problems arise (Schapel & Chadwick, 1996). Children on tiagabine with below-normal intelligence, especially post-encephalitis, may gain seizure control but experience impulsive control problems and violent, destructive rage reactions (Beran & Gibson, 1998; Kaufman *et al.*, 1999).

Tiagabine is reputed to be an antianxiety drug and an antidepressant. Improved moods may occur with tiagabine monotherapy. There may be occasional benefits in bipolar disorders (Ettinger *et al.*, 1999b). Tiagabine can cause nervousness (12%) and depression (5%) (Numberger *et al.*, 1986; Leppik, 1995; Leach & Brodie, 1998; Stephen & Brodie, 1998; Schmitz, 1999; Lambert & Robertson, 1999). The incidence of psychoses (2%) is not increased significantly, although postictal psychoses and, rarely, an alternative psychosis or a withdrawal psychosis may occur (Schmitz, 1999).

Topiramate

Topiramate is a powerful drug that acts in three ways: by inhibiting sodium or calcium channels, potentiating GABA-mediated chloride currents, and decreasing the release of excitatory amino acids. Topiramate is an antianxiety drug and possibly an antidepressant, but it can cause depression in some patients. Nearly 12% of patients experience psychiatric side effects. Topiramate may cause mood disorders (5%), anxiety (0.25%), irritability, behavior problems (6%), and psychoses (1.3%) (Abou-Khalil & Fakhoury, 1998; Betts *et al.*, 1997; Betts *et al.*, 1998; Dohmeier *et al.*, 1998; Shorvon, 1998; Tassari *et al.*, 1996). A neuropsychiatric history may be a significant predictor of adverse reactions in patients on topiramate (Kanner *et al.*, 2000; Kanner & Balabanov, 2002).

Although originally disputed (Ryback *et al.*, 1997; Schaffer & Schaffer, 1997), it has been found that topiramate may cause depression, with diffuse, dose-dependent affective problems seen at an incidence of 9% and 19% at low and high doses, respectively (Janssen-Cilag, 1996). When the drug is discontinued, mood improves (Sziklas *et al.*, 1999). Topiramate may be helpful in treating both manic and depressive phases of bipolar disorders (Marcotte, 1998; Suppes *et al.*, 1998).

In children started on topiramate, behavior changes include mood swings (3%), aggression (1.5%), irritability (1.5%), visual hallucinations (1.5%), and school difficulties (6%). Withdrawal of the drug results in partial to complete resolution of these problems. The behavioral changes are not related to the rate of dosage change (Hamiwka *et al.*, 1999). Retarded patients may benefit from topiramate and may experience improvement in adverse behavior (24%), although 8% experience behavior worsening and 20% show cognitive slowing (Doherty & Gates, 1999).

Since the clinical introduction of topiramate, psychiatric disorders including psychoses have been reported (Betts *et al.*, 1998), including rare psychoses, forced normalization, and schizophrenia, after several months on therapy. These disappear after discontinuing the drug (Luef & Bauer, 1996; Schmitz, 1999).

Vigabatrin

Vigabatrin is an irreversible inhibitor of GABA transaminase, resulting in an increase in GABA levels (Reynolds *et al.*, 1988). Vigabatrin is mood-stabilizing and antimanic (Schmitz, 1999). There is no relationship between mood changes and seizure control. Vigabatrin is associated with aggression, depression, a withdrawal syndrome, ADHD, an encephalopathy, and an alternative psychosis, especially in patients with subnormal intelligence (Beran & Gibson, 1998; Schmitz, 1999).

Vigabatrin may induce adverse psychiatric events, including psychoses (Sander *et al.*, 1991a; Sander *et al.*, 1991), especially with severe epileptic disorders, a sudden reduction in seizure frequency, and a past history of psychoses (Dulac *et al.*, 1991; Ettinger & Steinberg, 2001) or depressive illness (Brodie, 1996; Schmitz, 1999). It was thought initially that the incidence of psychiatric complications was 7%, including acute encephalitis, complex partial status epilepticus, bipolar affective psychosis, and manic episodes (Reynolds, 1990). However, the incidence dropped with further study to about 3.4%, which is about the same as with other antiepileptics (Ferrie *et al.*, 1996). There are three patterns to the appearance of psychoses: forced normalization, postictal psychosis following seizure cluster after initial control, and withdrawal psychosis (Thomas *et al.*, 1996). The most common serious adverse effect is behavioral disturbances, including agitation, confusion, hyperactivity, stupor, depression, and psychoses. No preceding history of psychoses is noted (77%). The psychoses occur after a marked change in the habitual pattern of the seizures (69%) or after a period of seizure freedom followed by a cluster of seizures (31%). Other patients remain seizure-free but then develop psychoses. The psychosis resolves after discontinuing the drug (Sander *et al.*, 1991b).

There is an incidence of depression in 5–10% of patients (Sander *et al.*, 1991b; Brodie, 1996b) within a few weeks of starting or increasing the dose of vigabatrin, especially in patients with a past history of psychiatric disturbances (Reynolds, 1990; Sander *et al.*, 1991b; Ring *et al.*, 1994; Lambert & Robertson, 1999).

In children, the most common psychiatric side effects are agitation, excitation, hyperkinesias, and aggression, much like those seen with the barbiturates. The incidence of behavior disorders in children is about 14% (Ferrie *et al.*, 1996). Hyperactivity may be worsened in children (Dulac *et al.*, 1991; Ettinger & Steinberg, 2001). A few patients with subnormal intelligence show similar aggressive reactions to vigabatrin, tiagabine, and other antiepileptic drugs (Beran & Gibson, 1998).

Zonisamide

Children with physical disorders not involving the brain or brain function show rate of emotional disturbances (11.5%) almost twice that seen in normals people (6.6%). Children with brain damage show a greater incidence of emotional disturbance (34.3%). Correlated factors such as low IQ and seizures add to the risks. A specific behavior such as hyperactivity or an emotional syndrome associated with brain damage has not been seen (Faight, 2001).

Psychiatric medications

Most antidepressants, tranquilizers, and many other drugs used to treat behavior disorders may cause seizures in a few (2%) patients seen for seizures. This is seen especially if the drug is introduced rapidly at high dosage (up to 9%), compared with low dosage (0.5%), and in seizure-prone individuals (Lambert & Robertson, 1999; Hauser & Hersdorffer, 2001).

Stimulants

The use of stimulant drugs in individuals with epilepsy is said to be safe, although such drugs have been incriminated with the precipitation of seizures. The incidence with methylphenidate hydrochloride is 1%. Barry (1998) reviewed the treatment of attention and affective disorders. Amphetamines lower the seizure threshold, but this is rarely clinically significant in lower dosages. Methylphenidate hydrochloride at low dosage appears to be relatively safe in patients with epilepsy. When on methylphenidate hydrochloride few, if any, seizure-free patients have a seizure. Three of five patients with continued seizures have exacerbations (Barry, 1998).

Mood elevators/antidepressants

Most non-monoamine oxidase inhibitor antidepressants can produce seizures (0.1–4%) (Rosenstein *et al.*, 1993), although the newer drugs appear less prone to do so. Depression and antidepressants may adversely affect memory and other cognitive functions (Cole & Zarit, 1984; Thompson, 1991). The older tricyclic antidepressants are more apt to have such effects than SSRIs. Seizure risks relate to higher dosage, rapid dose escalation, reduced frequency, and overdose, especially early in the first weeks of therapy. If seizures occur, the drug should be changed to a less epileptogenic medication (Edwards, 1985; Rosenstein *et al.*, 1993). Trazodone is thought to have the lowest epileptogenic potential, even at toxic dosages. Isolated reports of seizures with the newer antidepressants are rare. Some have been associated with hyponatremia related to inappropriate secretion of antidiuretic hormone, seen with all SSRIs.

Monoamine oxidase inhibitors

Irreversible monoamine oxidase inhibitors inhibitors are less proconvulsant than the tricyclic antidepressants, especially amoxapine and clomipramine (Lambert & Robertson, 1999).

Selective serotonin reuptake inhibitors

Exacerbation of seizure frequency or intensity is uncommon with the SSRIs. With low to moderate doses, seizure control may be improved (33%), unchanged (44%), or worsened (23%). Drugs to avoid in epileptic patients include amoxapine, bupropion (amfebutamone), and clomipramine. The lowest risk is with nefazodone and mirtazapine. Other SSRIs are of intermediate risk (Devinsky, 1998). Bupropion, a monocyclic antidepressant, has a seizure incidence of around 0.4% and can cause agitation, insomnia, and nausea.

Tricyclic antidepressants

Tricyclic drugs are proconvulsant (Jick *et al.*, 1983). Imipramine given 100 mg intravenously, but not orally, may produce seizures about one to two hours later in patients not on anticonvulsants. Oral imipramine in daily doses over 150 mg may occasionally produce seizures. Use of antidepressants in modest doses may be more tolerated and are far less apt to produce seizures. In tricyclic antidepressant overdosage, 6.2–8.4% of patients develop seizures (Frommer *et al.*, 1987). A family history of epilepsy or a condition that predisposes to epilepsy a potential risk for antidepressant-induced epilepsy (Edwards, 1985).

Convulsions have occurred in children on imipramine for nocturnal enuresis and hyperactivity due to organic brain disease (Fromm *et al.*, 1971; Fromm *et al.*, 1972; Fromm *et al.*, 1978). The overall convulsive risk, especially with tricyclics, appears to be 0.1–0.5%. The incidence of seizure induction is 0.4–1.4% for imipramine, 3.5% for clomipramine, 0.6% for amitriptyline, and 0.85% for buspirone (Edwards, 1985).

Tranquilizers

Tranquilizers, especially the older established drugs, may precipitate seizures. Chlorpromazine especially, but also thioridazine and, to a lesser degree, perphenazine, fluphenazine, trifluoperazine, thiothixene, and haloperidol, alter the seizure threshold. The route of administration is important: intravenous administration is most apt to produce seizures and EEG epileptiform changes (Trimble, 1986). In a study of overdosage of neuroleptics, 1.5% of patients develop seizures with phenothiazine overdosage. None developed seizures on risperidone overdosage. Clozapine may induce seizures when used in high therapeutic doses.

Surgery

Uncontrolled seizures may lead to worsening of the seizures and thus to greater memory and emotional problems. For patients with medication-resistant partial seizures, surgery may be an option. A full assessment should include a psychiatric/behavioral preoperative evaluation and a postoperative psychosocial rehabilitation approach over at least the first year (Rausch, 1991).

Preoperative evaluation

Trimble (1994) and Manchanda *et al.* (1996) reviewed the psychiatric findings in epilepsy surgery patients. They found psychopathology in 47.3–57% of the surgical candidates. Problems included 18–20% each with personality or psychosocial disorders, 11–20% with anxieties, 3–20% with depressive syndromes, and 4.3% with schizophrenia. Manchanda found slightly more psychiatric disorders in the generalized group (53.8%), including schizophrenia (7.7%). Anxieties were highest in the non-temporal partial group (16.3%). A schizophrenia-like psychosis personality disorder (18%) with dependence and avoidance problems may occur. Delusional, hallucinatory, and psychotic problems, but not neurotic problems, are seen more often in temporal lobe patients, with no laterality differences noted.

Postoperative status

Three types of psychological changes may follow seizure surgery. There may be postoperative transient anxiety and depression in the first year. There may be changes in the family, non-family, social, and academic relationships, especially with a marked seizure reduction. Rarely, a psychosis may emerge postoperatively, usually in adults who have a long history of seizures (Rausch, 1991). Trimble (1994) noted that new psychiatric disorders arising post-resection are seen in about one-third of patients and are exacerbated in three-quarters of patients. These disorders are easily controlled.

Trimble (1994) noted that immediately after surgery, the frequency of emotional problems is twice that noted preoperatively, possibly related to discontinuance of some medication, such as valproate, which may be suppressing a preceding depression. (It may be wise not to change anticonvulsants for a period of time.)

At six weeks, the overall psychopathology declines, but anxiety increases in 42% and some patients become depressed. By three months, the emotional reactions are less prominent. Depression may be more prominent in 37%, as anxiety fades. At six months, the depression is also fading away. At one year, 71–74% are free of any psychopathology. At this time, about 24% of patients continue to have psychosocial personality disorders, related only partially to seizure control. Only a few are still depressed (3%) or anxious (3%). Seizure freedom does not protect against psychopathology, although there is an increase in psychopathology, with less seizure control.

Postoperative anxiety may lead to conversion symptoms, acute panic reactions, and non-epileptic seizures, which may be misdiagnosed as a return of the seizures, especially if the patient is not well prepared to return to a seizure-free existence. These symptoms may be misdiagnosed as a seizure recurrence, i.e. presumed surgery failure, leading to further medication. The better postoperative quality of life depends on seizure relief and particularly on a better preoperative psychosocial status. Emotional problems are more apt to occur if an entire lobe of the brain is removed.

The postoperative period may be most important for emotional aspects of the changes ongoing in the brain's adjustments to the surgery. It is important to follow up the patient for psychopathology, perhaps at six weeks, three months, and one year. The six-week and three-month visits are most apt to pick up the commonest emergence of psychopathology.

Minimal behavior gains may be anticipated in children after successful temporal lobectomy. Impairments are dictated by factors other than seizure status. Children operated on for complex partial epilepsies may show a subsequent improvement in behaviors. Children before surgery and those not operated on have been stated to show more aggressive and bizarre behaviors, including promiscuity, thieving, provoked antisocial behavior, and tempers, often triggered by teasing. For such problems, early surgery may be worth considering (Davidson & Falconer, 1975).

Predictive variables

Good predictive outlooks include a lack of preoperative psychopathology and, especially, a good family support system, which leads to a very high chance of improvement.

Resultant behavior problems

Despite significant improvement in seizure status after temporal lobectomy, 34% of patients report clinically significant depressive symptoms one year later. More aggressive treatment of depression is needed before and after epilepsy surgery (Ryan *et al.*, 1999). When patients do not get adequate help before surgery, they are more prone to have emotional problems afterwards. Limited rehabilitation resources may establish the preoperative abnormal dysphoria. Postoperatively, the person must learn to live without epilepsy as part of the recovery plan.

Corpus callosotomy

In corpus callosotomy in children, most (80%) improve in attention, with only 7% becoming worse. In overall functioning, 60% improve, 20% are unchanged, and 20% become worse.

Stimulators

Vagal stimulation has been used for uncontrolled seizures in both adults and children. Nearly 40% experience significant improvements. Occasionally, the improvement relapses after about two years Morris & Mueller, 1999. Effects on behavior may not be dependent on seizure control (Vassilyadi *et al.*, 2000).

Before vagal stimulation, adults with intractable seizures have higher rates of depression, anxiety, and fatigue and a diminished quality of life. Changes in affect, quality of life, and seizure frequency occur after initiation of vagal stimulation (Ettinger, 1999b). Patients experience improved mood and less depression (Ravdin *et al.*, 2000). In children, mood improvement is seen in 22% (Helmers *et al.*, 1999).

Less than 9% of patients with vagal nerves stimulation develop significant psychiatric complications several months later in relation to at least a 75% reduction in seizure frequency. Some patients may become severely dysphoric, occasionally developing psychotic symptoms. It may be that psychiatric complications of treatment emerge when inhibitory mechanisms have become predominant, i.e. forced normalization (Alexander *et al.*, 1999).

Diets

Parents and physicians often anticipate compliance to a special diet to be a great source of child–parent strife. However, when the diet is effective and tolerated, the child often proves to be most compliant.

REFERENCES

Abou-Khalil, B. & Fakhoury, T. (1998). Neuropsychiatric profile of high-dose topiramate. *Epilepsia* **38** (suppl 8): 207.

Alexander, A., Blumer, D., & Davies, K. G. (1999). Psychiatric complications associated with vagus nerve stimulation. *Epilepsia* **40** (suppl 7): 208.

Barabas, G. & Matthews, W. (1988). Barbiturate anticonvulsants as a cause of severe depression. *Pediatrics* **82**: 284–5.

Barlow, C. F. (1978). Risk Factors of infancy and childhood: interrelationships of seizure disorders and mental retardation. In *Mental Retardation and Related Disorders*, pp. 768–76. Philadelphia: F. A. Davis.

Barry, J. (1998). Treatment of affective and attention deficit disorders. Presented at the American Epilepsy Society Conference, 1998.

Bensch, J., Blennow, G., Ferngren, H., *et al.* (1977). A double-blind study of clonazepam in the treatment of therapy resistant epilepsy in children. *Dev. Med. Child Neurol.* **19**: 335–42.

Beran, R. G. & Gibson, R. J. (1998). Aggressive behavior in intellectually challenged patients with epilepsy treated with lamotrigine. *Epilepsia* **39**: 280–82.

Betts, T., Crawford, P. & Trimble, M. R. (1998). Topiramate and psychoses. 3rd European Congress of Epileptology. *Epilepsia* **39** (suppl 2): 3.

Betts, T., Smith, K. & Khan, G. (1997). Severe psychiatric reactions in topiramate. *Epilepsia* **38** (suppl 3): 64.

Brent, D. A. (1986). Overrepresentation of epileptics in a consecutive series of suicide attempters seen at a children's hospital 1978–1983. *J. Am. Acad. Child Psychiatry* **25**: 242–6.

Brent, D. A., Crumrine, P. K., Varma, R. R., *et al.* (1987). Phenobarbital treatment and major depressive disorder in children with epilepsy. *Pediatrics* **80**: 909–17.

Brodie, M. J. (1996). Monotherapy with vigabatrin. Presented at the Second European Congress of Epileptology, The Hague, the Netherlands, 1996.

Brodie, M. J., Richens, A. & Yuen, A. (1995). Double-blind comparison of lamotrigine and carbamazepine in newly diagnosed epilepsy. *Lancet* **345**: 458–76.

Browne, T. R., Penry, S. K., Porter, R. S., *et al.* (1974). Responsiveness before, during, and after spike-wave paroxysms. *Neurology* **24**: 660–65.

Camfield, C. S., Chaplin, S., Doyle, A. B., *et al.* (1979). Side effects of phenobarbital in toddlers: behavior and cognitive aspects. *Pediatrics* **95**: 351–65.

Cole, K. D. & Zarit, S. H. (1984). Psychological deficits in depressed medical patients. *J. Nerv. Ment. Dis.* **172**: 150–55.

Corbett, J. A., Trimble, M. R. & Nichol, T. C. (1985). Behavioral and cognitive impairments in children with epilepsy: the long-term effects of anticonvulsant therapy. *J. Am. Acad. Child Psychiatry* **24**: 17–23.

Curran, H. V., Java, R. & Luder, M. H. (1991). Cognitive and psychomotor effects of oxcarbamazepine. 9th International Epilepsy Congress. *Epilepsia* **32** (suppl 10): 56.

Dalby, M. A. (1975). Behavioral effects of carbamazepine. In *Complex Partial Seizures and their Treatment*, ed. J. K. Penry & D. D. Daly, Vol. II, pp. 331–43. New York: Raven Press.

Davidson, S. & Falconer, M. A. (1975). Outcome of surgery in 40 children with temporal lobe epilepsy. *Lancet* **1**: 1260–63.

Devinsky, O. (1998). What should the neurologist remember on the psychopharmacology of epilepsy? Presented at the American Epilepsy Society Conference, 1998.

Dodrill, C. B., Arnett, J. L., Shu, V., *et al.* (1998). Effects of tiagabine monotherapy on abilities, adjustment and mood. *Epilepsia* **39**: 33–42.

Doherty, K. T. & Gates, J. R. (1999). Use of topiramate in the cognitively impaired. *Epilepsia* **40** (suppl 7): 62.

Dohmeier, C., Kay, A. & Greathouse, N. (1998). Neuropsychiatric complications of topiramate therapy. *Epilepsia* **39** (suppl 6): 189.

Drake, M. E. & Peruzzi, W. T. (1986). Manic state with carbamazepine therapy of seizures. *J. Natl. Med. Assoc.* **78**: 1105–7.

Dreifuss, F. (1983). Pediatric Epileptology. Boston, MA: John Wright PSG.

Dulac, O., Chiron, C., Luna, D., *et al.* (1991). Vigabatrin in childhood epilepsy. *J. Child Neurol.* **6**: 2830–37.

Edwards, J. G. (1985). Antidepressants and seizures: epidemiology and clinical aspects. In *The Psychopharmacology of Epilepsy*, ed. M. R. Trimble, pp. 119–39. New York: John Wiley & Sons.

Ettinger, A. B. & Steinberg, A. L. (2001). Psychiatric issues in patients with epilepsy and mental retardation. In *Psychiatric Issues in Epilepsy*, ed. A. B. Ettinger & A. M. Kanner, pp. 181–200. Philadelphia: Lippincott Williams & Wilkins.

Ettinger, A. B., Bernal, O. G., Andriola, M. R., *et al.* (1999a). Two cases of nonvconvulsive status epilepticus in association with tiagabine therapy. *Epilepsia* **40**: 1159–62.

Ettinger, N. E., Vitale, S., Schindler, R. J., *et al.* (1999b). Changes in mood and quality of life in adult epilepsy patients treated with vagal nerve stimulation. *Epilepsia* **40** (suppl 7): 62.

Ettinger, A. B., Weisbrot, D. M., Saracco, J., *et al.* (1998). Positive and negative psychotropic effects of lamotrigine in epilepsy patients with mental retardation. *Epilepsia* **39**: 874–7.

Faight, E. (2001). Zonisamide. *Neurology* **67**: 1774–9.

Farrell, K., Jan, J. E., Julian, J. V., *et al.* (1984). Clobazam in children with intractable seizures. *Epilepsia* **25**: 657.

Favale, E., Rubino, V., Mainardi, P., *et al.* (1995). Anticonvulsant effect of fluoxetine in humans. *Neurology* **45**: 1925–7.

Ferrari, M., Barbaras, G. & Matthews, W. (1983). Psychologic and behavioral disturbances among epileptic children treated with barbiturate anticonvulsants. *Am. J. Psychiatry* **140**: 112–13.

Ferrie, C. D., Robinson, R. O. & Panaziotopoulos, C. P. (1996). Psychotic and severe Behavioural reactions with vigabatrin: a review. *Acta Neurol. Scand.* **93**: 1–8.

Fitton, A. & Goa, K. L. (1995). Lamotrigine. *Drugs* **50**: 691–713.

Freeman, T. W., Clothier, J. L., Pazaglia, P., *et al.* (2002). A double-blind comparison of valproate and lithium in the treatment of acute mania. *Am. J. Psychiatry* **149**: 108–11.

Friedman, D. L., Kastner, T. & Plummer, A. T. (1992). Adverse behavioral effects in individuals with mental retardation and mood disorders treated with carbamazepine. *Am. J. Ment. Retard.* **9**: 541–6.

Fromm, G. H., Amores, C. Y. & Thies, W. (1972). Imipramine in epilepsy. *Arch. Neurol.* **27**: 198–204.

Fromm, G. H., Rosen, J. A. & Amores, C. Y. (1971). Clinical and experimental investigation on the effects of imipramine on epilepsy. *Epilepsia* **12**: 282.

Fromm, G. H., Wessel, H. B., Glass, J. D., *et al.* (1978). Imipramine in absence and myoclonic seizures. *Neurology* **28**: 953–7.

Frommer, D. A., Kulig, K. W., Marx, J. A., *et al.* (1987). Tricyclic antidepressant overdose: a review. *JAMA* **257**: 521–6.

Gadow, K. D. (1982). School involvement in the treatment of seizure disorders. *Epilepsia* **23**: 215–24.

Ghaemi, S. N., Katzow, J. J., Desai, S. P., *et al.* (1997). Gabapentin treatment of mood disorders: a preliminary study. *J. Clin. Psychiatry* **59**: 426–9.

Gutierrez, A., Dreifuss, F. E., Santilli, N., *et al.* (1984). Psychiatric symptoms associated with progabide therapy. *Epilepsia* **25**: 657.

Hamiwka, L. D., Gerber, P. E., Connolly, M. B., *et al.* (1999). Topiramate-associated behavioral changes in children. *Epilepsia* **40** (suppl 7): 116.

Harden, C. (2001). Safety profile of levetiracetam: pharmacological treatment of epilepsy. *Epilepsia* **42**: (suppl 4): 36–9.

Hartlage, L. C., Stovall, K. & Kocack, B. (1980). Behavioral correlates of anticonvulsant blood levels. *Epilepsia* **21**: 185.

Hauser, W. A. & Hesdorffer, D. C. (2001). Psychoses, depression and epilepsy: epidemiological considerations. In *Psychiatric Issues in Epilepsy*, ed. A. B. Ettinger & A. M. Kanne, pp. 7–18. Philadelphia: Lippincott Williams & Wilkins.

Helmers, S., Wheless, J. W., Frost, M., *et al.* (1999). Vagus nerve stimulation (VNS) in children: quality of life and safety. *Epilepsia* **40** (suppl 7): 121.

Herranz, J. L., Armijo, J. A. & Arteaga, R., (1988). Clinical side effects of phenobarbital, primidone, phenytoin, carbamazepine and valproate during monotherapy in children. *Epilepsia* **29**: 794–804.

Herranz, J. L., Arteaga, R. & Armijo, J. A. (1982). Side effects of sodium valproate in monotherapy controlled by plasma levels: a study of 188 pediatric patients. *Epilepsia* **23**: 203–14.

Holdsworth, L. & Whitmore, K. (1974). A study of children with epilepsy attending ordinary schools. I: their seizure patterns, progress, and behavior in schools. *Dev. Med. Child Neurol.* **16**: 746–58.

Holmes, G. L. (1987). Psychosocial Factors in Childhood Epilepsy, In *Diagnosis and Management of Epilepsy in Children*, pp. 112–24. Philadelphia: W. B. Saunders.

Janssen-Cilag. (1996). *Topomax*. Product monograph.

Jeavons, P. M. (1977). Choice of drug therapy in epilepsy. *Practitioner* **219**: 542–56.

Jick, H., Dinan, B. J., Hunter, J. R., *et al.* (1983). Tricyclic antidepressants and convulsions. *J. Clin. Psychopharmacol.* **3**: 182–5.

Kanner A. M. & Balabanov, A. (2002). Depression and epilepsy: how closely related are they? *Neurology* **58** (suppl 5): 27–39.

Kanner, A. M., Faught, E., French, A. J., *et al.* (2000). Psychiatric adverse events caused by topiramate and lamotrigine: A post marketing prevalence and risk study. *Epilepsia* **41** (suppl 7): 169.

Kasumakar, V. & Yatham, L. N. (1997). An open study of lamotrigine in refractory bipolar depression. *Psychiatry Res.* **19**: 145–8.

Kaufman, K. R., Kugler, S. L., Sachdeo, R. C., *et al.* (1999). Tiagabine in the management of post-encephalitic epilepsy and impulse control disorders. *Epilepsia* **40** (suppl 7): 57.

Kendrick, A. M., Duncan, J. S. & Trimble, M.R. (1993). Effects of discontinuation of individual antiepileptic drugs on mood. *Hum. Psychopharmacol.* **8**: 263–70.

Ketter, T. A., Nalow, B. A., Flamini, R., *et al.* (1994). Anticonvulsant withdrawal-emergent psychopathology. *Neurology* **44**: 55–61.

King, J. A. (1994). Increased incidence of adverse behavioral side effects associated with the addition of felbamate (FBM) to antiepileptic drug (AED) regimens in the mentally retarded (MR) population. *Epilepsia* **36**: (suppl 8): 94.

Kinsbourne, M. & Caplan, P. J. (1979). Cognitive power disorders. In *Children's Learning and Attention Problems*, p. 232 Boston, MA: Little Brown & Co.

Knoll, J. Stegman, K. & Suppes, T. (1998). Clinical experience using gabapentin adjunctively in patients with a history of mania or hypomania. *J. Affect. Disord.* **49**: 229–33.

Kossoff, E. H., Bergey, G. K., Freeman, J. M., *et al.* (2002). Levetiracetam psychosis in children with epilepsy. *Epilepsia* **42**: 1611–13.

Kulig, B. M. (1980). The evaluation of the behavioral effects of antiepileptic drugs in animals and man. In *Epilepsy and Behavior '79*, ed. B. M. Kulig, H. Meinardi & G. Stores, pp. 47–61. Lisse: Swets & Zeitlinger.

Lambert, M. V. & Robertson, M. M. (1999). Depression in epilepsy: etiology, phenomenology and treatment. *Epilepsia* **40** (suppl 10): 21–47.

Landolt, H. (1958). Serial electroencephalographic investigations during psychotic episodes in epileptic patients during schizophrenic attacks. In *Lectures on Epilepsy*, ed. L. DeHass. London: Elsevier.

Leach, J. P. & Brodie, M. J. (1998). Drug profile: tiagabine. *Lancet* **351**: 203–7.

Lee, D. O., Steingard, R. J., Cesena, J. M., *et al.* (1995). Behavioral side effects of gabapentin in children. *Epilepsia* **37**: 87–90.

Leppik, E. (1995). Tiagabine: the safety landscape. *Epilepsia* **36** (suppl 6): 10–13.

Loiseau, P., Psestre, M., Dartigues, J., *et al.* (1983). Long-term prognosis in two forms of childhood epilepsy: typical absence seizures and epilepsy with rolandic (centrotemporal) EEG foci. *Ann. Neurol.* **13**: 642–8.

Loiseau, P., Strube, E., Torr, U. J., *et al.* (1998). Evaluation neuropsychologique et therapeutique du stirpentol dans, l'epilepsie. *Rev. Neurol.* **144**: 165–77.

Luef, G. & Bauer, G. (1996). Topiramate in drug-resistant partial and generalized epilepsies. *Epilepsia* **37** (suppl 4): 69.

Manchanda, R., Miller, H., McLachlan, R. S., *et al.* (1996). Psychiatric disorders in candidates for surgery for epilepsy. *J. Neurol. Neurosurg. Psychiatry* **61**: 82–9.

Mandlebaum, D. E., Kugler, S. L., Wenger, E. C., *et al.* (2001). Clinical experience with levetiracetam and zonisamide in children with uncontrolled epilepsy. *Epilepsia* **42** (suppl 7): 183.

Marcotte, D. (1998). Topiramate in the treatment of mood disorders. *Proceedings of the 151st Annual Meeting of the American Psychiatric Association*. Toronto: American Psychiatric Association.

Mayeux, R., Brandt, J., Rosen, J., *et al.* (1980). Interictal memory and language impairment in temporal lobe epilepsy. *Neurology* **30**: 120–25.

McDanal, C. E. & Bolman, W. M. (1975). Delayed idiosyncratic psychosis with diphenylhydantoin. *JAMA* **231**: 1063.

McElroy, S. L., Soutullo, C. A., Keck, P. E., *et al.* (1997). A pilot trial of adjunctive gabapentin in the treatment of bipolar disease. *Ann. Clin. Psychiatry* **6**: 99–103.

Meador, K. J., Loring, D. W., Ray, P. G., *et al.* (2001). Differential cognitive and behaivoral effects of carbamazepine and lamotrigine. *Neurology* **56**: 1177–83.

Morris, G. L. & Mueller, W. M. (1999). Long-term treatment with vagus nerve stimulation in patients with refractory epilepsy. *Neurology* **53**: 1731–5.

Nemeroff, C. B., DeVane, C. L. & Pollock, B. G. (1995). Newer antidepressants and the cytochrome P450 system. *Am. J. Psychiatry* **153**: 311–20.

Numberger, J. I., Jr, Berrettini, W. H., Simmons-Alling, S., *et al.* (1986). Intravenous GABA administration is anxiolytic in man. *Psychiatry Res.* **19**: 113–17.

Ozdirim, E., Renda, Y. & Eupur, S. (1978). Effects of phenytoin and phenobarbital on the behavior of epileptic children. In *Advances in Epileptology 1977: Psychology, Pharmacotherapy and New Diagnostic Approaches*, ed. H. Meinardi & A. Rowan, pp. 120–23. Amsterdam: Swets & Zeitlinger.

Perrine, K. & Congett, S. (1994). Neurobehavioral problems in epilepsy. In *Neurology Clinics*, ed. O. Devinsky, pp. 129–252. Philadelphia: W. B. Saunders.

Pollack, M. H., Matthews, J. & Scott, E. L. (1998). Gabapentin as a potential treatment for anxiety disorders. *Am. J. Psychiatry* **155**: 992.

Post, R. M., Ketter, T. A., Denicoff, K., *et al.* (1996). The place of anticonvulsant therapy in bipolar illness. *Psychopharmacology* **128**: 115–29.

Pratt, J. A., Jenner, P., Johnson, A. L., *et al.* (1984). Anticonvulsant drugs alter plasma tryptophan concentrations in epileptic patients: implications for antiepileptic actions and mental function. *J. Neurol. Neurosurg. Psychiatry* **47**: 1131–3.

Rausch, R. 1991 Effects of temporal lobe surgery on behavior. In *Neurobehavioral Problems in Epilepsy, Advances in Neurology*, ed. D. B. Smith & D. B. Treiman, Vol. 55, pp. 279–92. New York: Raven Press.

Ravdin, L. S. D., Harden, C. L., Correa, D. D., *et al.* (2000). Memory and mood following vagus nerve stimulation for intractable epilepsy. *Epilepsia* **41** (suppl 7): 136.

Reynolds, E. H. (1990). Vigabatrin. *Br. Med. J.* **300**: 277–8.

Reynolds, E. H. & Travers, R. D. (1974). Serum anticonvulsant concentrations in epileptic patients with mental symptoms. *Br. J. Psychiatry* **124**: 440–45.

Reynolds, E. H, Chanaurin I, Milner G., *et al.* (1966). Anticonvulsant therapy, folic acid and Vitamin B12 metabolism and mental symptoms. *Epilepsia* **7**: 261–70.

Reynolds, E. H., Ring, H., & Heller, A. (1988). A controlled trial of gamma-vinyl-GABA (vigabatrin) in drug-resistant epilepsy. *Br. J. Clin. Pract. Suppl.* **61**: 33.

Ring, H. A., Moriarty, J. & Trimble, O. (1998). A prospective study of the early postsurgical psychiatric associations of epilepsy surgery. *J. Neurol. Neurosurg. Psychiatry* **64**: 601–4.

Ring, H. A., Trimble, M. R., Costa, D. C., *et al.* (1994). Striatal dopamine receptor binding in epileptic psychoses *Biol. Psychiatry* **356**: 375–80.

Rivinus, T. M. (1982). Psychiatric effects of the anticonvulsant regimens. *J. Clin. Psychopharmacol.* **2**: 165–92.

Robertson, M. M., Trimble, M. R. & Townsend, H. R. A. (1987). Phenomenology of depression in epilepsy. *Epilepsia* **28**: 364–72.

Rodin, E. A., Choon, S. R., Kitano, H., *et al.* (1976). A comparison of the effectiveness of primidone versus carbamazepine in epileptic outpatients. *J. Nerv. Ment. Dis.* **163**: 41–5.

Rogers, D., Bird, J. & Eames, P. (1993). Complex partial status after starting vigabatrin. *Seizure* **2**: 155–6.

Rosenstein, D. L., Nelson, J. C. & Jacobs, S. C. (1993). Seizures associated with antidepressants: a review. *J. Clin. Psychiatry* **54**: 289–99.

Ryan, L. M., Malamut, B. L., O'Connor, M. J., *et al.* (1999). Incidence of depression before and after temporal lobectomy for medically intractable epilepsy. *Epilepsia* **4** (suppl 7): 58–9.

Ryback, R. S. & Ryback, L. (1995). Gabapentin for behavioral dyscontrol. *Am. J. Psychiatry* **152**: 1399.

Ryback, R. S., Brodsky, L. & Mansifi, F. (1997). Gabapentin in bipolar disorder. *J. Neuropsychiatry Clin Neurosci.* **9**: 301.

Sander, J. A. S., Hart, Y. M, Trimble, M. R., *et al.* (1991a). Behavioral disturbances associated with vigabatrin therapy. 19th International Epilepsy Congress. *Epilepsia* **32** (suppl 1): 12.

Sander, J. A. S. Hart, Y. M., Trimble, M. R., *et al.* (1991b). Vigabatrin and psychosis. *J. Neurol. Neurosurg. Psychiatry* **54**: 435–9.

Schaffer, C. B., Schaffer, L. C. (1997). Gabapentin in the treatment of bipolar disorder. *Am. J. Psychiatry.* **15**: 491–2.

Schain, R. J. (1983). Carbamazepine and cognitive functioning. In *Antiepileptic Drug Therapy in Pediatrics*, ed. P. Morselli, C. E. Pippinger & J. K. Penry, pp. 189–92. New York: Raven Press.

Schapel, G. & Chadwick, D. (1996). Tiagabine and non-convulsive status epilepticus. *Seizure* **5**: 153–6.

Schmidt, D. (1992). *Epilepsien and epileptische Anfdlle*. Stuttgart: Thieme.

Schmitz, B. (1999). Psychiatric syndromes related to antiepileptic drugs. *Epilepsia* **40** (suppl 10): 65–70.

Schmitz, B. & Trimble, M. R. (1995). Carbamazepine and PIP-syndrome in temporal lobe epilepsy. *Epilepsy Res.* **22**: 215–20.

Sherard, E. S., Jr, Steiman, G. S. & Couri, D. (1980). Treatment of childhood epilepsy with valproic acid: results of the first 100 patients in a 6 month trial. *Neurology* **30**: 31–5.

Sheth, R. D., Goulden, K. J. & Penney, S. (1992). Catastrophic behavior outbursts requiring discontinuation of clobazam in children. *Epilepsia* **33** (suppl 3): 100.

Shorvon, S. D. (1998). Safety of topiramate: adverse events and relationships to dosing. *Epilepsia* **37** (suppl 2): 18–22.

Silverstein, F. S., Parrish, M. A. & Johnston, M. V. (1982a). Clinical and laboratory observations – adverse behavioral reactions in children treated with carbamazepine (Tegretol). *J. Pediatr.* **101**: 785–7

Silverstein, F. S., Parrish, M. A. & Johnston, M. V. (1982b). Adverse reactions to carbamazepine (Tegretol) in children with epilepsy. *Ann. Neurol.* **12**: 198.

Small, J. G., Klapper, M. H., Milstein, V., *et al.* (1991). Carbamazepine compared with lithium in the treatment of mania. *Arch. Gen. Psychiatry* **48**: 915–21.

Smith, K. R., Goulding, P. M., Wilderman, D., *et al.* (1994). Neurobehavioral effects of phenytoin and carbamazepine in patients recovering from brain trauma: a comparative study. *Arch. Neurol.* **51**: 653–60.

Sonnen, A. E. H., Zelvelder, W. H. & Bruens, J. H. (1975). A double blind study of the influence of dipropylacetate on behavior. *Acta Neurol. Scand.* (suppl) **60**: 43–7.

Sporn, J. & Sachs, G, (1997). The anticonvulsant lamotrigine in treatment resistant manic depressive illness. *J. Clin. Psychopharmacol.* **17**: 185–9.

Stagno, S. J. (1993). The epidemiology of epilepsy. In *The Treatment of Epilepsy: Principles and Practice,* ed. E. Wyllie, pp. 1149–62. Philadelphia: Lea & Febiger.

Stephen, L. J. & Brodie, M. J. (1998). New drug treatments for epilepsy. *Prescr. J.* **38**: 98–106.

Stoll, A. L., Banov, M., Kolbrener, M., *et al.* (1994). Neurologic factors predict a favorable valproate response in bipolar and schizoaffective disorders. *J. Clin. Psychopharmacol* **14**: 311–13.

Stores, G. (1975). Behavioral effects of anti-epileptic drugs. *Dev. Med. Child Neurol.* **17**: 647–58.

Stores, G. (1976). The investigation and management of school children with epilepsy. *Lond. Publ. Health.* **90**: 171–7.

Stores, G. (1981). Problems of learning and behavior in children with epilepsy. In *Epilepsy and Psychiatry*, ed. E. H. Reynolds & M. R. Trimble, pp. 33–48. New York: Churchill Livingstone.

Suppes, T., Brown, E. S., McElroy, S. L., *et al.* (1998). A pilot trial of adjunctive topiamate in the treatment of bipolar disorder. *Proceedings of the 37th Annual Meeting of the American College of Neuropsychopharmacology* pp. 306.

Sziklas, V. G., Montour-Proutz, I., Andermann, F., *et al.* (1999) Cognitive effects of topiramate therapy in patients with intractable partial epilepsy. *Epilepsia* **40** (suppl 7): 56.

Tallian, K. B., Nahata, M. C., Lo, W., *et al.* (1996). Gabapentin associated with aggressive behavior in pediatric patients with seizures. *Epilepsia* **37**: 501–6.

Tassanari, C. A., Michelucci, R., Chauvel, P., *et al.* (1996). Double-blind, placebo-controlled trila of topiramate (600 mg daily) for the treatment of refractory partial epilepsy. *Epilepsia* **37**: 763–8.

Theodore, W. H. & Porter, R. J. (1983). Removal of sedative hypnotic antiepileptic drugs from the regimens of patients with intractable epilepsy. *Ann. Neurol.* **13**: 320–24.

Thomas, L., Trimble, M. R., Schmitz, B., *et al.* (1996). Vigabatrin and behavior disorders: a retrospective survey. *Epilepsy Res.* **25**: 21–7.

Thompson, P. J. (1991). Memory function in patients with epilepsy. In *Neurobehavioral Problems in Epilepsy*, ed. D. Smith, D. Treiman & M. Trimble, Vol. 55, pp. 369–84. New York: Raven Press.

Thorn, I. (1975). A controlled study of prophylactic long-term treatment of febrile convulsions with phenobarbital. *Acta Neurol. Scand. Suppl.* **60**: 67–73.

Trimble, M. (1980). Anti-epileptic drugs and behavior – discussion notes. In *Epilepsy and Behavior '79*, ed. B. M. Kulig, H. Meinardi & G. Stores, pp. 76–9. Lisse: Swets & Zeitlinger.

Trimble, M. (1982). Anticonvulsant drugs and hysterical seizures. In *Pseudoseizures*, ed. T. L. Riley & A. Roy, pp. 148–58. Baltimore, MD: Williams & Wilkins.

Trimble, M. R. (1983). Anticonvulsant drugs and psychosocial development: phenobarbitone, sodium valproate and benzodiazepines. In *Antiepileptic Drug Therapy in Pediatrics*, ed. P. Morselli, C. E. Pippinger & J. Penry, pp. 201–17. New York: Raven Press.

Trimble, M. R. (1986). The psychoses of epilepsy and their treatment. In *The Psychopharmacology of Epilepsy*, pp. 83–94. New York: John Wiley & Sons.

Trimble, M. R. (1994). Psychiatric illness in epilepsy: a psychiatrist's perspective. Presented at the American Epilepsy Society Conference, 1994.

Trimble, M. R. (1997). Neuropsychiatric consequences of pharmacotherapy. In *Epilepsy. A Comprehensive Textbook*, ed. J. Engel & T. A. Pedley, pp. 2161–70. Philadelphia: Lippincott-Raven.

Trimble, M. R. (1998). Forced normalization and the role of anticonvulsants. In *Forced Normalization*, ed. M. R. Trimble & B. Schmitz, pp. 169–78. Petersfield, UK: Wrightson Biomedical.

Trimble, M. R. & Cull, C. (1990). Children of school age: the influence of antiepileptic drugs on behavior and intellect. *Epilepsia* **29** (suppl 3): 13–19.

Trimble, M. R. & Reynolds, E. H. (1976). Anticonvulsant drugs and mental symptoms: a review. *Psychol. Med.* **6**: 169–78.

Vaintrub, M. Y. (1998). Initial psychiatric and other disorders due to AED treatment. 3rd European Congress of Epileptology. *Epilepsia* **39** (suppl 2): 122.

Vassilyadi, M., Strawburg, R. H., Weber, A. M., *et al.* (2000). Vagal nerve stimulation at the children's hospital medial center. *Epilepsia* **41** (suppl 7): 136.

Vickery, B. G., Hayes, R. D., Graber, J., *et al.* (1992). A health-related quality of life instrument for patients reevaluated for epilepsy surgery. *Med. Care.* **30**: 299–319.

Vining, E. P. G. (1990). Cognitive and behavioral side effects of antiepileptic drugs. *Int. Pediatr.* **5**: 182.

Vining, E. P. G., Mellits, E. D., Dorsen, M. M., *et al.* (1987). Psychologic and behavioral effects of antiepileptic drugs in children: a double-blind comparison between phenobarbital and valproic acid. *Pediatrics* **80**: 165–74.

Weisbrot, D. M. & Ettinger, A. B. (1998). Psychiatric aspects of pediatric epilepsy. *Primary Psychiatry* **June**: 51–67.

Wilner, A. (2002). Antiepileptic reduces seizures in children. *CNS News* **4**: 15.

Wolf, P. (1991). Acute behavioral symptomatology at disappearance of epileptiform EEG abnormality: paradoxical or "forced" normalization. In *Neurobehavioral Problems in Epilepsy: Advances in Neurology*, ed. D. Smith, D. Treiman & M. Trimble, pp. 127–42. New York: Raven Press.

Wolf, S. & Forsythe, A. (1978). Behavior disturbances, phenobarbital and febrile seizures. *Pediatrics* **61**: 728–31.

Wolf, P., Inoue, Z., Roder-Wanner, U. U., *et al.* (1984). Psychiatric complications of absence therapy and their relation to alteration of sleep. *Epilepsia* **25**: 56–9.

Wolf, S. M., Shinnar, S., Kang, H., *et al.* (1995). Gabapentin toxicity in children manifesting as behavioral changes. *Epilepsia* **36**: 1203–5.

Young, L. T., Robb, J. C., Patelis-Siotis, I., *et al.* (1997). Acute treatment of bipolar depression with gabapentin. *Biol. Psychiatry* **42**: 851–3.

39

Helping with psychiatric problems

Devinsky (1998) noted that to be treated, behavior problems in epilepsy must be diagnosed. Often, they are overlooked or underappreciated, for they may not be reported spontaneously may not be asked about, or may be noted but considered to be minor. Behavior changes do not necessarily follow DSM-4 psychiatric nosology. Changes may be negative or positive. They differ from defined groups. Affect may be preserved in a psychosis. Problems may be undefined and impairing. Problems may exist in recognition of social cues or as a deficient comprehension of the emotions of others. Diagnosis should not be confined by the psychiatric classification. It is far easier to catch a problem early and intervene than to wait until the symptoms are blatant challenges that can no longer be ignored.

Approaching the young patient

The physician should take care not to neglect the younger patient or talk only with the parents. The physician should spend part of the time discussing and explaining pertinent information with the child. The discussion should include talking about the seizure, the tests, the drugs, and other therapeutic approaches. Questions and complaints should be encouraged and answered. The visit might begin with a brief chat with the child about the seizures and how things are going before the physician turns to the parents to get their full report. The examination should end with a reassuring explanation to the child of what has been determined and what is to be done. Some children are delighted to look at their X-rays, EEG, or CT scan images as the doctor explains them. If the physician can make the patient feel important, they are more apt to gain the patient's confidence, cooperation, and involvement, as well as the support of the parents.

Counseling and behavioral approaches

A wealth of behavioral support is available but underused. Counseling, including individual, family, and group approaches, is often needed. Behavior-management approaches include biofeedback and behavioral modification; stress-management approaches and behavioral intervention therapy for seizures may be considered for specific problems that arise.

Family therapy

Many of the problems of children with epilepsy involve the entire family, not just the young patient. Family therapy becomes an important part of the care approach. The therapist can start with the family's concerns and questions, but the therapist must also assess the family's attachment, affection, respect or lack thereof of family members for each other, expectations, closeness or distance, attitudes toward discipline, attitudes towards school performance (is this a family that values education?), the maturity of the parents (are they able to put their children's needs ahead of their own most of the time?), family encouragement of freedom of expression versus repressiveness, the family members' ability to enjoy one another's company, and their anxiety or tension levels.

Pharmacologic approaches

The management of behavior disorders begins with the identification of possible causes, biological, psychosocial, or both. The antiepileptic drugs in use should be reviewed. An effort should be made to reduce polypharmacy. Drugs prone to inducing psychiatric disturbances should be discontinued, although nearly all drugs may exhibit this potential. Drugs known to benefit behaviors may replace adverse drugs. If psychosocial causes appear to be more relevant, then supportive therapy or a combination of formal psychotherapies in association with medication may be considered. Low-dose psychopharmacologic medications may be considered in more severe situations (Torta & Keller, 1999).

Anticonvulsants

Ettinger (1998) noted that if seizures are intractable, then the associated behavior disorder is more severe and difficult to control. When selecting an anticonvulsant or when assessing behaviors in patients on such drugs, the potential positive and negative psychotropic effects of each agent should be reviewed (Smith et al., 1986; Dodrill et al., 1998).

The mechanisms of antiepileptic psychotropic actions include the effects on neurotransmitters, especially on the GABA system. If bipolar disorders are due to deceased GABAergic neurotransmission, then GABA enhancers may correct this. Negative effects may be direct or indirect, the latter as a reaction to altered cognition or an alternating psychosis (Smith et al., 1986; Dodrill et al., 1998).

Older antiepileptic drugs

Traditionally, antiepileptic selection has been by reputation, i.e. barbiturates and phenytoin are avoided because of adverse side effects whereas carbamazepine, valproate, and clonazepam have found favor in psychiatry. The ideal medication provides both antiepileptic protection and behavior benefits.

Carbamazepine

Perales (1999) noted that carbamazepine has beneficial psychotropic effects in 90% of patients. It tends to decrease irritability, aggression, impulsivity, dysphoric episodes, and depression. It may take three months to be manifest overall. Blumer (1994) notes its usefulness for organic affective disorders and borderline personality disorders. Ettinger (1998) comments that it is used to facilitate rapid reduction of benzodiazepine and in acute alcohol withdrawal. Carbanazepine is effective in acute mania, psychosis with aggression and dyscontrol, impulse-control disorders, especially with borderline personality mood disorders and psychosis, although tolerance may develop. It does not help with panic disorders (Beydown & Passaro, 2001). Carbamazepine, like valproate, has mood-stabilization properties and thus may be used to treat bipolar affective disorders (Calabrese & Delucchi, 1990; Small *et al.*, 1991; Weisbrot & Ettinger, 1998), including unipolar and bipolar depression.

Valproate

Perales (1999) and Blumer (1994) note that valproate is used for intermittent explosive disorders, panic disorders, and rapid-cycling bipolar disorders. It has been found to be effective for acute mania and possibly for depression, as well as for acute mania with depressive symptoms. Valproate is used in prophylaxis of bipolar disorders, but its role in major depression is not yet established. Valproate may help with secondary mania. It may be effective in anxiety disorders (Beydown & Passaro, 2001). The benefits may be related to GABA enhancement. Valproate also helps with past-traumatic stress disorder, behavior dyscontrol, irritability, aggressiveness, and alcohol or benzodiazepine withdrawal, (Ettinger, 1998).

Clonazepam

Post (1994) noted that clonazepam has antianxiety and anti-panic effects. In children, side effects include sedation and behavior problems. As with other benzodiazepines, seizures and behaviors may be accentuated by tapering the dose. Clonazepam is seldom the first drug of choice.

New antiepileptic drugs

The new anticonvulsants show both beneficial and adverse behavioral effects. In a review on psychiatric aspects of epilepsy, Trimble (1994) noted that in patients with mood disorders, lamotrigine, tiagabine, and vigabatrin have been effective in psychiatry. In some patients with psychoses, topiramate and vigabatrin have been helpful.

Seizure freedom is the ultimate goal, but some patients who become seizure free develop an emotional disorder. Patients need to be warned of this and told that help is available. Early signs such as insomnia, agitation, or tearfulness need to be reported. The drugs must be started at low doses and increased slowly. Patients with past psychiatric history need to be followed carefully. Those who become seizure free also need to be monitored. Antidepressants or antipsychotics may be used briefly if necessary, or the antiepileptic drug load may be reduced. In general, be aware of potential psychopathology. Ask for appropriate assessments. Interventions include psychotropic agents and psychotherapy. With antiepileptic and psychopharmacologic medications, avoid polytherapy (Trimble, 1986; Trimble, 1991).

Felbamate
Felbamate is restricted severely due to hepatic and hematologic reactions. Its glutamate antagonist properties make it potentially anxiolytic, and thus it might be considered for refractory inhibited bipolars.

Gabapentin
Gabapentin is a relatively safe and well-tolerated drug believed to have some potential effects on GABA. It displays anxiolytic effects (Beydown & Passaro, 2001). Ettinger (1998) notes that gabapentin may benefit the agitation of dementia, anxiety, social phobia, pain, and schizoaffective disorders. It may facilitate drug withdrawal. It has a positive effect on mood and cognition. Gabapentin may be useful in reducing the agitation of mania (Ryback et al., 1997; Schaffer & Schaffer, 1997) and the depressive phase of bipolar disorders, especially types II and I (Young et al., 1995). The drug has been useful for behavioral dyscontrol syndromes, refractory mood disorders, aggression (Ryback, 1995; Weisbrot & Ettinger, 1998), temper behavior disorders, and self-injurious behaviors (McManaman & Tam, 1999), although Ettinger (1998) notes that in children with developmental disabilities, there is a risk of behavioral agitation, with aggravation of tantrums, aggression, hyperactivity, and defiance.

Lamotrigine
Lamotrigine is a mood stabilizer, beneficial for resistant bipolar disorders and rapid-cyclers. It helps with the rapid-cycle depressed phase, especially in patients with a refractive bipolar depression and those refractory to lithium. It helps with bipolar schizoaffective cases. There are positive psychotropic benefits, with improved mood, energy, and enhanced alertness. It is not an antidepressant per se (Trimble, 1986;

Trimble, 1991; Fogelson & Sternbach, 1997; Weisbrot & Ettinger, 1998; Brodie *et al.*, 1999; Beydown & Passaro, 2001; Kanner & Balabanov, 2002). Adverse effects seem to appear in patients who are retarded and with behavior problems, mostly aggression, irritability and hyperactivity, although some show improvement (Beran & Gibson, 1998; Weisbrot & Ettinger, 1998).

Tiagabine

Tiagabine is a GABA reuptake inhibitor, with benefits of improved mood and adjustment independent of the seizure control. Tiagabine is beneficial for depression and psychoses, although total seizure control may occur in only 2% of patients (Trimble, 1986; Trimble, 1991). Ettinger (1998) reports benefits in bipolar disorders. Both positive and negative potential psychotropic effects have been noted (Crawford, 1998; Dodrill *et al.*, 1998; Leppik, 1995).

Topiramate

Topiramate produces psychomotor slowing, especially with rapid dosing or polytherapy. It may show independent depression benefit and may be useful in treating bipolar disorder, treating both manic and depressive phases of bipolar disorders. The drug may benefit patients with psychoses (Calabrese *et al.*, 1998; Marcotte, 1998). Topiramate may also produce anxiety, irritability, behavioral problems, confusion, psychosis, and hallucinations (Dohmeier *et al.*, 1998; Ketter *et al.*, 1999; Beydown & Passaro, 2001).

Vigabatrin

Vigabatrin, a GABAergic antiepileptic, is effective in depression psychoses. It has been associated with psychotic emergence, but in a large number of patients this is a forced normalization phenomenon. Vigabatrin and gabapentin polypharmacy may result rarely in a vigabatrin encephalopathy, which improves with discontinuance of gabapentin (Trimble, 1986; Trimble, 1991). Ettinger (1998) notes that vigabatrin may bring out a genetic predisposition to depression. It exacerbates hyperactivity in children with static encephalopathies.

Psychiatric drugs

Devinsky (1998) notes that in selecting psychotropic drugs in epilepsy, the physician must address the seizure threshold, sleep time and efficiency, interactions with anticonvulsants, augmentation of antiepileptic side effects, and impairment of other cognitive or behavioral functions. Perales (1999) warns that adding a psychiatric medication occasionally may worsen seizure control, although psychotropic agents may be used safely in the majority of epileptic patients. The agent chosen should have the fewest epileptogenic properties. A conservative dose titration should be used, and the lowest effective dosage of the agent should be selected. The psychotropic agent chosen should be monitored by serum levels to identify poor metabolizers. When using a highly epileptogenic agents, antiepileptic drug therapy should be optimized (Weisbrot & Ettinger, 1998).

Perales (1999) emphasizes that neurologic drugs increase neuroleptic and stimulant levels. Phenytoin, carbamazepine, phenobarbital, and primidone tend to induce hepatic metabolism, which can result in a reduction of some common psychotropic agents. Valproic acid tends to inhibit hepatic metabolism. Gabapentin, lamotrigine, topiramate, and tiagabine have few effects on other agents. SSRIs inhibit some specific isoenzymes of the cytochrome P450 class of hepatic enzymes, leading to the potential for reducing the metabolism of concomitant drugs, and thus elevating drug levels (Nemeroff et al., 1995; Weisbrot & Ettinger, 1998). Cytochrome P450 affects substrates, inducers, and inhibitors. Carbamazepine affects levels of fluoxetine, sertraline, fluvoxamine, and nefazodone (Barry et al., 2001).

It was once thought that 2% of patients with epilepsy experienced seizures due to psychiatric drug toxicity, but it is now thought that this may relate to non-anticonvulsant drug sensitivity. Neuroleptics are associated with a slightly increased risk of seizures. With phenothiazines, 1.2% of patients develop seizures. The incidence is dose-dependent, being 0.5% with low doses and up to 9% with high doses. Seizures occur most often when initiating treatment or when the dose is increased (Hauser & Hersdorffer, 2001). Doxepine, trazodone, desipramine, and fluoxetine may reduce seizure frequency (Favale et al., 1995; Kanner & Balabanov, 2002).

Drug groups

Psychiatric drugs are grouped according to the type of psychiatric problem that they treat. The various families have differing effects on the brain, often related to specific neurotransmitters.

Antianxiety agents

SSRIs are often chosen to treat anxiety disorders as they are effective yet low in epileptogenic potential. Additive CNS depressant affects occur with anxiolytics, as with other drugs. The benzodiazepines have also been used for anxiety as they have a very high potency and a short half-life. However, they are associated with increased risks for withdrawal symptoms, including rebound anxiety and seizures. The benzodiazepines are prone to abuse (Swedo et al., 1994).

Antidepressants

The major classes of antidepressants include the tricyclics, the mono-, bi-, tetra-, and heterocyclics, the monoamine oxidase inhibitors, and the SSRIs, as well as several newer drugs in their own classes. Antidepressants can produce seizures in patients even without a history of epilepsy. SSRIs and tricyclics lower the seizure threshold but can be used safely in modest doses to treat mood and behavior disorders in people with epilepsy. At higher doses, many antidepressants lower the seizure threshold. Spontaneous seizures have been seen occasionally, especially with overdoses. The risk of antidepressant-associated seizures ranges from 0.1% to 0.6% (Rosenstein et al., 1993). Trazodone, a non-tricyclic antidepressant, has the least seizure risk and may be anticonvulsant. It tends to be sedative (Pisani & Oteri, 1999; Lambert & Robertson, 1999).

The SSRIs are used in anxiety, behavior problems, and depression. Some antidepressants may display antiepileptic effects, especially in low doses, in experimental models of epilepsy and in humans, by mechanisms that are largely unknown. Drugs that increase serotonergic transmission are less convulsant or even more anticonvulsant than others. The incidence of seizures is very low, at less than 1% (Favale et al., 1995; Prediville & Gale, 1993). For fluoxetine, the seizure incidence is about 0.2%, including overdosages. Fluoxetine in animals has shown some anticonvulsant action (Buterbaugh, 1978; Dayley et al., 1992; Leander, 1992; Prediville & Gale, 1993), so it has been considered as a potential adjunct therapy in temporal lobe epilepsy (Favale et al., 1995; Troisi et al., 1995).

The SSRIs appear to be the best drugs for patients with epilepsy and depression (Pisani & Oteri, 1999; Barry et al., 2001; Kanner & Balabanov, 2002). Isolated reports of seizures with the newer antidepressants have been rare. Some have been associated with hyponatremia. All the SSRIs have been associated with inappropriate secretion of antidiuretic hormone. The SSRIs and mirtazapine do not impair memory processes (Lambert & Robertson, 1999).

The monoamine oxidase inhibitors are used in patients with depression, anxiety, rejection, oversensitivity, vegetative symptoms, and chronic therapy-resistant phobias. Monoamine oxidase inhibitors carry a very low seizure risk (0.1–0.2%) and may even have anticonvulsant properties. They are generally safe in patients with epilepsy. These drugs do not seem to be associated with seizures in non-epileptic patients. Theoretically, some monoamine oxidase inhibitors may interact with carbamazepine to cause a hypertensive episode or episodes of agitation, shivering, and muscle twitching (Stoudemire & Fogel, 1993; Lambert & Robertson, 1999; Barry et al., 2001; Kanner & Balabanov, 2002).

The tricyclics have been used commonly, especially in children, for anxiety, depression, ADHD, and enuresis. Seizures have been precipitated, especially in seizure-prone individuals, particularly if the drug is given with rapid increases, at higher dosages, with intravenous dosing, in overdosage, with concurrent use of other proconvulsant drugs, and in slow metabolizers. Seizure-prone individuals include those with a personal or family history of seizures, an abnormal pretreatment EEG, brain damage, alcohol or substance abuse or withdrawal, and concurrent use of

CNS-active medications (Lambert & Robertson, 1999; Barry *et al.*, 2001; Kanner & Balabanov, 2002). The incidence of tricyclic-induced seizures at normal dosages is around 0.6%, in at-risk patients around 3%, and in overdosage up to 8.4% (Frommer *et al.*, 1987). In children, fatal heart arrhythmias have been reported with higher dosages. Tricyclics may produce cognitive impairments and memory deficits, as may depression (Cole *et al.*, 1983). Recent studies suggest little difference in effectiveness between the tricyclics and placebo (Robertson, 1997; Robertson, 1998).

The mono-, bi-, tetra-, and heterocyclics are often used less in depressed patients with epilepsy. These drugs significantly lower the seizure threshold and therefore are not drugs of choice (Alldredge & Simon, 1992), even at low therapeutic dosage. The risk range is from 1.25–4.4% (Lambert & Robertson, 1999), rising to 15.6% for some (Barry *et al.*, 2001; Kanner & Balabanov, 2002).

Lithium is used for bipolar affect disorder and as an antidepressant. Lithium lowers the seizure threshold and may occasionally trigger de novo seizures. There are risks of sodium depletion and hypokalemia. Carbamazepine, valproate, clonazepam, and gabapentin are better alternatives. Used in combination with carbamazepine, lithium can cause an encephalopathy (Swedo *et al.*, 1994; Barry *et al.*, 2001).

Antipsychotics

Devinsky (1998) notes that antipsychotic drugs, including the classic tranquilizers, may lower seizure thresholds. The seizure tendency of antipsychotics tends to be dose-related. In choosing drugs, one must address the seizure threshold, sleep time and efficiency, interactions with anticonvulsants, augmentation of anticonvulsant side effects, and impairment of other cognitive or behavioral functions. Kanner (1998) noted that even at lower dosages but especially at higher dosages, the EEGs of patients on antipsychotics show background slowing and the appearance of paroxysmal activity. The incidence of dose-related seizures ranges from 1% to 6% with conservative dosages up to 9% with higher dosages.

Benzodiazepines have been used as alternatives to antipsychotics. They are effective but they may cause dependancy and tolerance. The dosage is variable and withdrawal is difficult. Behavioral and cognitive side effects exist.

Stimulants

Amphetamines have drug interactions with tricyclics, phenytoin, and phenobarbital. Stimulants are not very useful for treatment-resistant depression. The main role of these drugs appears to be as supplementary therapy for more complicated ADHD, although the incidence of seizures in patients treated with stimulants is around 1%.

Treatment approaches to psychiatric conditions
ADD and ADHD (ADDH)

Stimulant drugs such as the amphetamines and methylphenidate remain the adjunct drugs of choice once the diagnosis is confirmed. Antidepressants have been effective for short periods and tranquilizers have helped in out-of-control situations, but the patient on such drugs may be rendered an automaton (Szondi, 1963).

Anxiety disorders

Carbamazepine has been shown to be effective in anxiety disorders of epilepsy. Panic disorders and obsessive–compulsive disorder (OCD) are responsive to SSRIs. Paroxetine has a seizure incidence of 0.1%. The monoamine oxidase inhibitors have also been shown to be effective (Scicutella, 2001). Benzodiazepines have also been used for anxiety in children. For brief situational anxiety, a short-acting benzodiazepine may be useful; for more chronic problems, a long-acting preparation must be considered. Benzodiazepines have the risk of inducing withdrawal seizures as well as relapse anxieties. Alprazolam and clonazepam have been especially useful. Older children may benefit more from chlordiazepoxide and diazepam (Swedo et al., 1994). For performance anxiety, propranolol may be considered. Lorazepam may be used for episodic anxiety. Buspirone and tricyclics are effective but epileptogenic. Perales (1999) advises that anxiolytic drugs are best used only for short periods.

Panic reactions may be seen in preadolescents and adolescents; 25% of such reactions begin before age 15 years. Paroxetine is a fairly safe drug in children and teens with epilepsy. In the past, desipramine and imipramine were used, but more recently alprazolam or clonazepam alone or with imipramine at low dosage have been used. Tricyclics and benzodiazepines are useful for childhood panic (Swedo et al., 1994). Alprazolam may have antidepressant properties at higher doses in patients with panic disorders.

OCD, including self-injurious behaviors, may be treated effectively with clomipramine and fluoxetine. These drugs may also be helpful in the management of impulsive, aggressive, and self-destructive behaviors in some emotionally labile patients with brain damage and personality disorders (Perales, 1999). Personality traits of temporal lobe disorders have been referred to as part of the OCD spectrum and may respond to serotonergic agents, such as clomipramine and the SSRIs (Ravizza et al., 1991; Torta & Keller, 1999). Clomipramine, fluoxetine, sertraline, and paroxetine have been useful in children (Swedo et al., 1994). Fluvoxamine reduces pediatric OCD symptom severity, especially in younger children (Riddle et al., 2001). Serrtaline has also been released for the treatment of OCD in children.

Behavior disorders

Perales (1999) reports that most psychotropic medications can be used to treat behavior disorders in children and adolescents with epilepsy. Risperidone has been effective in managing aggressive children with conduct disorders. Carbamazepine has beneficial psychotropic effects, with psychotropic effects in 90% and seizure control in 60%. It tends to decrease irritability, aggression, impulsivity, dysphoric episodes, and depression and to improve intellectual capacity, attention, and concentration. It may take three months to be fully effective.

Aggression in children has often been treated with clonidine, which has an antiadrenergic effect. Clonidine provides a blockade of central antihypertensive effects. Clonidine can increase the levels of tricyclics, carbamazepine, leading to neuroleptic side effects. Death from cardiac irregularities has been reported with clonidine. Valproate and carbamazepine have been useful in aggression. For acute episodes, lorazepam may be useful. Of the SSRIs, fluoxetine and norfluoxetine have long half-lives, so paroxetine may be best in combination with anticonvulsants. Tranquilizers such as haloperidol, thioridazine, and risperidone have been used in aggression but occasionally they may trigger seizures. Intravenous or oral haloperidol may reduce ictal or interictal violence. All agents may occasionally produce a paradoxical exacerbation of aggression. Propranolol is effective for violent outbursts in patients with brain damage, but it may cause depression.

Agitation, especially intermittent agitation associated with organic brain diseases, has responded to carbamazepine, fluoxetine, trazodone, and buspirone.

Impulse-control disorders may respond to SSRIs such as fluoxetine. These drugs may be useful in impulsiveness and aggression (Torta & Keller, 1999; Youdofsky *et al.*, 1995). SSRIs and tricyclics show increased risk towards worsening of seizures at higher dosages (Torta & Keller, 1999). Tranquilizers are thought to be helpful in patients with impulse-control disorders, but they tend to aggravate seizures. Tricyclics have not been shown to be effective in the control of episodic moodiness and outbursts of rage (Blumer, 1977; Ounsted *et al.*, 1968). Both carbamazepine and tiagabine have helped with anger outbursts. Haloperidol, benzodiazepines and propranolol have been used in some cases. Phenothiazines, haloperidol, and stimulants may accentuate the problems (Kaufman *et al.*, 1999).

For explosive rages, various drugs have been tried, with some successes, including carbamazepine, valproate, lithium, and beta-blockers. Benzodiazepines may be useful if obsessive tendencies are seen. Alprazolam or lorazepam may be beneficial.

Rebellious resentful attitudes are treated primarily by behavioral therapy, not medication. There is no drug to promote good behavior or to stop rebellion.

Conduct and oppositional behaviors in children often have been treated with risperidone, which has been effective in managing aggressive children Risperidone shows a low seizure risk.

Mood disorders

When a person with epilepsy presents with a mood disorder, the physician must consider the relationships to epilepsy and the various causes. Dysphorias may be preictal, ictal, postictal, or interictal. One has to address social and psychological bases and biological problems such as the lesion and the epilepsy, as there may be possible left-sided focal hypometabolism. With some patients, there may be an inverse relationship between seizures and psychiatric disorders.

If the patient presents with a mood disorder, then the antiepileptic medication should be reviewed and optimized. Trimble (1994) notes that some antiepileptics may produce a dysphoria and some may treat mood disorders. Drugs that may cause depression include barbiturates, benzodiazepines felbamate, ethosuximide, tiagabine, topiramate, and vigabatrin. Conservative polytherapy and the new drugs may also help with mood disorders. Carbamazepine has been shown to be effective in patients with epilepsy and depression, especially with bipolar depression. Carbamazepine and valproate are most effective in affective disorders, but are less effective in psychotic disorders. Carbamazepine is the best drug to suppress the amygdalar after-discharge. Devinsky (1998) notes that in adults, lamotrigine and gabapentin may be helpful as adjunct drugs in treating depression but not effective when used alone.

Blumer advises that when depression emerges, it should be treated early to lessen both its impact and its duration. If the dysphoria persists, it should be treated. When a dysphoric mood is provoked by seizures or by the remission of seizures, it may take six to 18 months for the mood to dissipate. Psychotropic agents may be used safely in the majority of epileptic patients.

Physicians often hesitate to use antidepressant drugs in patients with epilepsy because of the concern that the drugs may cause seizures (Pisani & Oteri, 1999). Most antidepressants at therapeutic dosages exhibit in non-epileptic patients a seizure risk close to that reported for the first spontaneous seizure in the general population, which is less than 0.1% (Rosenstein *et al.*, 1993). SSRIs and monoamine oxidase inhibitors are safe to use in patients with epilepsy. Trazodone, fluoxetine, and fluvoxamine are the least apt to trigger seizures (Pisani & Oteri, 1999), with a risk of 0.1–0.2% (Barry *et al.*, 2001). In some patients, transient increases in seizure frequencies may be seen, but this settles down. Tricyclics with rapid titration, high dosage, or intravenous dosing are apt to trigger seizures, especially those that are rapid hydroxylators, in slow-metabolizing patients, and in patients with CNS pathology, abnormal EEG, or a personal or family history of epilepsy (Kanner & Balabanov, 2002).

SSRIs such as fluoxetine, sertraline, paroxetine, citalopram, and fluvoxamine (Pisani & Oteri, 1999) appear to be the drugs of choice for individuals with epilepsy and depression (Kanner & Balabanov, 2002), although tricyclics are often used. The incidence of seizures is very low (less than 1%) (Favale *et al.*, 1995; Prediville &

Gale, 1993; Barry *et al.*, 2001). Drug-resistant depression in epileptic patients may be helped by a tricyclic supplement, especially desipramine or nortriptyline in low dosage. Levels must be monitored because of tricyclic/SSRI interactions.

Antidepressants must be chosen for their efficacy, side-effects profile, safety, drug-interactions profile, and non-epileptogenic properties. Doses should be titrated conservatively, and the lowest effective dosage used. For selective psychotropic agents, serum levels must be monitored to identify poor metabolize's; the dose can then be adjusted accordingly. When treatment with a highly epileptogenic agent is required, antiepileptic drug therapy must be optimized (Weisbrot & Ettinger, 1998).

Anticonvulsants that utilize the cytochrome P450 system, such as phenytoin, carbamazepine, and the barbiturates, depress antidepressant levels, especially tricyclics and paroxetine. Some antidepressants, such as fluoxetine, may increase the anticonvulsant effects of phenytoin and carbamazepine, resulting in increased seizure control in some patients but increased toxicity in others (Leander, 1992).

Seizures tend to occur early in treatment or after dose increments, especially if titrated rapidly (Lambert & Robertson, 1999). Deterioration of behavior following the use of a psychotropic agent requires immediate attention and checking of the serum levels for any toxicity. Antidepressant therapy should be short-term. Carbamazepine may be useful in treating antidepressant-induced seizures (Trimble, 1991).

Blumer (1994), Devinsky (1998), and Trimble (1994) have all reviewed approaches to the treatment of mood disorders. The present first-line approach is to begin with a SSRI, such as paroxetine or fluoxetine, and build up the dose by increments every two weeks. The response rate is remission in 70%, improvement in 10%, and only transient relief in about 20%. In the past, the approach was to begin with a non-sedative tricyclic as the initial drug because of the broad spectrum of benefits for irritably, fears, and anxieties and quick effectiveness within days, but there are concerns over exacerbating seizure frequency and intensity, which may occur in up to 12% of patients. If the tricyclic was not effective, an SSRI was then added and the tricyclic dose reduced.

Electroshock therapy (ECT) is used for severely depressed adults who do not respond to other approaches. Some reports state that ECT improves physical and psychiatric states in patients with epilepsy. ECT has been used for intractable epilepsy and as a means of clearing prolonged postictal clouding of consciousness. During ECT therapy, the seizure threshold increases. There is an increased risk of unprovoked seizures following ECT in adults. Following ECT, 1.89% of patients demonstrate unprovoked seizures (Hauser & Hersdorffer, 2001).

Bipolar disorders

Acute mania may require an atypical antipsychotic or butyrophenone, while the depressive phases will require antidepressant therapy or ECT (Trimble, 1991). Post

(1994) noted that bipolarity appears to be a balance between depression and mania. Primary manic depressive illnesses tend to worsen and regress, with fewer inter-attack normal periods, much like the evolution of seizures.

The depressive phase is treated primarily with SSRIs. The manic phase is treated with neuroleptics. The equilibrium between the manic and depressive phases is treated with lithium and carbamazepine as mood stabilizers, and with ECT. Rapid cyclers do not respond well to lithium.

Blumer (1994) observed that anticonvulsants are effective in bipolar disorders. Patient selection for treatment with antiepileptic drugs for bipolar disorders usually includes those with organic affective disorders, especially children, patients who are lithium-refractory or rapid cycling, patients with mood swings, and patients with lithium non-compliance due to side effects. Lithium has less than a 50% benefit.

Carbamazepine and valproate have been helpful in maniac depressive disorders. Clonazepam and acetazolamide have been tried in combinations. Intravenous diazepam and phenytoin have also been tried, with equivocal results. Carbamazepine helps rapid cyclers, continuous cyclers, and patients with severe mania, a family history of mania, severe depression, and less chronic depression. Carbamazepine is better in prophylactic response to bipolar disorders than in the acute depressive state. There may be a loss of effectiveness. The tendency to speed up the rate of cycling is seen, as is the build-up of tolerance. Carbamazepine appears to induce a cross-tolerance to valproate. It has been found that seizures induce later affecter genes, which alter benzodiazepine genes and others, leading to cross-tolerance. If the drug is withdrawn for a period, some of the endogenous mechanisms may recover and respond again some time later.

Trimble (1994) notes that valproate is useful for rapid-cycling bipolar disorders, with a 50–60% response rate in manic-depressive disorders in general. Response to one anticonvulsant does not predict response to another. Some patients respond to valproate but not carbamazepine. Some respond to both in combination. The response with depression, unlike that with seizures, is not proportional to the blood level of the anticonvulsant, so the psysician must adjust the dose according to the clinical response. The valproate range is the same for both epilepsy and depression; milder cases need lower levels and severer ranges need high therapeutic levels.

The mania phase may respond to lithium, valproate, carbamazepine, and, perhaps, clonazepam and acetazolamide. Valproate is a good antimanic drug (Beydown & Passaro, 2001), with some benefit also in the depressive phase. Clonazepam may be primarily antimanic, but tolerance appears to develop rapidly and adverse reactions are prominent. Gabapentin, topiramate, and potentially tiagabine may be effective. In manic depressive illnesses, ECT helps all phases.

Carbamazepine is both an antidepressant drug and an antimanic drug equal to lithium. The antimanic effect lessens over time. The rate of response to the drug averages four to nine days for mania and one to three weeks for depression. Blumer (1994) notes that predictors of an antimanic response to carbamazepine include increased severity of mania, dysphoria, anxiety, and a rapidity of cycling in light of an absence of family history of affective disorders. The carbamazepine response is best with more hypermetabolic temporal lobes during the manic phase, whereas temporal (and frontal) hypometabolism is associated with poor drug responses, especially to carbamazepine. Patients with more psychosensory symptoms do better with lithium, showing a poor response to carbamazepine.

The depressive phase may respond to carbamazepine, especially in more severe cases that do not respond to other drugs. Carbamazepine appears to potentiate lithium. Carbamazepine is less of an antidepressant than ECT. For depression, a valproate–lithium combination is effective. Lamotrigine and, to a lesser degree, gabapentin and topiramate, may be helpful. Tiagabine has the potential to be beneficial. Alprazolam works well for depression. Tricyclics, monoamine oxidase inhibitors, and dopamine agnostics help with depression but may drive emotions to the other extreme. In children and adolescents with a bipolar presentation, lithium or carbamazepine have been used. If prominent depressive symptoms persist, an antidepressant is often added, including an SSRI such as fluoxetine Diazepam may help (Emslie *et al.*, 1995).

Psychoses

Blumer (1994) and Trimble (1994) note that psychoses are not uncommon in epilepsy. Mental changes in epilepsy may be secondary to inhibition. Patients with epilepsy develop their psychoses at least one to two years after the onset of seizures. Many tranquilizer may also produce seizures. Indeed, most drugs used to treat behavior disorders may cause seizures in some individuals, especially those who are seizure-prone.

Consider the circumstances of the psychoses in determining therapy. In paranoid and schizophrenic states, the presentation should be evaluated in terms of the onset in relationship to the seizure frequency and according to whether the problem is episodic or chronic (Trimble, 1986; 1991).

A peri-ictal psychosis is treated with anticonvulsants. If the psychotic episodes appear ictal, then seizure control may be the primary treatment of the psychoses. Ictal psychoses, including various status states, are treated with an appropriate increase in the anticonvulsant medications. If the psychotic state is due to a drug reaction, then discontinuing the aggravating drug should stop the psychosis. If the psychoses appear to be driven by the seizures and the seizures originate from a temporal lobe, then surgery may be of benefit. Postoperatively, there may be a risk for the development of a postoperative psychosis. Psychiatric follow-up will be required. A postictal psychosis should be recognized and treated early. Prompt symptomatic treatment with psychotropic medication, such as a benzodiazepine and antipsychotic agent, is needed on a short-term basis. Haloperidol given intravenously or intramuscularly may be of benefit in the agitated stage. When the psychosis has resolved, the psychopharmacologic agent should be tapered slowly, and not used chronically (Trimble, 1991).

An interictal psychosis requires specific psychotropic medication, perhaps with a reduction of the antiepileptic medication. Psychoses must be treated because of the high morbidity and mortality of interictal psychoses. Seizure clusters should be prevented. Interictal psychoses in the absence of epilepsy should be managed as a psychiatric disorder.

If the psychosis appears when the seizures are controlled, then a cautious reduction of the anticonvulsant may cause the psychotic behavior to disappear as a few seizures reappear. If the anticonvulsant is increased rather than decreased, the psychotic state may be made worse. With this so-called alternating (with seizures) psychosis, the EEG is the most normal when the psychosis is the most active. If there appears to be a direct relationship, especially if it is inverse, then possibly reducing antiepileptic therapy even to the point of allowing a few seizures to break through may alleviate the psychosis. Generally, chlorpromazine may be a logical clinical choice in these patients (Trimble, 1986; Trimble, 1991).

Consider the epilepsy and the antiepileptic management. Kanner (1998) emphasizes that when considering a neuroleptic drug in patients with epilepsy, it is important to first rule out that the psychosis is not the expression of an underlying problem or a drug. Devinsky (1998) notes that a psychosis may be associated with the institution of a new anticonvulsant as a reaction to the drug or to derived control over the seizures. A psychosis may be dose-related. Alterations in the balance of glutamatergic and GABAergic activity can also cause psychoses under predisposing conditions, as shown by several new antiepileptics, such as vigabatrin, topiramate, and tiagabine (Monaco, 1996; Monaco et al., 1997; McConell & Duncan, 1998). Polytherapy may worsen the mental status. If the psychosis appears to be related to a change in drug then the change should be reversed and the offending antiepileptic drug removed. Temporary treatment of the psychoses will probably be needed during the drug change period.

Devinsky (1998) advised that no antiepileptic medication treats psychoses. Psychotherapy is the desired treatment for epileptic psychoses, especially chronic psychoses, but usually in combination with medications. Perales (1999) noted that carbamazepine and valproate and possibly the newer antiepileptics have been used in patients with schizophrenia on neuroleptics. Carbamazepine may aggravate an alternating psychosis, but often it is helpful in other psychotic reactions, especially when used in combination with antipsychotic medication. The antipsychotic medications, such as the major tranquilizers, if used alone may trigger seizures. It may be that the benefit of the tranquilizer in an alternating psychosis is to activate the seizure enough to allow the psychosis to disappear. It is best to use an anticonvulsant along with the antipsychotic medication. A balanced combination of an anticonvulsant and an antipsychotic drug along with active psychotherapy is the desired management, especially for episodic psychoses. Antipsychotic drugs, especially those associated with reduced consciousness, appear to reduce restlessness. Paranoid symptoms may improve but seldom disappear completely.

If no relationship between the seizures and the psychosis exists, then consideration of a neuroleptic drug that is less apt to precipitate seizures would seem appropriate (Trimble, 1986; Trimble, 1991). All neuroleptic drugs can lower the seizure threshold; the estimated seizure rate is 0.1–0.2%. The epileptogenicity of a neuroleptic is related not only to a dopamine blockage but also to the agent's antihistaminergic activity (Oliver *et al.*, 1982). Kanner (1998) advises that certain risk factors for developing seizures should be sought, including high serum drug concentrations, high doses of neuroleptics, and recent rapid escalation in doses, especially if there is a history of epilepsy, other CNS disturbances, prior EEG abnormalities, or a family history for epilepsy. It is important to remember that enzyme-inducing antiepileptic drugs will lower the neuroleptic levels and thus may precipitate recurrence of psychotic symptoms. This must be heeded, especially when changing antiepileptic medications.

The benefits of dopamine agonists in the management of epilepsy are well known. Multiple dopamine receptor families sometimes mediate opposing influences on neuronal excitability. The effects of anticonvulsant action on dopamine have been attributed to D2 receptor stimulation of the forebrain. Seizures may be precipitated as a consequence of treating other neurologic disorders with D2 antagonists (neuroleptics) or D1 agonists (Burke *et al.*, 1990). Dopamine receptor antagonists such as neuroleptics can facilitate amygdaloid kindling (Torta & Keller, 1999).

Blumer (1994) advises an overall approach to psychoses of epilepsy, similar to the mood disorders of epilepsy. First, the anticonvulsant regimen should be optimized. A non-sedative tricyclic antidepressant should then be selected, starting at a low dosage and increasing slowly by small increments over a few days to weeks, not exceeding a modest dosage. This may have a rapid, broad-spectrum therapeutic effect within days. If needed and tolerated, further increments can be made cautiously. If this is not effective, as in 10% of patients, then a longer-acting SSRI such as paroxetine or fluoxetine can be added and increased modestly over weeks. As needed, risperidone may help, especially in children. A small dosage of trifluoperazine may be added to the antidepressant if needed.

A low dosage of haloperidol or olanzapine added slowly as monotherapy may be useful in patients with acute psychotic episodes (Trimble, 1986; Trimble, 1991). Haloperidol and probably risperidone are safe (Trimble, 1991). Paranoid states and schizophreniform psychoses may respond to chlorpromazine. There appears to be a clear biological link between the suppression of seizures and the development of psychoses. ECT may be effective (Trimble, 1986; Trimble, 1991).

The treatment of psychoses should involve more than just medication. As in all psychiatric problems, psychopharmacological management alone will not suffice. It is important to acknowledge that the patient with a psychosis and epilepsy has a double burden to bear. There remains perplexity and embarrassment over the psychoses and the fear of future bouts. With chronic psychoses, there may be further disintegration over years to be avoided. It is important to involve the family as well as the individual in ongoing counseling and therapy, with emphasis on compliance in the comprehensive care (Trimble, 1991).

Neurosurgical approaches

Surgery may be considered in the face of compelling cognitive and psychosocial issues that argue for avoiding delays in instituting early interventions (Duchowny et al., 1997). Studies show that severe psychosocial dysfunction may develop in children with intractable temporal lobe seizures, with marked improvements being seen in those who undergo temporal lobectomy (Lindsay et al., 1984; Weisbrot & Ettinger, 1998). A temporal lobectomy can have many beneficial effects on learning and behavior problems. Not only is the seizure control often improved, but aggressive traits are often reduced and depressed sexuality tends to normalize. There is little change in the religious and philosophical drives, the repetitive behaviors, perseverative deliberate thinking trends, or the psychoses themselves.

Preoperative status

Blumer (1994) emphasizes that in patients referred for epilepsy surgery, psychotic disorders may be frequent but intermittent. A short evolution may not reveal sufficient information about the patient. People with epilepsy characteristically vary day to day. Common complaints are frequent, including depression, lack of energy, sleep problems, pains, wide mood swings, irritability, mistrust, hallucinations, worries/anxieties, and fear of certain situations. The emotional aspects of patients facing surgery need to be explored in detail. The physician needs to be ready to help in these areas as well as to provide surgical relief for the seizures (Trimble, 1986; Trimble, 1991). A relationship established before surgery renders postoperative follow-up help for the emotional changes of the surgery much easier to provide.

Preoperative psychosocial status is a better predictor of a postoperative psychosocial outcome than is the seizure frequency. The strongest predictors of the functional and emotional outcomes may be the evaluation of mood. Full preoperative psychosocial testing should be performed. If any problems are identified, then the establishing of counseling before surgical referral is desirable for postoperative follow-up. The physician should be cautious in stopping any anticonvulsant drugs at the time of surgery. The patient must be prepared for a possible seizure-free existence

Postoperative changes

Blumer (1994) reports that following temporal lobectomy, there may appear de novo psychotic episodes (15%), de novo dysphoric disorders (15%), de novo severe depressive episodes (6%), and exacerbations of dysphoria (9%). Roughly 39% of patients thus experience postoperative psychiatric complications.

Discharging seizure-controlled patients postoperatively without any psycho-social rehabilitation does the patient no benefit. It is important to check for post-operative symptoms before discharge and at each revisit. The patient must be made aware of the risks of possible postoperative transient problems, such as anxiety, de-pression, other emotional problems, and potential memory problems. The patient should be aware of the physician's availability should any problems arise. Follow-up visits at six weeks, three months, and one year at least should be done, as well as at any time of problem occurrence, in order to pick up the commonest emergence of emo-tional problems before they become severe. Counseling should be re-established if problems emerge. Short-term antianxiety or antidepressant medication may be used temporarily if necessary.

The best surgery may halt or at least significantly reduce the seizure frequency, but often it does not remove pre-existing psychiatric conditions, especially those of exogenous origin. Epilepsy surgery may be followed by a transient period of anxiety and then a longer period of depression, both of which eventually fade. Occasionally, seizure surgery may halt the seizures but unleash a major behavioral reaction, such as a psychosis as a forced normalization phenomena. Early seizure surgery may prevent problems from developing, although it does not cure problems that have already developed. Surgery does not remove the need for psychiatric intervention; it only changes the substrate. Some patients and their families may need to be counseled in how to return to a normal life, having lost the excuse of epilepsy. Some families are not prepared to accept the family member as an equal member rather than a patient to be cared for. Family therapy may need to be a part of the surgical approach and thereafter, until the patient has totally recovered in all aspects.

Vagal nerve stimulation

Various brain stimulators are under evaluation for potential positive psychotropic benefits. Vagal nerve stimulation may help with depression in adults, but it has not been shown to help with other dysthymic symptoms (Weisbrot & Ettinger, 1998; Harden *et al.*, 1999).

Beyond pills and scalpels

The emphasis is now not only on seizure frequency but also on quality of life. Compliance is important, extending beyond just taking medication; it also requires compliance in lifestyle. In light of managed healthcare pressures, psychosocial areas will need to fight to survive. Strategies towards meeting this need must be developed. The specialist needs to be ready to respond to primary care physician needs. Mental health and epilepsy physicians need to work together, not just refer back and forth, as part of comprehensive care.

REFERENCES

Alldredge, B. K. & Simon, R. P. (1992). Drugs that can precipitate seizures. In *The Medical Treatment of Epilepsy*, ed. S. R. Resor & H. Kutt, pp. 497–523. New York: Marcel Dekker.

Barry, J., Lembke, A. & Huynh, N. (2001). Affective disorders in epilepsy. In *Psychiatric Issues in Epilepsy*, ed. A. B. Ettinger & A. M. Kanner, pp. 45–72. Philadelphia: Lippincott Williams & Wilkins.

Beydown, A. & Passaro, E. A. (2001). Anticonvulsants and psychiatric disorders. In *Psychiatric Issues in Epilepsy*, ed. A. B. Ettinger & A. M. Kanner, pp. 251–60. Philadelphia: Lippincott Williams & Wilkins.

Blumer, D. (1977). Neuropsychiatric aspects of psychomotor and other forms of epilepsy in childhood. In. *Comprehensive Management of Epilepsy in Infancy, Childhood and Adolescence*, ed. S. Livingston, pp. 486–97. Springfield, IL: Charles C. Thomas.

Blumer, D. P. (1994). Treatment of psychiatric illness in epilepsy patients. Presented at the American Epilepsy Society Conference, 1994.

Brodie, M. J., Overstall, P. W. & Giorgi, L. (1999). UK Lamotrigine Elderly Study Group. Multicenter, double-blind randomized comparison between lamotrigine and carbamazepine in elderly patients with newly diagnosed epilepsy. *Epilepsy Res.* **37**: 81–7.

Burke, K., Chandler, C. J., Starr, B. S., *et al.* (1990). Seizure promotion and protection by D-1 and D-2 dopaminergic drugs in the mouse. *Pharmacol. Biochem. Behav.* **36**: 729–33.

Buterbaugh, G. G. (1978). Effect of drugs modifying central serotonergic function on the response of extensor and nonextensor rats to maximal electroshock. *Life Sci.* **23**: 2393–404.

Calabrese, J. R. & Delucchi, G. A. (1990). Spectrum of efficacy of valproate in 55 patients with rapid cycling bipolar disorders. *Am. J. Psychiatry* **147**: 431–4.

Calabrese, J. R., Shelton, M. D., III, Keck, P. E., Jr, *et al.* (1998). Pilot study of topiramate in acute severe treatment-refractory mania. In *Proceedings of the 151st Annual Meeting of the American Psychiatric Association*, p. 306. American Psychiatric Association.

Cole, J. O., Branconnier, R., Salomon, M., *et al.* (1983). Tricyclic use in the cognitively impaired elderly. *J. Clin. Psychiatry* **44**: 14–19.

Crawford, P. (1998). An audit of topiramate use in a general neurologic clinic. *Seizure* **7**: 217–21.

Dayley, J. W., Yan, Q. S. & Mishra, P. K. (1992). Effects of fluxetine on convulsions and on brain serotonin as detected by microdyalisis in genetically epilepsy-prone rats. *Pharmacol. Exp. Ther.* **250**: 533–40.

Devinsky, O. (1998). What should the neurologist remember on the psychopharmacology of epilepsy? Presented at the American Epilepsy Society Conference, 1998.

Dodrill, C. B., Arnett, J. L., Shu, V., *et al.* (1998). Effects of tiagabine monotherapy on abilities, adjustment, and mood. *Epilespia* **39**: 33–42.

Dohmeier, C., Kay, A. & Greathouse, N. (1998). Neuropsychiatric complications of topiramate therapy. *Epilepsia* **39** (suppl 1): 189.

Duchowny, M. S., Harvey, S., Sperling, M. R., *et al.* (1997). Indications and criteria for surgical intervention. In *Epilepsy: A Comprehensive Textbook*, ed. J. Engel & T. A. Pedley, pp. 1677–85. Philadelphia: Lippincott-Raven.

Emslie, G. J., Kennard, B. D. & Kowatch, R. A. (1995). Affective disorders in children: diagnosis and management. *J. Child. Neurol.* **10** (suppl 1): 42–9.

Ettinger, A. B. (1998). Antiepileptic drugs with positive and negative psychotropic properties. Presented at the American Epilepsy Society Conference, 1998.

Favale, E., Rubino, V., Mainardi, P., *et al.* (1995). Anticonvulsant effect of fluoxetine in humans. *Neurology* **45**: 1926–7.

Fogelson, D. & Sternbach, H. (1997). Lamotrigine treatment of refractory bipolar disorder. *J. Clin. Psychiatry* **58**: 271–3.

Frommer, D. A., Kulig, K. W., Marx, J. A., *et al.* (1987). Tricyclic antidepressant overdose: a review. *JAMA* **257**: 521–6.

Harden, C. L., Pulver, M. C., Mikolov, B., *et al.* (1999). Effects of vagus nerve stimulation on mood in adult epilepsy patients. *Neurology* **52** (suppl 2): 238A.

Hauser, W. A. & Hesdorffer, D. C. (2001). Psychoses, depression and epilepsy: epidemiological considerations. In *Psychiatric Issues in Epilepsy*, ed. A. B. Ettinger & A. M. Kanner, pp. 7–18. Philadelphia: Lippincott Williams & Wilkins.

Kanner, A. K. (1998). Treatment of psychiatric disorders of epilepsy with neuroleptic drugs. Presented at the American Epilepsy Society Conference, 1998.

Kanner, A. M. & Balabanov, A. (2002). Depression and epilepsy: how closely related are they? *Neurology* **58** (suppl 5): 27–39.

Kaufman, K. R., Kugler, S. L., Sachdeo, R. C., *et al.* (1999). Tiagabine in the management of post-encephalitic epilepsy and impulse control disorders. *Epilepsia* **40**: (suppl 7): 57.

Ketter, T. A., Post, R. M. & Theodore, W. H. (1999). Positive and negative psychotropic effects of antiepileptic drugs in patients with seizure disorders. *Neurology* **64** (suppl 1): 52–66.

Lambert, M. V. & Robertson, M. M. (1999). Depression in epilepsy: etiology, phenomenology, and treatment. *Epilepsia* **40** (suppl 10): 21–47.

Leander, J. D. (1992). Fluoxetine, a selective serotonin-uptake inhibitor enhances the anticonvulsant effects of phenytoin, carbamazepine and ameltolide. *Epilepsia* **33**: 573–6.

Leppik, I. E. (1995). Tiagabine: the safety landscape. *Epilepsia* **36**: 1–13.

Lindsay, J. J., Glaser, G., Richards, P., *et al.* (1984). Developmental aspects of focal epilepsies in children treated by neurosurgery. *Dev. Med. Child Neurol.* **26**: 574–87.

Marcotte, M. (1998). Topiramate in the treatment of mood disorder. In *Proceedings of the 151st Annual Meeting of the American Psychiatric Association*, pp. 121–2. American Psychiatric Association.

McConell, H. W. & Duncan, D. (1998). Treatment of psychiatric comorbidity in epilepsy. In *Psychiatric Comorbidity in Epilepsy*, ed. H. W. McConnell & P. J. Snyder, pp. 245–62. Washington, DC: American Psychiatric Press.

McManaman. J. & Tam, D. A. (1999). Gabapentin for self-injurious behavior in Leisch–Nyhan syndrome. *Pediatr. Neurol.* **20**: 381–2.

Monaco, F. (1996). Cognitive effects of vigabatrin, a review. *Neurology* **47** (suppl 1): 6–11.

Monaco, F., Torta, R., Cicolin, A., *et al.* (1997). A lack of association between vigabatrin and impaired cognition. *J. Int. Med. Res.* **26**: 296–301.

Nemeroff, C. B., DeVane, C. L. & Pollock, B. G. (1995). Newer antidepressants and the cytochrome P450 system. *Am. J. Psychiatry* **153**: 311–20.

Oliver, A. P., Luchins, D. J. & Wyatt, R. J. (1982). Neuroleptic-induced seizures. An in vitro technique for assessing relative risk. *Arch. Gen. Psychiatry* **39**: 206–9.

Ounsted, C., Lindsay, J. & Norman, R. (1968). *Biological Factors in Temporal Lobe Epilepsy.* London: Spastics Society and Heinemann.

Perales, M. (1999). Psychiatric management in epilepsy. Presented at the Via Christi Epilepsy Conference, Wichita, KS, 1999.

Pisani, E. & Oteri, G. (1999). Antidepressant drugs and seizure susceptibility: from in vitro data to clinical practice. *Epilespia* **30** (suppl 1): 38–56.

Post, R. (1994). Psychiatric effects of antiepileptic drugs. Presented at the American Epilepsy Society Conference, 1994.

Prediville, S. & Gale, K. (1993). Anticonvulsant effect of fluoxetine on focally evoked limbic motor seizures in rats. *Epilepsia* **34**: 381–4.

Ravizza, L., Maina, G., Torta, R., *et al.* (1991). Are serotoninergic antidepressants more effective in episodic obsessive-compulsive disorders? In *Serotonin-system Related Psychiatric Syndromes, Clinical and Therapeutic Links*, ed. G. B. Casano & H. S. Akiskal, pp. 61–5. London: Royal Society of Medicine.

Riddle, M. A., Reeve, E. A., Yaryura-Tobias, J. A., *et al.* (2001). Fluvoxamine for children and adolescents with obsessive-compulsive disorder: a randomized controlled multicenter trial. *J. Am. Acad. Child Adolesc. Psychiatry* **40**: 222–9.

Robertson, M. M. (1997). Depression in neurological disorders. In *Depression and Physical Illness*, ed. M. M. Robertson & C. L. E. Katona, pp. 305–40. Chichester, UK: John Wiley & Sons.

Robertson, M. (1998). Mood disorders associated with epilepsy. In *Psychiatric Comoirbidity in Epilepsy, Basics mechanisms, Diagnosis and Treatment*, ed. H. W. McConnell & P. J. Sander, pp. 132–67. Washington, DC: American Psychiatric Press.

Rosenstein, D. L., Nelson, J. C. & Jacobs, S. C. (1993). Seizures associated with antidepressnts: a review. *J. Clin. Psychiatry* **54**: 289–99.

Ryback, L. (1995). Gabapentin for behavior dyscontrol. *Am. J. Psychiatry* **152**: 1399.

Ryback, R. S., Brodsky, L. & Munasilfi, F. (1997). Gabapentin in bipolar disorder. *J. Neuropsychiatry Clin. Neurosci.* **9**: 301.

Schaffer, C. B. & Schaffer, L. C. (1997). Gabapentin in the treatment of bipolar disorder. *Am. J. Psychiatry* **154**: 291–2.

Scicutella, A. (2001). Anxiety disorders in epilepsy. In *Psychiatric Issues in Epilepsy*, ed. A. B. Ettinger & A. M. Kanner, pp. 95–110. Philadelphia: Lippincott Williams & Wilkins.

Small, J. G., Kałapper, M. H., Milstein, V., *et al.* (1991). Carbamazepine compared with lithium in the treatment of mania. *Arch. Gen. Psychiatry* **48**: 921–51.

Smith, D. B., Craft, B. R., Collins, J., *et al.* (1986). Behavioral characteristics of epilepsy patients compared to normal controls. *Epilespia* **27**: 760–68.

Stoudemire, A. & Fogel, B. S. (1993). *Psychiatric Care of the Medical Patient.* New York: Oxford University Press.

Swedo, S. E., Leonard, H. L. & Allen, A. J. (1994). New developments in childhood affective and anxiety disorders. *Curr. Probl. Pediatr.* **24**: 12–38.

Szondi, L. (1963). *Schicksalsanalytische Therapie.* Bern: Hans Huber.

Torta, R. & Keller, R. (1999). Behavioral, psychotic and anxiety disorders in epilepsy: etiology, clinical features and therapeutic implications. *Epilepsia* **50** (suppl 10): 2–20.

Trimble, M. R. (1986). The psychoses of epilepsy and their treatment. In *The Psychopharmacology of Epilepsy*, ed. M. R. Trimble, pp. 83–94. New York: John Wiley & Sons.

Trimble, M. R. (1991). Treatment of epileptic psychoses. In *The Psychoses of Epilepsy*, pp. 150–64. New York: Raven Press.

Trimble, M. R. (1994). Psychiatric illness in epilepsy. A psychiatrist's perspective. Presented at the American Epilepsy Society Conference, 1994.

Troisi, A., Vicario, E., Nuccetelli, F., *et al.* (1995). Effects of fluoxetine on aggressive behavior of adult patients with mental retardation and epilepsy. *Pharmacopsychiatry* **28**: 73–6.

Weisbrot, D. M. & Ettinger, A. B. (1998). Psychiatric aspects of Pediatric Epilepsy. *Primary Psychiatry* **June**: 51–67.

Youdofsky, S. C., Silver, J. M. & Hales, R. E. (1995). Treatment of aggressive disorders. In *Textbook of Psychopharmacology*, ed. A. F. Schatzberg & C. B. Nemeroff, pp. 735–52. Washington, DC: American Psychiatric Press.

Young, G. B., Chandara, P. C., Blume, W. T., *et al.* (1995). Mesial temporal lobe seizures presenting as anxiety disorder. *J. Neuropsychiatry Clin. Neurosci.* **7**: 352–7.

40

Epilog

The mere listing of an increased association of a particular language, learning, or behavior deviation with a seizure type does not signify that it will always appear with every person who has that type of seizure. Fortunately, only a few people are handicapped with any such problems, but for those patients the handicap may surpass the seizures in severity. In light of the vast array of variables, more time is spent in debate than in determing why such problems are increased in certain seizure syndromes.

If a minority of patients experience a language, learning, or emotional problem, but still that small occurrence is significantly greater than expected, then a correlation exists and needs to be understood. Even with a low incidence, to the person who has the disorder the incidence is 100%. To understand such relationships is to learn how to prevent or at least lessen the impact.

Comprehensive concern and care involves treating the whole person, not just the epileptic events, EEG deviations, or medication levels.

If there are any set rules on how to treat epilepsy, then they should consist of the following five basic commandments:

1 Treat the whole patient (and family), not just the seizures.
2 Treat the patient's needs, not just your own particular interests.
3 Treat as a team member, because no physician is able to know all or do all that is needed by the epileptic patient and their family.
4 Help others to treat the epileptic patient appropriately.
5 Continue to treat the patient, not just the seizures, until the epilepsy and all its complications are overcome.

Index